fourth edition

CRITICAL CARE CERTIFICATION

Preparation, Review, & Practice Exams

Thomas Ahrens, RN, DNS, CS, CCRN
Clinical Specialist in Critical Care
Barnes-Jewish Hospital
St. Louis, Missouri

Donna Prentice, RN, MSN(R), CS, CCRN, TNS
Clinical Specialist in Critical Care
Barnes-Jewish Hospital
St. Louis, Missouri

Appleton & Lange
Stamford, Connecticut

Prentice Hall International (UK) Limited, *London*
Prentice Hall of Australia Pty. Limited, *Sydney*
Prentice Hall Canada, Inc., *Toronto*
Prentice Hall Hispanoamericana, S.A., *Mexico*
Prentice Hall of India Private Limited, *New Delhi*
Prentice Hall of Japan, Inc., *Tokyo*
Simon and Schuster Asia Pte. Ltd., *Singapore*
Editora Prentice Hall do Brasil Ltda., *Rio de Janeiro*
Prentice Hall, *Upper Saddle River, New Jersey*

Library of Congress Cataloging-in-Publications Data
Ahrens, Thomas.
    Critical care certification : preparation, review, & examination /
Thomas Ahrens, Donna Prentice. — 4th ed.
      p.   cm.
    Rev. and combined ed. of 2 separately published works: Critical
care, certification preparation & review. 3rd ed. / Thomas Ahrens,
Donna Prentice. c1993, and Critical care : certification practice
exams / Thomas Ahrens, Donna Prentice. 3rd ed. c1993.
    Includes bibliographical references and index.
    ISBN 0-8385-1474-X (pbk. : alk. paper)
    1. Intensive care nursing—Examinations, questions, etc.
I. Prentice, Donna. II. Ahrens, Thomas. Critical care,
certification preparation & review.   III. Ahrens, Thomas.   Critical
care. IV. Title.
    [DNLM: 1. Critical Care—nurses' instruction.   2. Critical Care—
examination questions. WY 18.2 A287c 1997]
RT120.I5A39 1998
610.73'61—DC21
DNLM/DLC
for Library of Congress
                                  97-15239
                                    CIP

Acquisitions Editor: David P. Carroll
Production Editor: Elizabeth C. Ryan
Designer: Libby Schmitz
Production Service: Tage Publishing Service Inc.

PRINTED IN THE UNITED STATES OF AMERICA

ISBN 0-8385-1474-X

9 780838 514740

90000

As always, I owe all my success to my wife, Pat. She is patient beyond my gratitude, always supportive and loving during my endeavors. TA

To my parents, James H. and Edna Prentice, thank you for giving me all the love, encouragement, and guidance that I have ever needed. (Proverbs 22:6) Michael, thanks for your continued love and support and to Alex and Nicole, your precious smiles make anything possible. DP

Contents

Contributors

Patricia A. Ahrens, RN
Staff/Charge Nurse—Emergency Department
St. Mary's Medical Center
St. Louis, Missouri

Karen Sudhoff Allard, RN, MSN(R), CS, CCRN
Clinical Specialist—Critical Care
University Hospital
Cincinnati, Ohio

Pamela Becker-Weilitz, RN, MSN(R), CS
Clinical Specialist—Pulmonary
Specialist in Critical Care
Director of Nursing Practice
Barnes-Jewish Hospital
St. Louis, Missouri

Deborah Klein, RN, MSN, CCRN
Clinical Specialist—Critical Care
Metro Health Medical Center
Cleveland, Ohio

Nelda K. Martin, RN, MSN, CS, CCRN
Clinical Specialist—Cardiology
Barnes-Jewish Hospital
St. Louis, Missouri

Donna S. McCormick, RN, MSN(R), CS, CCRN
Adult Nurse Practitioner
Private Practice
Seymour Medical Center
Knoxville, Tennessee

Cathy Powers, RN, MSN, CCRN
Formerly CNS Critical Care
Barnes-Jewish Hospital
St. Louis, Missouri

Lynn Schallom, RN, MSN, CCRN
Adjunct Faculty
Maryville University

Staff Nurse
Cardiovascular Recovery Unit
Missouri Baptist Medical Center
St. Louis, Missouri

Preface

This edition marks a major change in the history of this text. In this fourth edition of the book, which originally started from Dot Langfit's efforts, we have combined the test questions with the text. We did this with the intent of making it easier to prepare for the CCRN exam without having to purchase a second book to practice taking the test. You can now read a section and then take a test on that material to give you an idea of how prepared you are in that particular section. Two realistic CCRN exam tests are included at the end of the book. This allows you to take one exam to test your knowledge base. You can study the areas where you need further development and then take the second exam.

We have kept the book simple, with relatively short chapters, to aid in your reading. Like prior editions, this is a survey book, designed to help you strengthen areas in which you already have some knowledge by providing a refresher rather than starting from the beginning. In-depth information can be found in the books and articles listed in the references.

This text closely follows the CCRN blueprint. Every major section on the CCRN test is included in this book. The chapters have been prepared by expert clinicians, with our editorial assistance. The chapters are relatively consistent in their format with all key CCRN components addressed by the authors.

Remember, to pass the CCRN exam, you need to begin preparing in advance. This is best accomplished if you study *and* use the information in clinical practice. This reinforces the material far better than if you just read the content in this (or any) book. We have included tips to help take the test at the beginning of the practice CCRN exams.

Good luck in preparing for the exam and in using this book to guide your clinical practice. You will find passing the CCRN exam to be one of the most satisfying moments of your professional career. You can be proud of this accomplishment.

ACKNOWLEDGMENTS

We wish to thank Nancy Tune, RN, MSN, CCRN; Marilyn Shatz, RN, MSN, CCRN; Susan M. Camfield, RN, BSN; and Karen Gross, MSN, RN, CCRN, for their help in preparing and reviewing this manuscript for accuracy.

Test-taking Tips

The following are some general test-taking tips. Follow them as you prepare for the examinations in this text and on the CCRN examination. They can make the difference in several points on the examination.

1. Answer all questions. Unanswered questions are counted as incorrect.

2. Be well rested before the examination. Get a good night's sleep before the examination. Do not try to "cram" the morning of the test; you may confuse yourself if you study right before the test.

3. Have a good but light breakfast. You will be taking the test for perhaps 4 hours. Eat food that is not all carbohydrates to make it through the examination without becoming hungry or getting a headache.

4. Do not change answers unless you are absolutely sure: most first impressions are accurate.

5. Go through the test and answer all questions. Mark on a piece of scrap paper questions that are difficult. Then go back and review the difficult questions. Do not be discouraged if there are many hard questions.

6. Do not expect to answer all questions correctly. If you really do not know the answer, make a guess and go on. Do not let it bother you because you know you missed a few. You really do not have a good perception of how you did until you get the results.

7. Do not let the fact that other people finish early (or that you finish before others) disturb you. People work at different rates without necessarily a difference in results.

8. If you feel thirsty or need to go to the restroom, ask permission from the monitor. Always try to maintain your physiological status at optimal levels. An aspirin (or similar analgesic) may be in order if a headache develops during the test.

9. Do not try to establish patterns in how the items are written (for example, "Two B's have occurred, now some other choice is likely.") The AACN Certification Corporation has excellent test-writing mechanisms. Patterns in test answers, if they occur, would be coincidental.

I

CARDIOVASCULAR

Thomas S. Ahrens / Nelda K. Martin / Cathy Powers / Donna Prentice

Cardiovascular Anatomy and Physiology

EDITORS' NOTE

Although basic anatomy is not commonly addressed in the exam, an understanding of principles of anatomy may help your perception of more specific questions regarding cardiovascular concepts. The following chapter is a brief review of key anatomic and physiological cardiovascular concepts that should prove useful in preparing for the test. This chapter also addresses background information on cardiovascular concepts sometimes found on the CCRN exam. If you do not have a strong background in anatomy and physiology, study this section closely. You may want to review the cardiovascular sections of physiology textbooks as well.

The CCRN test places the most emphasis on the cardiovascular component, with approximately 39% of the test questions in this content area. While many nurses are relatively strong in cardiovascular concepts, do not take this part of the exam lightly. The better you perform in any one area, the greater your chances of overall success on the exam.

NORMAL LOCATION AND SIZE OF THE HEART

The heart lies in the mediastinum, above the diaphragm and surrounded on both sides by the lungs. If one looks at a frontal (anterior) view, the heart resembles a triangle (Fig. 1–1). The base of the heart is parallel to the right edge of the sternum, whereas the lower right point of the triangle represents the apex of the heart. The apex is usually at the left midclavicular line at the fifth intraclavicular space. The average adult heart is about 5 inches long and 3½ inches wide, about the size of an average man's clenched fist. The heart weighs about 2 g for each pound of ideal body weight.

NORMAL ANATOMY OF THE HEART

The heart is supported by a fibrous skeleton (Fig. 1–2) composed of dense connective tissue. This fibrous skeleton connects the four valve rings (annuli) of the heart: the tricuspid, mitral, pulmonic, and aortic valves. Attached to the superior (top) surface of this fibrous skeleton are the right and left atria, the pulmonary artery, and the aorta. Attached to the inferior (lower) surface of the fibrous skeleton are the right and left ventricles and the mitral and tricuspid valve cusps.

The heart can be studied as two parallel pumps: the right pump (right atrium and ventricle) and the left pump (left atrium and ventricle). Each pump receives blood into its atrium. The blood flows from atria through a one-way valve into the ventricles. From each ventricle, blood is ejected into a circulatory system. The right ventricle ejects blood into the pulmonary circulation, while the left ventricle ejects blood into the systemic circulation. Although the right and left heart have differences, the gross anatomy of each is similar. Structural features of each chamber are discussed below.

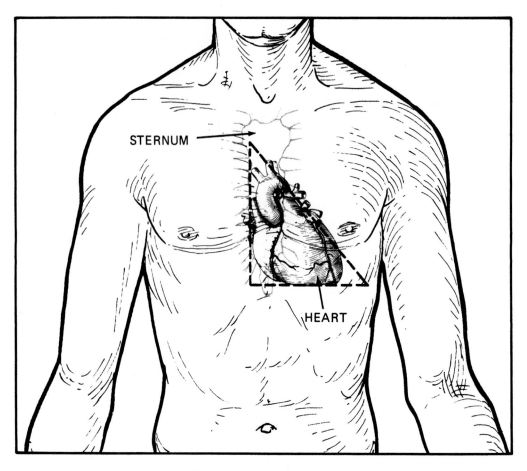

Figure 1–1. Frontal view of the heart.

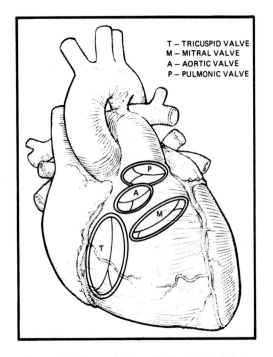

T – TRICUSPID VALVE
M – MITRAL VALVE
A – AORTIC VALVE
P – PULMONIC VALVE

Figure 1–2. Fibrous skeleton of the heart (frontal view).

STRUCTURE OF THE HEART WALL

The heart is enclosed in a fibrous sac called the pericardium. The pericardium is composed of two layers. The fibrous pericardium is the outer layer that helps support the heart. The inside layer is a smooth fibrous membrane called the parietal pericardium.

Next to the parietal serous layer of the pericardium is a visceral layer, which is actually the outer heart surface. It is most often termed the epicardium. Between the epicardium and the parietal pericardium is 10 to 20 ml of fluid, which prevents friction during heart contraction and relaxation.

The myocardium is the muscle mass of the heart composed of cardiac muscle, which has characteristics of both smooth and skeletal muscles. The endocardium is the inner surface of the heart wall. It is a membranous covering that lines all of the heart chambers and the valves.

Papillary muscles originate in the ventricular endocardium and attach to chordae tendineae

(Fig. 1–3). The chordae tendineae attach to the inferior surface of the tricuspid and mitral valve cusps to enable the valves to open and close. The papillary muscles are in parallel alignment to the ventricular wall.

CARDIAC MUSCLE CELLS

The information in this section regarding cellular aspects of cardiac muscle anatomy and physiology is not likely to be on the CCRN test. Any questions on this area are infrequent. However, the concepts addressed in this section form the basis for myocardial dysfunction and pharmacologic intervention. Read this section with the intent of becoming familiar with the concepts but not necessarily focusing on memorizing specific details.

The sarcomere (Fig. 1–4) is the contracting unit of the myocardium. The outer covering of the sarcomere is the sarcolemma, which surrounds the

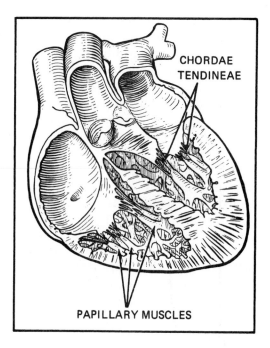

Figure 1–3. Papillary muscles and chordae tendineae.

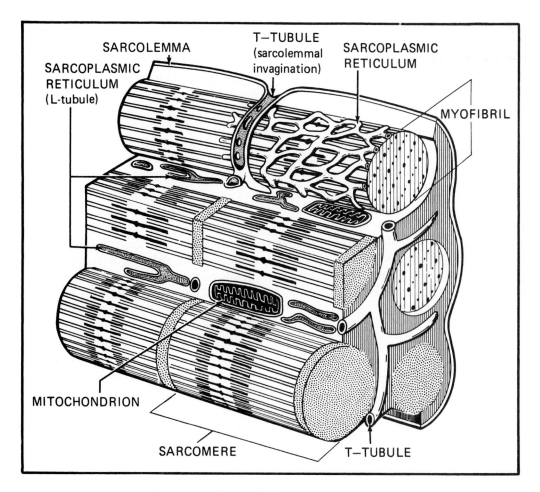

Figure 1–4. The sarcomere.

muscle fiber. The sarcolemma covers a muscle fiber that is composed of thick and thin fibers often collectively called myofibrils. Sarcomeres are separated from each other by a thickening of the sarcolemma at the ends of the sarcomere. These thickened ends, called intercalated discs, are actively involved in cardiac contraction. Each sarcomere has a centrally placed nucleus surrounded by sarcoplasma.

The sarcolemma invaginates into the sarcomere at regular intervals, resulting in a vertical penetration through the muscle fibrils coming into contact with both the thick and thin fibrils. These invaginations form the T tubules. Closely related to, but not continuous with, the T-tubule system is the sarcoplasmic reticulum. The sarcoplasmic reticulum (containing calcium ions) is an intracellular network of channels surrounding the myofibrils. These channels comprise the longitudinal (L-tubule) system of the myofibrils.

Myofibrils are thick and thin parts of the muscle fiber. Thick fibrils are myosin filaments. They have regularly placed projections that form calcium gates to the thick myofibrils. The thin myofibrils are actin. The myosin and actin myofibrils are arranged in specific parallel and hexagonal patterns (Fig. 1–5). This arrangement of fibers forms a syncytium that results in all of the fibers depolarizing when even one fiber is depolarized. This is known as the "all or none" principle—all fibers will depolarize or no fibers depolarize.

Troponin and tropomyosin are regulatory proteins attached to or affecting actin. These thick and thin myofibrils slide back and forth over each other, resulting in contraction and relaxation of the sarcomeres and, thus, the heart.

The study of physiology of the cardiac cycle examines the means by which the heart pumps blood and the various mechanisms that control the heart pump. Before looking at the heart as a whole, let us examine the contraction of a single sarcomere.

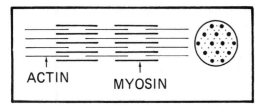

Figure 1–5. Arrangement of myosin and actin myofibrils.

CONTRACTION OF THE SARCOMERE

The sarcomeres are much like striated muscles, but they have more mitochondria than do striated or smooth muscles. The mitochondria provide the energy for the sarcomeres to contract. This energy is released by converting adenosine triphosphate (ATP) into adenosine diphosphate (ADP). In addition, the mitochondria are crucial in the storing of energy through the formation of ATP from ADP. The adding of a phosphate molecule to ADP to form ATP is called phosphorylation. This formation of ADP from ATP normally takes place in the presence of oxygen (aerobic metabolism) and is referred to as oxidative phosphorylation. Energy can be produced without oxygen (anaerobic metabolism) but not as efficiently as during aerobic metabolism. Cardiac muscle cells are highly dependent on constant blood flow to maintain adequate supplies of oxygen for the formation of ATP.

In the sarcomere, thick (myosin) and thin (actin) fibrils are arranged side by side in parallel rows. The myosin fibrils have projections that make contact with actin at specific points. These contact points are referred to as calcium gates (Fig. 1–6). During cardiac contraction, the myosin and actin slide together and overlap to as great an extent as possible (Fig. 1–7). (In the normal resting state, there is some overlapping of the myosin and actin fibrils.) Troponin and tropomyosin are protein rods interwoven around the actin fibril, having a regulatory effect upon the actin and its ability to connect with the calcium gates in the presence of calcium ions.

At the start of cellular excitation leading to a contraction, calcium ions (Ca^{++}) attach to troponin molecules around the actin fibril. This enables the projections (calcium gates) of the myosin fibril to attach to the actin. These projections twist around, causing a sliding of the fibers over each other. The calcium is removed from the calcium gates by calcium pumps located throughout the sarcoplasmic reticulum. As soon as the calcium is removed, the myosin and actin fibers slide back to their original position. This process repeats, causing contraction and relaxation of the cardiac cell.

It is important to remember that calcium initiates and regulates the sarcomere depolarization and repolarization. The role of calcium in the contraction and relaxation of the cardiac muscle cell serves as the basis for several cardiac therapies, including the use of calcium channel blocking agents and the

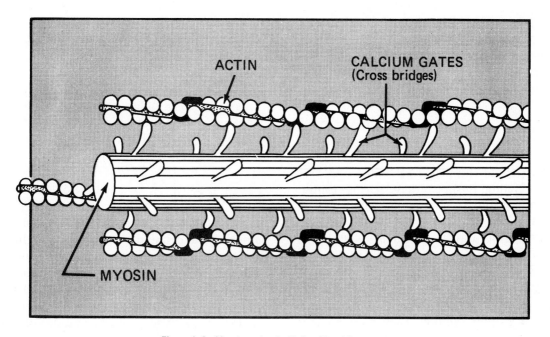

Figure 1–6. Myosin and actin fibrils with calcium gates.

potential inotropic (strength) value in administering calcium.

Even though calcium ions initiate the sliding movement of the fibrils, calcium alone is not able to cause the contraction. In addition to the presence of calcium, an exchange of ions (creating electrical energy) must occur during phases of depolarization and repolarization. This ionic exchange is mainly between sodium and potassium, and creates an ionic action potential. The exchange of chemical elements occurs across the semipermeable cell membrane in three ways: filtration, osmosis, and diffusion (active or passing).

ACTION POTENTIAL OF THE CARDIAC CELL

There are five phases of activity during the cardiac cell cycle; each phase is described below. The exchange and concentration of ions differ in each phase. Mainly four ions are involved: sodium (Na^+), potassium (K^+), calcium (Ca^{++}), and chloride (Cl^-). Normally, there is more sodium, calcium, and chloride outside the cell and more potassium inside the cell. Since all ions have an electrical charge, an electrical gradient is established. When a state of ionic electrical neutrality exists, there is a relative imper-

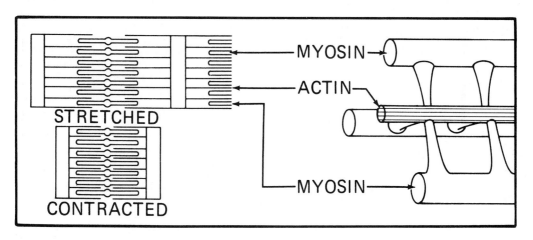

Figure 1–7. Contraction of the myosin and actin fibrils.

meability of the cell membrane, a period known as the resting potential. The presence of an electrical and chemical (ion) gradient plus membrane selectively establishes an action potential consisting of five phases, phase 0 through phase 4.

Phase 0

As a result of the presence of sodium and potassium outside and inside the cell, respectively, an electronegative gradient occurs. A depolarizing stimulus is caused by afflux of potassium from the cell, increasing the cell permeability for sodium. Calcium ions in the T-tubule and L-tubule systems of the sarcomere are at Ca^{++} gates on the cell membrane and "open" the gates for the influx of sodium. When this gradient reaches about –90 millivolts (mV) inside the cell, there is a rapid increase of the action potential (zero in Fig. 1–8). The result of the depolarization stimulus is an increase in the cell permeability for sodium. As the sodium threshold (the point at which sodium moves most freely) is reached (about –55 mV), sodium rushes into the cell and depolarizes it. Actually, more sodium rushes in than the amount required to reach electrical neutrality (zero). The

cell becomes electropositive at about +20 to 30 mV, causing a spike on the action potential diagram.

Phase 1

This is the spike phase of positive electrical charge. There is a brief period of rapid repolarization (tip of spike to #1 in Fig. 1–8), which is probably due to a flow of chloride ions into the cell.

Phase 2

This is a plateau phase of repolarization. Calcium entering the cell and potassium leaving the cell balance each other, so there is no net electrical change and thus a flat line (plateau) appears. Sodium entry into the cell is almost completely inactivated. A slow movement on calcium into the cell begins (phase 2 in Fig. 1–8). Also, a small amount of potassium begins leaving the cell at this point.

Phase 3

This is a rapid decline phase of repolarization (phase 3 in Fig. 1–8). Potassium loss from the cell is greatest

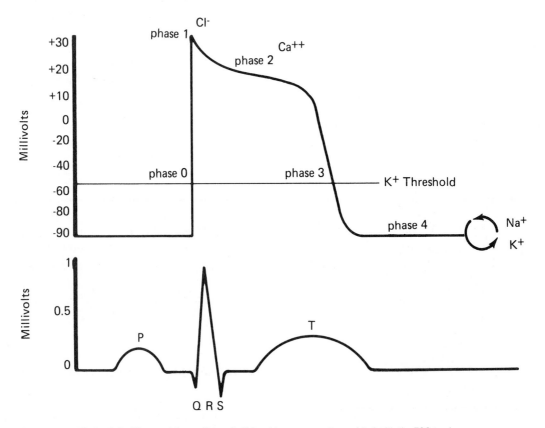

Figure 1–8. Phases of the cardiac potential and ion movement correlated with the ECG tracing.

in this phase. This potassium loss returns the cell to electronegativity. Sodium and calcium currents are completely inactivated.

Phase 4

This is the resting interval between action potentials (phase 4 in Fig. 1–8). The sodium/potassium pumps (diffusely spread throughout the sarcomere) are the most active here in effecting an exchange of position of potassium for sodium across the cell membrane. Potassium continues to leave the cell, and when electronegativity reaches –90 mV, phase 0 starts again if a stimulus occurs.

HEART CHAMBERS

There are four chambers in the heart (Fig. 1–9). The atria are superior to the ventricles and are separated from the ventricles by valves. The right atrium and ventricle are separated from the left atrium and ventricle by the atrial and ventricular septum.

Right Atrium

The right atrium is a thin-walled chamber exposed to low blood pressures. Systemic venous blood from the head, neck, and thorax enters the right atrium from the superior vena cava. Systemic venous blood from the remainder of the body enters from the inferior vena cava. Venous blood from the heart enters the

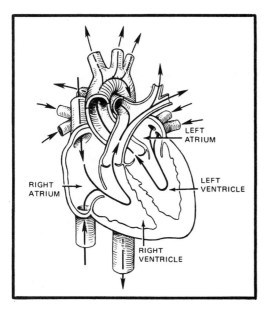

Figure 1–9. Four chambers of the heart.

right atrium through the thebesian veins, which drain into the coronary sinus. The coronary sinus is located on the medial right atrial wall just about the tricuspid valve.

Right Ventricle

The right ventricle is the pump for the right heart. The right ventricle contracts to pump venous blood into the pulmonary artery and to the lungs. The lungs are normally a low-pressure system. The right ventricle is shaped and functions like a bellows to propel blood out during contraction.

Left Atrium

The left atrium, just like the right, is thin walled. Blood flowing passively from the low-lung-pressure area does not stress the walls of the left atrium. The left atrium receives oxygenated blood from the four pulmonary veins.

Left Ventricle

The left ventricle is the major pump for the entire body. As such, it must have thick, strong walls. To overcome the high pressure of the systemic circulation, the left ventricle is shaped like a cylinder. As it contracts (starting from the apex), it also narrows somewhat. This cylindrical shape provides strong physical force to propel blood into the aorta with sufficient force to overcome the high systemic pressure (resulting from the requirement to pump the blood to distant body areas).

HEART VALVES

There are two types of valves in the heart: the atrioventricular and the semilunar valves. All valves in the heart are unidirectional, unless they are diseased or dysfunctional. Normally the valves provide very little resistance to cardiac contractions. If the valves become narrow (stenotic) or allow blood to flow past when the valves should be closed (regurgitation), the work of the heart will substantially increase.

Atrioventricular Valves

The atrioventricular (AV) valves of the heart are the tricuspid and the mitral valves. These valves allow blood to flow from the atria into the ventricles during atrial contraction and ventricular diastole. Mnemonics may help you remember which valve is on which side of the heart. Consider the following: "L" and "M" come together in the alphabet and in the heart. The left heart contains the mitral valve. Likewise, "R" and "T" are close in the alphabet. The right heart contains the tricuspid valve. Both the mitral and the tricuspid valves have two large opposing leaflets and small intermediary leaflets at each end.

Mitral Valve

The mitral valve's two large leaflets are not quite equal in size (Fig. 1–10). The chordae tendineae from adjacent leaflets are inserted upon the same papillary muscles. This physical feature helps to ensure complete closure of the valve. When the mitral valve is open, the valve, chordae tendineae, and papillary muscle look like a funnel. Of all the valves, the mitral is most commonly involved in clinical conditions of valvular dysfunction. Mitral regurgitation is the most common clinical valvular disturbance. Clinically, mitral regurgitation may be insignificant (subclinical) or represent a life-threatening situation (papillary muscle rupture). The key factor influencing the significance of any valvular disturbance is the effect on stroke volume (amount of blood the heart pumps with each contraction).

Tricuspid Valve

The tricuspid valve differs from the mitral valve in that it has one larger leaflet than the mitral valve and has three papillary muscles instead of two. Otherwise, the structures and functions of the two valves are similar. Tricuspid dysfunction is not as much of a clinical problem as is mitral dysfunction.

Semilunar (Pulmonic and Aortic) Valves

The semilunar valves (Fig. 1–11) of the heart are the aortic and the pulmonary valves. Each has three symmetrical valve cusps to provide for complete opening without stretching of the valve. The pulmonary valve is located between the right ventricle and the pulmonary artery. The aortic valve is located between the left ventricle and the aorta.

Pulmonary valve dysfunction will potentially affect the performance of the right ventricle. Aortic valve disturbance can affect the performance of the left ventricle.

Physical Assessment of the Cardiac Valves

Cardiac valves can be assessed to some extent through auscultation. Heart sounds can be identified partially based on specific valve functioning. The heart normally generates two sounds, referred to as S_1 and S_2. S_1 is the sound generated through the closure of the mitral (M_1) and tricuspid (T_1) valves. M_1 is best heard at the fifth intercostal space (ICS) in the left mid-clavicular line. T_1 is best heard the fourth ICS at the left sternal border. S_1 is produced during ventricular contraction. S_1 can be identified

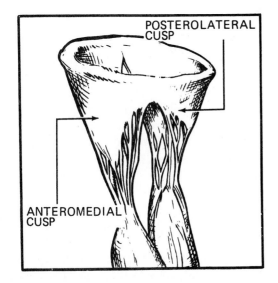

Figure 1–10. Side view of the mitral valve.

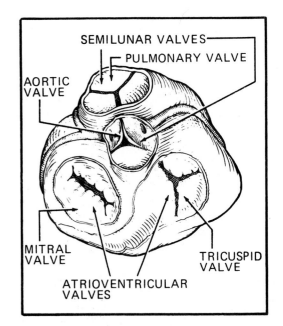

Figure 1–11. The semilunar valves and the AV valves (posterior view).

by listening (it normally is the loudest of the two cardiac sounds at the fourth ICS, left sternal border or the fifth ICS, left midclavicular line) or by comparing the sounds to the electrocardiogram (ECG). The S_1 sound occurs immediately after the QRS complex (which indicates ventricular depolarization and contraction).

S_2 is produced by the closure of the aortic (A_2) and pulmonic (P_2) valves. A_2 is best heard at the second ICS, just to the right of the sternum. The P_2 sound is heard best at the second ICS, just to the left of the sternum. S_2 can also be identified by listening (it is loudest in the locations described above) or by comparing to the ECG. Normally, the S_2 sound occurs during diastole (when aortic and pulmonary blood pressures are higher than ventricular pressures, forcing the aortic and pulmonary valves to close). The S_2 sound normally appears during the T wave or slightly before the QRS complex.

Abnormal Heart Sounds
Heart valves normally produce sound during closure. Four common abnormal situations exist when other sounds might develop. These situations are valve regurgitation, stenosis, ventricular or atrial failure, or disturbances of electrical conduction.

Valve Regurgitation
When a valve becomes regurgitant (sometimes referred to as insufficient), blood flows past the valve, which is normally closed. This produces a sound usually described as a murmur. Murmurs are sounds that are described in several ways, such as blowing and swishing. Murmurs are graded in degree from I to VI. A grade I murmur (written as I/VI) is a very soft sound. A grade VI murmur (written as VI/VI) is so prominent that it can be heard with the stethoscope held about 1 inch from the chest wall. The other grades of murmurs are subjectively described as between I and VI. It is frequently up to the clinician to grade a murmur, since there are no clear objective criteria for grading murmurs.

Mitral and tricuspid regurgitation will produce a murmur that occurs during systole (normally the mitral and tricuspid valves close during systole). Aortic and pulmonic regurgitation will produce a diastolic murmur.

Valvular Stenosis
A stenosis of a valve produces a murmur that may sound like a regurgitant murmur. However, the reasons for the murmur are different. A mitral or tricuspid stenosis produces a murmur during diastole (normally atrial contraction does not meet resistance to pushing blood past the mitral or tricuspid valve). An aortic or pulmonic stenosis can produce a systolic murmur.

Valves can be dysfunctional in isolation (such as a mitral regurgitation) or in multiples. The clinician attempts to identify the cause of the murmur through auscultation and clinical history.

Ventricular and Atrial Failure
During ventricular failure, an increased pressure builds in the ventricles and atrium. After systole, when blood enters the ventricles from the atrium, the high atrial pressure may force blood into the ventricles with considerable force. This increased flow of blood into the ventricles may produce a sound, the S_3 sound. The S_3 sound occurs immediately after the S_2 sound and can be found after the T wave on the ECG. S_3 sounds are not always abnormal but should be considered significant, particularly in the presence of tachycardia. The combination of a tachycardia and S_3 produces a characteristic "gallop" sound associated with left ventricular (congestive heart) failure.

Another heard sound associated with high pressures is the S_4 sound. The S_4 sound is thought to be an atrial sound, associated with high atrial pressures. It can be found immediately before the QRS complex and after the P wave when compared with an ECG tracing.

Electrical Conduction Defects
When there is an electrical conduction defect, such as a bundle branch block, the potential exists for the valves to fail to function in unison. When this occurs, a split in the heart sound will occur. For example, a right bundle branch block causes a delay in right ventricular contraction. The result is that the pulmonic valve closes slightly after the aortic valve. The S_2 sound now becomes softer and produces two sounds instead of one. The split S_2 can aid in the diagnosis of a right bundle branch block.

Pulsus Paradoxus and Change in Heart Sounds
Heart sounds can be diminished in intensity if air (as in chronic obstructive pulmonary disease) or fluid (pericardial effusion or tamponade) is between the heart and the stethoscope. In tamponade, fluid fills the pericardial sac and limits sound transmission. In addition, the increased fluid restricts ventricular expansion and can dangerously drop the cardiac output. If tamponade occurs, the inability of the ven-

tricle to distend will produce diminished heart sounds, equalizing chamber pressures (e.g., central venous and pulmonary capillary wedge pressures begin to equalize), venous distension develops, and pulsus paradoxus may occur. Pulsus paradoxus is the decreasing of blood pressure during inspiration. A decrease in systolic blood pressure of more than 10 mm Hg is characteristic of pulsus paradoxus. The blood pressure decreases because of the increase in blood entering the atrium during inspiration, further increasing the pericardial pressure. The added pericardial pressure further decreases stroke volume and systolic blood pressure.

Heart sounds can be useful clinical parameters, but they require frequent practice in order to become proficient. More accurate tests are replacing their clinical use. If valve dysfunction is thought to exist, echocardiography is the test of choice. If conduction defects exist, electrocardiography is more accurate in detecting abnormalities. For the purpose of the CCRN test, the basic information provided above will help identify the essential information. Be prepared for questions in which a heart sound is given and you must then identify a clinical condition. However, be aware of the more accurate methods for assessing cardiac function, as they may also be addressed on the test.

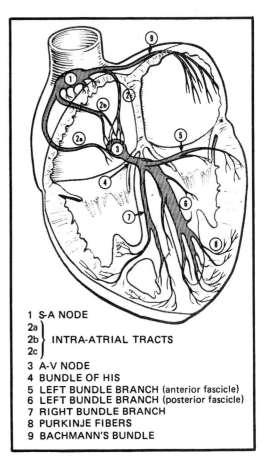

1 S-A NODE
2a
2b } INTRA-ATRIAL TRACTS
2c
3 A-V NODE
4 BUNDLE OF HIS
5 LEFT BUNDLE BRANCH (anterior fascicle)
6 LEFT BUNDLE BRANCH (posterior fascicle)
7 RIGHT BUNDLE BRANCH
8 PURKINJE FIBERS
9 BACHMANN'S BUNDLE

Figure 1–12. Conduction system of the heart.

THE NORMAL CONDUCTION SYSTEM OF THE HEART

The conduction of an electrical impulse normally follows an orderly, repetitive pattern from the right atrium, through the ventricles, and into the myocardium, where the impulse usually results in ventricular contraction (Fig. 1–12).

The sinoatrial (SA) node is at the junction of the superior vena cava and the right atrium. The SA node is a group of specialized heart cells that are self-excitatory. All self-excitatory cells have automaticity; that is, if the cells can excite themselves, they require no stimulus and may excite themselves at will. This is termed inherent automaticity or spontaneous depolarization. The SA node excites itself faster than any other cardiac cells under normal conditions. For this reason, the SA node becomes the heart's normal pacemaker.

Once the impulse originates in the SA node, it spreads through the atria along three paths called internodal tracts. The impulse continues from the internodal tracts into the AV junction. The AV node is located at the superior end of the junctional tissue, near the tricuspid valve ring just above the ventricular septum. There is a slight pause in the impulse at the upper portion of the AV node to allow for completion of atrial contraction. The impulse traverses the AV node and the junctional tissue, and then reaches the bundle of His. The bundle of His carries the impulse to the bundle branches. The bundle of His divides into right and left bundle branches.

The left bundle branch continues along the ventricular septum, dividing into two subdivisions called fascicles. The anterior fascicle excites the anterior and superior surfaces of the left ventricle. The posterior fascicle excites the posterior and inferior surfaces of the left ventricle. The right bundle branch continues as a single branch to innervate the right ventricle.

Having passed through the bundle of His and the bundle branches, the impulse arrives at the Purkinje fibers, which spread into the ventricular myocardium. The impulse spread usually is followed by ventricular contraction, and thus the cycle repeats.

Disturbances in this conduction system will be reviewed as to the specific resulting dysrhythmias. The current CCRN format requires a good understanding of the electrical system of the heart and the ability to interpret dysrhythmias and 12-lead ECGs. While specific sections are provided on dysrhythmias and 12-lead analysis, understanding the basic anatomy and physiology of the electrical conduction system is important.

CIRCULATORY SYSTEMS OF THE BODY

Circulatory paths can be remembered by the mnemonic that "a" for artery means "a" for away. *All* arteries carry blood, either oxygenated or deoxygenated (pulmonary), *away* from the heart. Conversely, all veins carry blood, either oxygenated or deoxygenated, to the heart.

There are two circulatory systems in the body, the pulmonary and the systemic. The heart must pump blood through these two systems in the amount needed by the body to maintain optimal function. In addition, the coronary circulation (a branch of the systemic circulation), the pulmonary circulation, and the systemic circulation have some features helpful to note for the purpose of the CCRN exam.

The Pulmonary Circulation

The pulmonary system is unique in that it is the only system (excluding the fetal) in which the pulmonary artery carries unoxygenated blood away from the heart to the lungs, and the four pulmonary veins carry oxygenated blood from the lungs to the left atrium. The right ventricle sends venous blood into the main pulmonary artery, which divides into the right and left pulmonary arteries. These arteries follow the normal blood vessel path, that is, arteries to arterioles to capillaries (where the blood becomes oxygenated) to venules to veins.

The Systemic Circulation

The aorta is the only artery that the left ventricle normally ejects blood into; it arches over the pulmonary artery. The aorta gives off many branches as it traverses down the body to bifurcate into the iliac arteries. In the capillaries, the blood surrenders oxygen and picks up carbon dioxide. The inferior and superior venae cavae are the final veins returning blood to the right atrium.

The Coronary Circulation

The coronary circulatory system begins with the inflow of oxygenated blood into the coronary arteries. The openings of these arteries are located near the cusps of the aortic valve. These arteries fill during ventricular diastole.

The right coronary artery supplies the posterior and inferior myocardium with oxygenated blood. The left coronary artery starts at the valve cusp as the left main coronary artery and bifurcates to form the left anterior descending (LAD) and the circumflex arteries. The LAD artery supplies the anterior and septal myocardium. The circumflex artery supplies the lateral myocardium. These arteries then follow the normal sequence of becoming arterioles, capillaries, venules, and veins as they course through the myocardium. The veins empty into thebesian veins, which in turn empty into the coronary sinus. Blood from the coronary sinus joins the venous blood in the right atrium.

Autonomic Regulation of Peripheral Vessels

The sympathetic nervous system has an adrenergic effect upon peripheral vessels. The norepinephrine released by the sympathetic system causes vasoconstriction. This vasoconstriction prevents pooling of blood in the peripheral vessels and augments the return of blood to the heart.

The parasympathetic nervous system has a cholinergic effect upon peripheral vessels. Acetylcholine is released by the parasympathetic nervous system. This causes a vasodilatation of peripheral vessels. With dilation, more blood can remain in the peripheral vessels, and less blood is returned to the heart.

Baroreceptor Control

Baroreceptors are also called pressoreceptors or stretch receptors since these areas respond to a stretching of arterial and venous vessel walls. These receptors are specialized cells located in the aortic arch, carotid sinus, atria, venae cavae, and pulmonary arteries. These receptor sites are responsive to mean arterial pressure greater than 60 mm Hg. When stimulated by an elevated pressure, these receptors send signals to the medulla oblongata in the brain. The medulla then inhibits sympathetic nervous system activity, which allows the vagus nerve of the parasympathetic nervous system to assume control. This results in vasodilatation of peripheral vessels and a decreased heart rate. Under normal circumstances, this will allow the blood pressure to return to normal.

Conversely, if pressure is low, vagal tone is decreased, which allows the sympathetic nervous system to assume control. This results in vasoconstriction of the peripheral vessels and an increased heart rate. Under normal circumstances, this will allow the blood pressure to return to normal.

Vasomotor Center of Regulation

There are two areas of vasomotor control in the medulla oblongata: a vasoconstrictor area and a vasodilator area. The vasomotor center responds to baroreceptors and chemoreceptors in the aortic arch and carotid sinus.

If the vasoconstrictor area is stimulated, normally an increased heart rate, stroke volume, and cardiac output will result because of peripheral vasoconstriction. As the peripheral vessels constrict, more blood is forced from these vessels and returned to the heart. This normally restores arterial blood pressure.

If the vasodilator area is stimulated (by inhibition of the vasoconstrictor area), a decrease in stroke volume and cardiac output will normally occur. The vasodilatation allows for more blood to remain in peripheral vessels; therefore, less blood is returned to the heart. The normal end result will be a decrease in blood pressure. This partially explains the bradycardia seen in patients who are hypertensive.

Chemoreceptors are activated by decreased oxygen pressures, an increased carbon dioxide level, and/or a decreased pH. Once activated, the chemoreceptors stimulate the vasoconstrictor area. The events that normally occur with such stimulation are then set into action.

HEART RATE

The other regulator of cardiac output, heart rate, can be used as a guide to therapy and assessments. The heart rate is regulated by the autonomic nervous system through sympathetic (adrenergic) and parasympathetic (cholinergic) mechanisms. Sympathetic regulation occurs through alpha and beta receptors located in the cardiovascular system. There are two types of alpha and beta cells: $alpha_1$ and $alpha_2$, and $beta_1$ and $beta_2$. Parasympathetic effect is primarily through the vagus nerve.

When a bradycardia exists, treatment is based on the factors that control the heart rate. For example, parasympathetic stimulation has a stronger effect on the heart than does sympathetic stimulation. The stronger parasympathetic effect is the rea-

son atropine is the first drug given to treat a bradycardia. Isoproterenol, a sympathetic stimulator, is the second choice.

The heart rate is a valuable diagnostic tool in that it is the first compensatory response to a decrease in stroke volume. A sinus tachycardia frequently heralds a decrease in stroke volume. The other reason an increase in the heart rate may occur is an increase in metabolic rate. The increase in metabolic rate requires an increase in cardiac output, generally met by increasing both heart rate and stroke volume.

Heart rate elevations, e.g., sinus tachycardia, by themselves are not generally dangerous. Although the increase in heart rate will increase myocardial oxygen consumption (MVo_2), the reason for the development of the tachycardia is more important. A clinical clue to investigate is the origin of a sinus tachycardia, followed by treating the cause of the tachycardia rather than the tachycardia itself.

RELATIONSHIP OF BLOOD FLOW AND PRESSURE IN CARDIAC CYCLE

The pressure of a fluid in a chamber depends upon the size of the chamber, the amount of fluid, the distensibility of the chamber, and whether the chamber is open or closed.

The atria (both right and left) are open chambers. The venae cavae in the right atrium and the pulmonary veins in the left atrium are always open. Thus, pressures in these chambers will remain low unless something occludes the openings or prevents them from emptying.

The anatomic structure of the right ventricle contributes to its low pressure. The right ventricle normally empties into a low-pressure system, the lungs.

The left ventricle has a high pressure. Its anatomic structure contributes to the high pressure. It empties into a high-pressure, closed system, the aorta. Trace the flow of blood through the chambers and examine its relationship to the cardiac valves and the chamber pressures. These relationships are shown in Fig. 1–13.

Atrial Pressure Curve

Throughout diastole, pressure slowly increases in the atria because of the influx of blood. The volume of blood increases in relation to the chamber size (resulting in a V wave on the atrial waveform). With atrial contraction (first curve on the atrial line in

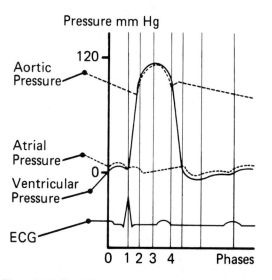

Figure 1–13. Blood flow and pressure during the cardiac cycle.

The normal atrial pressures generate three waves: A, C, and V (Fig. 1–14). The A wave is the result of atrial contraction and can be found in the PR interval. One exception to the location of the A wave is in regard to the pulmonary capillary wedge pressure (PCWP). The PCWP is found slightly later, in the QRS, because of the time it takes the wave to travel from the left atrium to the pulmonary catheter. The importance of the A wave is that the mean of the A wave is the parameter used to estimate the central venous pressure (CVP) and PCWP values.

The C wave is due to closure of the tricuspid and mitral valves. The V wave is due to atrial filling and the bulging of the tricuspid and mitral valves into the atrium. Large V waves can develop with noncompliant atria and mitral or tricuspid regurgitation (Fig. 1–15).

Fig. 1–13), there is a sudden increase in pressure (producing an A wave in the atrial waveform) since the contraction decreases the size of the atrium. During atrial contraction, pressure is greater in the atrium than in the ventricle. This higher pressure causes the AV valves to open. Atrial blood flows through the open AV valves into the ventricles.

As the ventricles begin the systolic phase, blood flow is reversed. As soon as the blood flow reverses, the blood completely closes the partially closed AV valves. The ventricular pressure increase is so sudden that the AV valves bulge into the atria, increasing the intra-atrial pressure (second curve on atrial line in Fig. 1–13). Following this second curve, there is a sharp fall in atrial pressure. Gradually, the atrial pressure rises again during the next period of diastole, and the cycle repeats.

Ventricular Pressure Curve

During diastole, the ventricular pressure is less than the atrial pressure. Just before atrial systole occurs, the AV valves open and blood flows into the ventricles. As soon as the ventricles fill, the blood flow reverses and closes the AV valves. At this point, the ventricles become closed chambers. The ventricle walls contract against the volume of blood in the ventricle. Since the ventricle is a closed chamber, pressure rises rapidly. Aortic pressure during diastole has fallen to about 80 mm Hg. The period during which ventricular pressure builds from near zero to 80 mm Hg is termed the isometric contraction phase (ventricle curve between lines 1 and 2 in Fig. 1–13). The left ventricle continues to contract strongly, and the pressure rises to about 110 mm Hg. Since left ventricular pressure exceeds the aortic pressure of 80

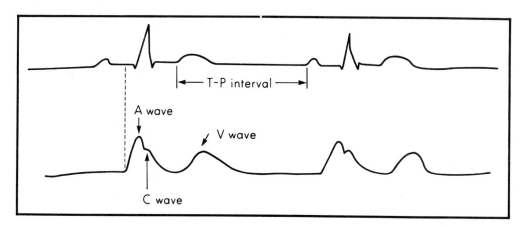

Figure 1–14. Normal atrial waveforms.

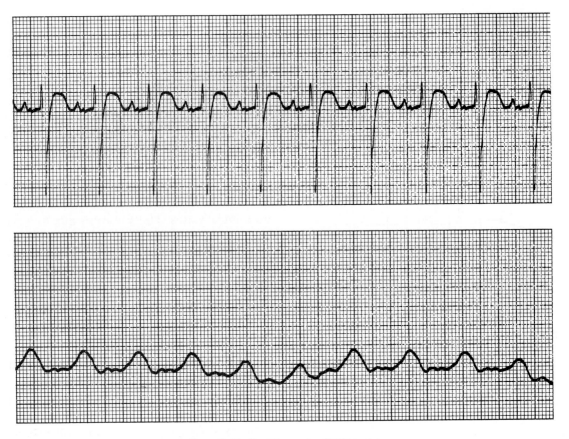

Figure 1–15. Giant V waves in a PCWP tracing.

mm Hg, the aortic valve is forced open, and blood is ejected into the aorta. These same mechanisms are occurring concurrently in the right ventricle, only under much lower pressures. This is called the rapid ejection phase (ventricle curve between lines 2 and 3 in Fig. 1–13). Pressure begins to drop in the ventricle because blood is being ejected faster than the ventricle is contracting. This is called the reduced-ejection phase (ventricular curve between lines 3 and 4 in Fig. 1–13). Ventricular contraction ceases, and the ventricle relaxes. Since the ventricular pressure has dropped rapidly, the blood flow starts to reverse at about 80 mm Hg in the aorta. This backward flow closes the aortic valve. The ventricle again becomes a closed chamber, but since no blood is entering, the pressure does not rise. The fall of pressure in the ventricle continues until it is less than the atrial pressure. Then the cycle begins again.

Diagnosis and Treatment of Cardiovascular Disorders

INVASIVE AND NONINVASIVE DIAGNOSTIC TESTS

EDITORS' NOTE

There is no section specifically on testing in the CCRN exam. However, several questions either directly or indirectly address cardiovascular assessment via diagnostic tests. In this short section, cardiac diagnostic tests are categorized according to what they do and when they are indicated. Depending on the importance of the test, they will also be covered in chapters on specific cardiac conditions later in this book. This section should help you familiarize yourself with the tests which will potentially be on the exam.

Cardiac Isoenzyme and Protein Level

Following trauma or hypoxia, enzymes and proteins leak from damaged cells. These isoenzymes and proteins are used in the identification of myocardial injury, most commonly myocardial infarction. Any myocardial injury, however, including cardiopulmonary resuscitation, cardiac contusion, and cardiac surgery, will elevate cardiac enyzmes and proteins. Some tests are better than others at avoiding confounding factors. The most common cardiac enzymes and proteins are listed in Table 2–1.

Electrocardiography

The electrocardiogram (ECG) is the most commonly used noninvasive diagnostic test for patients with known or suspected cardiac disease. The ECG is defined as a graphic tracing of the electrical forces produced by the heart. A 12-lead ECG provides information beyond the bedside monitor. The bedside monitor is primarily used to assess heart rate, rhythm, and life-threatening dysrhythmias. The 12-lead ECG provides more information in terms of myocardial injury and ischemia, conduction disturbances, axis orientation, and heart size.

It is important to note that, although the ECG's simplicity makes it very useful, it is of limited accuracy and should be used in conjunction with other information, such as physical assessment and laboratory tests. The ECG is not simple to interpret, despite its simplicity of use. Many factors alter the ECG's appearance and many of these factors are not clinically significant. However, it is essential for the ICU nurse to be able to identify the important changes on the ECG since many times it is the bedside nurse who is responsible for interpreting the ECG.

Echocardiography

Echocardiography (echo) is excellent at identifying structural changes in the heart. Echocardiography uses pulses of reflected ultrasound to evaluate cardiac structure and function. Different types of echocardiography exist, including two-dimensional and transesophageal techniques. Transesophageal echocardiography is more specific, but requires the patient to swallow a device which resembles a nasogastric tube.

Echocardiography can detect valve disturbances, septal defects, the presence of pericardial fluid, and abnormalities of ventricular muscle movement. In conditions such as myocardial infarction and contusion, it can detect what part of the heart is

TABLE 2–1. COMMON CARDIAC ENZYME AND PROTEIN DETERMINATIONS USED IN DIAGNOSING CARDIAC INJURY

Cardiac Test	Purpose
(CPK) Creatine phosphokinase	Nonspecific muscle enzyme, found in muscle and heart tissue. Some studies have indicated that the greater the rise in the CPK, the greater the damage to the heart. This test is less useful when muscle damage is also present.
CPK-MB	A more specific cardiac muscle enzyme. The most common test used in diagnosing myocardial injury. Highly specific for cardiac injury, although it also can rise with muscle damage.
(LDH) Lactic dehydrogenase	A nonspecific muscle enzyme whose chief value in cardiac diagnostics is its slow rise and persistent elevation. It is used to detect MIs which may be more than 24 hr old. Will likely be replaced by troponin I in the near future.
Subforms of CPK-MB	Cardiac isoenzyme subforms (CPK-MB$_1$ and -MB$_2$) may be the fastest changing of myocardial enzymes. Evidence exists that MIs can be identified within 2 hours of occurrence if these forms are measured and (CPK-MB$_2$ > CPK-MB$_1$) the short-lived CPK-MB$_2$ is found to exceed CPK-MB$_1$.
Troponin I	A very specific cardiac muscle protein, one of the first of a new generation of diagnostic tests for cardiac assessment. It rises rapidly like CPK-MB but stays elevated for about 8 days. Is likely to replace LDH measurements in cardiac assessments.
Myoglobin	A very specific cardiac muscle protein which elevates and returns to normal rapidly. May be useful in rapid detection, with a higher precision than before, of myocardial injury.

damaged by noting dysfunctional movement in the muscle of the heart. It is an essential aspect of identifying disturbances in physical properties of the heart. Since it is noninvasive, it is one of the diagnostic tests of choice of many cardiologists.

Radionuclide Imaging

Radionuclide imaging detects pathologic cardiac conditions through the external detection of photons emitted from the body after the administration of radioisotopes. This is useful in detecting abnormalities in left ventricular wall motion, as well as ventricular size, volume, and ejection fraction. Radionuclide imaging is increasingly used to detect disturbances in cell function and blood flow.

The thallium scan is a radionuclide imaging technique which is used to evaluate regional myocardial perfusion and viability. Thallium scans can be performed with the patient at rest or during exercise. For those patients unable to exercise, dobutamine and dipyridamole thallium scanning ARC is used to increase coronary blood flow in place of exercise.

Positron emission tomography (PET) scanning is a sophisticated imaging technique which measures specific radioisotopes injected into the body via the blood. PET scans may be used to determine the exact part of the heart that is threatened by a loss of oxygen. It is capable of distinguishing dysfunctional but viable myocardium from areas of infarction.

Cardiac Catheterization

Cardiac catheterization involves insertion of catheters into cardiac chambers and blood vessels to measure intracardiac pressures, oxygen saturation, and coronary blood flow. Angiography, a part of the cardiac catheterization procedure, is used specifically to examine the blood vessels by injection of measureable contrast material. Coronary angiography generally involves the injection of radiopaque contrast medium into the chambers of the heart, coronary arteries, and great vessels. The passage of the contrast dye is followed and filmed as the heart beats spontaneously. The moving pictures of the coronary circulation are called cineangiograms.

Cardiac catheterization is usually performed to evaluate the presence and severity of coronary artery atherosclerosis. Virtually all patients undergoing cardiac surgery have cardiac catheterization before surgery. Cardiac catheterization is also evolving into a variety of treatments, including percutaneous transluminal coronary angioplasty and intracoronary stent placement.

Electrophysiology Studies

Electrophysiology studies (EPS) are used to assess the conduction of electricity through the heart, with much more specificity than surface ECG. EPS provide definitive diagnostic information on cardiac dysrhythmias, such as premature ventricular contractions (PVCs), and help direct proper therapies. EPS are similar to cardiac catheterization and are commonly performed in the same area. Intracardiac catheters placed under fluoroscopic guidance are used to record intracardiac electrical activity. They are often used to provoke cardiac dysrhythmias under a controlled, treatment-ready setting. Treatment plans for various dysrhythmias often emerge from the results of EPS. Many hospitals are not equipped to perform EPS and patients need to be referred to more specialized settings.

PHARMACOLOGICAL TREATMENT

EDITORS' NOTE

You can expect several questions, perhaps as many as 10, that directly or indirectly address pharmacological treatments for abnormal hemodynamics. It is not necessary or desirable to review all therapies while preparing for the CCRN exam. However, it is critical to understand the most common therapies and how they work. The focus of this section is essential pharmacological therapy used in the treatment of abnormal hemodynamics. More specific therapies, such as thrombolytics and antidysrhythmics, are covered in other chapters. If you have a good understanding of this section, you should be well prepared for the CCRN exam questions on this content.

Treatment of abnormal hemodynamics centers on improving either cardiac output or systemic vascular resistance (SVR). In the treatment of inadequate cardiac output, the components of stroke volume (preload, afterload, and contractility) are the most commonly manipulated parameters. A large number of cardiac therapies are available to treat hemodynamic abnormalities.

Treatment of Low Cardiac Output States

Treatment of conditions which cause low stroke volume and low cardiac output usually centers on the left ventricle. Normally, low cardiac output is caused by weakening of the left ventricle [due, for example, to congestive heart failure (CHF), myocardial infarction (MI), or cardiomyopathy] or inadequate blood volume (hypovolemia). If the problem is a weak left ventricle, therapies which might be used include (1) preload reduction; (2) afterload reduc-

tion; and (3) increasing contractility. There are also a few physical interventions, such as allowing the patient to sit up or attempting to reduce anxiety, as well as mechanical support of the heart with intra-aortic balloon pumping and ventricular assist devices. The majority of therapies, however, focus on pharmacological support. It is this treatment modality that is most important for the bedside clinician to understand.

Improving the Strength of the Heart

In the patient presenting with symptoms of left ventricular dysfunction, relief is obtained by improving the strength of the heart. This is also referred to as inotropic therapy. Inotropic therapy increases the strength of the cardiac contraction. As a consequence of the improved strength, an increase in ejection fraction, stroke volume, cardiac output, and, ideally, tissue oxygenation occur.

Many inotropes are available (Table 2–2). These include dobutamine (Dobutrex), dopamine, amrinone, milrinone, epinephrine, and digoxin. The most common inotrope used is dobutamine. Dobutamine acts by stimulating beta cells of the sympathetic nervous system, which in turn strengthens contraction (positive inotropic response) and makes the heart beat faster (positive chronotropic). Since beta stimulation also causes smooth muscle relaxation, blood vessels dilate. This results in a drop in preload (pulmonary capillary wedge pressure and central venous pressure) and afterload (SVR).

Dopamine is also used, particularly in moderate dosages (2–10 μg/kg/min). However, dopamine stimulates alpha cells of the sympathetic nervous system, causing vasoconstriction (increased SVR). This vasoconstriction might increase the blood pressure but it also causes an increase in myocardial work.

There are times when sympathetic stimulation cannot provide any more improvement in contractility. At this time, drugs having different mechanisms of action, such as the phosphodiesterase inhibitors amrinone and milrone, might be used. These drugs increase the availability of intracellular calcium and the strength of the heart.

Digitalis preparations such as digoxin are not used in acute situations. These drugs might be used in chronic ventricular dysfunction but not in acute failure.

TABLE 2–2. COMMON INOTROPIC (CONTRACTILITY) DRUGS

	Dose	Onset	Route	Drip conc.
Dobutamine (Dobutrex)	2.5–10 µg/kg/min	1–2 min	IV	250 mg/100 ml D$_5$W or NS
Dopamine (Intropin) Beta adrenergic	2–10 µg/kg/min	<5 min	IV	400 mg/250 ml D$_5$W or NS
Amrinone (Inocor)	Loading 0.75 mg/kg over 2–3 mins. Maintenance is 5–10 µg/kg/min.	5–10 min	IV	200 mg/100 ml NS
Milrinone (Primicor)				
Digoxin (IV) (Lanoxin)	Loading 10–15 µg/kg in divided doses over 12 to 24 hr q 6–8 hr.	5–30 min	IV	NA
Digoxin (PO) (Lanoxin)	Loading 0.5 mg × 1 then 0.25 mg q 6 hr until desired effect or total digitalizing dosage is achieved. Maintenance 0.125–0.25 mg/day.	1–2 hr	PO	NA

D$_5$W, 5% dextrose in water; NS, normal saline; NA, not applicable.

Improving Cardiac Strength Through Preload Reduction

The strength of the heart might be improved if overstretched myocardial muscle fibers can be allowed to shrink back to normal. Preload reduction can accomplish this goal. Preload reduction is done through vasodilation or with diuretics.

Diuretics are commonly used for preload reduction, mainly because they help reduce the excess fluid in the circulatory system that results

TABLE 2–3. DIURETICS

	Dose	Onset	Route	Drip conc.
Mild				
Mannitol (Osmotic diuretic)	12.5–200 g/day	Within minutes	IVP (filter) or IV drip	50 g in NS or D$_5$W to 250 ml final volume
Spironolactone (Aldactone) (K$^+$ sparing class)	25–2100 mg/day	24–48 hr	PO	NA
Moderate				
Chlorothiazide (Diuril) (Thiazide class)	500–2000 mg/day	1–2 hr	PO/IV	NA
Hydrochlorothiazide (Hydrodiuril) (Thiazide class)	25–200 mg/day	2 hr	PO	NA
Metolazone (Zaroxolyn, Microx) (Nonthiazide)	2.5–20 mg/day	1 hr	PO	NA
Strong				
Furosemide (PO) (Lasix) (Loop diuretic)	20–600 mg/day	1 hr	PO	NA
Furosemide (IV) (Lasix) (Loop diuretic)	≥20 mg/day	5 min	IV	1 g in NS or D$_5$W to 250 ml final volume
Ethacrynic acid (PO) (Edecrin) (Loop diuretic)	25–400 mg/day	30 min	PO	NA
Ethacrynic acid (IV) (Edecrin) (Loop diuretic)	50–100 mg/day	5 min	IV	No standard drip
Bumetanide (PO) (Bumex) (Loop diuretic)	0.5–10 mg/day	30 min	PO	NA
Bumetanide (IV) (Bumex) (Loop diuretic)	0.5–10 mg/day	Within minutes	IV	No standard drip

NA, not applicable.

TABLE 2-4. VASODILATORS

	Dose	Onset	Route	Drip conc.
Nitroglycerin (IV) (Tridil, Nitrostat IV) (Nitrate vasodilator)	5–160 μg/min. Titrate to desired effect; at high dose becomes afterload-reducing agent.	1–2 min	IV	50 mg in D₅W or NS to a final volume of 250 ml
Nitroglycerin (SL) (Nitrostat)	0.15–0.6 mg q 5 min × 3	1–3 min	SL	NA
Diltiazem (IV) (Cardizem) (Calcium channel blocker)	20 mg (average) bolus over 2 minutes. May repeat with 25-mg bolus then start drip.	1–2 min	IV	125 mg in D₅W or NS to a final volume of 125 ml
Diltiazem (PO) (Cardizem) (Calcium channel blocker)	Tablets: 120–360 mg total daily dose in 3–4 divided doses Sustained-release: 120–360 mg/day in 1–2 divided doses	30–60 min	PO	NA
Nifedipine (PO) (Procardia, Procardia XL, Adalat) (Calcium channel blocker)	Capsules: 30–180 mg total daily dose in 3–4 divided doses Sustained-release: 30–120 mg/day in once-daily dosing	Capsules: 5–10 min Sustained-release: 20 min	PO	NA

NA, not applicable.

from renal compensation for decreased blood flow through the kidneys. Many types of diuretics are available (Table 2–3). All diuretics work by blocking reabsorption of sodium and water. They usually produce a rapid increase in urine output. How effective the diuretic is depends on the improvement in the cardiac performance.

Preload reduction can also occur with vasodilation. Drugs such as nitroglycerin, diltiazem, and morphine can reduce preload through vasodilation (Table 2–4). Vasodilation causes an "internal phlebotomy" by reducing the amount of blood returning to the heart.

Increasing Cardiac Strength Through Afterload Reduction

One of the best methods for improving cardiac performance is to reduce the work the heart does to eject blood. This can be accomplished by afterload reduction. Afterload reduction can be achieved with many different drugs (Table 2–5). However, only a few of these drugs are common in critical care.

The use of afterload reducers is common in two situations: during hypertensive episodes and when the cardiac output is low and the SVR is high. The principles of their use are similar in both situations.

While potentially dangerous, the most common drug to reduce resistance is nitroprusside. Nitroprusside acts quickly and is effective only with continuous administration. Once stopped, its effect

will wear off in minutes. It is very effective at reducing resistance and is frequently used in ICUs. Nitroprusside use has two disadvantages. First, it breaks down into cyanide. Cyanide levels therefore need to be monitored daily in patients on nitroprusside. Second, it acts as a nonselective arterial dilator. This dilation can open flow into areas which do not need more oxygen. However, as more flow enters these areas, some areas which need more oxygen (ischemic myocardium) might have flow diverted from them. This is called the "coronary steal" phenomenon.

In order to avoid the problems with nitroprusside, other afterload reducers, such as calcium channel and beta blocking agents, are used. While these drugs reduce afterload, they unfortunately also tend to weaken the heart. If calcium channel blockers (e.g., nicardipine) or beta blockers (e.g., labetalol) are used, their effect on both SVR and cardiac output must be monitored.

Other afterload reducers exist, most notably the angiotensin converting enzyme (ACE) inhibitors. ACE inhibitors are most often used in the management of nonacute forms of cardiac failure because they do not activate compensating neurohumoral responses like other afterload reducers. This makes them attractive for long-term use in such situations as CHF. They tend to reduce SVR without increasing cardiac output. The net effect

TABLE 2–5. AFTERLOAD REDUCERS

	Dose	Onset	Route	Drip conc.
Sodium Nitroprusside (Nipride, Nitropress)	0.5–10 μg/kg/min	30–60 sec	IV	50 g in D₅W to a final volume of 250 ml
Hydralazine (IV) (Apresoline)	10–40 mg prn	10–20 min	IV, IM	NA
Diazoxide (Hyperstat)	50–150 mg	1–2 min	IV	NA
Nitroglycerin (IV) (Tridil, Nitrostat IV) (Nitrate vasodilator)	5–160 μg/min. Titrate to desired effect	1–2 min	IV	50 mg in D₅W or NS to a final volume of 250 ml
Nitroglycerin (SL) (Nitrostat)	0.15–0.6 mg q5 min × 3	1–3 min	SL	NA
Alpha Inhibitors				
Prazosin (Minipress)	1–20 mg total daily dose in 2–3 divided doses	30 min–3 hr	PO	NA
Phentolamine (Regitine)	0.1–2 mg/min	Immediate	IV	No standard drip
Clonidine (Catapres)	0.1–2.4 mg total daily dose in 1–2 divided doses	30–60 min	PO	NA
Methyldopa (PO) (Aldomet) (Loop diuretic)	250 mg–3 g total daily dose in 2–4 divided doses	2 hr	PO	NA
Methyldopa (IV) (Aldomet) (Loop diuretic)	250 mg–1 g q6h	2 hr	IV	NA
Trimethaphan (Arfonad) (Ganglionic blocker)	3–4 mg/min up to 6 mg/min	1–2 min	IV	500 mg in D₅W 500 ml
Calcium Channel Blockers				
Diltiazem (IV) (Cardizem)	20 mg (average) bolus over 2 min. May repeat with 25-mg bolus then start drip	1–2 min	IV	125 mg in D₅W or NS to a final volume of 125 ml
Diltiazem (PO) (Cardizem)	Tablets: 120–360 mg total daily dose in 3–4 divided doses. Sustained-release: 120–360 mg/day in 1–2 divided doses	30–60 min	PO	NA
Nifedipine (PO) (Procardia, Procardia XL, Adalat)	Capsules: 30–180 mg total daily dose in 3–4 divided doses. Sustained-release: 30–120 mg/day in once daily dosing	Capsules: 5–10 min. Sustained-release: 20 min	PO. SL	NA
Nicardipine (IV) (Cardene)	5 mg/hr Maximum dose 15 mg/h	1–5 min	IV	25 mg/250 ml D₅W or NS
Nicardipine (PO) (Cardene)	20–60 mg bid–tid		PO	
Ace Inhibitors (Most common agents in use)				
Captopril (PO) (Capoten)	25–450 mg total daily dose in 2–3 divided doses	15–30 min	PO	NA
Enalapril (PO) (Vasotec)	2.5–40 mg qd	1 hr	PO	NA
Enalapril (IV)	1.25–5 mg q6h	15 min	IVP	NA
Lisinopril (Zestril/Prinivil)	10–40 mg qd	1 hr	PO	NA
Beta Blockers				
Atenolol (PO) (Tenormin)	50–200 mg qd		PO	NA
Metoprolol (PO) (Lopressor)	100–450 mg total daily dose in 4 divided doses		PO	NA
Metoprolol (IV) (Lopressor)	5 mg q 2 min × 3 (for a total dose of 15 mg)		IV	NA
Propranolol (PO) (Inderal)	120–240 mg in divided doses		PO	NA
Esmolol (Brevibloc)	1–3 mg		IV	NA
Labetolol (PO) (Normodyne or Trandate)	200–2400 mg total daily dose in 2–3 divided doses	2–4 hr	PO	NA
Labetalol (IV) (Normodyne or Trandate)	0.25 mg/kg q 10 min initially to a total dose of 50–300 mg	5 min	IV	200 mg in D₅W or NS to a final volume of 200 ml

NA, not applicable.

is a substantial reduction in myocardial oxygen consumption.

Management of Hypovolemia

When hypovolemia is present, the circulating blood volume has to be replenished by one of three therapies: blood (e.g., whole blood, packed cells), crystalloids (normal saline, lactated Ringer's solution), and colloids (hetastarch, albumin). The choice of therapy is dependent upon the clinical situation. General guidelines for fluid replacement are as follows:

1. Blood is used when the patient is actively bleeding and the hemoglobin levels are in the range of 7–8 g/dl. Blood is the only fluid replacement that actually carries oxygen.
2. Crystalloids are used when volume depletion does not have to be corrected rapidly, when depletion of more than vascular volume is suspected, or when hypovolemia is suspected but is not a clear diagnosis.
3. Colloids are used when rapid volume expansion is necessary but the use of blood is not indicated or blood is not available.

Considerable controversy exists regarding the proper fluid replacement therapy. Generally crystalloids are the first agent used in suspected hypovolemia (Table 2–6). They are inexpensive and do not cause any allergic reactions. However, they take longer to expand the vascular volume than either colloids or blood.

Treatment of Low Systemic Vascular Resistance

Many hemodynamic problems are a result of disturbances of blood flow. In sepsis, one of the most common of these disturbances, SVR is abnormally low. Other conditions can cause this situation as well, including hepatic disease and neurogenic shock. The key to all treatment is reversal of the underlying problem. For example, in sepsis, antibiotics might be the primary treatment, and hemodynamic interventions are viewed primarily as supportive therapies.

The primary hemodynamic therapies are aimed at achieving three goals: (1) maintaining circulating blood volume with volume expansion; (2) increasing blood flow with inotropic therapy; and (3) maintaining blood flow with agents to increase the SVR.

Maintaining blood flow with volume expansion and inotropic therapy has already been discussed. Maintaining blood flow with agents to increase the SVR is done with one of four agents (Table 2–7). All of these agents work by stimulating the alpha-1 cells of the sympathetic nervous system. These drugs produce vasoconstriction and some also increase the cardiac output. These are potent drugs which should elevate blood pressure and blood flow. However, they must be used with caution because they might

TABLE 2–6. VOLUME EXPANDERS

	Dose	Onset	Route	Drip conc.
Hetastarch (Hespan)	100–500 ml maximum 150 ml/day	30 min	IV	NA
Albumin	25 g initially maximum 250 g/48 hr	Varies	IV	NA
Crystalloids	100–500 ml/30 min	30 min	IV	Titrate to effect
Normal saline	NA	NA	IV	NA
Lactated Ringer's solution	NA	NA	IV	NA

NA, not applicable.

TABLE 2–7. COMMON VASOPRESSORS

	Dose	Onset	Route	Drip conc.
Dopamine (Intropin) Alpha adrenergic	10–20 μg/kg/min	<5 min	IV	400 mg/250 ml D$_5$W or NS
Epinephrine (Adrenaline)	1–4 μg/min	<5 min	IV	5 mg/500 ml or 4 mg/100 ml D$_5$W or NS
Norepinephrine (Levophed)	2–10 μg/min 1–20 μg/min to effect	1–2 min	IV	8 mg/500 D$_5$W
Phenylephrine (Neosynephrine)	10–100 μg/min	1–2 min	IV	10 mg/250 ml D$_5$W or NS

elevate the SVR and blood pressure but not increase tissue oxygenation.

Alpha stimulants cause marked vasoconstriction. These drugs are so potent that they are given centrally to avoid the tissue damage that would result in the event of infiltration during peripheral intravenous administration.

Specific Cardiovascular Drugs

Drugs which are specific to clinical conditions are discussed in chapters about those conditions. For example, thrombolytics are presented in the chapter on myocardial infarction and antidysrhythmics are covered in that on dysrhythmias. This section was designed for a general review of treatment of hemodynamic disturbances. For more information on specific drug therapy, locate the specific condition of interest.

IMPLICATIONS OF CARDIOVASCULAR DYSFUNCTION ON OTHER ORGAN SYSTEMS

EDITORS' NOTE

The cardiovascular system will affect every organ system as it fails. The majority of these effects will be covered in chapters on specific organ systems in this book. It is not likely the CCRN exam will address the specific effects of cardiovascular dysfunction on other organs directly. More likely, the exam will have a few questions which integrate the cardiovascular system into the dysfunction of other systems. Read this short section with the intent of familiarizing yourself with the general effects of the cardiovascular system on other organs. In order to simplify the contents of this section, all pertinent information is listed in the tables.

When assessing the effect of cardiovascular dysfunction on other organs, it is helpful to understand the blood flow from each ventricle, since the effects of dysfunction are different in each ventricle. For example, left ventricular dysfunction results in a failure to move blood to the tissues adequately. This threatens every organ's ability to maintain its normal metabolic activity. Since any threat to circulation threatens oxygen delivery, all tissues are at risk when left ventricular function is disturbed. In addition, a backup of blood into the lungs will eventually occur, causing pulmonary symptoms such as orthopnea (Table 2–8).

Right ventricular dysfunction results in a loss of blood flow through the lungs and a backup of blood into the venous system, causing symptoms such as venous engorgement (Table 2–9).

Since any organ can be affected, symptoms of dysfunction may be found in any organ. Table 2–10 shows the effects of ventricular dysfunction on each organ.

TABLE 2–8. LEFT VENTRICULAR DYSFUNCTION: HEMODYNAMIC AND SYSTEMIC EFFECTS

Increased preload	Reduced subendocardial perfusion
	Decreased renal perfusion
	Antidiuretic and aldosterone released, causing sodium and fluid retention
	Increased blood volume
	Fluid overload
Increased afterload	Catecholamines and angiotensin II released, causing vasoconstriction via the renin-angiotensin-aldosterone compensatory mechanism
	Impaired vascular smooth muscle relaxation
	Increased systemic vascular resistance
Impaired contractility	Decreased cardiac output due to reduced left ventricular reserve
	Decreased skeletal muscle blood flow
	Decreased exercise capacity
	Poor forward blood flow
	Increased backward pressure into the pulmonary vasculature

TABLE 2–9. RIGHT VENTRICULAR DYSFUNCTION: HEMODYNAMIC AND SYSTEMIC EFFECTS

Increased preload	Passive organ congestion
	Hepatic engorgement
	Hepatojugular reflux
	Coagulopathies
	Elevated liver enzymes
	Gastric congestion
	Dependent, peripheral edema
	Distended neck veins
	Decreased cardiac output due to the reduced forward flow from the right ventricle (see Table 2–8)

TABLE 2-10. END-ORGAN EFFECTS OF VENTRICULAR DYSFUNCTION

Left Ventricular Failure	Right Ventricular Failure	Organ System	Effect	Clinical Presentation
+	+	Central nervous system	Reduced cerebral perfusion due to decreased cardiac output	Altered level of consciousness Disorientation Confusion Lethargy Anxiety Insomnia Dizziness/syncope
			Deceased skeletal muscle perfusion	Fatigue Deceased exercise capacity
+	+	Renal system	Reduced renal perfusion, causing Na$^+$ retention and fluid accumulation	Fluid overload Increased SVR Oliguria during day Nocturia Metabolic acidosis Weight gain Peripheral edema Hyponatremia Hypokalemia due to diuretic therapy Dark, concentrated urine
	+	Hepatic system	Passive congestion and reduced perfusion of liver due to elevated systemic venous pressure cause liver damage and dysfunction and deficiencies in coagulation factors	Hepatomegaly Abdominal distention Hepatojugular reflex Elevated liver enzymes (SGOT, SGPT, LDH, GGT, lipase, etc.) Elevated PT, PTT, INR
	+	Gastrointestinal system	Passive congestion of gut slows due to visceral edema	Nausea/vomiting Anorexia Ascites Nutritional deficiencies Poor oral medication absorption Cachexia
+		Pulmonary system	Backward pressure due to poor left ventricular systolic function; causing pulmonary edema	Gravity-dependent crackles Wheezes Orthopnea Dyspnea on exertion Paroxysmal nocturnal dyspnea Low Pao_2/Sao_2/pH Use of accessory muscles Cheyne–Stokes respirations Productive cough of blood-tinged, frothy sputum
+		Cardiovascular system	Fluid overload of left ventricular Stretching of myocardium and valvular radius	S3 and/or S4 Systolic murmur of mitral regurgitation PMI shifts to the left
			Poor left ventricular contractility	Pulsus alternans Deceased pulse pressure Cold/discolored extremities Cool, clammy skin Deceased capillary refill Diaphoresis
+	+		Reduced subendocardial perfusion	Ischemic symptoms Dysrhythmias Atrial or ventricular bundle branch block
	+		Fluid overload	Jugular vein distention Pulsus paradoxus Pedal edema

PT, prothrombin time; PTT, partial thromboplastin time; PMI, point of maximal impulse; Pao$_2$, arterial oxygen pressure; Sao$_2$, arterial oxygen saturation.

The Normal ECG

EDITORS' NOTE

Generally, the CCRN exam requires interpretation of fewer than three rhythm strips but may have several questions regarding 12-lead ECG analysis.

In this chapter, a review of normal and preferred ECG leads, as well as the normal components of ECG waves, is provided. Generally only a few questions will be based on material taken directly from this chapter, however, content from this chapter is used for dysrhythmia analysis and 12-lead ECG interpretation. Review this chapter carefully if ECG monitoring is not one of your strengths.

COMPONENTS OF THE NORMAL ECG

The electrocardiograph is a machine that records the electrical activity of the heart on special paper. The result is an electrocardiogram (ECG or EKG). The electrical activity measured by the ECG is the electrical potential between two points on the body, a positive pole and a negative pole. When one is monitoring patients in critical care, all monitoring leads have one negative and one positive pole. For example, in lead I, the right arm is negative and the left arm is positive. Electrical activity in the heart is monitored by these two poles. Electrical activity that is directed toward the positive pole results in an upright deflection. Activity heading toward the negative pole is upside down. The sum of all cardiac electrical activity (referred to as cardiac vectors) is generally in a direction that is inferior and to the left. The leftward direction of cardiac electrical activity is primarily due

to the size and therefore electrical activity of the left ventricle.

The 12-lead ECG is the graphic recording of the electrical output of the heart from 12 different positions. A 12-lead ECG can be diagnostic in drug toxicity, conduction disturbances, electrolyte imbalances, ischemia, and infarction, and can aid in determining the size of the heart chambers and axis orientation of the heart.

Cardiac monitoring uses rhythm strips to assess heart rate, rhythm, and dysrhythmias. Rhythm strips may be run on any one of the 12 leads used in a 12-lead ECG and several other special leads.

The most common leads used to monitor patients are leads II and MCL_1. Lead II is a standard lead with the negative pole attached to an electrode placed on the upper chest near the right arm and the positive pole attached to an electrode placed on the lower left side of the chest. Lead II normally sees electrical activity in the heart in an upright ECG pattern, since its positive electrode is on the left side of the body. Lead II is especially useful in assessing P waves and QRS complexes that have a small amplitude. It is not, however, the ideal monitoring lead. MCL_1 is a better routine monitoring lead.

MCL_1 is a modified chest lead representative of V_1 of the 12-lead EKG. In MCL_1, the negative pole is attached to an electrode placed on the upper left chest and the positive pole is attached to an electrode placed to the right of the sternum at the fourth intercostal space (Fig. 3–1). Since the MCL_1 positive electrode is placed to the right of the sternum, it views the cardiac electrical activity as heading away from it and therefore sees the QRS complex as primarily upside down.

MCL_1 gives more information on conduction defects such as right and left bundle branch blocks than do other routine monitoring leads. As such, it is the routine lead employed to identify most

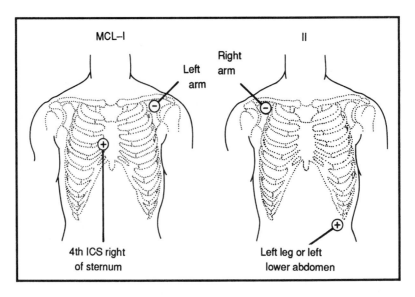

Figure 3–1. Normal placement for MCL₁ and lead II.

dysrhythmias, particularly aberrant atrial premature contractions from premature ventricular contractions. The one situation for which MCL₁ is not as useful is with newer monitoring systems that employ ST-segment analysis. ST-segment analysis operates better when large R waves are sensed. If large R waves are desired, lead II, MCL₅, or MCL₆ is employed.

When monitoring dysrhythmias, develop the practice of using multiple leads. Use of a single lead for all situations limits your ability to interpret complex dysrhythmias.

A key ingredient to accurate dysrhythmia analysis is the correct application of lead placement. While the CCRN exam generally does not ask specific questions on lead placement, such questions are possible. More importantly, accurate lead placement has an effect on correct rhythm and 12-lead analysis. Studies have indicated significant changes in QRS morphology with incorrect lead placement.

ECG Paper

The CCRN exam will not ask questions about the ECG paper. However, you must know the time grids within the ECG paper to make interpretations of dysrhythmias and 12-lead analysis.

The ECG paper has a series of horizontal lines exactly 1 mm apart (Fig. 3–2).

The horizontal lines represent voltage (or amplitude). ECG paper also has vertical lines that represent time. Each vertical line is 0.04 sec apart. To help in measuring waveforms, every fifth line is darker than the other lines, both horizontally and vertically. The intersection of these lines produces both small boxes (the lighter lines) and large boxes (the darker, bolder lines). Horizontally, each small box represents 1 mm (0.1 mV) and each large box represents 5 mm (0.5 mV). (Note that each large box is made up of five small boxes.) Vertically, each small

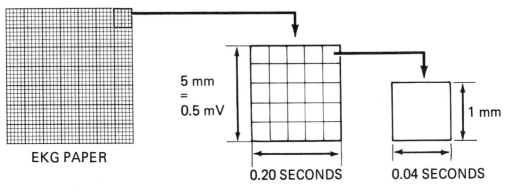

Figure 3–2. ECG paper.

box represents 0.04 sec and each large box represents 0.20 sec. Because of the design of ECG paper, one can measure the duration of impulses (wavelengths) and the amplitude (height) of impulses. All waves will be either isoelectric (no net electrical activity = flat), positively deflected (upright, toward the positive pole), or negatively deflected (downward, toward the negative pole).

COMPONENTS OF A CARDIAC CYCLE

Before a rhythm strip can be labeled, a systemic analysis of each portion of the strip and the relation of each wave to the electrical activity in the cardiac cycle is made. The interpretations will be made using lead II or MCL$_1$ in this text. It is conventional to label the components of the cardiac cycle P, QRS, and T. (There is no reason why these specific letters were chosen.)

There are three prominent deflections in the ECG: the P wave, the QRS complex, and the T wave (Fig. 3–3).

P Wave

This represents the generation of an electrical impulse and depolarization of the atria (Fig. 3–4). The P wave is important in determining whether the impulse started in the SA node or elsewhere in the atrium.

QRS Complex

The QRS complex is composed of three separate waveforms which represent ventricular depolarization (Fig. 3–5). Multiple variations exist in the shape of the QRS complex. A Q wave is the first negative

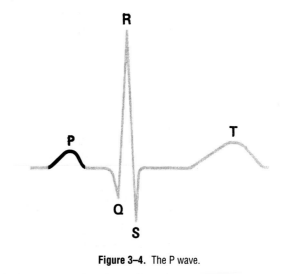

Figure 3–4. The P wave.

deflection and may or may not be present. A large Q wave may be indicative of myocardial death. To be clinically significant, the Q wave should be greater than 0.04 sec and the depth should be greater than one third the height of the R wave.

The R wave is the first positive deflection in the complex. The R wave is usually large in leads where the positive electrode is on the left (I, II, III, avL, avF, V$_5$, V$_6$) and small in leads where the positive electrode is on the right (MCL$_1$, V$_1$, V$_2$, avR).

The S wave is the negative deflection following the R wave. The S wave can be useful in interpreting terminal electrical activity in the heart.

T Wave

The T wave is the third major deflection in the ECG (Fig. 3–6). It represents repolarization of the ventricles. In most lead II of a healthy heart, the T wave is

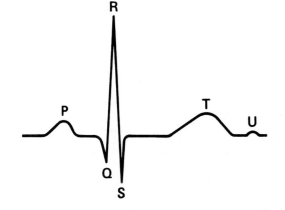

Figure 3–3. The normal PQRST deflections, lead II.

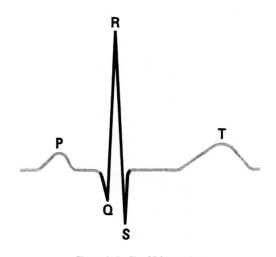

Figure 3–5. The QRS complex.

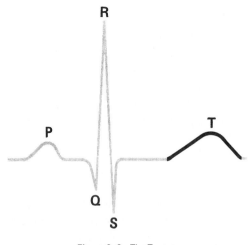

Figure 3–6. The T wave.

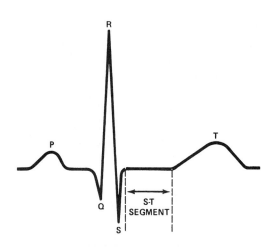

Figure 3–8. The ST segment.

positively deflected. In ischemia or infarction, the T wave may be inverted.

Intervals and Segments

There are four other intervals and segments of a rhythm strip and an ECG that must be identified.

PR Interval

The PR interval (Fig. 3–7) represents the time for the electrical impulse to spread from the atrium to the atrioventricular (AV) node and His bundle. It is measured from the beginning of the P wave to the beginning of the QRS complex. Normally, this interval is 0.12 to 0.20 sec.

ST Segment

The ST segment (Fig. 3–8) represents the time from complete depolarization of the ventricles to the

beginning of repolarization (recovery) of the ventricles. In the healthy heart, the ST segment is flat or isoelectric. Since no net electrical activity is present during the recovery phase of the cardiac cycle, the wave is not deflected in either direction. In myocardial injury, the segment may be elevated. In ischemia, the ST segment is depressed.

PR Segment

This segment (Fig. 3–9) represents the normal delay in the conduction of the electrical impulse in the AV node. It is normally isoelectric and is measured from the end of the P wave to the beginning of the R wave. Duration of the PR segment varies. Clinically, the PR segment is not usually addressed.

QT Interval

This interval (Fig. 3–10) represents the total period of time required for depolarization and repolarization (recovery) of the ventricles. It is measured from the

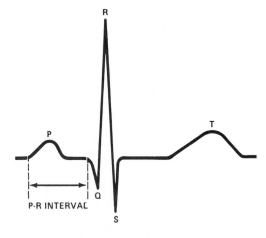

Figure 3–7. The PR interval.

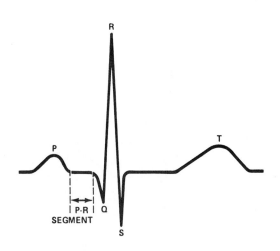

Figure 3–9. The PR segment.

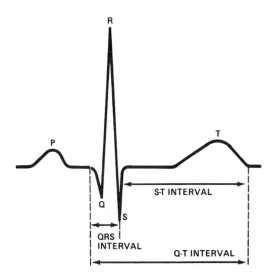

Figure 3–10. The QRS, ST, and QT intervals.

beginning of the QRS complex to the end of the T wave. It is normally less than 0.40 sec, but is dependent upon heart rate, sex, age, and other factors.

Occasionally another wave is seen after the T wave and before the next P wave. This is called a U wave (Fig. 3–11). Some authorities believe that it represents repolarization of the Purkinje fibers. It may or may not be seen.

INTERPRETATION OF A RHYTHM STRIP

Five basic steps are followed in analyzing a rhythm strip (or an ECG) to aid in the interpretation and identification of a rhythm. Each step should be followed in sequence. Eventually this will become a habit and will enable one to identify a strip correctly, accurately, and quickly.

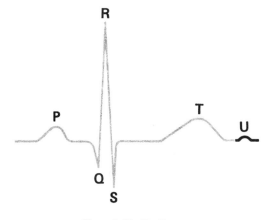

Figure 3–11. The U wave.

Step 1

Determine the rates at which the atria and the ventricles are depolarizing. The rates may not be the same. To count the rate of the atria, count the number of P waves present in the 6-sec rhythm strip and multiply by 10. (Each mark at the top edge of the ECG paper represents 3 sec, and each inch of the ECG paper equals 1 sec.) This gives the atrial rate per minute.

Count the number of QRS complexes in a 6-sec strip and multiply by 10. This gives the ventricular rate per minute.

For regular rhythms, another method may be used. Determine the rate by counting the number of small boxes between each P wave and divide into 1500 or count the number of large boxes between each P wave and divide into 300. Do the same thing to determine the ventricular rate by counting QRS complexes.

Step 2

Determine whether the rhythm is regular or irregular. The most accurate method is to measure the interval from one R wave to the next R wave. (Set one point of the cardiac calipers on the tip of the first R wave and the other point on the tip of the next R wave.) Then move the cardiac calipers from R to R. If the measurement is the same (or varies less than 0.04 sec between beats), the rhythm is regular. If the intervals vary by more than 0.04 sec, the rhythm is irregular. Often one can tell by simply looking at the strip that the rhythm is irregular. However, if it looks regular, it is best to measure the R-to-R intervals to be certain.

Step 3

Analyze the P waves. A P wave should precede every QRS complex. All of the P waves should be identical in shape. The normal P wave is fairly sharply curved, less than 3 mm in height, and less than 0.1 sec in width in lead II. If the P wave is abnormally shaped or varies in shape from wave to wave, the stimulus may have arisen from somewhere in the atrium other than in the sino-atrial (SA) node. Almost all impulses that originate in the SA node will meet the "normal" shape and size previously stated if heart function is normal. A biphasic P (a single P wave moves above and below the baseline) may indicate left atrial enlargement; a peaked P may indicate right atrial enlargement, and both of these P waves originate in the SA node. If there is no P wave or if the P wave does not precede the QRS complex, the impulse did not originate in the SA node.

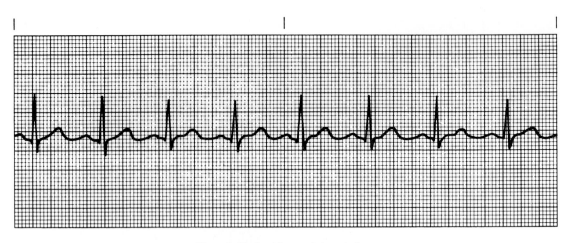

Figure 3–12. Lead II normal sinus rhythm.

Step 4

Measure the PR interval. This is measured from the beginning of the P wave to the beginning of the QRS complex. It should measure between 0.10 and 0.20 sec. Intervals outside this range indicate a conduction disturbance between the atria and the ventricles.

Step 5

Measure the width of the QRS complex. This is measured from the beginning of the Q (if present, otherwise the R) to the end of the S wave. The normal duration is 0.06 to 0.12 sec. A QRS measurement of greater than 0.12 sec indicates an intraventricular conduction abnormality.

Figure 3–12 is a 6-sec, lead II rhythm strip. Let us analyze this rhythm strip by applying the five steps just mentioned.

- Step 1: The atrial rate is 80 (eight P waves in 6 sec). The ventricular rate is 80 (eight R waves in 6 sec). The heart rate is 80.
- Step 2: There is less than a 0.04-sec variation from R wave to R wave, so the rhythm is regular.
- Step 3: The P waves are all the same shape, size (in height), and duration. Each P wave appears immediately before a QRS complex. These factors indicate that the impulse starts in the SA node.
- Step 4: The PR interval is about 0.16 sec. This is within the normal duration range, indicating normal conduction of the impulse from the SA node to the AV node.
- Step 5: Each QRS complex is less than 0.10 sec in duration, which is normal.
- Interpretation of the strip: Normal sinus rhythm.

The 12-Lead ECG

The CCRN exam can include questions that require an understanding of the 12-lead electrocardiogram (ECG). With the recent increased emphasis on cardiovascular concepts, the CCRN exam may include 12-lead ECGs for you to interpret. Other typical questions involving the 12-lead ECG usually focus on conditions such as left and right ventricular hypertrophy, left and right bundle branch blocks, differentiation of aberrant atrial premature contractions from premature ventricular contractions (PVCs), and identification of myocardial infarction patterns. This chapter provides the information necessary to interpret these conditions.

The 12 monitoring leads used to assess myocardial conduction patterns are listed in Table 4–1. When assessing patterns of injury, hypertrophy, or axis deviations, noting the views of the heart from different leads is essential. Whenever available, a prior 12-lead ECG can help interpret questionable results.

IDENTIFYING MYOCARDIAL INFARCTION AND ISCHEMIA

EDITORS' NOTE

The most important aspects of the ECG to understand have to do with identifying myocardial ischemia and injury. Your understanding of how to identify evidence of infarction or ischemia on an ECG will be tested on the CCRN exam. However, these concepts are not as difficult as they sometimes seem. This is particularly true of trying to identify whether a patient might be having a myocardial infarction.

When reviewing the 12-lead ECG for infarction and ischemic injury patterns, it must be kept in mind that the ECG is not foolproof. In a small but substantial percentage of patients who have a myocardial infarction (MI), the ECG will show no evidence of damage. Changes in cardiac isoenzyme levels are more accurate, but they take longer to determine. The speed with which one can obtain an ECG is the primary reason why ECGs still have clinical value.

The first step in identifying MI is to look at the ST segment. It is one of the first parts of the ECG to change with MI. Typically, if MI is occurring, the ST segment will be elevated (Fig. 4–1). Elevation of the ST segment is a strong warning sign of cardiac injury. The ST segment may be depressed if only ischemia of the heart exists (Fig. 4–2). To identify changes in the ST segment, examine where the ST segment is .08 sec (two small blocks) from the end of the QRS (Fig. 4–3).

The ST segment in the area opposite the MI might show depression, a concept referred to as reciprocal change (Fig. 4–4). Whether these changes indicate ischemia in the area or just repolarization abnormalities due to the MI is controversial. Currently, it is believed that the ST changes opposite the MI are relatively benign.

The T wave may also indicate cardiac ischemia and may change before the ST segment. It usually becomes inverted with cardiac ischemia (Fig. 4–5).

Q-wave formation is the primary indication that a patient has had an MI. Q waves are negative deflections in front of R waves (Fig. 4–6). They are considered significant if they are wide (greater than .04 sec) and large (greater than one-third the height of the R wave). Q waves indicate cardiac muscle death. Because they take about 24 hr to form, if a Q wave is present, one can estimate that the MI occurred at least 1 day

TABLE 4–1. 12-LEAD ECG LEADS

Lead	View of the heart
I	Lateral wall
II	Inferior wall
III	Inferior wall
avR (augmented vector of the right)	
avL (augmented vector of the left)	Lateral wall
avF (augmented vector of the foot)	Inferior wall
V_1	Ventricular septum
V_2	Anterior wall
V_3	Anterior wall
V_4	Anterior wall
V_5	Lateral wall
V_6	Lateral wall

earlier. From a nursing perspective, we would want to determine whether cardiac damage is occurring before the muscle actually dies. To do this, we look for ST-segment changes before the formation of a Q wave. If the Q wave is present, you know that the MI is too old for some treatments, such as thrombolysis.

When reading a 12-lead ECG, it is necessary to identify the location of any injury. The heart is nor-

mally divided into 4 parts, each identified with different ECG leads.

Part of the Heart	Leads
Anterior/septal MI	V_1–V_4
Lateral MI	I, avL, V_5, V_6
Inferior MI	II, III, avF
Posterior MI	V_1, V_2
Right ventricular MI	V_{3R}, V_{4R}, V_{5R}, V_{6R}

Anterior MIs are usually the most dangerous, because of the amount of muscle damaged and the injury to the ventricular conduction system. This usually represents obstruction of the left anterior descending artery. Lateral MIs might accompany anterior MIs or occur alone. Lateral MIs usually occur with obstruction of the circumflex artery. Inferior MIs are the second most dangerous type. They frequently produce dysrhythmias such as second-degree heart block. Inferior MIs are associated with obstruction of the right coronary artery. Inferior MIs are also commonly associated with right

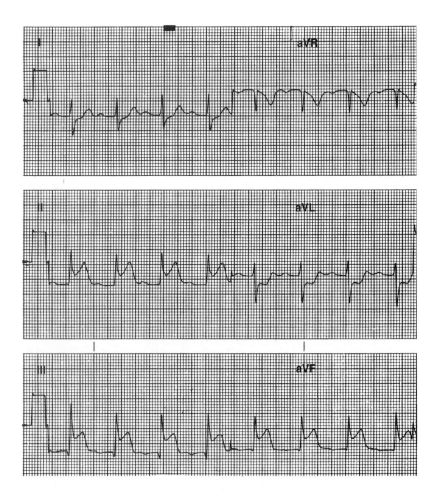

Figure 4–1. ST-segment elevation during MI.

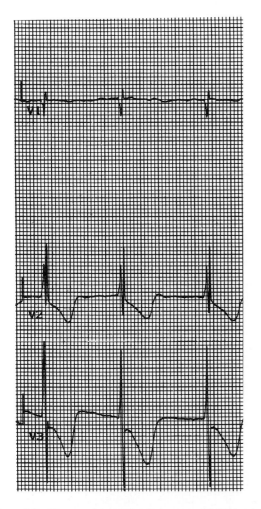

Figure 4–2. ST-segment depression during myocardial ischemia.

wave indicate an MI, the presence of a large R wave in V_1 and V_2 (the mirror test) might indicate a posterior MI. A posterior MI can be the result of obstruction of either the circumflex or the right coronary artery.

Injury Patterns

The more areas of the heart that are damaged, the more dangerous the MI becomes. For example, an anterior/lateral MI is more dangerous than either one individually. Common patterns include anterior/lateral, inferior/posterior, and anterior/septal.

AXIS DEVIATION

EDITORS' NOTE

....

Understanding the axis of the heart is necessary to interpret a 12-lead ECG. However, it is unlikely the CCRN exam will have a question regarding axis deviation. But, to be safe, this section has been included. Read this section if you want to be thoroughly prepared for the exam and feel you know most areas well enough to allow some more in-depth reading.

....

ventricular (RV) MIs. RV MIs are identified by using right-sided precordial chest leads, specifically V_{3R}–V_{6R}. Posterior MIs are difficult to see with the normal ECG. When the V_1 and V_2 leads are used to examine the back of the heart the criteria for cardiac death are usually reversed. Instead of having a Q

Axis calculation refers to identifying the source of major electrical activity in the heart. This is done by using vectors. A vector is a quantity that has magnitude and direction. Cardiac vectors represent electrical activity and force, and are identified by arrows. If a cardiac vector is headed toward a positive lead on an ECG, it is represented by an upright arrow. If it is headed away from the positive electrode, it is viewed

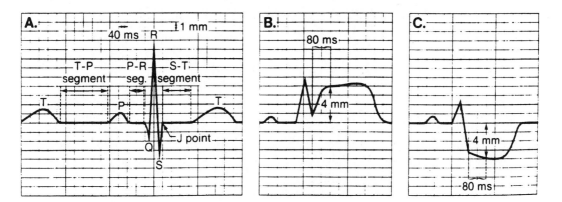

Figure 4–3. Correct location for measuring ST-segment changes.

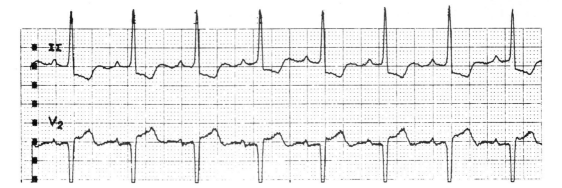

Figure 4–4. Reciprocal changes in the ECG during MI.

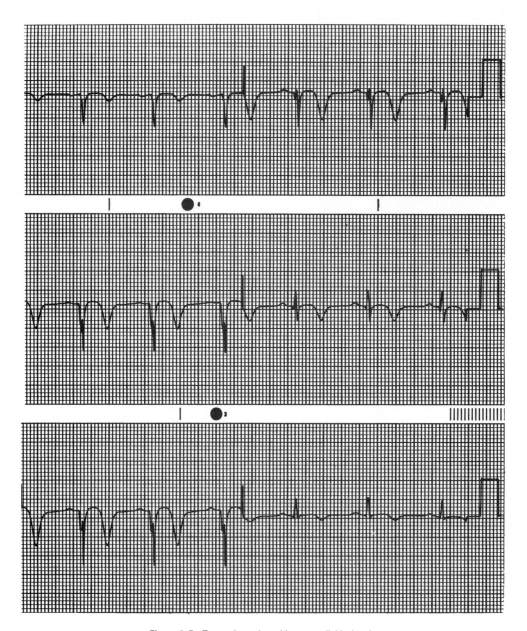

Figure 4–5. T-wave inversion with myocardial ischemia.

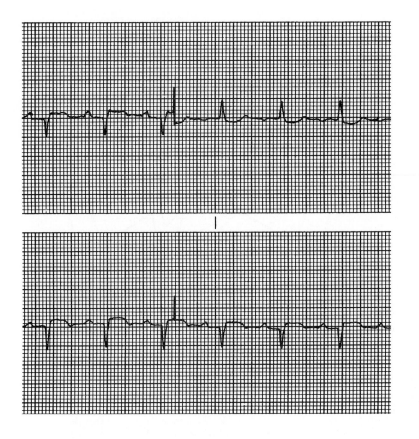

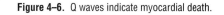

Figure 4–6. Q waves indicate myocardial death.

as negative. Normally, the mean cardiac vector is directed inferiorly and to the left (Fig. 4–7). If all the electrical activity in the heart were averaged, the net direction of electrical impulses would be toward the area of largest muscle concentration, that is, the left ventricle.

Vectors are usually represented on a circular diagram known as the hexaxial reference system (Fig. 4–8). As Figure 4–8 shows, the circle is divided into 30° segments. Each lead is represented, separated by 30° increments. The axis is indicated by the number to which the major cardiac vector is pointing.

The axis can deviate. Typically these deviations are classified as right axis deviation, left axis deviation, and extreme right axis deviation (Fig. 4–9) (or indeterminate). Causes for these changes are listed in Table 4–2.

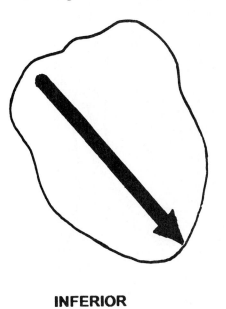

LEFT

INFERIOR

Figure 4–7. Representation of the mean cardiac vector.

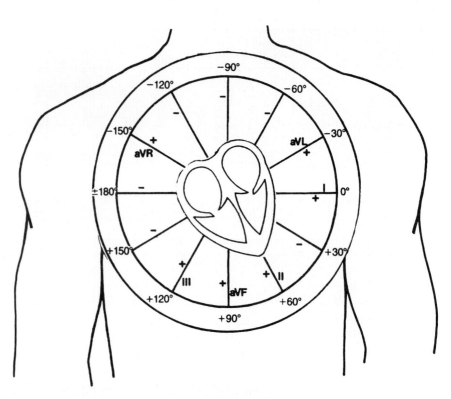

Figure 4–8. Geometric circle for vector measurement.

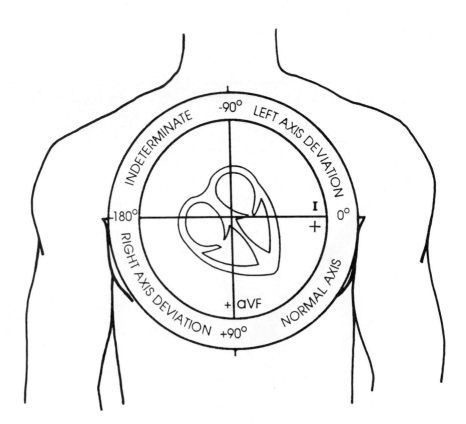

Figure 4–9. Normal and abnormal axes.

TABLE 4–2. COMMON CAUSES FOR AXIS DEVIATIONS

Left axis deviation	Anterior hemiblock
	Left ventricular hypertrophy
	PVCs
Right axis deviation	Posterior hemiblock
	Right ventricular hypertrophy
Extreme right axis deviation	PVCs

Determining if an axis is normal or not can be done by examining the largest QRS complex in the frontal plane leads, i.e., I, II, III, avR, avL, and avF. The largest QRS complex is the result of the cardiac vector heading directly toward or away from the positive electrode.

Using Figure 4–10 as an example, we can calculate the axis as follows. Note the locations of the positive and negative electrodes in each lead. Then observe the QRS complex in the 12-lead ECG. Note that lead III has the largest deflection. This means the vector is 90°. In Figure 4–11, avL has the largest QRS. This means the vector is –30° (330°).

This is a very brief explanation of axis calculation. For simple ECG interpretation, and for the purposes of preparing for the CCRN exam, this explanation should be all you need to know.

BUNDLE BRANCH BLOCKS

EDITORS' NOTE

Bundle branch blocks may be on the CCRN exam. It is possible that at least two questions addressing this area might be included. It is helpful to have a basic understanding of this topic.

Interpreting bundle branch blocks focuses on identifying changes in the QRS complex. Normally, the QRS complex has small Q and S waves. Conduction

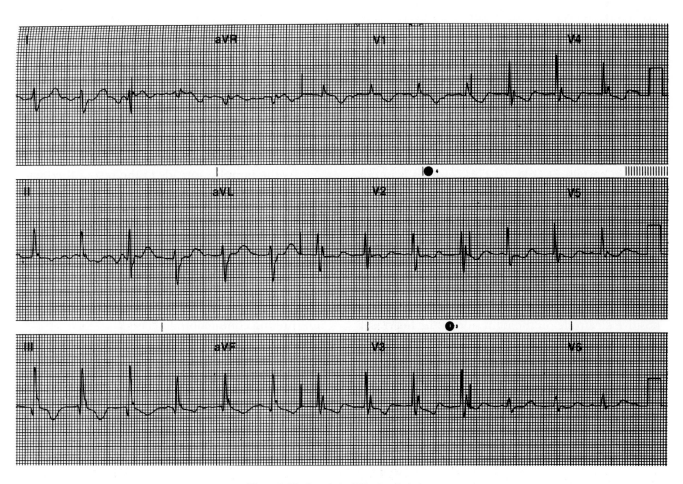

Figure 4–10. Sample lead III axis calculation.

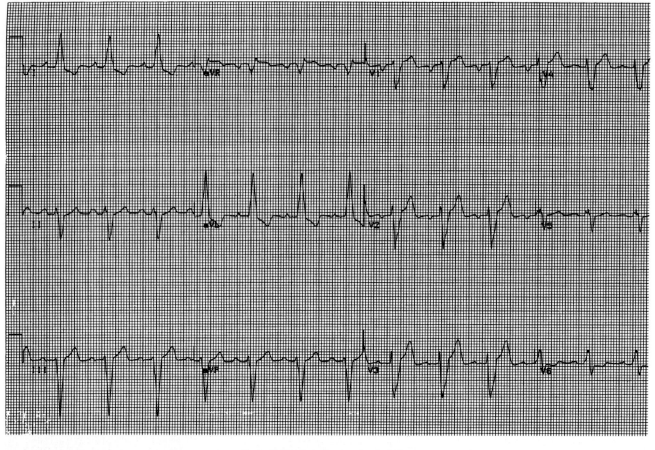

Figure 4–11. Sample avL axis calculation.

blocks can change this appearance. Bundle branch blocks are usually preceded by normal P waves and PR intervals. The primary difference is seen in the QRS complexes. However, these changes may only occur in certain ECG leads. This is why it is important to monitor leads correctly.

To understand conduction blocks, it is important to understand how the ventricles depolarize. Normally, the ventricles depolarize in the following manner: As the impulse spreads from the bundle of His, the left bundle depolarizes slightly ahead of the right. This causes the ventricular septum to be depolarized from a left to right direction. Leads with a positive electrode on the right side of the heart view this depolarization wave (vector) as coming toward it, creating an R wave (Fig. 4–12). Leads with a positive electrode on the left side of the heart view this wave as heading away from it, creating a Q wave.

As the impulse spreads to the rest of the heart, the main depolarization wave is directed inferiorly and to the left (Fig. 4–13). This is due to the influence of the large left ventricle. Depolarization in this manner creates a S wave for right-sided leads and an R wave for left-sided leads.

With conduction disturbances, these normal depolarization waves can be altered. Understanding the changes in depolarization waves is the key to interpreting conduction defects.

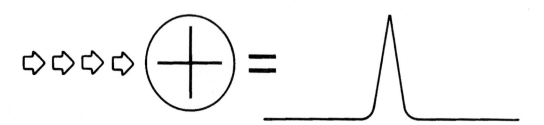

Figure 4–12. Depolarization occurring toward the positive electrode.

right bundle is blocked, a delayed rightward vector is created. This causes a third wave heading toward the positive electrode in V_1, resulting in a triphasic pattern. It simultaneously produces a wave headed away from the positive electrode in lead I. This causes a deep S wave in lead I. It will also cause a deep S wave in other lateral leads, such as V_6.

A RBBB might have a widening of the QRS but usually by no more than .14 sec. P waves are usually visible in front of the rsR′ pattern, although they might be lost in the preceding T wave. Variations of the rsR′ pattern are occasionally found, however the CCRN exam is not likely to cover complex variations from these common conduction patterns.

Left Bundle Branch Block

A left bundle branch block (LBBB) also has two common characteristics, a QS wave in lead V_1 and a wide, notched R wave in lead I (Fig. 4–15). With a LBBB, the normal initial septal depolarization is altered. The first vector created is from the right bundle, creating a rightward directed depolarization

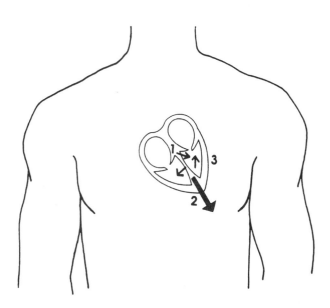

Figure 4–13. Ventricular depolarization vectors.

Right Bundle Branch Block

A right bundle branch block (RBBB) has two common characteristics, a triphasic pattern (rsR′) in lead V_1 and a deep S wave in lead I (Fig. 4–14). Since the

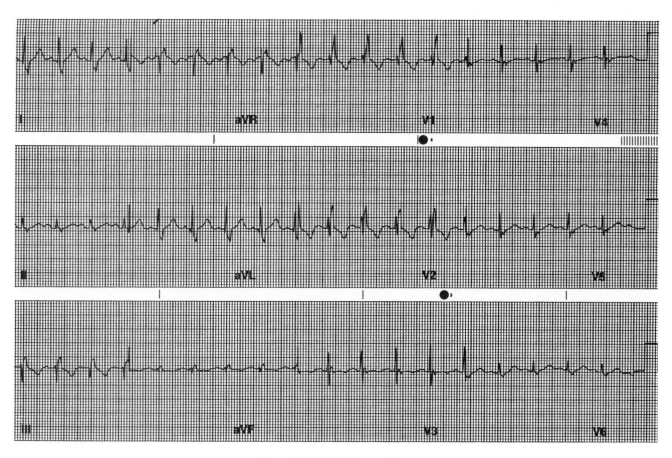

Figure 4–14. RBBB characteristics.

wave. This is seen by right-sided chest leads (like V_1) as headed away from it, creating a Q wave. Left-sided chest leads see this as an R wave (lead I).

Left bundle branch blocks are almost always wide (greater than .12 sec) and frequently notched. P waves are usually visible but can be lost in the preceding T wave. As with RBBBs, there are some variations from these patterns, but they are not as common.

Anterior Hemiblocks

An anterior hemiblock occurs when the anterior portion of the left bundle is obstructed (Fig. 4–16). The result is a shift in axis forces to the left (usually greater than –60°). This left axis deviation also causes leads II, III, and avF to become inverted. Small Q waves may be noted in leads I and avL. There may or may not be a prolongation of the QRS complex.

Posterior Hemiblocks

A posterior hemiblock occurs when the posterior portion of the left bundle is obstructed. The result is a shift in the axis to the right. The vector in this direction causes large R waves in II, III, avF (Fig. 4–17). Small r waves with deep S waves are present in I and avL. There may or may not be a prolongation of the QRS.

LEFT AND RIGHT VENTRICULAR HYPERTROPHY

Left ventricular hypertrophy (LVH) causes more electrical forces to be generated on the left side of the heart. This can understandably lead to left axis deviation. The leads viewing the heart on the left side (such as V_5 and V_6), will reflect the increased electrical activity by having large R waves. Leads on the right side show large S waves, the opposite of large R waves. The most common criterion for diagnosing LVH is a combination of right and left precordial chest leads. For example, if the height of the R wave in V_5 combined with the depth of the S wave in V_1 exceeds 35 mm, then the voltage criterion for LVH is present (Fig. 4–18).

Right ventricular hypertrophy (RVH) is better noted from right precordial leads. Leads V_{3R} and V_{4R} are better able to pick out changes in right

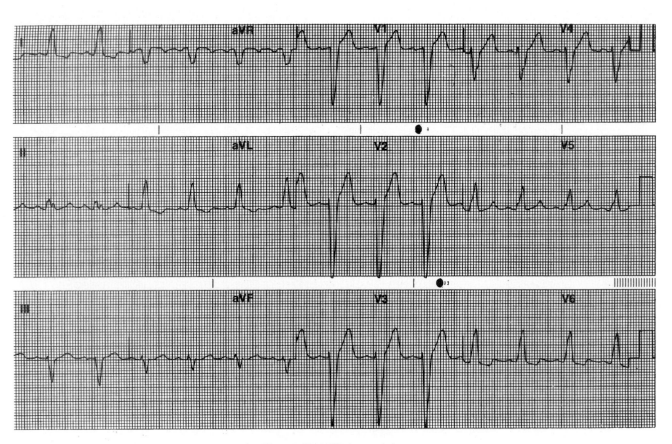

Figure 4–15. LBBB characteristics.

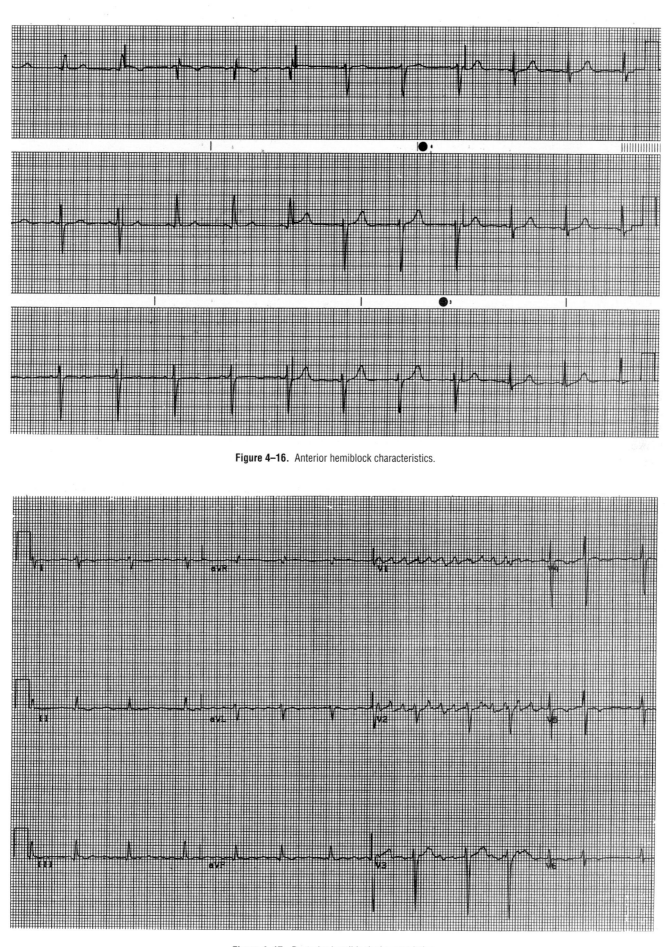

Figure 4–16. Anterior hemiblock characteristics.

Figure 4–17. Posterior hemiblock characteristics.

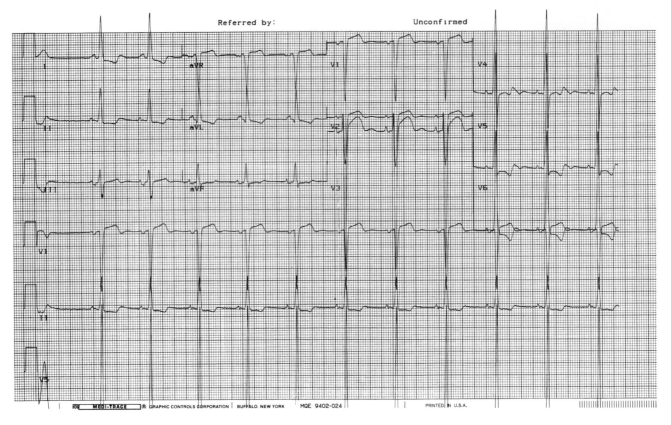

Figure 4–18. Left ventricular hypertrophy.

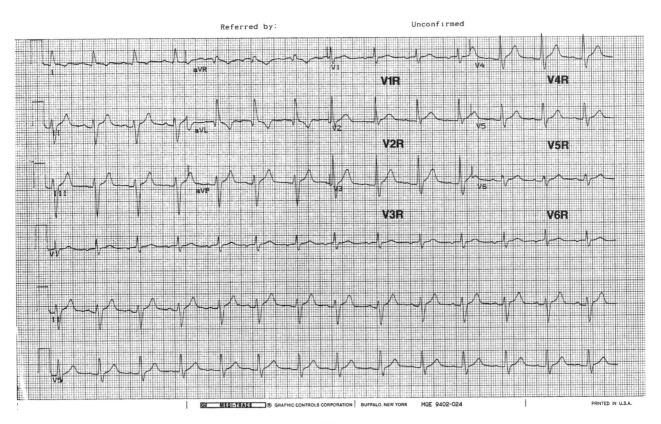

Figure 4–19. Right precordial leads.

ventricular size through the presence of large R waves (R:S ratio > 1). Figure 4–19 illustrates right precordial leads. In addition to possible right axis deviation, the best criteria for RVH include a large R wave in V_1 and V_2 and a deep S in V_5 and V_6. Table 4–3 lists criteria for left and right ventricular hypertrophy.

SUMMARY

If you understand the concepts briefly presented in this chapter, you should do well on the CCRN 12-lead questions. It is more likely that questions will be oriented toward infarction and ischemia, although an occasional question on other areas may appear. However, if they do appear, there will not be many of them.

TABLE 4–3. CRITERIA FOR LEFT AND RIGHT VENTRICULAR HYPERTROPHY

Condition	Leads and Criteria
Left ventricular hypertrophy	S wave in V_1 + R wave in V_5 > 35 mm $R_1 + S_3$ > 26mm
Right ventricular hypertrophy	V_{3R} and V_1 and V_2, R > S V_{4R}, R:S ratio > 1:1

Hemodynamic Monitoring

EDITORS' NOTE

The purpose of this chapter is to review the concepts associated with hemodynamic monitoring, discuss the technology utilized in hemodynamic monitoring, and present methods for interpreting hemodynamic parameters. It is essential that nurses who are planning to take the CCRN exam understand the content of this chapter. There will be several questions taken directly from material covered in this chapter. Normally, the questions focus on interpreting hemodynamic data. There will be few, if any, questions on hemodynamic technology. However, to be safe, key concepts in hemodynamic monitoring, in terms of both interpretation and technology, are presented.

MONITORING HEMODYNAMIC DATA

Cardiac Output and Stroke Volume

The key parameters obtained from the pulmonary artery catheter are cardiac output and stroke volume. These blood flow parameters are the first to be assessed when monitoring hemodynamic data. If these parameters are adequate, tissue oxygenation is generally adequate; if they are abnormal, a threat to tissue oxygenation may exist. Normal hemodynamic parameters are given in Table 5–1.

Cardiac Output and Index

Normal cardiac output is usually in the range of 4–8 L/min. The cardiac index, which is an adjustment of cardiac output based on the size of the person, is another commonly used descriptor of blood flow. A normal cardiac index is 2.5–4 $L/min/m^2$. Levels

below 2.2 $L/min/m^2$ indicate a threat to tissue oxygenation and require that consideration be given to beginning treatment.

Generally, the cardiac index is a better parameter to use than the cardiac output. Some patients tolerate a low cardiac index without clinical problems. Tracking trends in the cardiac index is more useful than monitoring single data points since temporary changes in values may not be clinically significant. Monitoring both cardiac index and tissue oxygenation parameters, such as mixed venous oxyhemoglobin (SvO_2), together will increase one's accuracy in identifying a clinically dangerous event.

Cardiac output is determined by two factors, heart rate and stroke volume. Understanding heart rate and stroke volume is essential for knowing how to treat abnormal cardiac output. Abnormal cardiac output is most commonly related to a problem with stroke volume.

Stroke Volume, Stroke Index, and Ejection Fraction

Stroke volume is defined as the amount of blood ejected with each heart beat. The stroke index, like the cardiac index, is a more useful measure that individualizes the stroke volume based on the patient's size.

The ejection fraction is defined as the amount of blood pumped with each contraction in relation to the amount of blood available to be pumped. For example, assume the left ventricular (LV) end diastolic volume (LVEDV), the amount of blood left in the heart just before contraction, is about 100 ml and that the stroke volume is 80 ml. Since 80 ml of the possible 100 ml in the ventricle is ejected, the ejection fraction is 80%. A normal ejection fraction is usually 60% or more.

In any condition in which the heart begins to malfunction, the stroke volume/index will decline; however, in certain circumstances, such as LV failure

47

TABLE 5–1. NORMAL HEMODYNAMIC PARAMETERS

Parameter	Normal Level	Consider Intervention
Stroke volume	50–100 ml/beat	<50 ml
Stroke index	25–45 ml/m2	<25 ml
Cardiac output	4–8 L/min	<4 L/min
Cardiac index	2.5–4 L/min/m2	<2.2 L/min/m2
Ejection fraction	>60%	<40%
Wedge pressure (PCWP or PAOP)	8–12 mm Hg	<8 (hypovolemia)* >18 (LV failure)*
Central venous pressure	2–5 mm Hg	<2 (hypovolemia)* <10 (RV failure)
Pulmonary artery pressure	25/10	>35/20 (pulmonary hypertension)

*If stroke volume is low. PCWP, pulmonary capillary wedge pressure; PAOP, pulmonary artery oxygen pressure.

and sepsis, the stroke volume may not initially decline because of the heart's compensatory mechanisms. If a patient with coronary artery disease begins to have LV dysfunction, the left ventricle will dilate, causing the LVEDV to increase. Although the increase in LVEDV might prevent a drop in stroke volume, dysfunction can still be detected by observing a drop in the ejection fraction. For example, assume a patient starts with the following:

LVEDV	90 ml
Stroke volume	65 ml
Ejection fraction	72% (65/90)

Over time, the same patient begins to have LV dysfunction with dilation of the left ventricle. Although the heart muscle begins to weaken, the stroke volume is maintained by the increase in LVEDV:

LVEDV	150 ml
Stroke volume	65 ml
Ejection fraction	43% (65/150)

Notice that the stroke volume is maintained but the ejection fraction falls and LVEDV rises, reflecting early LV dysfunction. Because changes in the ejection fraction (and end diastolic volumes) can provide early warning of ventricular dysfunction, they are ideal monitoring parameters. Unfortunately, monitoring of these parameters is not routinely available, due to limitations in technology.

The stroke volume or index thus becomes the single most important piece of information regarding cardiac function in the absence of ejection fraction monitoring. The stroke volume is extremely important because it will typically fall once blood volume becomes too low (hypovolemia) or the left ventricle becomes

too weak (LV dysfunction) to eject blood. In some cases, such as with exercise or in clinical conditions such as sepsis, the stroke volume can be increased; however low stroke volume is more commonly found during hemodynamic monitoring. For the diagnosis of hypovolemia or LV dysfunction to be made, there generally must be a reduced stroke volume.

Regulation of Stroke Volume

Three factors regulate stroke volume: preload, afterload, and contractility. Definitions of preload, afterload, and contractility are presented in Table 5–2. Preload is concerned with factors which affect the stretch of myocardial muscle, including the pressure and volume in the ventricle as well as the compliance (ability to stretch) of the muscle.

According to Starling's law, the more a muscle stretches, the more forceful the contraction. If the muscle stretches too much, however, the contraction becomes weaker. It is difficult to actually measure preload in clinical practice, and so we estimate it from the ventricular filling pressure. If the ventricular filling pressure increases beyond normal (normal LV diastolic filling pressure is about 8–12 mm Hg), it is assumed the left ventricle is weakening. If the pressure exceeds about 18 mm Hg, the ventricle is assumed to be near failure level (the point where the muscle is stretching excessively). Conversely, when the ventricular filling pressure is too low (less than 8 mm Hg), then it is assumed the blood volume is low (hypovolemia).

This estimate is frequently inaccurate since pressure alone does not determine preload. However, the assumption used to estimate preload is important to understand since it is widely used in critical care. To increase the accuracy of assessments based on pres-

TABLE 5–2. DETERMINANTS OF STROKE VOLUME

Preload	Amount of stretch in a muscle just before contraction	Estimated by the PAOP for LV assessment and by the CVP for RV assessment
Afterload	Resistance a muscle faces as it attempts to contract	Estimated by the SVR for LV resistance by the PVR for RV resistance
Contractility	Strength of the muscle contraction	Estimated by SV and PAOP or CVP. If the stroke volume is low and the PAOP or CVP is high, then the heart is assumed to be weakened.

PAOP, pulmonary artery occlusive pressure; SVR, systemic vascular resistance; PVR, pulmonary vascular resistance.

sure alone, pressure measurements should always be compared with the stroke volume or stroke index. As the filling pressures elevate, they should decrease the stroke index if they are clinically significant. If the filling pressures are low, the stroke index must be low as well before one can assume that hypovolemia exists. Combining the stroke index with filling pressure is essential in order to avoid misinterpreting the filling pressure.

Heart Rate

The heart rate needs to be evaluated in order to detect early changes in hemodynamics. Since cardiac output is a product of stroke volume multiplied by heart rate, any change in stroke volume will normally produce a change in the heart rate. If the stroke volume is elevated, the heart rate may decrease (as seen in adaptation to exercise). The exception to this guideline is during an increase in metabolic rate, in which both the stroke volume and the heart rate increase.

If the stroke volume falls, the heart rate normally increases; thus evaluation of tachycardias becomes an essential component of hemodynamic monitoring. Generally, bradycardia and tachycardia are significant because they may reflect a potentially dangerous interference in cardiac output. Bradycardia which develops suddenly is almost always reflective of a threat to cardiac output. Tachycardia, a more common clinical situation, also may indicate a threat to cardiac output.

Sinus tachycardia develops for three reasons:

1. an increase in metabolic rate (as with a temperature elevation);
2. a psychological factor (anxiety, fear); or
3. a reduction in stroke volume.

All three factors need to be considered when evaluating a rapid heart rate. For example, if a patient has a heart rate of 120 beats/min, the clinician must rule out a fever or anxiety or pain before assuming the heart rate is increased due to a reduced stroke volume.

If the heart rate is increased and a raised metabolic rate or a psychological factor does not appear to be the cause, then a low stroke volume is indicated and an investigation into its cause is necessary. The two most common reasons for a low stroke volume are hypovolemia and LV dysfunction. Both causes of low stroke volume can produce an increased heart rate if no abnormality exists in regulation of the heart rate (such as autonomic nervous system dysfunction or use of drugs which interfere with the sympathetic or parasympathetic nervous system).

An increased heart rate can compensate for a decrease in stroke volume, although this compensation is limited. The faster the heart rate, the less time there is for ventricular filling. As an increased heart rate reduces diastolic filling time, the potential exists to eventually reduce the stroke volume. There is no specific heart rate at which diastolic filling is reduced so severely that stroke volume decreases. However, it should be remembered that as the heart rate increases stroke volumes can be negatively affected.

Another important concept regarding heart rate has to do with the effect it has on myocardial oxygen consumption (MVo_2). The higher the heart rate, the more likely the heart will consume more oxygen. Typically, the MVo_2 can only be estimated because direct measurement is not easy. Since heart rate is not the only determinant of oxygen consumption (contractility and vascular resistance are also determinants), heart rate alone will not predict MVo_2. Keeping heart rates as low as possible, particularly in patients with altered myocardial blood flow, is one way of protecting myocardial function.

Hemodynamic Pressures

Hemodynamic pressures are some of the most common parameters monitored in critical care. Blood pressure, central venous pressure (CVP), and pulmonary artery and pulmonary capillary wedge pressures (PCWP or PAOP) are routinely monitored in the care of critically ill patients.

Interpreting Arterial Pressures

The arterial pressure is one of the most commonly used parameters to assess the adequacy of blood flow to the tissues. Blood pressure is determined by two factors, cardiac output and systemic vascular resistance (SVR). This fact is critical to the interpretation of blood pressure. Blood pressure will not reflect early clinical changes in hemodynamics because of a compensatory mechanism by which cardiac output and SVR interact to maintain adequate blood pressure. While this interaction is not always predictable, it works as follows: If the cardiac output decreases, the SVR will increase just enough to overcome the fall in cardiac output and maintain blood pressure at near normal levels (Table 5–3). Conversely, if the SVR falls, the cardiac output will increase to offset the fall in SVR.

In addition, the cardiac output is maintained by the heart rate and stroke volume. These two interact with each other to keep the cardiac output normal. If the stroke volume begins to fall because of loss of vol-

TABLE 5–3. REGULATION OF BLOOD PRESSURE

Cardiac Output	Systemic Vascular Resistance	Blood Pressure
Normal	Normal	Normal
Decreased	Increased	Remains near normal
Increased	Decreased	Remains near normal
Increased	Increased	Rapidly elevates
Decreased	Decreased	Rapidly falls

ume (hypovolemia) or dysfunction (LV failure), the heart rate will increase to offset this decrease in stroke volume. The net effect will be to maintain the cardiac output at near normal levels. If the cardiac output does not change, there will be no change in the blood pressure.

The key point to the above interactions is that the blood pressure cannot signal early clinical changes. If a patient begins to bleed postoperatively, the blood pressure will generally not reflect this event until it becomes so severe that an increase in the heart rate and SVR no longer compensates. This is also the case for patients who have congestive heart failure or myocardial infarction.

Blood pressure is typically defined as normal if it falls within the following parameters: systolic 90–140 mm Hg, diastolic 60–90 mm Hg, mean 60–110 mm Hg. Blood pressure is considered normal if two problems can be ruled out: hypotension, which is associated with inadequate blood flow to the tissues, and hypertension, which is associated with excessive pressure and damage to the peripheral circulation.

Hypotension is probably present if there is evidence of tissue oxygenation deficits. Blood pressure therefore needs to be assessed along with measures of tissue oxygenation, such as SvO_2 and lactate levels. The implication of the interaction between tissue oxygenation and blood pressure is that blood pressure cannot be viewed in isolation.

Hypertension is more difficult to identify since there are fewer clinical parameters to indicate when peripheral circulatory changes are occurring. However, pressure alone is an important determinant of circulatory damage. As such, it is a little more reliable as a parameter in hypertension than in hypotension. Studies of hypertension-induced injury have not shown clearly what blood pressure produces actual injury. As a guideline, however, a systolic blood pressure of 140 mm Hg or higher is considered potentially injurious to the circulation.

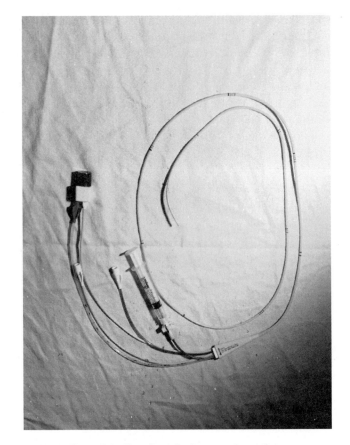

Figure 5–1. Flow-directed pulmonary artery catheter.

Interpreting Pulmonary Artery Pressures

Pulmonary artery and cardiac pressures are typically obtained from a flow-directed catheter inserted into a major vein and directed into the heart and pulmonary artery (Figs. 5–1 and 5–2). Since the pulmonary vasculature is normally a low-resistance system, the pulmonary artery blood pressure is generally approximately 25/10 mm Hg. If the pressure in the pulmonary vasculature elevates, the capillary hydrostatic pressure exceeds capillary osmotic pressure and fluid is forced out of the vessels. Interstitial and alveolar flooding can then occur with resulting interference in oxygen and carbon dioxide exchange.

The pulmonary artery pressures can be helpful in diagnosing many clinical conditions. Pulmonary artery pressure greater than 35/20 mm Hg is considered pulmonary hypertension.

Interpreting the Central Venous Pressure

Determining intracardiac pressure frequently centers on measurement of atrial pressure. Atrial pressure is used to estimate ventricular end diastolic

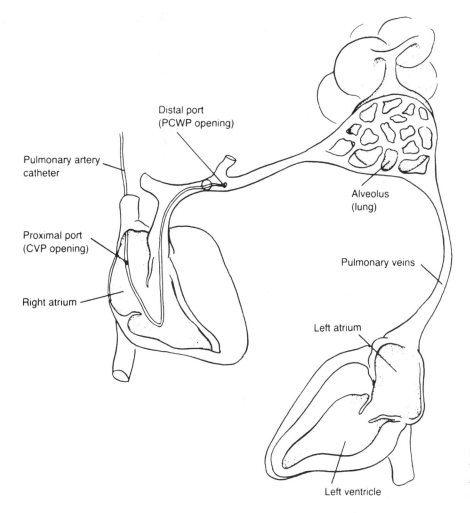

Distal port
(PCWP opening)

Pulmonary artery
catheter

Proximal port
(CVP opening)

Right atrium

Alveolus
(lung)

Pulmonary veins

Left atrium

Left ventricle

Figure 5–2. Pulmonary artery catheter in place within the pulmonary artery. (Adapted from Ahrens, T. S. (1993). *Hemodynamic Waveform Recognition*. Philadelphia: W.B. Saunders.)

pressures. Ventricular end diastolic pressure is potentially useful since it partially reflects preload. Right atrial pressure is also referred to as the central venous pressure (CVP) and left atrial pressure is referred to as the pulmonary capillary wedge pressure (PCWP) or pulmonary artery occlusive pressure (PAOP).

The CVP is an estimate of right ventricular (RV) end diastolic pressure (RVEDP) and is used to assess the performance of the right ventricle. The guidelines for interpreting the CVP have traditionally been relatively simple. The CVP is normally between 2 and 6 mm Hg. If the CVP is low, hypovolemia is assumed to exist. If the CVP is normal, normovolemia is present. If the CVP is high, RV dysfunction is present. While this traditional interpretation of hemodynamics is somewhat simplistic, it is adequate for CCRN qualification. However, the best way to interpret pressure values is to compare them to another parameter, such as the stroke index. If both the CVP and the stroke index are low, then hypo-

volemia is likely. However, if the CVP is low and the stroke index is normal, then hypovolemia may not be present. The opposite is also true, that is, if the CVP is high and the stroke index is low, RV dysfunction is probable. However, if the CVP is high and the stroke index is normal, then RV dysfunction may not be present (or clinically significant). Perhaps the most difficult part of interpreting pressures is that normal pressures do not indicate normal cardiac functioning.

While the CVP is useful in assessing RV function, the assessment of LV function is generally more important. If the left ventricle dysfunctions (such as with myocardial infarction or cardiomyopathies), then a threat to tissue oxygenation and survival may exist.

Interpreting the Pulmonary Capillary Wedge Pressure

Assessment of LV preload is commonly performed by obtaining the PCWP (PAOP). The use of the

PCWP to estimate left ventricular end diastolic pressure (LVEDP) is based on the assumption that a measurement from an obstructed pulmonary capillary will reflect an uninterrupted flow of blood to the left atrium since there are no valves in the pulmonary arterial system. A second assumption is that when the mitral valve is open, left atrial pressure reflects LVEDP. As long as these assumptions are accurate, the use of the PCWP to estimate LVEDP is acceptable. The guidelines for interpreting the PCWP are relatively simple and similar to those of CVP interpretation. Normal PCWP is about 8–12 mm Hg. If the PCWP is low, hypovolemia is assumed to be present. If the PCWP is normal, normovolemia is present. If the PCWP is high, LV dysfunction is present. However, PCWP interpretation has the same limitations as CVP interpretation, plus a few more. As with the CVP, the PCWP should not be interpreted in isolation. When analyzing the PCWP, always use the stroke index to help interpret the value. If the PCWP is low and the stroke index is low, then hypovolemia is probable. If the PCWP is low and the stroke index is normal, then hypovolemia is not likely. Use care when interpreting high PCWP values as well. If the PCWP is high and the stroke index is low, LV dysfunction is probable. However, if the PCWP is high and the stroke index is normal, then LV dysfunction may not be present (or clinically significant).

TABLE 5–4. NORMAL DERIVED HEMODYNAMIC PARAMETERS

Parameter	Normal Level	Consider Intervention
Mean arterial pressure (MAP)	70–110 mm Hg	<60 mm Hg
Mean pulmonary arterial pressure (MPAP)	15–25 mm Hg	>25 mm Hg
Systemic vascular resistance (SVR)	900–1300 dynes/sec/cm^5	<800 dynes/sec/cm^5
		>1500 dynes/sec/cm^5
Pulmonary vascular resistance (PVR), where	40–150 dynes/sec/cm^5	>200 dynes/sec/cm^5

$$MAP = \frac{(2 \times DBP) + SBP}{3}$$

$$MPAP = \frac{(2 \times DPAP) + SPAP}{3}$$

$$SVR = \frac{MAP - CVP \times 80}{CO}$$

$$PVR = \frac{MPAP - PAOP \times 80}{CO}$$

DBP/SBP, diastolic/systolic blood pressure; DPAP/SPAP, diastolic/systolic pulmonary artery pressure; CO, cardiac output.

Derived Parameters

Several hemodynamic parameters are derived or calculated from other variables. Some common derived hemodynamic parameters are listed in Table 5–4. Most bedside monitors will perform the calculations necessary to attain these values. However, it is essential for the critical care nurse to know which variables are included in the calculation. This knowledge is essential to understanding how hemodydnamics interact and to interpreting the derived parameters.

Systemic and Pulmonary Vascular Resistance

One of the most common derived parameters is vascular resistance. Vascular resistance is frequently assumed to represent afterload, or the resistance the ventricles face during ejection of blood. It is important to keep in mind that afterload is not measured by vascular resistance alone. Afterload is also influenced by blood viscosity and valvular resistance. While these values can change, vascular resistance can be used to estimate afterload since viscosity and valvular resistance tend to change less often than blood vessel resistance.

In clinical practice, this formula is:

$$SVR = \frac{\text{Mean arterial pressure} - \text{right atrial pressure}}{\text{Cardiac output}}$$

The value obtained from this formula is then multiplied by a factor of 80 to generate a value measured in dynes/sec/cm^5.

Two types of vascular resistance are commonly measured, systemic and pulmonary vascular resistance. Systemic vascular resistance (SVR) reflects LV afterload, whereas pulmonary vascular resistance (PVR) reflects RV afterload.

Normal SVR is about 900–1300 dynes/sec/cm^5. If the SVR is elevated, the left ventricle will face increased resistance to the ejection of blood. The SVR commonly rises for two reasons. It can increase in response to primary systemic hypertension or secondary systemic hypertension (peripheral vascular disease), or to compensate for a low cardiac output, such as would occur in shock states. It is important for the clinician to know why the SVR is elevated. If the SVR is elevated because of systemic hypertension, then afterload-reducing agents are a critical part of the therapy. However, if the SVR is elevated in compensation for low cardiac output, then therapy is directed at improving the cardiac output more than reducing SVR.

If the SVR is low, the left ventricle meets with lower resistance to the ejection of blood. Generally, the SVR does not lower except as a pathologic response to inflammation. The SVR can also be reduced in hepatic disease (because of increased collateral circulation) or neurogenic-induced central vasodilation. If the SVR is reduced, attempts to increase the resistance center on vasopressors. More important to consider, though, is the treatment of the underlying condition. If the underlying condition is not treated, the use of vasopressors will provide only short-term success.

Pulmonary vascular resistance reflects the work the right ventricle faces as it attempts to contract. The PVR is normally between 40 and 150 dynes/sec/cm^5. The PVR elevates for one of three reasons: (1) primary pulmonary hypertension; (2) secondary active pulmonary hypertension; and (3) secondary passive pulmonary hypertension. In primary pulmonary hypertension, the cause is unknown and the PVR is markedly elevated. No known cure exists for this condition. In secondary active pulmonary hypertension, a cause is known but the condition is not very responsive to treatment. For example, chronic obstructive pulmonary disease or pulmonary emboli can cause this type of pulmonary hypertension. Secondary passive pulmonary hypertension is the result of LV dysfunction. In this case, the pulmonary arterial pressure decreases as the LV function improves. It is the most responsive pulmonary hypertension in terms of treatment. Also, this form of pulmonary hypertension can be identified by noting the close correlation between the PCWP and the pulmonary artery diastolic pressure (normally the pulmonary artery diastolic pressure is slightly higher than the PCWP).

Oxygenation and Hemodynamics

It is critical to understand that the human cardiopulmonary system exists only to provide nutrients to the tissues, the primary nutrient being oxygen. Subsequently, hemodynamics need to be viewed in terms of the adequacy of tissue oxygenation.

Several parameters reflect tissue oxygenation (Table 5–5). However, the most helpful in terms of real-time monitoring is the mixed venous oxyhemoglobin (SvO_2) measurement. SvO_2 values are obtained in two ways:

1. Sampled directly from the distal port of the pulmonary artery catheter. When measuring

TABLE 5–5. MEASURES OF TISSUE OXYGENATION

Parameter	Normal Level	Consider Intervention
SvO_2	60–75%	<60% or >75%
Lactate	1–2 mmol/L	>4 mmol + pH <7.25

the SvO_2 in this way, you should draw the sample slowly so as not to aspirate pulmonary capillary blood (producing an arterial-like blood sample).

2. Continuously measured via fiberoptics in the pulmonary artery catheter (Fig. 5–3). This technique has the obvious advantage of providing a continuous reading of SvO_2, avoiding the expense of blood gases and loss of blood as well as the risk of exposure of the nurse to blood.

The value of measuring SvO_2 centers on the concept that the amount of oxygen returning to the lungs is an accurate reflection of tissue oxygenation. Consider that oxygen is normally removed from hemoglobin as it passes through

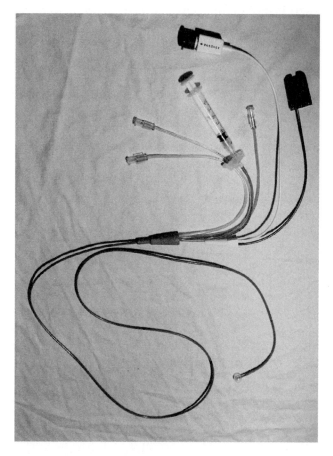

Figure 5–3. Fiberoptic pulmonary artery catheter.

the capillary bed. Normally, about 25% of the oxygen in hemoglobin is removed. This means the amount of oxygen returning to the lungs still attached to hemoglobin should be about 75%. The oxygen that is in hemoglobin is the only oxygen reserve in the body. If the tissues are deprived of oxygen, either by too little delivery of oxygen (oxygen delivery, DO_2) or an increase in oxygen demand (oxygen consumption, VO_2), the tissues will extract more oxygen from hemoglobin. This extraction occurs as the tissue PO_2 falls, creating an increased oxygen tension gradient between the tissues and blood. In clinical situations, SvO_2 levels (the amount of oxygen still in hemoglobin when it returns to the lungs) are generally at least 60%. If they drop below this level, a potential threat to issue oxygenation has to be considered.

Deciding when a hemodynamic parameter, such as cardiac output or blood pressure, has changed in a clinically significant manner is one of the most important responsibilities facing the bedside clinician. The use of SvO_2 monitoring makes the decision-making process easier.

INTERPRETING HEMODYNAMIC WAVEFORMS

EDITORS' NOTE

Reading hemodynamic waveforms is the key to obtaining the pressures which are used in hemodynamic monitoring. Learning how to read waveforms for the CCRN exam is very easy and there are very few questions that address this content. It is unlikely you will actually have to read waveforms on the exam. Just read this section and understand the meaning of the waves and the principles of waveform interpretation.

Reading CVP and PCWP (Wedge) Waveforms

One critical point to remember when reading CVP and PCWP (or PAOP) tracings is that they are used to estimate ventricular end diastolic pressures. As such, only one part of the PCWP and CVP tracing correlates with ventricular end diastolic pressure. That part is just before closure of the mitral and tricuspid valves

prior to ventricular systole. In order to identify this point, the electrocardiogram (ECG) is used as the reference point. Since the mitral and tricuspid valves close just before ventricular contraction, the valves must still be open during the QRS complex (Fig. 5–4). For the CVP waveform, identify the point near the end of the QRS and draw a line straight down. The point at which this line intersects with the wave is the CVP value. For the PCWP waveform, the line is drawn about 0.08 sec after the QRS complex (Fig. 5–5). This difference from the CVP reflects the time needed for the wave to travel from the left atrium back to the pulmonary artery catheter.

A second method for reading the CVP and PCWP waveform involves averaging the A wave of the atrial waveforms.

Research has shown that bedside monitors are frequently inaccurate. Bedside monitors give an accurate reading in simple waveforms but become less accurate as the waveforms become more complex.

Abnormal CVP and PCWP Waveforms

Abnormal waveforms can make reading pressure values difficult. Fortunately, abnormal waveforms are easy to avoid by using the above techniques for obtaining CVP and PCWP values. Probably the two most common abnormal waves are large A and V waves. Large A waves occur when the atrium and ventricles contract simultaneously (as in third-degree heart block or premature ventricular contractions). Large V waves are common in conditions such as mitral or tricuspid regurgitation and ventricular failure (Fig. 5–6).

Arterial Waveforms

An arterial waveform has three common characteristics: (1) a rapid upstroke; (2) a dicrotic notch; and (3) a progressive diastolic runoff (Fig. 5–7). Diastole is read near the end of the QRS complex and systole is read before the peak of the T wave.

A ventricular waveform is similar to an arterial wave in that it also has three common characteristics (i.e., a rapid upstroke, a rapid diastolic drop, and an end diastolic pressure rise) (Fig. 5–8). Systole and diastole are read in the same manner as an arterial waveform. Normally a ventricular waveform is not monitored. This is unfortunate since a CVP value is less desirable than a RV waveform. If a ventricular waveform is present on the monitor, it is important to verify the correct location of the catheter. A catheter which is floating freely in the ventricle tends to cause premature ventricular contractions.

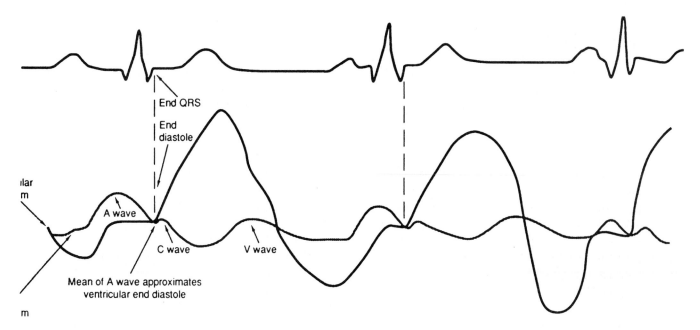

Figure 5–4. Correlation of ventricular end diastole with atrial pressure. (Used with permission. Ahrens T. S. & Taylor L. (1992). *Hemodynamic Waveform Analysis.* Philadelphia: W. B. Saunders.)

Respiratory Artifacts

Waveforms obtained from blood vessels in the chest are subject to artifact. This artifact is the result of the transducers' being referenced to atmospheric pressure, not pleural pressure. In order to avoid this artifact, respiratory waveforms are read at end expiration, the point at which atmospheric and pleural pressures are relatively close.

A spontaneous inspiration or a triggered ventilator inspiration produces a decrease in the waveform due to a fall in pleural pressure (Fig. 5–9). A ventilator inspiration will produce a positive deflection due to an increase in unmeasured pleural pressure (Fig. 5–10). To avoid artifact, find the point just before the inspiration (spontaneous, triggered ventilator, or unassisted ventilator) occurs. This will avoid most artifact (Fig. 5–11).

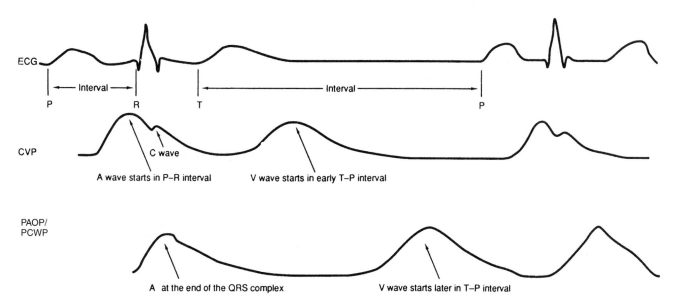

Figure 5–5. Reading CVP and PCWP waveforms. (Used with permission. Ahrens T. S. & Taylor L. (1992). *Hemodynamic Waveform Analysis.* Philadelphia: W. B. Saunders.)

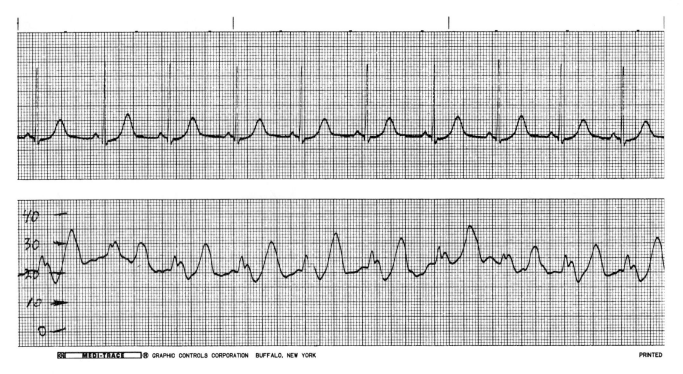

MEDI-TRACE ® GRAPHIC CONTROLS CORPORATION BUFFALO, NEW YORK   PRINTED

Figure 5–6. Abnormal V waves in a PWCP waveform.

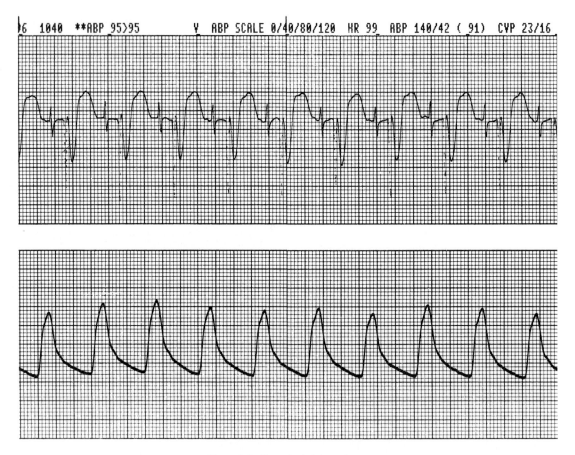

Figure 5–7. Normal arterial waveform.

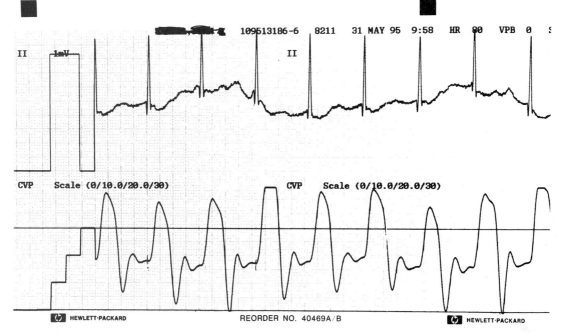

Figure 5–8. Normal ventricular waveform.

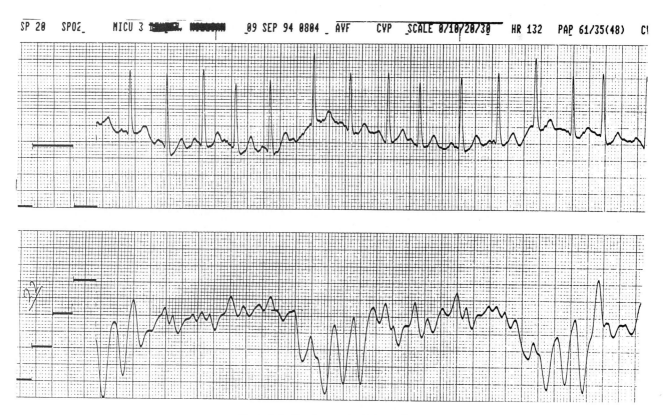

Figure 5–9. Spontaneous inspiratory artifact.

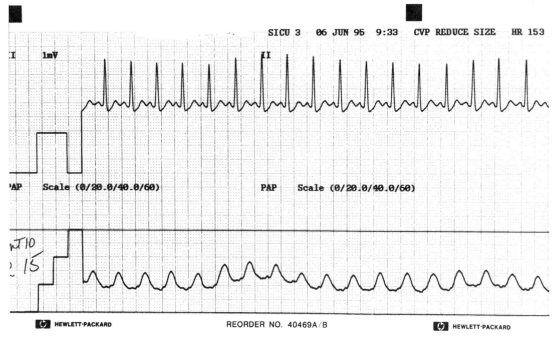

Figure 5–10. Respiratory artifact from mechanical ventilation.

OBTAINING ACCURATE HEMODYNAMIC VALUES

EDITORS' NOTE

The information obtained from hemodynamic monitoring technology must be verified for accuracy by the bedside clinician. However, the CCRN exam is unlikely to include many specific questions in this area. Only the steps necessary to obtain accurate values are provided. You might want to review this content for your own clinical practice and just to be safe for the exam.

Ensuring Accuracy

To obtain accurate values, five steps are necessary.

1. Set the transducer to zero (usually has to be done only once).
2. Ensure that the transducer is level (should be done whenever the patient or transducer moves from the original level position).
3. Read the waveform accurately.
4. Perform a square-wave test to verify the accuracy of the tubing and catheter.
5. Perform a calibration of the transducer (if necessary at all, it needs to be done only once).

"Zeroing" the Transducer and Leveling the Transducer to the Catheter Tip

"Zeroing" is done by exposing the transducer to air and pushing or activating a zero button (Fig. 5–12).

Leveling is the process of aligning the tip of the vascular catheter with a zero point, usually a stopcock in the pressure tubing. For example, leveling a pulmonary artery catheter is done by opening a stopcock at the level of the mid-axillary line (Fig. 5–13A). Leveling a radial artery catheter is done the same way but now the stopcock is opened to the radial artery (Fig. 7–13B).

Leveling is performed when obtaining the first set of hemodynamic information and then any time the patient or transducer has moved from the original position. When obtaining the first set of readings, zeroing and leveling are performed simultaneously. After this initial combined effort, only leveling needs to be performed and then only if the patient or transducer have moved from the original position.

Square-Wave Test

The square-wave test is done to ensure the tubing catheter system does not interfere with waveform transmission to the transducer. If an obstruction (such as air, blood, or stopcock connection) is

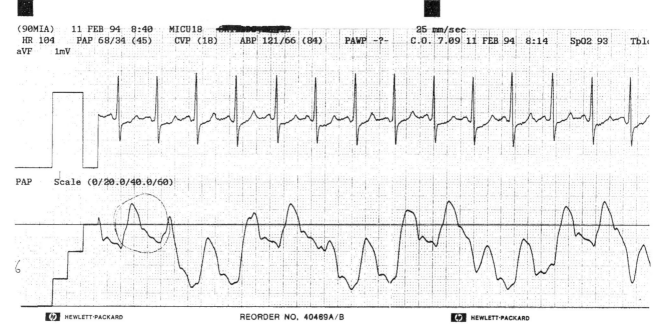

(90MIA)   11 FEB 94   8:40   MICU18   25 mm/sec
HR 104   PAP 68/34 (45)   CVP (18)   ABP 121/66 (84)   PAWP -?-   C.O. 7.09 11 FEB 94 8:14   SpO2 93   Tbl
aVF   1mV

PAP   Scale (0/20.0/40.0/60)

Figure 5–11. Avoiding inspiratory artifact in a patient with a respiratory rate greater than the ventilator rate.

present, it is said to be "**overdamped**" (Fig. 5–14). Overdamping decreases systolic pressures and increases diastolic pressures. If something increases the wave (such as excessive tubing), it is said to be "**underdamped**" (Fig. 5–15). Underdamping increases systolic pressures and decreases diastolic pressures.

The ideal square-wave test is called an "optimally damped" test (Fig. 5–16). It is important to remember that the square-wave test is the best method available to the clinician to check the accuracy of an arterial pressure reading. This test is more accurate than comparing an arterial pressure to a cuff pressure.

Calibration of the Transducer/ Amplifier System

All disposable transducers are precalibrated. This reduces the need for clinicians to perform calibration. If a calibration check is desired, the fluid col-

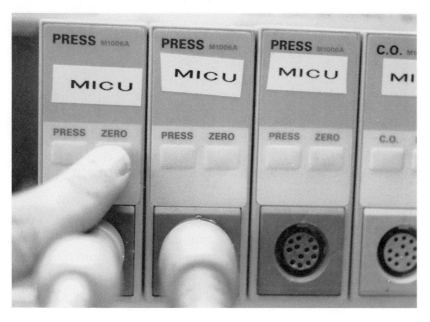

Figure 5–12. "Zeroing" a transducer.

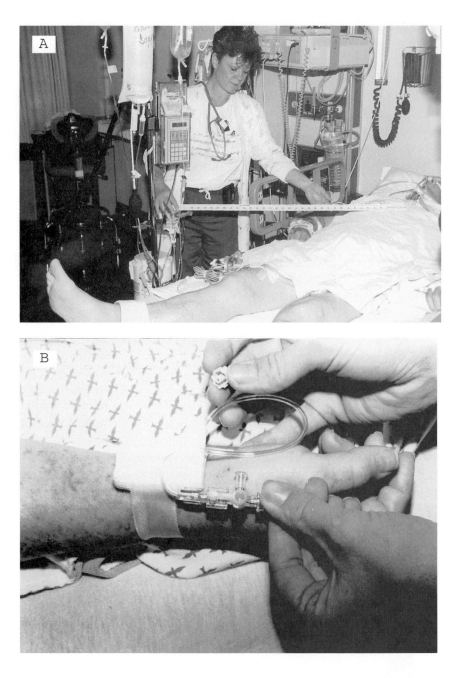

Figure 5–13. (**A**) Leveling a transducer to the catheter tip. (**B**) Leveling a radial artery catheter.

umn on the transducer can be used. A known height of the fluid column will reveal the weight of the fluid column. This known weight should be displayed on the monitor. If it is not, the clinician needs to adjust the monitor to display the correct pressure.

Factors to Consider During Hemodynamic Monitoring

Patient position during hemodynamic monitoring can be anywhere from flat to about 40° upper-body elevation. In this range, hemodynamic readings should be consistent. It is not necessary that patients lie flat in order to obtain hemodynamic values.

Measuring Cardiac Output

A few key points should be remembered while measuring cardiac output:

1. All outputs should be within 10% of each other.
2. Room-temperature ice injectates are both acceptable. Ice injectates might be preferable in low or high cardiac output states.

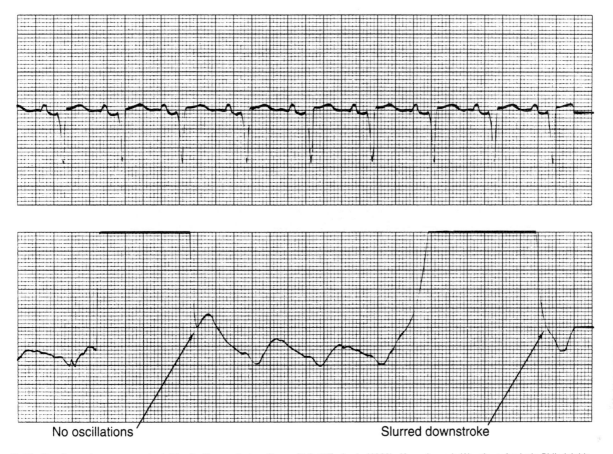

No oscillations   Slurred downstroke

Figure 5–14. Overdamped square-wave test. (Used with permission. Ahrens T. S. & Taylor L. (1992). *Hemodynamic Waveform Analysis.* Philadelphia: W. B. Saunders.)

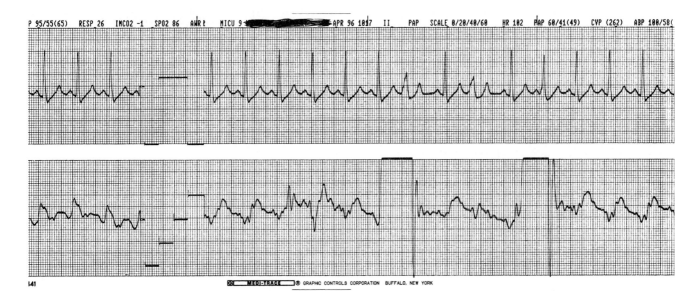

P 95/55(65)   RESP 26   IMCO2 -1   SP02 86   AWR ℓ   MICU 9▬▬▬▬▬▬▬▬APR 96 10:17   II   PAP   SCALE 0/20/40/60   HR 102   MAP 60/41(49)   CVP (262)   ABP 100/58(

141   MEDI-TRACE ® GRAPHIC CONTROLS CORPORATION BUFFALO, NEW YORK

Figure 5–15. Underdamped square-wave test.

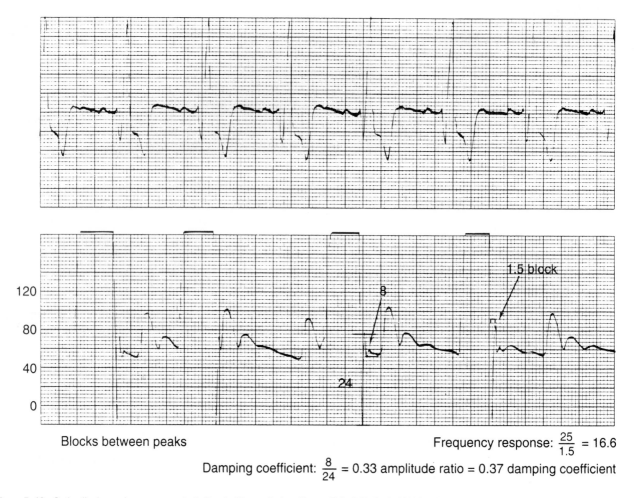

Blocks between peaks

Frequency response: $\frac{25}{1.5}$ = 16.6

Damping coefficient: $\frac{8}{24}$ = 0.33 amplitude ratio = 0.37 damping coefficient

Figure 5–16. Optimally damped square-wave test. (Used with permission. Ahrens T. S. & Taylor L. (1992). *Hemodynamic Waveform Analysis.* Philadelphia: W. B. Saunders.)

3. The presence of the following limit the accuracy of thermodilution measurements: ventricular or atrial septal defect, tricuspid regurgitation, or dysrhythmias.
4. Injecting at a consistent point in the respiratory cycle will help reduce variability in readings.
5. If the cardiac output measurements are inconsistent, use the Fick equation to measure cardiac output:

$$\text{Cardiac output} = \frac{\text{Vo}_2/10}{1.34 \times \text{Hgb} \times (\text{Sao}_2 - \text{Svo}_2)}$$

where (Vo$_2$) = oxygen consumption and $1.34 \times \text{Hgb} \times (\text{Sao}_2 - \text{Svo}_2)$ = arterovenous oxygen content difference. It is unlikely that the Fick equation will be on the CCRN test.

Angina Pectoris and Myocardial Infarction

EDITORS' NOTE

The CCRN exam can be expected to contain questions on assessing and treating coronary artery disease. This chapter provides brief but key concepts in the area of coronary artery disease. Expect several questions in the CCRN exam on the assessment, diagnosis, and treatment of angina and myocardial infarction.

Angina (including coronary artery vasospasm and unstable angina) and myocardial infarction (MI) are common test items on the CCRN exam. This chapter emphasizes the main features of the origin, symptomatology, and medical and nursing interventions associated with angina and MI. An understanding of the concepts in this chapter should aid in successfully answering questions regarding these conditions.

PATHOPHYSIOLOGY

A series of physiologic changes within the body and heart starts with arteriosclerosis and advances (without intervention) to coronary artery disease. A combination of lipid accumulation and endothelial injury with subsequent thrombosis formation probably forms the basis for obstruction of blood flow. While obstruction of blood flow is responsible for symptoms associated with coronary artery disease, the symptoms will vary depending on the develop-

ment of collateral circulation. The first symptoms of coronary artery disease may be those of angina pectoris, but they may also be MI or sudden death.

ATHEROSCLEROSIS

Classification

The CCRN exam has not traditionally included questions regarding the classification of atherosclerosis. For the purpose of this chapter, simple descriptions will be used for illustration. Normally (i.e., ideally), significant atherosclerosis is not present. However, almost all blood vessels have some degree of atherosclerosis.

Obstruction by atherosclerotic plaques may occur in any or all of the coronary arteries.

Etiology

Unalterable Risk Factors

1. Hereditary predisposition to the development of atherosclerosis seems to be a prime factor in developing atherosclerosis.
2. Age appears to influence the development of atherosclerosis, since it is more prevalent in older persons than in younger persons.
3. Sex seems to be a factor in the development of atherosclerosis, since the condition is more prevalent in men than in women (at least prior to menopause). Recent evidence suggests that postmenopausal women may have a higher incidence of myocardial disease than was previously estimated.

4. Race may influence atherosclerosis. It appears to be more common in Caucasians, although other factors, such as diet, may obscure the influence of race.

Medically Alterable Risk Factors

1. Hypertension has been shown to be related to the development of atherosclerosis. Close medical treatment of hypertension may retard the development of atherosclerosis.
2. Diabetics develop atherosclerosis more often than nondiabetics. Close medical treatment and control of diabetes may reduce the atherosclerotic process.
3. Hyperlipidemia, when accompanied by high serum cholesterol levels, may have a bearing on the development and/or progression of atherosclerosis. The presence of low-density lipoproteins appears to be a precursor to the development of atherosclerosis. Medical treatment of hyperlipidemia may help retard the atherosclerotic process.

Personal Alterable Risk Factors

These factors can be altered by the individual to decrease the possibility or progression of atherosclerosis.

1. Weight control can be beneficial in reducing the risk of coronary artery disease.
2. Cigarette smokers have a higher incidence of heart disease than do nonsmokers. Elimination of smoking will reduce the risk of MI.
3. Emotional tension and stress may be influential in the development of myocardial disease. The exact role of emotional stress is not as clear as the physical factors contributing to coronary disease.
4. Sedentary life styles predispose one to developing atherosclerosis. Exercising three to four times per week for 30 minutes of activity that pushes the heart rate into the target heart rate zone for aerobic exercise will reduce the rate of coronary artery disease.
5. Moderate alcohol intake may reduce the risk of coronary artery disease. However, the limitation to moderate intake is difficult in many people, and the risk of alcoholism may outweigh the benefit of this factor.

If an individual is sufficiently motivated, these last five risk factors can be incorporated into a personal life style.

Prognosis

One cannot change some risk factors, one can alter other risk factors with medical treatment, and one can eliminate some risk factors if so motivated. If risk factors are not modified, atherosclerosis may progress from the development of angina and ischemia to MI, congestive heart failure, or sudden death. Despite the prognosis with alterable risk factors, coronary atherosclerosis is still one of the leading causes of deaths in the United States. However, the incidence of coronary artery disease has decreased over the last 30 years.

ANGINA PECTORIS

Angina can result from a reduced blood flow, low oxygen content, or myocardial oxygen demand in excess of supply. No actual injury to the myocardial muscle occurs during most types of angina. Autopsy results of patients with angina have demonstrated frequent total occlusion of coronary vessels with subsequent development of extensive collateral circulation. The development of collateral circulation has allowed maintenance of coronary perfusion and no permanent injury to the myocardium even when cardiac catheterization results have indicated total occlusion. Differing types of lesions are noted during cardiac catheterization (Fig. 6–1).

Causes of reduced blood flow to the myocardium include atherosclerosis, valvular dysfunction, hypoten-

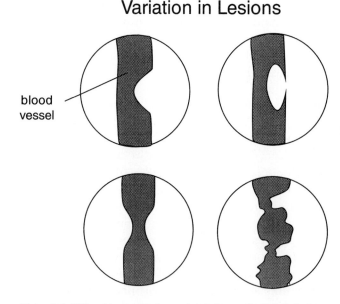

Variation in Lesions

blood vessel

Figure 6–1. Different types of lesions noted during cardiac catheterization.

sion, and coronary vasospasm. Low oxygen content can also precipitate anginal episodes. Causes of low oxygen content include reduced hemoglobin and low oxygen pressure/saturation (PaO_2/SaO_2) levels. Causes of excessive oxygen demands relative to perfusion include hypertension, exercise, and increased metabolic rates. Many predisposing factors can precipitate a reduced blood flow, decreased oxygen content, or increased myocardial oxygen demands.

The occurrence of angina is variable, depending substantially on the degree of collateral circulation that has developed to reduce blood and oxygen flow. Angina can be suddenly precipitated by any event that increases oxygen demand (such as anxiety, stress, eating, or exercise) or reduces blood flow (smoking).

Clinical Presentation

Pain is the primary symptom. It may be described as burning, squeezing in a tight band, or extreme heaviness or pressure on the lower sternum. It may radiate to the neck, jaws, shoulders, arms, and stomach.

Characteristically, the pain begins after eating or physical activity and subsides with rest. The pain usually lasts 1–4 min, but it may require as long as 10 min to subside completely. Anginal pain should always last less than 30 min. Pain for more than 30 min suggests MI and the need for immediate treatment. Not all coronary artery disease will present with anginal symptoms. Some patients can have evidence of ischemia without symptoms. This possibility of ischemia without pain serves as a clue in the education of patients with angina and MI. Frequent evaluation of cardiac status, such as with exercise testing, can detect symptoms earlier than waiting for an anginal episode to indicate ischemia.

Diagnosis

Diagnosis of angina is based on history and electrocardiogram (ECG) findings. Cardiac isoenzymes are usually normal. The 12-lead ECG usually has depressed ST segments over the affected area. ST segment elevation (Prinzmetal's angina) can occur but is less common.

Treatment

Vasodilators, such as sublingual nitroglycerin, usually relieve the angina within 1½ min. Nitroglycerin taken before an activity may prevent an attack. Alteration of one's life style to eliminate the alterable risk factors may help decrease the severity and frequency of attacks. If the angina attacks increase in frequency or intensity (crescendo angina), stress testing and/or cardiac catheterization to determine the extent of the disease is indicated. Nitrates, beta blockers, and calcium channel blockers may be used alone or in combination to resolve anginal episodes. The patient may be a candidate for transluminal angioplasty or coronary artery bypass surgery, which will stop the angina and decrease the risk of MI. The patient is advised to exercise within the limits of pain and obtain adequate rest. Coronary artery bypass grafting (CABG) is the treatment for failure of medical intervention. CABG has demonstrated the potential for alleviating symptoms of angina although not necessarily prolonging life.

Unstable Angina

Several variations of angina exist, the most prevalent of which is unstable angina. Unstable angina differs from stable angina in that it is more easily initiated. Unstable angina usually involves crescendo angina, may occur at rest, and is characterized by increasing severity in the past few months. Clinically, the patient may complain of reduction in activities that precipitate anginal episodes and an increase in severity of symptoms.

Treatment of unstable angina usually requires additional medical therapy. Beta blockers (e.g., propanolol) are helpful in reducing myocardial oxygen consumption. Calcium channel blockers (e.g., nifedipine) may be useful in reducing afterload and myocardial oxygen use.

Another type of angina is Prinzmetal's angina. In this form of angina, the origin is thought to be both coronary vasospasm and stenosis. The patient presents with symptoms most often including pain at rest and other symptoms of angina. The ECG shows reversible ST segment elevation rather than depression.

Calcium channel blockers have more effect in reducing the anginal episode than do beta blockers, probably because they reduce vasospasm to a greater extent. Diltiazem and nifedipine are both effective in reducing episodes of Prinzmetal's angina. If medical therapy fails, both unstable angina and Prinzmetal's angina may require CABG or angioplasty.

Coronary Artery Vasospasm

Coronary artery vasospasm, a form of variant angina, is a transient narrowing of a large coronary artery.

The origins are unclear but could include sympathetic stimulation, prostaglandin mediation, or pharmacological stimulation. Treatment is similar to that for angina, with more emphasis on calcium channel blockers as well as nitroglycerin.

ACUTE MYOCARDIAL INFARCTION

Myocardial infarction is the actual necrosis, or death, of myocardial tissue because of reduced blood supply (loss of oxygen) to a specific area of the heart (Fig. 6–2).

Etiology

In most MIs, atherosclerotic heart disease is present. The remaining incidences of MIs are likely due to coronary artery spasm in which the artery spasms sufficiently to prevent blood from reaching the myocardium.

Most MIs have been demonstrated to be the result of coronary thrombosis formation on top of an atherosclerotic plaque. The rapid identification of MI is crucial to treatment. Within 6 hr of onset, myocardial muscle becomes generally irreversibly damaged. While this time period can vary and some tissue can be salvaged at later times, the earlier the treatment, the more likely recovery will take place.

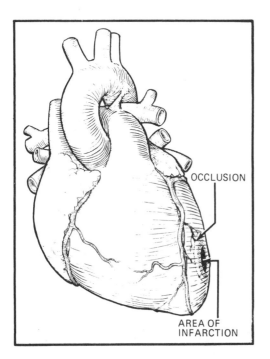

OCCLUSION

AREA OF INFARCTION

Figure 6–2. Myocardial infarction.

Diagnosis and Clinical Presentation

Chest pain with nausea (and maybe vomiting), diaphoresis, and weakness are the most common symptoms of an MI. The infarct pain differs from anginal pain. With an MI, the chest pain is constant, severe, and not relieved with nitroglycerin. The location of the pain is similar to that for anginal pain. It is, however, not relieved with rest or lying down. The duration of pain exceeds 30 min without relief. In fact, it often occurs at rest without a clear precipitating event. As the pain, nausea, weakness, and diaphoresis continue, patients become dyspneic and often develop severe apprehension that may be accompanied by a sense of impending doom.

However, MIs may present without any symptoms or with only mild signs, such as indigestion. These "silent" MIs are extremely difficult to treat since the signs are not severe enough to prompt a visit to the hospital or physician.

The 12-lead ECG reveals initial T-wave inversion followed quickly by ST segment elevation in the affected area. Q-wave formation, indicating cellular death, occurs after 24 hr and is considered more diagnostic of myocardial infarction. Areas of the heart and their corresponding ECG leads for MI interpretation are presented in Table 6–1. Figure 6–3 gives an example of MI of the anterior septal region; Fig. 6–4 gives an example of an inferior MI.

Cardiac isoenzyme level abnormalities are the most diagnostic criteria for MIs, specifically, creatine phosphokinase (CPK) isoenzymes. CPK isoenzymes include MM, MB, and BB bands. The CPK-MB band is more specific for cardiac muscle. If the CPK-MB band elevates more than 12 IU, MI can be diagnosed (Table 6–2). Other enzymes, such as

TABLE 6–1.   AREAS OF THE HEART AND THEIR CORRESPONDING ECG LEADS FOR INTERPRETATION OF MYOCARDIAL INFARCTION

Location	ECG Location	ECG Changes
Anterior	V2–V4	Q waves, ST segment elevation
Inferior	II, III, avF	Q waves, ST segment elevation
Lateral	I, avL, V5, V6	Q waves, ST segment elevation
Right ventricular	V3R–V6R	ST segment elevation
Posterior	V1, V2	Large R wave
Septal	V1	Q waves, ST segment elevation

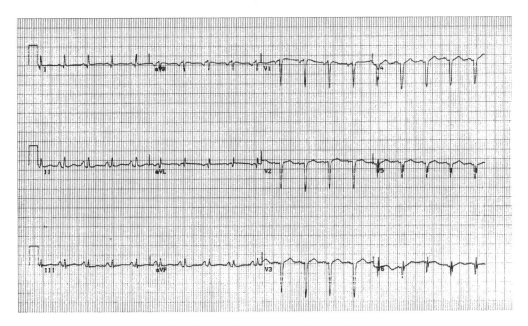

Figure 6–3. Anterior septal myocardial infarction.

lactic dehydrogenase (LDH) isoenzyme, might be used. When LDH isoenzymes are used, the LDH 1 isoenzyme, indicative of cardiac muscle, elevates. LDH 1 is normally lower than LDH 2; in an MI, LDH 1 exceeds LDH 2, resulting in a "flip" of LDH 1 and 2.

The potential value of LDH in MI is the slower elevation of the LDH isoenzymes. CPK isoenzymes elevate within hours of injury, peaking within 24 hr. LDH rises more slowly and may not peak until 48 to 72 hr. The slower rise in LDH may be useful in the patient who delays coming to the hospital after the onset of symptoms.

Newer diagnostic techniques for MI are under evaluation. For example, an isoform of the CPK-MB might be a more rapid indicator of an MI. If the MB_2 isoform is greater than the MB_1 (ratio 1.5:1 or above), then MI is highly likely. This test is available within 2 hr and could decrease ICU admissions to rule out MI.

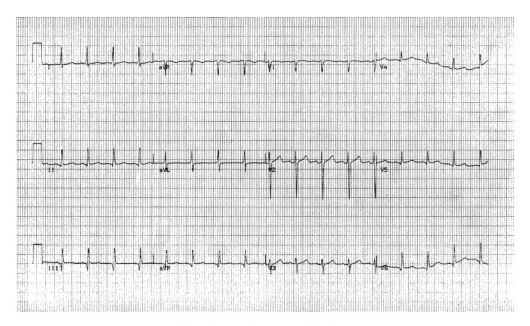

Figure 6–4. Inferior myocardial infarction.

TABLE 6–2.   CARDIAC ENZYMES AND PROTEINS USED IN THE DIAGNOSIS OF MYOCARDIAL INFARCTION

CPK	30–200 IU	Not specific by itself for MI; the size of MI is referenced to the degree of total CPK elevation (i.e., the higher the CPK, the greater the size of the MI)
CPK-MB	<5 ng/ml	>8 ng/ml suggests MI
Ratio of lactic dehydrogenase (LDH) 1 to LDH 2	LDH 1: 18–28 LDH 2: 25–35 LDH 1:2 ratio is normally <1	LDH 1:2 ratio > 1 suggests MI. Used if MI is suspected to be more than 24 hr old. Is being replaced by troponin levels
Troponin I	<0.6 ng/ml	>1.5 ng/ml suggests MI—elevates within 4 hours of MI and remains elevated for up to 8 days

Other cardiac-specific enzymes such as troponin I and T could improve identification of MIs, but may not be any faster at revealing MIs than CPK-MB. However, troponin I remains elevated for more than 8 days and likely will replace LDH levels.

Other diagnostic tests include the use of two-dimensional echocardiography and radionuclide imaging. Echocardiography reveals MIs by identifying defects in regional wall motion. Negative results also help rule out MIs.

Location of Infarction

Occlusion of the right coronary artery results in an inferior MI. Inferior MIs have a lower mortality rate than anterior MIs. Symptoms associated with an inferior MI include more mild AV node dysrhythmias, such as first- and second-degree type I blocks.

Occlusion of the left anterior descending coronary artery results in an anterior MI. Anterior MIs have higher mortality rates and are associated with more serious dysrhythmias. Rhythm disturbances are more likely to include second- and third-degree blocks.

Less serious MIs are lateral and posterior, each with lower mortality rates than inferior or posterior MIs. More dangerous MIs are those which affect multiple regions, such as anterior-lateral MIs. When more than 40% of the left ventricle is acutely damaged, mortality is extremely high.

Right ventricular (RV) MIs are less common but are associated with obstruction of the right coronary or left circumflex artery. Mortality is lower with RV MIs. Diagnosis is made from the ECG indicating a posterior MI pattern (large R waves in V_1 and V_2) and ST segment elevation in the right precordial leads (e.g., V_{4R} and V_{6R}).

Symptoms include elevated central venous pressure (CVP) despite normal pulmonary capillary wedge pressure (PCWP). Venous congestion, the result of the high CVP from RV failure, is the primary symptom. Treatment centers on maintaining CVP values higher than normal, up to 25 mm Hg, in order to improve blood flow through the right ventricle. In severe RV failure, less blood is pumped into the lungs, and a drop in PCWP results.

Treatment and Complications

The goals of treating an infarction are to increase coronary blood flow and decrease oxygen demand. These goals should prevent death or extension of injury to the myocardium and control or correct dysrhythmias that occur.

Pain relief is a prime objective and is usually accomplished with intravenous analgesics such as morphine sulfate (drug of choice), hydromorphone hydrochloride (Dilaudid), or meperidine hydrochloride (Demerol). Vasodilators such as nitroglycerin are also likely to reduce pain.

Thrombolytic Therapy

If the patient presents within 4 hr of onset of symptoms, thrombolysis is the treatment of choice. Controversy exists as to the agent of choice, either a tissue plasminogen activator (tPA) or streptokinase. tPA has more specific clot resolution activity than streptokinase but is much more expensive.

Several large studies have suggested that tPA is more useful in hemodynamically unstable cases (Table 6–3). tPA has a slight advantage in reducing mortality than streptokinase, but also has a slightly higher incidence of cerebral bleeding. The risks of tPA are balanced against the patient's need for thrombolysis. Thrombolytics require clear evidence of MI before they are administered. Usually at least

TABLE 6–3. THROMBOLYTIC THERAPIES USED IN TREATING MYOCARDIAL INFARCTIONS

Drug	Common Dose	Advantages
Alteplase tPa (Activase)	100 mg over 1 hr	Improved survival, particularly in patients with anterior MI
Streptokinase (Streptase)	1.5 million U over 30–60 min	Much less expensive

ST segment elevation or a new left bundle branch block is required for treatment.

Nursing care of the patient with thrombolytic therapy centers around reducing potential episodes of bleeding. Only arterial punctures and venipunctures that are absolutely necessary should be performed. Finger oximetry should be employed, for example, rather than drawing blood gases to obtain a PaO_2 level. If venipuncture must be performed, extra time spent holding the site will be necessary to achieve hemostasis.

Assessment of the patient for signs of bleeding is important. Hypotension, tachycardia, or specific organ changes (i.e., reduced level of consciousness) are indicators of possible bleeding.

Reperfusion dysrhythmias are common. Bradycardias are frequently seen after infusion of thrombolytic agents. Ventricular tachycardias are also common.

Cardiac catheterization is performed as soon as possible, perhaps even during the acute MI episode. Angioplasty, athrectomy, or surgery (CABG) may be performed at this time.

Angioplasty

Angioplasty is the dilatation of a stenotic coronary artery through the insertion of a catheter into the coronary artery. Once the catheter is inserted, the stenotic area (identified by cardiac catheterization) is compressed by expanding a balloon on the end of the catheter. Angioplasty has the benefit of avoiding CABG while maintaining good results with expanding the stenotic area.

Several criteria for angioplasty must be met: (Table 6–4). One-vessel coronary artery disease, stable angina of less than 1 yr, no prior MI, lesion that is easy to reach (proximal) and discrete, and normal left ventricular function; a patient meeting these criteria is a candidate for CABG if necessary.

TABLE 6–4. CRITERIA FOR ANGIOPLASTY IN MYOCARDIAL INFARCTION PATIENTS

Clear Criteria
Cardiogenic shock, < 75 years old
Myocardial failure (e.g., Killip class III or IV)
Prior Q wave in another region of the heart
Patient is not a candidate for thrombolytic therapy

Uncertain Criteria
Clinical appearance of MI but not clear based on ECG
Patient presents > 6 hr after onset of symptoms
Prior CABG
Cardiogenic shock but age > 75 years

Nursing care of the patient with angioplasty includes care of the cardiac catheterization insertion site (bedrest and site compression for several hours) and observation for signs of reocclusion (dysrhythmias). If the stenosis recurs, chest pain or symptoms of decreased cardiac output may occur.

Intracoronary Stents

A technique which is increasing in popularity is the use of intracoronary stents. A stent is a device which holds open the coronary artery in a place where narrowing has occurred. Stents are continuing to evolve in design. In the most current design a balloon is used to inflate the stainless steel stent, which after the balloon is deflated stays in place (Fig. 6–5).

The most common problem following stent placement is the development of reocclusion. Anticoagulation is necessary following stent placement.

Athrectomy

A newer therapy is athrectomy, or the removal of the atherosclerotic plaque by excision. This technique is still developing, but essentially involves cutting the narrowed area after it has been identified from cardiac catheterization. While reocclusion still occurs,

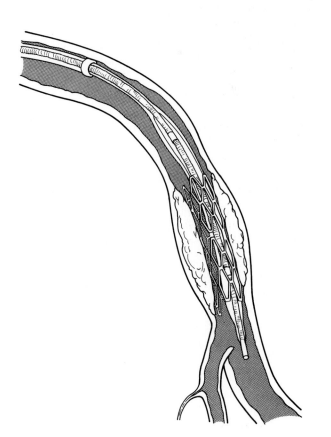

Figure 6–5. Stainless steel stent inflated by a balloon.

the technique has the potential for improving long-term patency of the coronary artery.

Medical Therapy

If cardiac support is necessary, dobutamine is the therapy of choice to improve inotropic (strength) properties of the heart. Dopamine is reserved for episodes of hypotension or at low doses (less than 5 μg/kg min) to improve renal blood flow. If medical support is not adequate, intra-aortic balloon pumping has been demonstrated to effectively increase hemodynamic performance.

Vasodilators, such as nitroglycerin or nitroprusside, may be cautiously employed in an attempt to reduce preload and afterload. Continuous hemodynamic monitoring is necessary to accurately manipulate many of the cardiac medications. Reduction in myocardial work is critical to avoiding episodes of congestive heart failure. Use of angiotensin converting enzyme (ACE) inhibitors (enalapril) has become a key aspect of post-MI treatment because of their ability to reduce afterload (systemic vascular resistance) without increasing cardiac output. Other therapies, such as beta blockers (labatelol), also may be used. However, beta blockers should be used with caution in patients who already have congestive heart failure. Beta blockers have negative inotropic (weakening) effects on the heart.

Continuous cardiac monitoring is used to provide for the early identification and intervention of dysrhythmias. If the patient survives the initial infarction and subsequently dies, death is usually due to a shock syndrome. Dysrhythmias of all types, including conduction disturbances, occur.

Oxygen therapy is usually started to ensure that sufficient oxygen content is available for myocardial needs. An intravenous line is started for use in emergency situations. Food, usually low in sodium, is given as tolerated. Many cardiac care units prohibit foods containing caffeine (a mild cardiac stimulant).

Hemodynamic monitoring must be continuous for early intervention in congestive heart failure, ventricular failure with pulmonary edema, and cardiogenic shock. Bedrest and emotional support of the patient are necessary for healing the injured myocardium. Use of platelet inhibitors to decrease clotting is part of standard therapy. Currently, low-

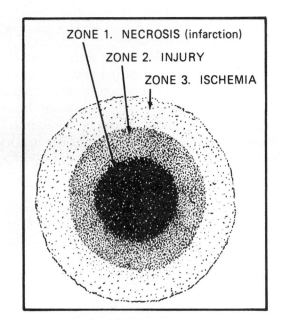

Figure 6–6. The development of scar tissue following myocardial infarction.

dose aspirin (325 mg) appears adequate to avoid early reocclusion.

Long-term immobility may result in venous pooling, with an increased risk of thromboembolism. Passive and active range-of-motion exercises and support hose help reduce this risk.

Less common but equally lethal complications of an MI include pericarditis, papillary muscle rupture, ventricular aneurysm, and ventricular rupture. Sudden death commonly occurs with the last three of these complications.

Recovery

Recovery begins as soon as myocardial injury and necrosis stop. Scar tissue develops (Fig. 6–6) at the necrotic area. This process takes 6 to 8 weeks to complete.

Emotional support of the patient and family is a key factor in recovery. Patients often feel that their active and productive lives are over. It is not uncommon to see the patient and family members going through the stages of grief following an MI. Education of the patient and family in ways of changing their life styles to eliminate alterable risk factors is an essential role of the nurse and helps the patient and family work through the emotional grieving process.

Conduction Blocks

FIRST-DEGREE BLOCK

Etiology

First-degree atrioventricular (AV) junctional block may be caused by arteriosclerotic heart disease (ASHD), acute myocardial infarction, AV node ischemia, and drugs that act at the AV node (e.g., digitalis). The AV node delays the progression of the impulse from the sinoatrial (SA) node for an abnormal length of time (Fig. 7–1).

Identifying Characteristics

The rate is normal. The rhythm is regular. P waves are normal. The PR interval is prolonged beyond 0.20 sec. The QRS complex is normal. Conduction is normal except for the prolonged delay at the AV node.

Risk

First-degree block is not a serious dysrhythmia itself. It may progress to a second-degree type I block and less commonly to a second-degree type II or third-degree block.

Treatment

If the PR interval is less than 0.25 sec and if it does not increase, no treatment may be required. The length of the PR interval is not as significant as the effect on stroke volume and heart rate. No treatment is indicated unless a bradycardia results.

Nursing Intervention

Document the dysrhythmia with a rhythm strip. Monitor the patient closely for progression to a slower heart rate or a worsening block. If progression develops, document with a rhythm strip and notify the physician immediately.

SECOND-DEGREE BLOCK—TYPE I AND TYPE II

The terms Mobitz I and Wenckebach (named after cardiac physiologists in the early twentieth century) are frequently used instead of type I. Mobitz II is also used in place of type II. These terms will not be used in this section, although it is helpful to remember that you may see them on the exam or in clinical practice.

Both type I and type II are AV junctional blocks. The AV node delays the progression of the SA node impulse for a longer than normal time. The characteristics, treatment, and prognosis for these two forms of second-degree AV block differ. The type I form of second-degree block will be considered first.

SECOND-DEGREE TYPE I

Etiology

Conduction arises normally from the SA node and progresses to the AV node. With each succeeding

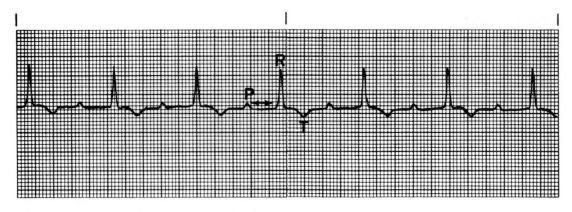

Figure 7–1. First-degree AV heart block.

impulse, it becomes more difficult for the AV node to conduct the impulse. Eventually, one impulse is not conducted and a QRS complex does not occur. The progression then begins again. Ischemia or injury to the AV node is the cause of this progression (Fig. 7–2).

Identifying Characteristics

The following are the key components of the second-degree type I heart block:

1. Progressive prolongation of the PR interval
2. Increment of conduction delay that is greatest between the first and second sinus beat in each cycle
3. Progressive decrease in succeeding increments of delay
4. Progressive shortening of the PR interval before each pause
5. Pause in the ventricular rhythm that is less than twice the PP interval or sinus cycle length

Risk

Second-degree type I is often a temporary block following an acute myocardial infarction. It may, however, progress to a complete (third-degree) block. For this reason, second-degree type I is considered a potentially dangerous dysrhythmia, although by itself it usually does not produce a clinical problem.

Treatment

Frequently, no treatment is indicated. If the ventricular rate is slow, atropine may increase AV conduction. Epinephrine may be used to increase the SA node rate and thus the overall rate. On occasion, an external pacemaker or temporary transvenous pacemaker may be inserted.

Nursing Intervention

Document the dysrhythmia with a rhythm strip. Monitor the patient, although this dysrhythmia is normally not clinically significant. If the ventricular

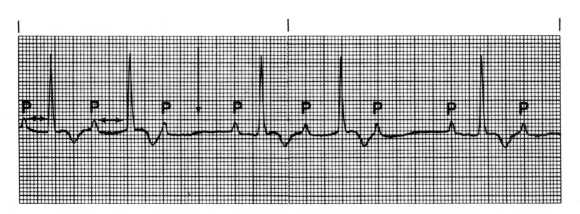

Figure 7–2. Second-degree AV block—type I (Wenckebach).

rate slows enough to produce symptoms, document it with a rhythm strip and notify the physician.

SECOND-DEGREE TYPE II

Etiology

An impulse originates in SA node and progresses normally to the AV node. Below the AV node in the common bundle or bundle branches, impulses are blocked on a regular basis with every second, third, or fourth impulse not being conducted. In this block, a QRS complex is regularly missing. More than one P wave is present for every QRS complex. This dysrhythmia is due to disease of the AV node, the AV junctional tissue, or the His-Purkinje system (Fig. 7–3).

Identifying Characteristics

Atrial rate may be normal. The ventricular rate is usually one-half or one-third of the atrial rate (referred to as 2:1 or 3:1 block). At times, the block rate may be even greater than 3:1. The ventricular rate depends on the frequency of the block. (In 4:1 block, there are four atrial beats to every one QRS complex.) The atrial rhythm is regular. Ventricular rhythm is regular or irregular, but slow. P waves are normal. The PR interval is constant. The QRS complex may be normal or widened. Conduction is normal in the atria and may be abnormal in the ventricles.

Risk

Type II block is unpredictable and may suddenly advance to complete heart block or ventricular standstill, especially common after inferior infarction. This is a dangerous warning dysrhythmia.

Treatment

If the ventricular response is slow, atropine or epinephrine may be tried. Because the condition is so unpredictable, a temporary pacemaker is often the treatment of choice. A permanent pacemaker is frequently necessary.

Nursing Intervention

Document the dysrhythmia with a rhythm strip. Determine the width of the QRS complex. The greater the width, the more dangerous the dysrhythmia. Monitor the patient closely for a widening of the QRS complex. The width of the QRS complex indicates the location in the conduction system of the block. The wider the complex, the lower the block is in the bundle branch system. Document the widening, if it occurs, with a rhythm strip, notify the physician immediately, and prepare for the insertion of a transvenous pacemaker or use of an external pacemaker. Assess the patient frequently for hemodynamic compromise if the ventricular response is slow (3:1 and 4:1 block).

While type I and II heart blocks are differentiated by the PR interval changes, another feature is important to bear in mind with these two types of dysrhythmias. Consider that the right coronary artery is responsible for feeding the AV node in 90% of the population. In addition, the right coronary artery supplies the inferior region of the left ventricle. Therefore, in inferior myocardial infarctions (MIs), a common dysrhythmia is AV block, specifically type I block. Clinically this is relevant since type I blocks may appear like II blocks (i.e., in 2:1 patterns). These 2:1 blocks generally are less dangerous, though, because the bundle branches remain intact. If a pacemaker is required, a temporary will usually suffice.

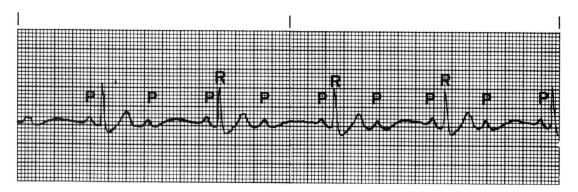

Figure 7–3. Second-degree AV block—type II.

Anterior MIs are different, however, in their effect on producing type II blocks. An anterior MI is usually the result of obstruction of the left anterior descending artery. This artery also feeds the left and right bundle branches. In the presence of an anterior MI, a type II block may also appear in a 2:1 pattern. This pattern is more dangerous with an anterior MI since the block is due to loss of ventricular conduction system, i.e., the left and/or right bundle system. Type II blocks in the presence of an anterior MI require more attention. Pacemakers for this dysrhythmia usually need to be permanent.

THIRD-DEGREE BLOCK—COMPLETE HEART BLOCK

Etiology

Ischemia or injury to the AV node, junctional tissue, or His-Purkinje tissue is the cause of complete heart block. The ischemia may be secondary to ASHD, acute MI, drug use (e.g., digitalis toxicity), systemic disease, or electrolyte imbalances (especially in renal patients) (Fig. 7–4).

Identifying Characteristics

Atrial rates are faster than ventricular rates. P waves are not conducted. The ventricular rate is 30 to 40 (unless there is a junctional escape mechanism). The rhythm is regular for both the atria and the ventricles even though they are depolarizing completely independently of each other. P waves are normal and not associated with a QRS complex. The PR interval is not constant. QRS complexes are close to normal if they arise near the AV node. The QRS complex may be wide and bizarre if the impulse arises from the ventricles. There is no AV conduction. The atrial

pacemaker controls the atria, and the ventricular pacemaker controls the ventricles.

Risk

The main danger of third-degree heart block is the potential bradycardia producing a decrease in cardiac output, leading to hypotension and myocardial ischemia. Third-degree heart block is a potentially lethal dysrhythmia.

Treatment

Immediate pacemaker insertion is the treatment of choice. A temporary pacemaker may be tried initially until the presence of the block has been determined to be permanent. Complete heart block may be temporary after MI, and pacing should be available for several days after the return of a normal sinus rhythm.

Nursing Intervention

Document the dysrhythmia with a rhythm strip and notify the physician immediately. Monitor the patient for signs of ventricular failure and hypotension. Hemodynamic status is compromised by the slow ventricular rate, and circulatory collapse is not uncommon.

ATRIOVENTRICULAR DISSOCIATION

Many conditions can be termed AV dissociation. Ventricular tachycardia and conduction defects where the atrial and ventricular rhythms do not match can all be examples of AV dissociation. Some clinicians make the mistake of using the term third-degree block synonymously with AV dissociation;

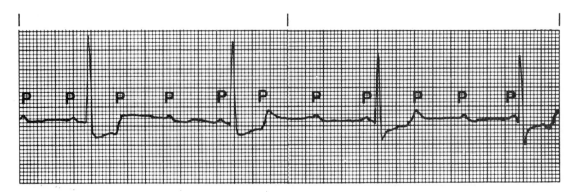

Figure 7–4. Third-degree (complete) AV block.

however, third-degree block is only one form of AV dissociation.

Etiology

The many causes of AV dissociation include anesthesia, medications, infections, acute MI, and ischemic heart disease (Fig. 7–5).

Identifying Characteristics

The PR interval is inconsistent since the atrial and ventricular pacemakers are independent of each other. The P wave, usually normal in form, may vary slightly in measurements. The P wave may fall immediately before, during, or after a QRS complex during the absolute refractory period of the ventricles (the period in which they cannot depolarize). The QRS complex may be normal or abnormal, depending on whether the ventricular pacemaker is at or below the bundle of His.

Risk

Atrioventricular dissociation by itself is significant since atrial and ventricular contractions are not in synchrony. The loss of synchrony can produce a substantial reduction in cardiac output. However, rather than treat AV dissociation, the underlying rhythm producing AV dissociation should be addressed.

Treatment

Treatment is dependent on the underlying rhythm and the effect on hemodynamics. Treatments range from pacemakers for bradycardias to antidysrhythmics for ventricular tachycardia.

Nursing Intervention

Monitor the patient closely for signs of cardiac decompensation and progression of the dysrhythmia. Document the dysrhythmia with a rhythm strip and notify the physician.

BUNDLE BRANCH BLOCKS
EDITORS' NOTE

The CCRN exam can have two to four questions on cardiac conduction defects. This section provides an overview of reading these conduction problems.

For more information on bundle branch blocks, see the complete review in Chapter 3.

Bundle branch blocks are also termed intraventricular conduction defects. There may be a right or left bundle branch block. In addition, the left bundle has two divisions, referred to as fascicles. These fascicles may also become blocked. Obstructions of the fascicles are termed hemiblocks. There may be a left anterior hemiblock of the anterior fascicle of the left bundle branch or there may be a left posterior hemiblock of the posterior fascicle of the left bundle branch. Trifascicular blocks involve both left bundle fascicles and the right bundle branch. Bifascicular blocks usually involve the right bundle branch and one fascicle of the left bundle branch, or both fascicles of the left branch. Bundle branch blocks *cannot* be diagnosed by a rhythm strip, only suspected. A 12-lead ECG is essential.

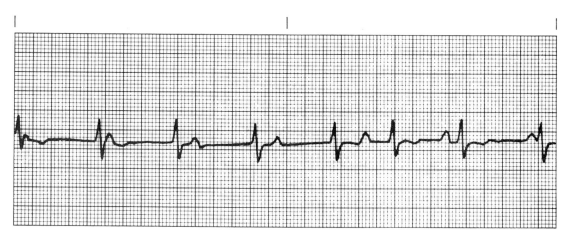

Figure 7–5. One type of AV dissociation.

Criteria for diagnosing conduction defects are listed in Table 7–1. Identification of conduction defects is useful for several reasons, ranging from identifying areas of disease in the heart to assessing the significance of injury patterns. In addition, interpretation of conduction defects, particularly right bundle branch blocks, is helpful in differentiating atrial premature contractions with aberrant conduction from PVCs.

Etiology

Three different factors may cause a bundle branch block. First, an acute MI may cause ischemia in the intraventricular conduction system. Second, chronic degeneration with fibrous scarring may permanently block the bundle branches. Third, bundle branch blocks may be congenital or rate dependent (i.e., they appear only at certain heart rates).

Identifying Characteristics

Bundle branch blocks cannot be diagnosed by a rhythm strip. Rate is usually normal, although it may vary if the bundle branch block varies. Rhythm is regular. P waves may be normal. The PR interval is normal. The QRS complex is wide (greater than 0.12 sec) and may be notched, depending upon the lead viewed.

Risk

The development of bundle branch blocks indicates marked ischemia of the intraventricular conduction system, and bundle branch blocks are potentially more dangerous than AV blocks since these blocks are subjunctional. The involvement of more than

one fascicle often progresses to complete heart block. In these instances, the prognosis is poor.

Treatment

It is not uncommon for the bundle branch block to cause no symptoms. Because of the lack of symptoms, most bundle branch blocks require no direct treatment. Many patients tolerate conduction defects such as bundle branch blocks for long periods of time without developing any problems. The potential danger of the bundle branch block, however, is that it can deteriorate into a more severe obstruction such as complete heart block. In this case, the treatment is focused on improving the heart rate, as with atropine or a pacemaker.

Nursing Intervention

The primary consideration is to identify the conduction defect and document the type of block. Notify the physician if the block is new. Monitor the rhythm and be aware of the potential for a bradycardia, such as complete heart block, to develop.

PACEMAKERS

There are many pathologic states that may be most efficiently treated by the use of an artificial pacemaker. Pacemakers may be particularly useful in the treatment of symptomatic bradycardias that have not responded to atropine or epinephrine.

Definition

A pacemaker is a system consisting of a lead and a pulse generator. The generator is capable of producing repeated, short (3–5 msec), and rhythmic bursts of electric current for a prolonged period of time. The bursts of electric current are of sufficient magnitude to initiate depolarization of the heart.

Modes of Pacing

There are two modes of pacing. Temporary pacing is one mode used mainly to manage emergencies such as acute heart block and cardiac arrest. Two types of temporary pacemakers exist: transvenous or transthoracic and transcutaneous (external). In the transvenous or transthoracic mode, the lead is inserted into the right atrium or ventricle. The pulse generator is external. Insertion routes include the

TABLE 7–1. CRITERIA FOR VENTRICULAR CONDUCTION DEFECTS

Condition	Lead	QRS Appearance
Right bundle branch block	V$_1$ (MCL$_1$)	rSR′
	I & V$_6$	Deep S wave
Left bundle branch block	I & V$_6$	Wide QRS (>0.12)
	I & V$_6$	Notched QRS
	V$_1$	QS wave
Anterior hemiblock	I, avF	Left axis > 30 degrees
	I, avL	Initial Q wave
	II, III, avF	Small R wave, deep S wave
Posterior hemiblock	I	Large S wave Right axis
	I, avL	Initial R wave
	II, III, avF	Large R wave

transvenous (brachial via cutdown), subclavian, femoral, or jugular (via percutaneous entry), post-surgery (endocardial), and transthoracic (needle through chest into heart muscle). The power supply for temporary pacing is external batteries (the pulse generator). For a specific insertion procedure, the nurse is referred to his or her institution policy.

Transcutaneous cardiac pacing has gained increasing acceptance in recent years. The principle of transcutaneous pacing is based on sending direct current transcutaneously between electrodes placed on the skin. The advantages of transcutaneous pacing are the ease of use (it can be applied in a matter of minutes) and the fact that no invasive equipment is necessary. The benefit of pacing is obtained through this method without the difficulty of inserting the transvenous or transthoracic pacing mode.

In the transcutaneous mode of pacing, the nurse must be aware of the potential for some discomfort for the patient due to the electrical stimulation. The electrical stimulation will cause superficial, as well as cardiac, muscle contraction. Some conscious patients, particularly if the milliampere setting is high, may complain of pain upon stimulation. Sedatives or analgesics may be required.

Permanent pacing with a fully implantable system is a second mode of pacing the heart. The pulse generator is implanted into the patient. The pulse generator contains the circuit for the specific pacing mode selected and a battery that provides energy to the circuit. The components are encased in a nonconductive plastic material that does not react with body tissue.

Indications for Pacing

The major indication for pacing is the development of second-degree type II or third-degree heart block. Pacemakers can be used for any bradycardia that is producing hypotension or signs of reduced cardiac output.

Chronic heart block of varied degrees may be treated by pacing if the patient has syncopal episodes, congestive heart failure, convulsions, or evidence of cerebral dysfunction.

Intermittent complete heart block (third degree) is often treated with a pacemaker. Usually, there is evidence of block in one or two of the three bundle branches (fascicles). Thus, these patients rely solely on the third fascicle, which may become dysfunctional at any time.

Complete heart block that develops in conjunction with an acute MI may be an indication for pacing.

If the infarction is anterior, the involved artery is usually the left anterior descending. This results in ischemia or necrosis of part of the ventricular septum, with damage to the intraventricular conduction system below the His bundle. These patients frequently die despite the insertion of a pacemaker because of the extent of myocardial damage. If the infarction is posterior or inferior, the artery involved is usually the right coronary (90% of the time) or the circumflex (10% of the time). The area of damage is the AV node area. Types I and II may be indications for pacing. Type I may progress into a type II (2:1) or higher block. Type II, due to the block occurring below the AV node, often progresses into third-degree heart block. A block that develops postinfarction is usually transient and responds to atropine or a brief period of time with a temporary pacemaker.

Conduction defects may occur after a cardiac surgical procedure. For this reason, most cardiac surgeries (e.g., coronary artery bypass grafting) have pacing wires attached to the epicardium for postoperative management. Some centers also use a pacing port through a pulmonary artery catherer.

Pacemakers may be used in other rhythm disturbances if bradycardia is a component of the dysrhythmia. Sick sinus syndrome indicates dysfunction of the SA node. This may occur as sinus bradycardia, sinus arrest, and/or brady-tachy syndromes.

Pacemakers may also be used to treat tachydysrhythmias, such as atrial or ventricular tachycardia. In these rhythmias, the pacemaker rate is increased to a level higher than the tachycardia. Once the pacemaker is controlling the rate, the rate is slowed to a more acceptable level.

Pacemakers may be used as a diagnostic aid to evaluate SA node function and AV node function. They may be used to eliminate multiple ectopic foci by overriding the rate of the foci, or they may be used to abolish reentry phenomena by delivering a premature stimulus that breaks the reentry pattern.

Types of Pacing Modes

Several types of pacing modes exist. These are categorized according to the Inter-Society Commission on Heart Disease (ICHD) nomenclature in Table 7–2. There are two codes, a simplified three-letter and more comprehensive five-letter code. Table 7–2 contains the five-letter code. As a rule, the CCRN exam requires one to remember only the simpler three-letter code.

The major concept to remember is that the pacemaker electrically paces a cardiac chamber (the

TABLE 7–2. FIVE-POSITION PACEMAKER CODE (ICHD)

I. Chamber Paced	II. Chamber Sensed	III. Mode of Response	IV. Programmability	V. Tachyrhythmia Functions
V = Ventricle		I = Inhibited	P = Programmable rate and/or output	B = Burst
A = Atrium		T = Triggered		N = Normal rate completion
D = Atrium and ventricle		D = Atrial triggered and ventricular inhibited	M = Multiprogrammability	S = Scanning
O = None			O = None	E = External
		O = None	C = Programmable with telemetry	

first letter), senses an electrical impulse in a cardiac chamber (the second letter), and discharges the impulse in either a triggered or inhibited manner (the third letter). In critical care, the inhibited manner is almost always used.

If a patient had a transvenous pacemaker inserted that would pace and sense only in the ventricle, the ICHD description would be a VVI. If the pacemaker paced both atrium and ventricle, but sensed only in the ventricle, then the pacemaker would be a DVI (AV sequential) pacemaker.

Nursing Care

The patient with a temporary pacemaker will need documentation as to the effectiveness of rhythm capture and sensing. The electrical signal indicating that a pacemaker impulse has occurred should be evident only immediately prior to capturing a paced beat (Fig. 7–6). If a pacemaker signal is present and the heart is not in a refractory mode, a captured beat should follow. If no beat occurs, this would be called failure to capture (Fig. 7–7). Failure to sense would be a paced

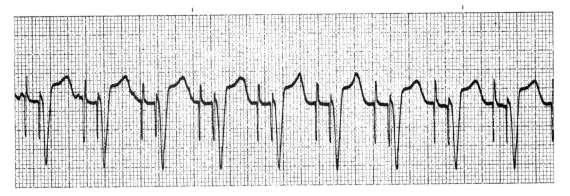

Figure 7–6. Normal pacemaker (DVI) electrical pattern.

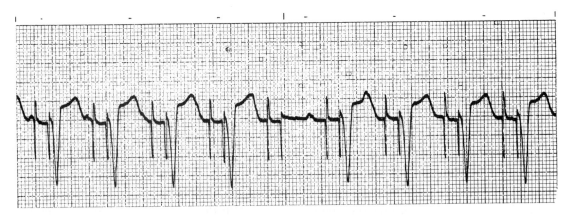

Figure 7–7. Failure of pacemaker to capture.

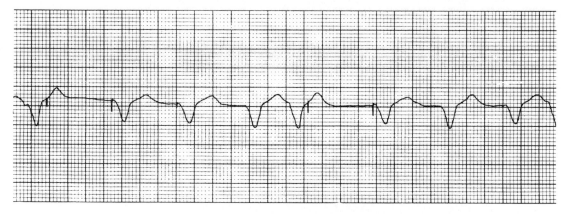

Figure 7–8. Failure of pacemaker to sense.

beat or pacemaker artifact occurring too soon after a spontaneous beat. The spontaneous beat should inhibit the next paced impulse; if it does not, failure to sense is present (Fig. 7–8). Notify the physician if either of these conditions occurs more than once.

Care of the pacemaker insertion site is the same as for any central intravenous catheter. Careful explanation of the purpose and duration of the pacemaker to the patient is important in order to avoid unnecessary anxiety.

Congestive Heart Failure, Pulmonary Edema, and Hypertensive Crisis

EDITORS' NOTE

The assessment of abnormal hemodynamics, particularly in regard to left and right ventricular failure, is a common topic for questions in the CCRN exam. This chapter reviews the major concepts normally employed in the assessment, as well as diagnosis and interventions associated with ventricular dysfunction. Expect several questions on the CCRN exam from this content area.

All forms of myocardial failure are based upon a disturbance in the relation BP = CO × SVR, where BP is blood pressure, CO is cardiac output, and SVR is systemic vascular resistance. Specifically, the problem lies in a disturbance of the cardiac output, although the SVR can affect the output. When studying the concept of myocardial failure, keep in mind the factors that regulate cardiac output, i.e., preload, afterload, and contractility. All myocardial failure can be assessed and treated through these three components. While ventricular failure can be assessed by noting each component of cardiac output, each ventricle is assessed slightly differently. For example, preload of the left ventricle is partially assessed by the pulmonary capillary wedge pressure (PCWP), while preload of the right ventricle is assessed by the central venous pressure (CVP). Other factors used to differentiate left and right ventricular influences are listed in Table 8–1.

The specific pressures frequently used in the assessment of ventricular preload are listed in Table 8–2. While these guidelines are general examples, the CCRN exam is likely to utilize values such as these when clinical scenarios are provided in situations describing ventricular failure. More sophisticated measures to estimate cardiac performance, such as radionucleotide ventriculography and echocardiography, are available. However, the basic guidelines listed in Tables 8–1 and 8–2 are fundamental to assessing cardiac performance in most clinical practice settings. Because of the common application of these concepts, it is helpful to understand their role in clinical assessment.

CONGESTIVE HEART FAILURE

Congestive heart failure (CHF) is the inability of the heart to pump blood through the systemic circulation in an amount sufficient to meet the body's needs. CHF normally refers to biventricular failure, although it is important to understand that each ventricle can fail independently of the other. Left ventricular (LV) failure is a common precursor to right ventricular (RV) failure and can precede RV dysfunction. RV failure is frequently associated with lung disease or dysfunction, or it may be the result of ischemia of the right-sided coronary circulation. RV failure will produce LV hypovolemia by failing to move blood through the lungs.

Chronic heart failure is the gradual inability of the heart to pump sufficient blood to meet the body's demands. Chronic heart failure can become acute without an obvious cause or may be precipitated by an acute ischemic cardiac event. The presence of RV failure in the face of LV failure usually indicates a more advanced disease state and worse prognosis.

TABLE 8–1. METHODS TO ASSESS LEFT AND RIGHT VENTRICULAR PERFORMANCE

Parameter	Right Ventricle	Left Ventricle
Preload	CVP	PCWP
Afterload	PVR	SVR
Contractility	Stroke volume	Stroke volume

CVP, central venous pressure; PCWP, pulmonary capillary wedge pressure; PVR, pulmonary vascular resistance; SVR, systemic vascular resistance.

Etiology

Unless specified otherwise, assume that the term congestive heart failure implies biventricular failure. On the CCRN exam, if only one ventricle is involved, the term will not likely be employed. Signs and symptoms of CHF result from both ventricles failing. However, even though signs and symptoms of CHF are biventricular in nature, the origin of the failure is usually the left ventricle. Factors commonly influencing the development of LV dysfunction and eventually causing CHF are listed in Table 8–3.

Left ventricular pump failure usually occurs before RV pump failure. The LV myocardium weakens to the extent that it cannot eject blood in the normal amount. This reduces the cardiac output secondary to a reduction in stroke volume. Before stroke volume decreases, however, two changes in myocardial function may take place. First, if the failure is slow, the left ventricle enlarges in both capacity (measured by end diastolic volume [EDV]) and muscle size. Second, the ability of the heart to eject blood (measured by the ejection fraction [EF]) is reduced but offset by the increased EDV.

Normally, about 70% of the EDV is ejected with each beat. The amount of blood ejected with each beat is the stroke volume. The amount of blood ejected (stroke volume [SV]) in comparison with the EDV is termed the ejection fraction (SV/EDV = EF). As the contractile ability of the heart worsens, the ejection fraction falls. As the ejection fraction levels

TABLE 8–2. USE OF THE PULMONARY CAPILLARY WEDGE PRESSURE (PCWP) AND CENTRAL VENOUS PRESSURE (CVP)

Value	SI	Condition Indicated
PCWP		
<8	<25	Hypovolemia
8–12	25–45	Normal
12–18	<35	Beginning failure or fluid overload
>18	<25	LV failure
CVP		
0–5	<35	Normal or hypovolemia
5–10	25–45	Beginning failure or fluid overload
>10	<25	RV failure

TABLE 8–3. CAUSES OF CONGESTIVE HEART FAILURE

Systemic hypertension
Coronary artery disease
  Myocardial infarction
  Angina
Aortic stenosis
Mitral regurgitation
Cardiomyopathy
Atrial and ventricular tachydysrhythmias

decrease to below 40%, exercise limitations become evident and progress to interfere with activities of daily living.

If the left ventricle cannot pump all the blood it receives from the atrium, a buildup of blood and pressure occurs in the left atrium. As the pressure increases in the left atrium, it becomes more difficult for blood to enter the atrium from the pulmonary veins. As the blood in the pulmonary veins becomes unable to flow into the left atrium, blood backs up in the lung vessels. When pressure in the pulmonary capillaries exceeds 18 to 25 mm Hg, fluid from the capillaries leaks into the interstitial spaces. Once this leaking of fluid into the pulmonary interstitial space exceeds the ability of the pulmonary lymphatics to drain the fluid, pulmonary edema may develop.

Systolic Dysfunction

Systolic dysfunction is characterized by a decrease in muscle strength. Forward blood flow falls, producing systemic hypoperfusion. Stroke volume and the ejection fraction also fall.

Systolic dysfunction also causes pulmonary congestion, but is more dangerous because of the potential to decrease forward blood flow.

Diastolic Dysfunction

Diastolic dysfunction is the inability of the ventricle to fully relax. The result is increasing pressure and volume in the ventricle. This produces pulmonary congestion as pressures "back up" the pulmonary veins.

Since the lung vasculature is distensible, it can accept a moderate amount of increased pressure and volume. However, without intervention, the pressure in the pulmonary capillaries increases to the point that the right ventricle cannot eject its blood into the lungs for oxygenation. As the backflow pressure increases, the right ventricle fails and the CVP increases. Then blood from the right atrium cannot drain completely, and consequently the right atrium cannot accommodate all of the blood entering from the venae cavae. Since venous blood flow to the heart is impeded, venous pooling and eventual organ congestion with venous blood occur.

Left Versus Right Heart Failure

Right heart failure is most commonly caused by left heart failure and then by all the factors that cause left heart failure. Right heart failure may also be caused by isolated right coronary ischemia, pulmonary emboli, essential pulmonary hypertension, and chronic obstructive pulmonary disease.

Left heart failure alone can occur from the same factors that cause CHF. Since left heart failure occurs before right heart failure in these cases, initial symptoms of left heart failure differ from those of CHF. Because of the potential for left heart before right heart failure, measures that formerly were used to estimate left heart function by right-sided measures (such as CVP) have been demonstrated to be inaccurate.

Clinical Presentation

Symptoms of left and right heart failure are presented in Table 8–4.

Complications

The major complications of heart failure are the progression of failure and loss of cardiac output and oxygen delivery. In addition, progression of cardiac failure can lead to the development of lethal dysrhythmias. It is also important to keep in mind that therapies to treat heart failure may cause drug toxicity (including oxygen toxicity) and fluid and electrolyte imbalances.

Treatment and Nursing Intervention

The goal of treating CHF is to improve ventricular function and to prevent the progression to right heart failure. Three methods of treatment exist, based on the factors regulating stroke volume.

TABLE 8–4. SYMPTOMS OF LEFT AND RIGHT VENTRICULAR FAILURE

Left Ventricle	Right Ventricle
Orthopnea	Distended neck veins
Dyspnea of exertion	Dependent edema
Crackles	Hepatic engorgement
Low $Pao_2/Sao_2/Spo_2$	Hepatojugular reflux
S_3, S_4	
Systolic murmur	

1. Improve contractility of the ventricle. This is attempted by drug therapy with positive inotropic agents such as dobutamine. Within the limits of Starling's law, this method of treatment is very effective. Only three inotropes are commonly used in acute clinical settings: dobutamine, dopamine, and amrinone. Indications for use of these inotropes are centered around low cardiac indices (less than 2.2 $L/min/m^2$) and high PCWP (over 18 mm Hg). In theory, these agents are the ideal treatment choice because of their ability to directly improve stroke volume, ejection fraction, and cardiac output. Unfortunately, no consistently effective oral inotrope has been demonstrated to be effective. Digitalis preparations, such as digoxin, have been used in the chronic control of CHF. Its role in acute CHF is less clear.

   Part of the reason for the less than optimal effectiveness of oral inotropes may involve a concept called down regulation. Down regulation refers to the lack of responsiveness of cardiac muscle to sympathetic stimulation. In chronic heart failure, sympathetic stimulation has been occurring for a long time. This chronic stimulation leads eventually to failure of the cardiac muscle to respond to further stimulation. Because of the failure of long-term oral inotropes in the presence of CHF, the current therapy emphasizes manipulation of preload and afterload to improve contractility.

2. Decrease afterload. Afterload is the resistance of the blood, valves, and blood vessels that the left ventricle must overcome to eject blood. Decreasing any of these factors will decrease afterload. Reduction in afterload (estimated by the SVR) eases the work of the left ventricle. Reduced work may allow for improved contractility, thereby increasing stroke volume and cardiac output. Afterload agents include vasodilators of several different pharmacological types, including nitroprusside, angiotensin-converting enzyme inhibitors (captopril and enalapril), calcium channel blockers (nifedipine and nicardipine), and many other agents.

3. Decrease preload. If one can lower the volume of blood entering the left atrium, the stress on the left ventricle is reduced.

Diuretic therapy (e.g., furosemide and thi-azides), venodilators (nitroglycerin), and fluid and sodium restrictions are examples of treatment of preload.

Close monitoring of the patient and his or her response to these treatments is very important in early detection of a deteriorating state requiring more aggressive therapy.

High-Output Failure

Some conditions are associated with high cardiac output. When associated with symptoms of CHF, these conditions are called high-output failure. Table 8–5 lists conditions commonly associated with high-output failure. Treatment of high-output failure is based on relieving the underlying condition, such as excess catecholamines and thyroid dysfunction.

PULMONARY EDEMA

Pulmonary edema is the most serious progression of CHF. Pulmonary edema may occur when pressure in the pulmonary vasculature exceeds 18–25 mm Hg. This results in extravasation of fluid from pulmonary capillaries into interstitial tissue and intra-alveolar spaces.

Etiology

Acute pulmonary edema is usually the result of fail-ure although noncardiac forms of pulmonary edema (e.g., adult respiratory distress syndrome) exist. Symptoms of CHF are exacerbated in pulmonary edema. Dyspnea and orthopnea become markedly pronounced; crackles may be heard throughout the lungs and be accompanied by blood-tinged, frothy sputum. Hypoxemia will worsen as lung function deteriorates from the increased fluid. Restlessness and anxiety precede changing level of consciousness as cerebral oxygenation falls.

Radiographic Changes

Changes due to pulmonary edema occur on roentgenograms in stages equal to the progression and/or severity of the pulmonary edema. The first

TABLE 8–5. CAUSES OF HIGH CARDIAC OUTPUT FAILURE

Hyperthyroidism	Thiamine deficiency
Severe anemia	Paget's disease
Arteriovenous fistula	

change is an enlargement of the pulmonary veins. As interstitial edema occurs, the vessels become poorly outlined and foggy. This is frequently referred to as hilar haze. As intra-alveolar edema develops, the roentgenogram shows a density in the inner middle zone. This gives the appearance of a "bat wing" or "butterfly" at the hilum.

Treatment and Nursing Intervention

The treatment for pulmonary edema is the same as for CHF, with a few exceptions. The goal of therapy is to resolve the pulmonary edema by improving cardiac function, which will improve renal function while sup-porting respiratory needs. The goal is to decrease pre-load, decrease afterload, and increase contractility.

Preload is reduced by diuretic therapy. Furosemide (Lasix) and ethacrynic acid are potent, fast-acting diuretics that may be used. Pulmonary edema responds well to Lasix, possibly because of its vasodilatory effect as much as its diuretic action. Morphine sulfate intravenously is used to both relieve anxiety and cause vasodilation to occur, resulting in a reduced afterload.

Cardiac function is immediately supported with dobutamine. If hypotension exists, mid-dose dopamine may be given. If no response from dobut-amine is seen, amrinone can be given.

Normally, hypoxemia is aggressively treated. Hypoxemia can be treated by increasing the fraction of inspired oxygen (FIO_2). Oxygen therapy is usually administered by a high-flow face mask system, with oxygen concentrations from 40 to 100% sometimes required. The addition of continuous positive airway pressure or intubation and implementation of posi-tive end expiratory pressure may be necessary for patients whose hypoxemia (PaO_2 levels below 60 mm Hg) does not respond to oxygen therapy. However, when positive pressure is applied, care must be taken to avoid a decrease in cardiac output.

Nursing intervention focuses on monitoring sig-nificant changes in preload, afterload, and contrac-tility. If the preload (PCWP) changes, the nurse must observe whether other parameters (e.g., stroke vol-ume and cardiac output) have changed. Trends in data analysis are more important than absolute num-bers. Monitoring treatments over several readings as opposed to a single data point is very important for accurately assessing clinical conditions.

Emotional support of the patient with pul-monary edema is made difficult by the patient's fear of shortness of breath. It is important to decrease this fear concurrently with providing treatment.

HYPERTENSIVE CRISIS

Hypertension is not a disease but rather a symptom of a disease. The "normal" blood pressure range is 110/60 to 140/80 mm Hg. Hypertension is considered present if systolic pressure is 140 mm Hg or higher (in the adult) and/or if the diastolic pressure is greater than 90 mm Hg.

Primary hypertension (idiopathic, or of unknown cause) is common in the general population, with up to 30% of the population being affected. Hypertensive crises, however, occur only in a small percentage of the hypertensive population.

Mean arterial pressure (MAP) is routinely lower in normal populations (MAP of between 60 and 120 mm Hg) than in chronic hypertensive patients (MAP commonly between 120 and 160). The fact that hypertensive patients have higher mean pressures is important when therapeutic end points are identified. The chronic hypertensive patient may tolerate a higher MAP, and rapid reduction to normal levels is generally not necessary.

The severity of the hypertensive disturbance can be identified along the guidelines of the Joint National Committee on Detection, Evaluation and Treatment of High Blood Pressure, published in 1992. Emergencies are blood pressure levels that need treatment within 1 hr; urgencies are blood pressure levels that need treatment within 1 day. Characteristics of emergencies are listed in Table 8–6.

Etiology

Hypertension may be classified by etiology.

1. Unknown origin accounts for 90% of all cases of hypertension identified. This is termed essential hypertension.
2. Adrenal origin results from a tumor (pheochromocytoma) secreting epinephrine and norepinephrine, Cushing's disease, or a brain tumor.
3. Renal origin is due either to an interruption of blood supply or to a disease state of the kidney itself (e.g., pyelonephritis).
4. Cardiovascular hypertension can either be in response to CHF or myocardial ischemia or act as their cause. Postoperative hypertension is common, particularly early in CABG recovery. The postoperative hypertension is probably due to excess catecholamine release.
5. The origin of obstetric hypertension is unclear, but the condition usually presents in the second trimester of pregnancy.

TABLE 8–6. CHARACTERISTICS OF EMERGENCY HYPERTENSION

Diastolic blood pressure >120 mm Hg
Presence of one of the following:
    Acute aortic dissection
    LV failure with or without pulmonary edema
    Myocardial ischemia
    Acute renal failure
    Cerebrovascular or subarachnoid bleed
    Hypertensive encephalopathy
    Head injuries
    Grade 3–4 Keith-Wagener-Barker retinopathy
    Toxemia of pregnancy
    Burns
    Medication interaction
    Pheochromocytoma crisis

6. Medications that cause vasoconstriction.
7. Lack of compliance with medical therapy in "known" hypertension or inadequate treatment in "known" hypertension. Also, certain drugs may cause hypertension.

Clinical Presentation

The most common symptom is severe headache accompanied by nausea, vomiting, restlessness, and mental confusion, which may rapidly advance to coma and/or convulsions. Signs of a specific organ injury may be present. For example, myocardial ischemia, cerebral vascular accident, hematuria, or retinopathy may become evident. Sudden elevations in blood pressure are more likely than gradual elevations to present with symptoms.

Treatment

Treatment of hypertensive crisis centers around reduction of blood pressure to safe levels without producing a subsequent hypotension. Remember, hypotensive symptoms can appear at higher than

TABLE 8–7. MEDICATIONS TO TREAT HYPERTENSIVE CRISIS

Most Common	Less Common	Chronic
Nitroprusside (Nipride)	Trimethaphan (Arfonad)	Clonidine
Esmolol (Brevibloc)	Diazoxide (Hyperstat)	Propanolol
Labetalol	Hydrazaline (Apresoline)	Captopril (Capoten)
Nifedipine (Procardia)	Phentoloamine (Regitine)	Prazosin (Minipress)
Nitroglycerin		Hydralazine
		Nicardipine
		Enalapril

expected pressures in the patient with chronic hypertension. Gradual reduction of the MAP to below 85 is generally safe. Therapeutic modalities to achieve the MAP reduction generally initially involve a rapidly acting agent, with conversion to an oral agent as soon as possible. A diuretic is frequently added to counter potential water and sodium disturbances resulting from normal renal compensatory mechanisms of the hypertension. Examples of rapidly acting and oral maintenance agents are listed in Table 8–7.

Cardiogenic Shock

EDITORS' NOTE

Expect a few questions addressing the assessment and treatment of cardiogenic shock. Understandably, hypovolemic monitoring will substantially assist in answering these questions.

ETIOLOGY

Cardiogenic shock produces the same cellular disruption of oxygen as does hypovolemic shock but with different causes. In cardiogenic shock, mortality is frequently greater than 80%. As with hypovolemic shock, mean arterial pressure (MAP) is less than 60 mm Hg, the cardiac index is less than 1.8, and tissue oxygenation parameters, like the SaO_2 level, are abnormal. Preload is elevated, characterized by a pulmonary capillary wedge pressure (PCWP) of greater than 18–25 mm Hg. As the left ventricle is unable to maintain forward flow of blood, pressure builds in the ventricle, causing an increased left ventricular (LV) end diastolic pressure (preload). Two primary manifestations of the reduced cardiac output are seen. The most dangerous manifestation is the development of systemic hypotension. In addition, pulmonary congestion secondary to the increased preload will occur, with a resulting increase in the intrapulmonary shunt (decrease in arterial oxygen pressure, PaO_2, and saturation, SaO_2, levels).

COMPENSATION MECHANISMS

Cardiogenic shock produces compensation mechanisms similar to those for hypovolemic shock. In an attempt to maintain tissue perfusion, several compensation mechanisms are activated. Two key compensation mechanisms for shock are as follows:

1. Sympathetic stimulation. Release of epinephrine acts to increase heart rate, improve contractility, and improve impulse transmission. Epinephrine has a mild vasoconstrictive effect as well. Norepinephrine, which has a strong vasoconstrictive effect, is released, with a resultant mild increase in heart rate, strength, and impulse transmission. The increased contractility and heart rate serve to increase the cardiac output. The increased vasoconstriction acts to maintain perfusion pressures and improve core organ blood flow.
2. Decrease of renal perfusion. Decreased renal perfusion activates the renin-angiotensin system, promoting sodium and water retention. This mechanism acts to increase an already normal or elevated total vascular volume compartment.

IDENTIFYING CHARACTERISTICS

The patient in cardiogenic shock will present with the symptoms listed in Table 9–1. In addition, the patient may present with hyperventilation brought on in an attempt to compensate for a lactic acidosis. The nurse should attempt to identify any potential risk factors to aid in identifying the types of shock involved.

TREATMENT

In a patient who presents with cardiogenic shock, myocardial function must be improved as rapidly as

TABLE 9-1. SYMPTOMS OF HYPOVOLEMIC AND CARDIOGENIC SHOCK

Symptoms	Hypovolemic	Cardiogenic
Common		
Blood pressure	Low	Low
Pulse	Tachycardia	Tachycardia
Urine output	Low (<0.5 ml/kg)	Low
Level of consciousness	Altered	Altered
Skin	Cool, clammy	Cool, clammy
Pulse quality	Weak	Weak
Differentiating		
Pao_2	Normal	Low
Sao_2	Normal	Low
Cyanosis	Absent	May be present
a/A ratio	Normal	Low
PCWP	Low (<10)	High (>18)
Orthopnea	Minimal	Present
Crackles	Minimal	Present
Dependent edema	Absent	Present

possible. Much of the current treatment centers on pharmacological or mechanical support of the heart.

Pharmacological Treatment

Improving Cardiac Output—Contractility
Improvement in cardiac output is most often achieved with the use of dobutamine, although amrinone and mid-dose dopamine may also be used.

Improving Cardiac Output—Preload Reduction
Diuretics and vasodilators (nitroglycerin, diltiazem) may be employed. The use of a pulmonary artery catheter may facilitate assessment of the effectiveness of these agents. The goal of preload reduction is to reduce preload and improve myocardial contractility while reducing pulmonary congestion.

Improving Blood Pressure
In the patient with severe hypotension, vasoconstrictors such as norepinephrine, phenylephrine, or dopamine may be employed. Use of these drugs is not without risk because of the increased myocardial oxygen consumption associated with their vasoconstrictive properties, but if the improvement in blood pressure is accomplished, an improved myocardial blood flow may offset the increased myocardial oxygen consumption. However, an improved blood pressure does not always cause an improved blood flow. Use of oxygenation parameters, such as venous oxygen saturation (SvO_2) values and lactate levels, will help determine whether an improvement in blood pressure has improved blood flow.

Adjuncts to Pharmacological Support

If the cardiogenic shock is due to a recent myocardial infarction, thrombolytic therapy may also be employed. In addition, angioplasty coupled with thrombolysis may reestablish blood flow and improve LV function. While this form of therapy is not standard, it does emphasize the importance of reestablishing blood flow rather than treating symptoms.

Use of mechanical support of the heart is increasing for the patient with cardiogenic shock. Mechanical support ranges from intra-aortic balloon pumping to LV and (RV) assist devices.

Protecting Ventilation

Intubation and aggressive oxygen therapy are frequently necessary in cardiogenic shock. Positive end expiratory pressure (PEEP) should be used cautiously, and the nurse should monitor cardiac output changes if PEEP is employed.

Treating Lactic Acidosis

Lactic acidosis will resolve if perfusion is reestablished. In the case of severe systemic pH disturbances (<7.20), small doses of sodium bicarbonate may be necessary. Despite the controversy over this measure, if the pH is below 7.20, bicarbonate administration to maintain pH levels over 7.20 may buy time in reestablishing blood flow.

Intra-Aortic Balloon Pump

Use of the aortic counterpulsation balloon, or the intra-aortic balloon pump (IABP), is increasingly available. The IABP reduces afterload of the left ventricle and increases blood flow into the coronary arteries, which makes it useful in treating refractive cardiac failure and cardiogenic shock and setup. IABP may be used as a supplement to medical treatment for cardiogenic shock or as a presurgery cardiac augmentation mechanism.

Insertion of the IABP
The IABP is inserted in the femoral artery (maybe a subclavian artery) after local anesthesia is achieved. It is advanced up the artery until it is in the descending thoracic aorta (Fig. 9-1). The IABP is synchronized with the patient's own heart rate and is timed

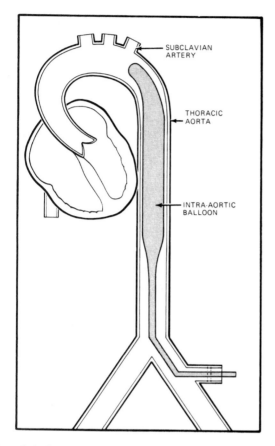

Figure 9–1. The intra-aortic balloon pump (IABP) in the thoracic aorta.

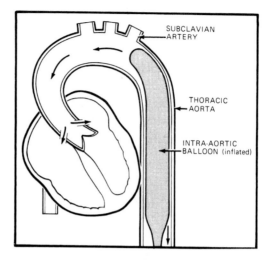

Figure 9–2. The IABP inflated during ventricular diastole.

to inflate immediately after aortic valve closure. Deflation occurs at variable points prior to the next QRS complex. The exact point varies from patient to patient to optimize afterload reduction.

Inflation should not occur until after the aortic valve closes due to the increased resistance the left ventricle would encounter. Blood may also be forced back into the left ventricle.

Deflation must occur before the end of the QRS complex to avoid balloon inflation during ventriculation contraction. Proper deflation will result in a reduction in afterload due to a "windkessel" effect.

Principles of the IABP

The IABP decreases strain on the left ventricle by lowering afterload in the aorta. With a reduced afterload, the ventricle does not have to contract as forcibly to expel its blood into the aorta.

During ventricular diastole, the balloon inflates to improve coronary blood flow. Blood is forced back into the coronary arteries with proper inflation (Fig. 9–2). The proper point for inflation is frequently near the dicrotic notch. Closure of the aortic valve is the event that produces the dicrotic notch on the arterial wave (Fig. 9–3). As discussed earlier, prior to ventricular systole (Fig. 9–4), the balloon deflates, decreasing the aortic afterload.

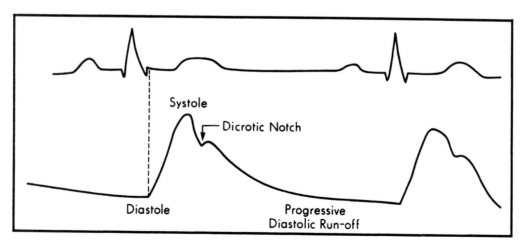

Figure 9–3. Normal arterial waveform.

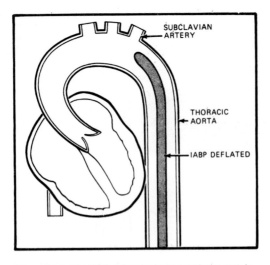

SUBCLAVIAN ARTERY

THORACIC AORTA

IABP DEFLATED

Figure 9–4. The IABP deflated prior to ventricular systole.

Complications of the IABP

There are two major issues associated with the use of the IABP.

1. Circulation to the leg inferior to the insertion site is compromised to varied degrees. Monitoring and documenting the pulses, temperature, and appearance of the leg below the insertion site is extremely important. A comparison with the opposite extremity should be made.

2. The patient is weaned off the IABP usually by changing the ratio of IABP function to cardiac function. The ratio with insertion is normally 1:1. To effect weaning, the ratio first becomes 2:1, then 4:1, and then 8:1, as the patient tolerates it. Weaning may also be achieved by decreasing balloon volume, depending upon the model of the IABP machine in use. There are times when the left myocardium is so severely damaged that it cannot function adequately without the support of the IABP. In any event, use of the IABP must be terminated at some point.

A complication of IABP therapy is balloon rupture. For this reason, a rapid-exchanging gas (e.g., helium) is used for the balloon.

Contraindications of IABP include the presence of aortic or ventricular aneurysms, ventricular septal defects, or aortic regurgitation.

Hemorrhagic (Hypovolemic) Shock

EDITORS' NOTE

The CCRN exam is likely to ask several questions that test your knowledge of treatment of the major forms of shock. In this chapter, a simple approach to understanding the forms of shock is presented. This approach should provide you with the information necessary to successfully answer questions on the concepts of shock.

Two major syndromes producing shock, hemorrhagic and cardiogenic shock, are both due to loss of cardiac output. One other syndrome commonly produces shock: a low systemic vascular resistance (SVR), as occurs in sepsis. In low-SVR shock, high cardiac output is more likely than low output. In this chapter, the emphasis is placed on identifying low cardiac output states and the symptoms associated with hemorrhagic and cardiogenic shock. The hemodynamic changes associated with sepsis are discussed in Chapter 5.

The CCRN exam can be anticipated to contain questions on each type of shock. The review presented here is designed to build on previous chapters and improve your ability to recognize and differentiate the types of shock that produce a low cardiac output state.

Shock occurs when a low mean arterial pressure (MAP) (less than 60 mm Hg) produces clinical symptoms of cellular hypoxia. Two common types of shock that can be readily identified based on differences in preload are hemorrhagic and cardiogenic. While causes of the various types of shock are markedly different, clinical differentiation is possible based on understanding the principles involved in the regulation of blood pressure.

Hemorrhagic shock is basically characterized by loss of blood volume due to active bleeding or chronic loss of vascular volume. For clinical purposes, the concept of hemorrhagic shock can also include hypovolemia from a number of causes. In the rest of this section, hypovolemic shock will replace the term hemorrhagic shock.

The causes of the loss of blood volume are wide ranging and include trauma, postoperative bleeding, and third spacing of fluid. Specific causes of hypovolemic shock are listed in Table 10–1. Both medical and surgical units are likely to see hypovolemic shock. Loss of vascular volume is probably the most common cause of loss of blood pressure, making this the most common reason for hypotension. When a patient is admitted with hypotension of unknown origin, hypovolemia must be suspected and treated before other forms of therapy are instituted.

ETIOLOGY

The loss of circulating blood volume leads to reduction in preload and eventually to reduction in stroke volume and cardiac output. The loss of stroke volume can be compensated for by an increase in heart rate. The increase in heart rate can be substantial enough to prevent reduction in blood pressure. The compensating increase in heart rate may result in early phases of hypovolemic shock not being reflected in blood pressure changes.

As the heart rate increase fails to compensate for the loss of stroke volume and cardiac output falls, SVR increases as a second compensatory mechanism. Again, the blood pressure does not change markedly until the SVR cannot regulate the blood pressure. At the same time that heart rate and SVR are compensating for loss of stroke volume, microcirculation

TABLE 10–1. CAUSES OF HYPOVOLEMIC AND CARDIOGENIC SHOCK

Hypovolemic	Cardiogenic
Trauma	Myocardial infarction
Postoperative bleeding	Atrial tachydysrhythmias (atrial tachycardia, flutter, fibrillation)
Gastrointestinal bleeding	Ventricular tachycardia, fibrillation
Burns	Congestive heart failure
Capillary leak syndromes	Papillary muscle rupture
	Septal or ventricular wall rupture
	Tension pneumothorax
	Pericardial tamponade

changes are occurring in an attempt to maintain organ blood flow.

The microcirculation is a group of blood vessels that act as an independent organic unit to regulate blood supply to the tissues (Fig. 10–1).

The components of the microcirculation are capillaries, which form the vascular system between arterioles and venules. The arterioles bifurcate at points called metarterioles or precapillary arterioles. Smooth muscle cells cover the metarterioles at the bifurcation but disappear as each metarteriole becomes a true capillary.

At the point of metarteriole bifurcation into true capillaries, there is a muscle sphincter. This precapillary sphincter acts as an autoregulatory system, dilating to allow increased perfusion when blood pressure is low or constricting when blood pressure is increased to adjust to the metabolic needs of the tissues in normal states.

The precapillary sphincter constricts in cases of shock and sympathetic nervous system stimulation to maintain perfusion of the vital organs. This constriction directs the available blood from nonessential tissues, such as the stomach, to vital organs, especially the heart and brain. This is the first major compensatory mechanism to be activated with the onset of shock.

Many chemical and humoral factors alter the regulation in the microcirculatory system. Some of these factors are listed in Table 10–2. Neurochemical controls provide a negative feedback response that results in adaptive responses to maintain cellular oxygenation. If the shock is mild and/or slow in developing, the negative feedback of the microcirculatory system will reverse the shock state. If the shock is severe or rapid in developing, this negative feedback of the microcirculatory system may not reverse the shock state. Failure to restore a hemostatic state allows a positive feedback system to develop. In this vicious cycle of positive feedback, inadequate tissue perfusion leads to a deterioration in cardiovascular function, which decreases tissue perfusion even more. Consequently, in these instances, the shock state precipitates an even more severe shock state, leading to death if not reversed.

The release of catecholamines (epinephrine and norepinephrine) in early shock results in vasoconstriction of the microcirculatory vessels at the precapillary sphincter level. The precapillary sphincter constriction is an attempt to increase venous return to the heart (by preventing blood flow in unnecessary tissues), which in turn improves cardiac output and tissue perfusion.

The hemodynamic mechanism to resolve shock is movement of fluid from the interstitial space into the vascular tree, causing an increase in plasma volume. This fluid shift occurs because a change in the hydrostatic pressure in the capillaries alters fluid exchange across the capillary membrane. With increased fluid shifting into the vascular tree, the plasma is diluted, decreasing plasma oncotic pressure and fostering more fluid movement into capillary beds. After hemorrhage, the liver synthesizes new proteins immediately to replace the lost plasma

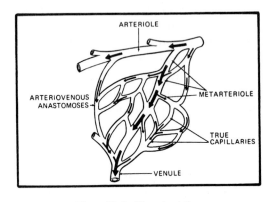

Figure 10–1. Microcirculation.

TABLE 10–2. REGULATION OF THE MICROCIRCULATORY SYSTEM

Chemical	C	D	Humoral	C	D
Hypoxemia		+	Catecholamines		
Hydrogen		+	Epinephrine	+	+
Potassium		+	Norepinephrine	+	
Hypercapnea	+		Dopamine	+	+
Hyperosmolarity	+		Amines		
			Serotonin	+	+
			Acetylcholine		+
			Histamine		+
			Polypeptides		
			Angiotensin	+	
			Kinins	+	
			Vasopressin		+

C, vasoconstriction; D, vasodilatation.

proteins in an attempt to force the fluid shift from the interstitium to the vascular tree and thus maintain adequate intravascular volume.

The renin-angiotensin-aldosterone cascade is activated by decreased renal blood flow. The renin is acted upon in several stages to convert it to angiotensin II. Angiotensin II is one of the most potent vasoconstrictors known. It augments the blood pressure and ideally increases blood flow in the process. Angiotensin II and the catecholamines (epinephrine and norepinephrine) increase vasoconstriction in all organs except the brain and heart. At the same time, aldosterone secretion is stimulated by angiotensin II. Aldosterone increases sodium retention by the kidneys, thereby increasing water reabsorption in the convoluted tubular system of the nephron. This additional retention of water helps increase intravascular volume.

A low cardiac output, secondary to hypovolemia, stimulates the neurohypophysis to increase release of the antidiuretic hormone (ADH). ADH promotes water reabsorption through its actions on the convoluted tubules and collecting ducts of the kidneys. ADH also has a vasoconstricting effect that further increases arterial pressure. Because of this action, ADH is sometimes called vasopressin.

Chronic hypovolemia can manifest physically in many ways. Acute hypovolemia, however, may be difficult to detect until hypotension develops. One method for assessing physical symptoms of hypovolemia is to apply the concept of preload. Preload (pulmonary capillary wedge pressure, PCWP) in hypovolemia is low, differentiating hypovolemic shock from congestive heart failure (CHF) and cardiogenic shock. The low preload does not produce any of the pulmonary or vascular congestion symptoms seen in CHF and cardiogenic shock. Specific symptoms of hypovolemic shock are given in Table 10–1.

Orthostatic blood pressure changes can indicate hypovolemia. These changes, which are measured by changing positions from supine to sitting, are defined by an increased heart rate (more than 10 beats/min) and a fall in systolic (less than 25 mm Hg) and diastolic blood pressure (less than 10 mm Hg).

Since initial symptoms of any shock are minimal, observation to detect subtle changes is important. A gradually increasing heart rate coupled with a downward trend in blood pressure may be a clue of impending hypovolemia. Initial intervention can result in much more favorable outcomes. If intervention is delayed, enough cellular damage may occur

that the shock becomes irreversible. Measurement of oxygenation principles will give an idea of the severity of the shock state. Lactate levels, for example, have been correlated with survival in patients with hemorrhagic shock. If lactate levels exceed 4 mmol/L and are associated with a pH decrease, the likelihood of survival drops markedly.

Systemic signs of hypovolemia include possible decrease in urine output (less than 30 ml/hr of 0.5 ml/kg), change in level of consciousness (LOC) or behavior (cerebral ischemia may develop when the cerebral perfusion pressure drops below 60 mm Hg), increase in respiratory rate, and change in pulse quality. These symptoms are highly variable in the initial stages of shock. As shock progresses, severe depression in LOC, cool clammy skin, oliguria, hypotension, and tachycardia are common.

COMPLICATIONS

Sustained tissue hypoxia will lead to tissue necrosis and release of endotoxins into the system. Brain damage secondary to stagnation or prolonged hypoperfusion occurs as glucose, the only substrate available for cerebral metabolism, is consumed. Coma, seizures, and intracerebral hemorrhage may occur.

Electrolyte disarrangement and acid-base alterations are a result of both the shock state and renal failure. Cardiac dysrhythmia may herald the onset of irreversible shock resulting in death. Systemic disturbances, such as adult respiratory distress syndrome, are possible complications as cellular hypoxia develops.

TREATMENT

The primary focus in hypovolemic shock is the replacement of lost vascular volume. The treatment modalities are controversial in the correction of hypovolemic shock, with the controversy centering on which type of plasma expander, crystalloid or colloid infusion, to use. This question is addressed below. In addition, if the patient has a decreased LOC, intubation and protection of the airway is the highest priority.

Often, whole blood and a crystalloid solution (e.g., normal saline or lactated Ringer's solution) are used to provide a balance between infusion of red blood cells, electrolytes, and fluid that would affect all three compartments (intravascular, intracellular, and extracellular). Interstitial and intracellular compartments are not replenished by blood or other colloidal agents. Blood administration increases vascular volume, osmotic pressure, and oxygen-carrying capacity.

Colloidal therapy is based on the administration of fluids that contain large-molecular-weight solutes, such as albumin or a glucose polymer (hetastarch). The proponents of colloidal agents claim that increasing the colloid osmotic pressure in the vascular tree will either "pull" interstitial fluids back into the vascular system or at least provide for a rapid volume expansion, since fluid will not leak out of the vascular compartment. Many authorities believe that acute hypovolemia can best be managed with use of colloidal agents; others feel that there is a greater risk of overtransfusion with colloids, which remain in the intact vascular tree, than with crystalloids, which can be absorbed into intracellular and interstitial spaces.

NURSING INTERVENTION

Monitoring hemodynamic parameters of shock usually involves a central venous pressure (CVP) line or ideally a pulmonary artery catheter in order to guide the effectiveness of treatment. Nursing procedures related to any CVP or pulmonary artery catheter are applicable to the shock patient.

Patients traditionally have been placed in the Trendelenburg position or positioned with use of "shock blocks." Research indicates that a supine position or elevation of only the legs provides adequate circulation to the brain. If a concurrent head injury exists, the head of the bed may be placed in a low Fowler's position. In cases of severe shock, a supine position with legs elevated 20° to 30° by pillows may increase venous return.

Cardiovascular status, in addition to hemodynamic monitoring, is continuously monitored for signs of dysrhythmias. Dysrhythmias due to electrolyte disturbance are common with massive blood transfusions and with inadequate vascular volume.

Vasomotor tone is normally controlled by constriction secondary to sympathetic and catecholamine factors. Sympathetic stimulants such as norepinephrine (Levophed) and dopamine may need to be administered to maintain blood pressure.

Acid-base disturbances may be severe, and mixed metabolic and respiratory acidosis is common. Respiratory acidosis is corrected by adequate ventilation. Metabolic acidosis may be corrected by reversing decreased organ blood flow. If the pH is severely reduced, i.e., below 7.20, sodium bicarbonate ($NaHCO_3$) may be used to raise the pH to tolerable levels (above 7.20). One milliequivalent per kilogram of body weight is an initial loading dose for sodium bicarbonate. Additional doses depend upon the arterial blood gas values. The use of sodium bicarbonate is controversial, however, and changes in the guidelines for its application may alter the above recommendations.

Renal function is monitored hourly, usually with an indwelling Foley catheter. Severe or sustained hypovolemia may result in acute tubular necrosis, although prerenal azotemia is the first renal response. The blood urea nitrogen (BUN) may rise disproportionately to the creatinine, creating an increased BUN/creatinine ratio (greater than 15:1).

Nutritional support is essential, since a shock state rapidly depletes glucose storage with a resulting negative nitrogen balance, and protein catabolism increases acidotic states. Hyperalimentation (total parenteral nutrition) may be instituted to provide adequate nutrition. If the shock state was not caused by gastrointestinal or esophageal bleeding, a small-bore duodenal tube may be inserted and a continuous drip infusion of commercial food substitutes (e.g., Ensure, Osmolite, and Jevity) is started.

Stress ulcers may occur secondary to necrosis of the gastric mucosa during the hypovolemic period. Intravenous H_2 blockers (e.g., ranitidine and cimetidine) are often used to help reduce the incidence of gastric ulcers.

Emotional support consists of reassurance and explanation of procedures. Short brief comments regarding the patient's condition and the use of monitoring equipment will help decrease anxiety. Explanations to family members about the patient's current status and nursing procedures usually console the family and the patient.

Interpreting Dysrhythmias

The CCRN exam can be expected to directly address either the interpretation or treatment of sinus and atrial dysrhythmias. There may be few or many questions, depending on the type of test. The most important concepts in this area are the correct interpretation of dysrhythmias and the treatment each would require. Most of this information is included in a basic ECG course, something most of us have already had. However, if dysrhythmia interpretation is not a strength for you, review this chapter carefully.

All dysrhythmias are caused by a disturbance in the formation of the cardiac impulse or a disturbance in the conduction of the impulse. Classification of dysrhythmias is shown in Table 11–1.

Every dysrhythmia has specific identifying characteristics. The first four dysrhythmias discussed in this chapter originate in the sinoatrial (SA) node. The next six dysrhythmias originate in the atrium, but not in the SA node. The final eight dysrhythmias originate from electrical impulses initiated in the junctional tissue around the atrioventricular (AV) node. (*Note:* All rhythm strips are 6 sec, lead II.)

SINOATRIAL NODE DYSRHYTHMIAS

Sinus Arrhythmia (or Sinus Dysrhythmia)

Etiology
Variations of impulse formation in the SA node are caused by the vagus nerve and changes in venous return to the heart. This results in an irregular rhythm with alternating fast and slow rates (Fig. 11–1).

Identifying Characteristics
The rate varies, usually between 60 and 100 beats/min. The rate increases with inspiration and decreases with expiration. Both atrial and ventricular rhythms are regularly irregular if the variation is due to a regular breathing pattern. The P waves are normal and the PR interval is within normal limits. The QRS complex is normal. The difference between normal sinus rhythm and sinus arrhythmia is the variation of the RR intervals. In sinus arrhythmia, the variation is at least 0.04 sec between the shortest and the longest RR intervals. The variation in normal sinus rhythm is less than 0.04 sec.

Risk
No risk exists for the patient because this dysrhythmia is a normal variant and causes no hemodynamic compromise.

Treatment
No treatment is needed.

Nursing Intervention
Document the dysrhythmia with a rhythm strip. This interpretation can be substantiated if the patient holds his or her breath and the rate stabilizes.

Sinus Bradycardia

Etiology
Parasympathetic (vagal) control over the SA node due to ischemia, pain, drugs, sleep, or athletic conditioning decreases the formation of electrical impulses (Fig. 11–2).

TABLE 11–1. CLASSIFICATION OF DYSRHYTHMIAS

Dysrhythmias Due to Disorders in Impulse Foundation or Accessory Pathway	Dysrhythmias Due to Conduction Disturbances

SA node dysrhythmias
  Sinus tachycardia
  Sinus bradycardia
  Sinus arrhythmia
  Wandering pacemaker
  SA arrest
Atrial dysrhythmias
  Premature atrial contractions
  Paroxysmal atrial tachycardia
  Atrial flutter
  Atrial fibrillation
AV nodal area (junctional) dysrhythmias
  Premature junctional contractions
  Junctional escape rhythm
  Paroxysmal junctional tachycardia
  Junctional tachycardia
Ventricular dysrhythmias
  Premature ventricular contractions
  Ventricular tachycardia
  Ventricular fibrillation
  Ventricular asystole
	SA block
	AV blocks
	  First-degree AV block
	  Second-degree type I AV block
	  Second-degree type II AV block
	  Third-degree (complete) AV block
	Intraventricular blocks
	  Left bundle branch blocks
	  Right bundle branch blocks
	  Bilateral bundle branch blocks

Identifying Characteristics

The rate is less than 60 but usually more than 40. Both atrial and ventricular rhythms are usually regular. P waves are normal. The PR interval is within the upper limits or is slightly prolonged. The QRS complex is normal. Conduction is normal.

Risk

This dysrhythmia may lead to syncopal attacks, angina, premature beats, ventricular tachycardia, congestive heart failure (CHF), and cardiac arrest. This is a serious warning dysrhythmia if the rate is low (about 40) and accompanied by hypotension (blood pressure below 90/60). Sinus bradycardia is generally benign but should be assessed for its effect on hemodynamics.

Treatment

No treatment may be necessary if the rate is close to 60 or if the patient is asymptomatic. If the rate is low and/or the patient is symptomatic (hypotensive or showing signs of CHF), atropine given intravenously is the drug of choice to increase the heart rate. If this treatment is unsuccessful, isoproterenol hydrochloride (Isuprel) by intravenous drip may be tried. An external or temporary pacemaker may be required if pharmacological management is unsuccessful.

Nursing Intervention

Document the dysrhythmia with a rhythm strip. Monitor and document the effectiveness of drug therapy. Do not administer drugs such as digitalis or propanolol (Inderal) that may further slow the heart

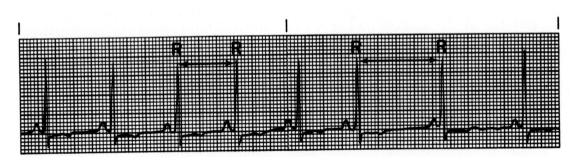

Figure 11–1. Sinus arrhythmia.

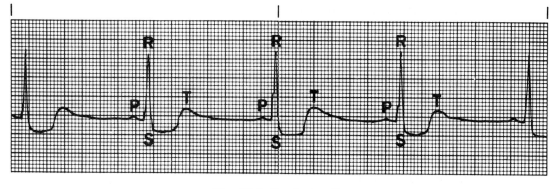

Figure 11–2. Sinus bradycardia.

rate. Be especially alert for premature ventricular contractions (PVCs). If PVCs occur, obtain a rhythm strip and notify the physician; do not treat with lidocaine or other agents that may eliminate the PVCs. PVCs associated with a bradycardia are generally treated with atropine or isoproterenol. As the heart rate increases, the PVCs usually disappear.

Sinus Tachycardia

Etiology

Cardiac decompensation (congestive heart failure, CHF) is the most serious cause of sinus tachycardia. The increase in heart rate during CHF is a compensatory response due to a reduced stroke volume. Sinus tachycardia may also be caused by any factor that stimulates the sympathetic nervous system, such as anxiety, exertion (physical), and fever (Fig. 11–3).

Identifying Characteristics

The rate is greater than 100 and is usually between 100 and 160. Both atrial and ventricular rhythms are regular. The P wave is normal but may be difficult to identify because of the rapid rate. (*Note:* Look for

the P wave superimposed on the T wave with fast rates.) The PR interval is usually at the lower limits of normal.

Risk

Regardless of the etiology, prolonged sinus tachycardia may precipitate CHF in patients with borderline cardiac function. The ability to tolerate a prolonged sinus tachycardia is dependent on the underlying cardiac function of the patient.

Treatment

Effective treatment depends upon controlling the underlying cause. Normally sinus tachycardia does not in itself require treatment. In a persistent sinus tachycardia that is compromising the cardiac output, pharmacological treatment may be required with therapies such as calcium channel blockers (e.g., verapamil), beta blockers (e.g., esmolol), or adenosine or digitalis preparations (e.g., digoxin).

Nursing Intervention

Document the dysrhythmia with a rhythm strip. Monitor the patient for signs of left ventricular (LV)

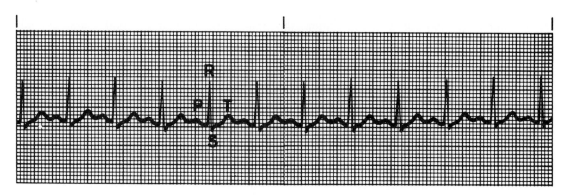

Figure 11–3. Sinus tachycardia.

failure (restlessness, orthopnea, cough, shortness of breath). Attempts to calm the patient and to decrease the patient's stress may be helpful.

Sinus Pause/Arrest, Sinoatrial Block

Etiology
Ischemic injury to the SA node is the most common and important cause of SA block. A technical, but not clinical, difference exists between sinus pause/ arrest and SA block. In the pause/arrest, the SA node does not form an electrical impulse. In SA block, the node initiates an impulse, but the impulse is prevented from leaving the node and thus it cannot be visualized. Regardless of this difference, the end result is that no impulse stimulates the atria or the ventricles. The terms pause and block are often used interchangeably. Sinus disease, vagal effect, digitalis toxicity, quinidine sulfate (Quinidine), and sympathetic stimulation may be causes of SA block (Fig. 11–4).

Identifying Characteristics
The rate is usually slower than normal. Rhythm (both atrial and ventricular) is generally regular

except for the arrest/block complex. P waves are absent in arrest and block for a specific time period. Otherwise, P waves are normal. The PR interval is absent in the arrest/block complex. The QRS complex may be normal or abnormal in arrest, depending on the escape site. No QRS complexes are seen during the block. Conduction depends on the escape site in arrest and is absent in sinus block for that specific interval.

Risk
The greatest risk is that both sinus pause/arrest and sinus block may proceed to a reduced cardiac output if the arrest or block is frequent. If the arrest or block is infrequent and self-limiting, it is not dangerous.

Treatment
If the arrest or block is rare, it does not require treatment. If the arrest is frequent, treatment is essential. If drugs are the underlying cause, they should be evaluated and stopped. Atropine and epinephrine may be effective in increasing the heart rate. If these are not effective and the patient is symptomatic, initially an external pacemaker could be applied, but long-term treatment will require a permanent pacemaker.

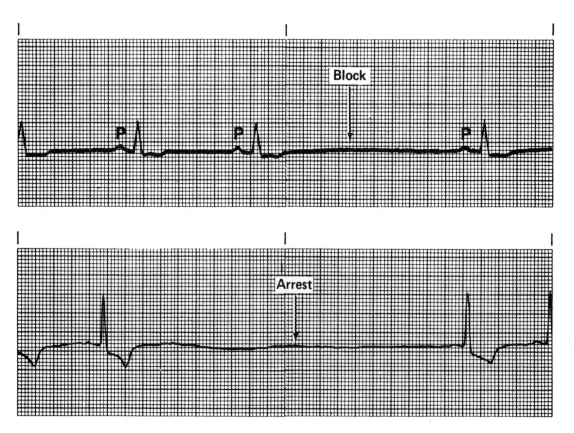

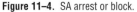

Figure 11–4. SA arrest or block.

Nursing Intervention

Document the dysrhythmia with a rhythm strip. If a drug is the possible underlying cause, withhold the drug until reordered. Monitor the patient closely to determine whether the frequency of arrest or block is increasing. If it is, document with rhythm strips and notify the physician; a pacemaker may be indicated.

ATRIAL DYSRHYTHMIAS

Paroxysmal Atrial Tachycardia

Etiology

Paroxysmal atrial tachycardia (PAT) is the term to describe several causes for a rapid atrial heart rate (Fig. 11–5). Another term, paroxysmal supraventricular tachycardia, is also used to describe this rhythm. In PAT, excessive sympathetic stimulation or abnormal conduction situations are present. Abnormal conduction situations include AV nodal reentry problems or the presence of accessory pathways.

Identifying Characteristics

Three characteristics are associated with PAT:

1. It starts suddenly.
2. It ends abruptly.
3. The ventricles respond to either every impulse created by the focus (1:1 conduction) or most impulses, creating a rapid ventricular response.

Both atrial and ventricular rates are usually between 150 and 250. The rhythm is regular. P waves are present but may be very difficult to identify. The P wave will not have the normal, smooth, rounded shape of a sinus P wave, since this impulse originates in the atrium. The PR interval varies. It may be within normal limits and is frequently greater than one expects for the rate. However, in some accessory pathway situations, the PR interval may be shortened. The QRS complex is usually normal. Once again, however, if the problem is due to an accessory pathway, an initial distortion in the QRS complex may be present. This distortion is sometimes seen as a delta wave, causing a slurring of the upstroke on the R wave of the QRS complex.

Risk

Paroxysmal atrial tachycardia frequently stops spontaneously. If it does not, the rapid rate may lead to myocardial ischemia and, eventually, cardiac decompensation. If PAT occurs post-myocardial infarction or in the patient with limited cardiac function, it may rapidly lead to increased myocardial ischemia and injury and LV failure.

Treatment

Vagal stimulation and other vagal maneuvers such as coughing and pressure on the eyes may terminate the dysrhythmia. Having the patient perform a Valsalva maneuver stimulates the vagus nerve. If this fails to terminate the rhythm, carotid massage by the doctor (or nurse, if allowed) often terminates PAT. If this fails and the patient is asymptomatic, drug therapy may be tried. Beta blockers such as esmolol or propanolol, digoxin, calcium channel blockers (verapamil or diltiazem), or adenosine intravenously may terminate PAT. If the patient is symptomatic (complains of angina, becomes diaphoretic, short of breath, and hypotensive), synchronized cardioversion may be used immediately. Cardioversion usually terminates PAT.

Surgical interventions and radiofrequency ablation are increasingly options for the patient with PAT. In order to surgically cut the accessory pathway

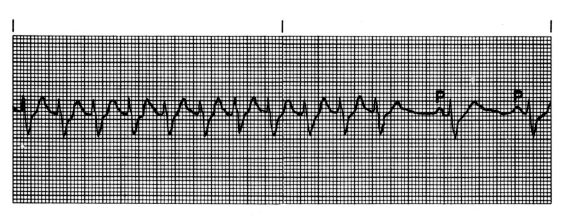

Figure 11–5. Paroxysmal atrial tachycardia.

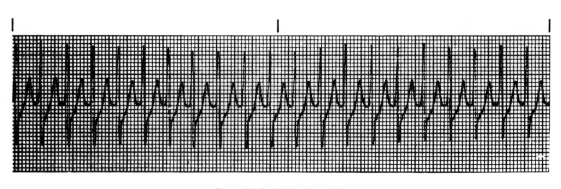

Figure 11–6. Atrial tachycardia.

(or eliminate the path with radiofrequency ablation), extensive electrical mapping of the heart in an electrophysiology lab is required in order to locate the origin of the abnormal pathway.

Nursing Intervention

Document the dysrhythmia with a rhythm strip. Assess and monitor the patient for signs of ischemia and decompensation. Medicate as ordered by the physician. Be prepared for synchronized cardioversion.

Atrial Tachycardia

The impulse of atrial tachycardia originates in the atrium. The rate of atrial tachycardia is constant. The difference between PAT and atrial tachycardia is only that PAT starts and stops suddenly. Atrial tachycardia is a constant rhythm, not irregular. All other parameters of PAT apply to atrial tachycardia (Fig. 11–6).

Premature Atrial Contractions

Note: Premature atrial contractions (PACs) are also called atrial premature beats.

Etiology

On occasion, an irritable focus in the atrium or an impulse through an accessory pathway causes an unexpected complex initiating depolarization. The irritable focus does not become the heart's pacemaker except for this single beat (Fig. 11–7).

Identifying Characteristics

The underlying rate is usually normal. The rhythm has an occasional irregularity due to the premature nature of the beat and a brief pause after the premature beat. The P wave is abnormally shaped for only the premature beat. The PR interval is usually prolonged but may be normal or shortened. The QRS complex is normal. PACs may be blocked or may have an aberrant (abnormal or wide QRS) conduction. Conduction below the atria (junctional and ventricular) is usually normal.

Risk

If PACs occur infrequently, there is no risk. If they occur six or more times per minute, they indicate atrial flutter, atrial fibrillation, or atrial tachycardia.

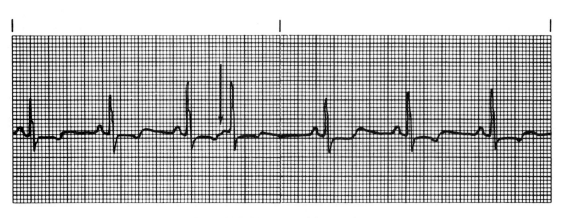

Figure 11–7. Premature atrial contraction.

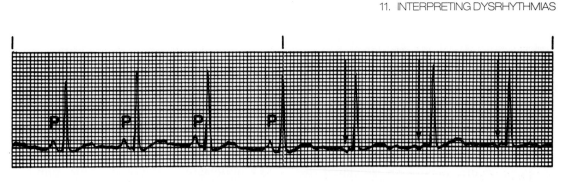

Figure 11–8. Wandering atrial pacemaker.

Treatment

Premature atrial contractions of fewer than 6/min do not need treatment. With more than six PACs per minute, the physician may elect to control them with digitalis or with calcium channel or beta blockers.

Nursing Intervention

Document the dysrhythmia with a rhythm strip. Monitor the patient for increasing frequency of PACs. Increasing PACs may cause anxiety, some hemodynamic compromise, hypotension, and dyspnea. Document an increase in frequency with rhythm strips and notify the physician of the increase.

Wandering Atrial Pacemaker

Etiology

Various foci within the atrium or from the AV node supersede the SA node as the pacemaker for a variable number of beats (Fig. 11–8).

Identifying Characteristics

Rate is usually normal but may be slow. Rhythm is frequently regular. P waves are abnormal and change in size, shape, and deflection. The PR interval may vary or may be constant. The QRS complex is normal. Conduction is abnormal in the atrium and sometimes in the AV node. Below the AV node, conduction is normal.

Risk

Generally there is no risk. The presence of a wandering atrial pacemaker is normally insignificant, although it may indicate the presence of SA disease.

Treatment

Usually no treatment is necessary. If the rhythm produced symptoms, the symptoms would be treated. For example, a bradycardia could be treated with atropine.

Nursing Intervention

Document the dysrhythmia with a rhythm strip. Monitor for an unacceptably low ventricular rate (below 50 beats/min) and treat as necessary.

Atrial Flutter

Etiology

An irritable atrial focus or accessory pathway may supersede the SA node and produce atrial flutter. This is a fairly common dysrhythmia in atherosclerotic heart disease and some congenital heart diseases (Fig. 11–9).

Identifying Characteristics

The atrial rate is rapid, usually 250 to 350 beats/min. Atrial rhythm is regular, and ventricular rhythm varies with the number of impulses transmitted through the AV node. The P wave is replaced by a

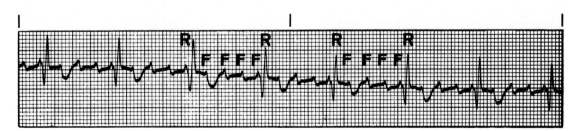

Figure 11–9. Atrial flutter.

flutter wave (F wave). Flutter waves have no isoelectric interval between the waves. The PR interval is usually prolonged although difficult to measure from a rhythm strip. The QRS complex is usually normal. Conduction is abnormal in the atria, and the AV node normally blocks many of the F waves.

Risk

Congestive heart failure may occur quickly if the patient has limited cardiac function and if the AV node conducts almost all of the F waves. There is the possibility of severe hemodynamic compromise. If the ventricular response is rapid, there is insufficient filling time for the ventricle. The rapid rate can cause a reduction in cardiac output. Rapid response of the ventricle increases myocardial oxygen demand, which cannot be met due to the decreased cardiac output. If severe, the hemodynamic compromise may lead to CHF.

Treatment

Digitalis preparations may be used in treating this dysrhythmia if the ventricular response is not fast (e.g., <150). If the ventricular response is rapid, synchronized cardioversion with low voltage is the preferred treatment.

Nursing Intervention

Document the dysrhythmia with a rhythm strip. Monitor the patient closely for signs of hemodynamic compromise. The physician should be notified when this dysrhythmia develops.

Atrial Fibrillation

Etiology

Many irritable foci develop in the atrium to the extent that normal atrial contraction is an impossibility. This condition may be caused by rheumatic heart disease, coronary disease, hypertension, thyrotoxicosis, and congenital heart disease (Fig. 11–10).

Identifying Characteristics

The atrial rate is not measurable but is probably greater than 300. The atrial rate is so high that the AV node cannot accept all of the stimuli it receives. Consequently, the atrial and ventricular rates are markedly different. The atrial and ventricular rhythms are irregular. P waves are nonexistent and are replaced by fibrillatory waves. There is no true PR interval. The QRS complex may be normal or abnormal. Ventricular response may be slow, normal, or very rapid. Conduction is abnormal in both the atria and the AV node. The number of impulses that the AV node transmits determines the degree of AV block.

Risk

There may be a rapid development of CHF. Atrial thrombi may form, leading to embolization. Marked hemodynamic disturbance is common if the rhythm is of recent onset. Angina and increased myocardial ischemia may occur.

Treatment

If the dysrhythmia is not causing hemodynamic compromise, digitalis preparations (digoxin) are commonly employed. If hemodynamic compromise develops, synchronized cardioversion is essential to reduce and control the ventricular response, provided the dysrhythmia has not been present for 72 or more hours. The risk of atrial thrombus development after 72 hr contraindicates the use of cardioversion to terminate the dysrhythmia, since it may produce embolization.

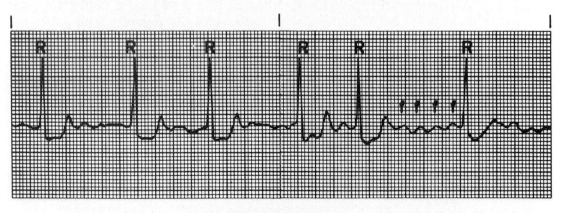

Figure 11–10. Atrial fibrillation.

If there is hemodynamic compromise within the first 72 hr, synchronized cardioversion is essential to reduce and control a rapid ventricular response. This is considered an acute form of atrial fibrillation.

A chronic form of atrial fibrillation is considered to exist if there is no hemodynamic compromise, if the dysrhythmia has been present for more than 72 hr, and if the patient is asymptomatic and has a ventricular response of greater than 50 complexes per minute but less than 100 complexes per minute. In these instances, treatment may not be needed.

Nursing Intervention

Document the dysrhythmia with a rhythm strip. Notify the physician if atrial fibrillation develops suddenly. Monitor the patient carefully for hemodynamic compromise and embolization. Contact the physician if rapid ventricular response develops or if an unacceptably low ventricular response develops (less than 50 beats/min).

ATRIOVENTRICULAR NODE AND VENTRICULAR DYSRHYTHMIAS

EDITORS' NOTE

The most common dysrhythmias likely to be addressed on the CCRN exam involve disturbances of the AV node (junctional rhythms and conduction blocks) and ventricular ectopy (premature ventricular contractions, ventricular tachycardia, and fibrillation). This section contains information that addresses several questions from the exam. Each of these areas can also be expected to contain information addressed on the CCRN exam. Once again, if dysrhythmias are not a strength for you, review this chapter carefully.

It was once thought that the AV node itself could initiate impulses. Such rhythms were termed nodal rhythms. Research has shown that the AV node itself does not initiate an electrical impulse but that an electrical impulse is initiated in the junctional tissue around the AV node. This finding has resulted in changing the term nodal rhythm to the more accurate term of junctional rhythm.

Junctional Rhythm

Etiology
This dysrhythmia is often due to an acute myocardial infarction, an SA block, digitalis toxicity, or treatment with drugs that slow the atrial rate (e.g., digitalis and procainamide) (Fig. 11–11).

Identifying Characteristics
The rate is usually 40 to 60 beats/min. The rhythm is usually regular. P waves are abnormal in shape and size and may precede or follow the QRS complex or be buried in it. If seen, the P wave is usually inverted (negatively deflected). This inversion is caused by the electrical impulse originating in junctional tissue and moving both down into the ventricles (a normal path) and back up into the atrium (retrograde movement, which is an abnormal path). The PR interval, if present, is less than 0.10 sec and often is immeasurable. The QRS complex is normal, unless a P wave is buried in it. Conduction to the atria is abnormal due to its retrograde depolarization of the atria.

Risk
The junctional impulse formation is slow. The junctional rhythm is normally a protective rhythm, taking over as the pacemaker of the heart when the SA node slows to rates below 40 to 60 beats/min. Hemodynamic balance may be compromised by a

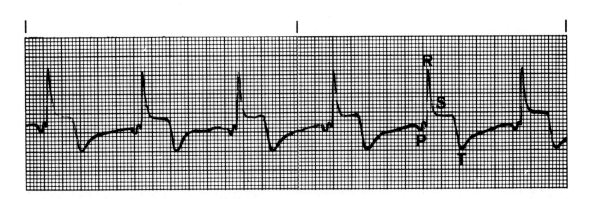

Figure 11–11. Junctional rhythm.

slow ventricular rate, leading to poor cardiac output and perhaps ventricular failure.

Treatment

Medications that increase the heart rate, such as atropine, would be considered if the bradycardia was associated with hypotension or CHF. If medications fail to work, pacemakers can be used to override the slow rate. If drug toxicity is the underlying cause, the drug should be stopped immediately.

Nursing Intervention

Document the dysrhythmia with a rhythm strip. Monitor the patient closely. PVCs may occur and do not respond well to lidocaine or other ventricular antidysrhythmic agents, since the PVCs are usually a result of decreased cardiac output. Increasing the heart rate is a more effective method for eliminating the PVCs. Monitor for signs of hemodynamic compromise. Notify the physician immediately if compromise occurs.

Premature Junctional Contraction

Etiology

An irritable focus in the junctional tissue initiates an impulse early. The impulse depolarizes the ventricles normally and the atria in a retrograde fashion. Coronary artery disease, acute myocardial infarction, and digitalis toxicity are frequent causes. Any factor that increases junctional ischemia may produce a premature junctional contraction (PJC) (Fig. 11–12).

Identifying Characteristics

The underlying rate may be normal or slow. The rhythm is regular except for the premature (early) beat. P waves are abnormal, inverted, and may precede, follow, or be buried in the QRS complex of the PJC. The PR interval varies with the position of the pacemaker and is frequently immeasurable.

The QRS complex is normal unless the P wave is buried in it or aberration occurs. Conduction is normal through the ventricles and retrograde through the atria.

Risk

Premature junctional contractions may lead to a supraventricular tachycardia if frequent. If rare, PJCs do not pose a threat for the patient.

Treatment

If PJCs are infrequent or the patient is asymptomatic, no treatment is necessary. If frequent, PJCs may be controlled by digitalis preparations or other atrial antidysrhythmics such as pronestyl.

Nursing Intervention

Document the dysrhythmia with a rhythm strip (to justify junctional origin rather than ventricular origin). Monitor the patient for increasing frequency of PJCs and notify the physician if the frequency does increase.

Paroxysmal Junctional Tachycardia

Etiology

Paroxysmal junctional tachycardia (PJT) is probably similar to PAT, both in origin and in treatment. The cause may be disease of the AV node or abnormal pathways, either anatomic or physiologic (Fig. 11–13).

Identifying Characteristics

The rate is usually 150 to 250 beats/min. The rhythm is usually regular. P waves are abnormal and inverted, and they may precede, follow, or be buried in the QRS complex. The PR interval, if present, is shortened or not measurable. The QRS complex is normal unless the P wave is buried in it or it is aberrantly conducted. Conduction of the QRS may be normal. Atrial conduction is retrograde. PJT may be

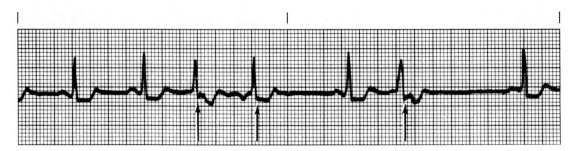

Figure 11–12. Premature junctional contraction.

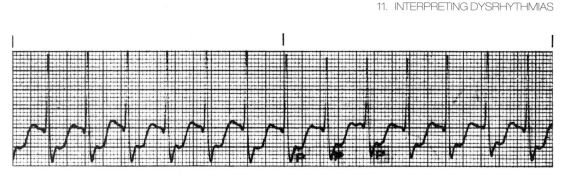

Figure 11–13. Paroxysmal junctional tachycardia.

difficult to distinguish from PAT. They are often called supraventricular tachycardia (SVT).

Risk

The danger associated with PJT is the same as for PAT. The faster the rate, the greater the likelihood of a decreased cardiac output. If the cardiac output is reduced enough, LV failure will result.

Treatment

The treatment is similar to that for PAT.

Nursing Intervention

Document the dysrhythmia with a rhythm strip. Assess the patient for hemodynamic compromise. If compromise occurs, notify the physician and medicate as the situation dictates.

Idioventricular Rhythm

Etiology

In this rhythm, there is no functioning pacemaker above the ventricles. A secondary pacemaker in the ventricles initiates an impulse in order to generate a

heart rate. Normally, a ventricular pacemaker is very slow, generally less than 40 beats/min. The terms idioventricular pacemaker (which means unknown ventricular pacemaker) and ventricular escape rhythm both apply to this dysrhythmia. All diseases and injuries that cause loss of function from the SA node down are etiologic factors (Fig. 11–14).

Identifying Characteristics

The ventricles initiate a rate at their inherent ability, usually 20–40 beats/min. The rhythm is regular but may slow as a "dying heart syndrome" progresses. There is no P wave. There is no PR interval. The QRS complex is wide and bizarre, measuring 0.12 sec or more.

Risk

The imminent danger is ventricular standstill. It is possible that the electrical event is not leading to an effective contraction, which means that electrical mechanical dissociation has developed. This rhythm is normally a protective or compensatory response. It may be the last natural pacemaker in the heart, so treatment becomes urgent.

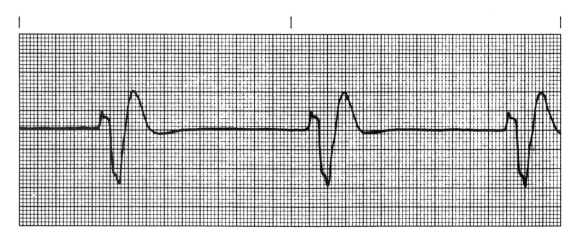

Figure 11–14. Idioventricular rhythm.

Treatment

A pacemaker is the only reliable and totally effective form of treatment. In a crisis until a transvenous or external pacemaker can be applied, atropine or iso-proterenol hydrochloride (Isuprel) may accelerate the heart rate.

Nursing Intervention

Document the dysrhythmia with a rhythm strip. Notify the physician immediately. Assess and treat the patient continuously for hypotension or signs of CHF. Prepare an external pacemaker for use or be prepared to assist in the insertion of a transvenous pacemaker.

Accelerated Idioventricular Rhythm

Etiology

The etiology is the same as for the idioventricular rhythm (Fig. 11–15).

Identifying Characteristics

These are the same as for an idioventricular rhythm with the exception that the rate is usually 60–100 beats/min.

Risk

The immediate risk is that the accelerated focus may cease and the dysrhythmia may convert to an idioventricular rate or cardiac standstill. The accelerated idioventricular rhythm is generally of no danger by itself.

Treatment

No treatment is indicated unless the patient demonstrates signs of hemodynamic compromise. Since the rate is normal, this dysrhythmia may generate an adequate cardiac output.

Nursing Intervention

Monitor the patient for signs of hypotension or CHF.

Premature Ventricular Contractions

Premature ventricular contractions (PVCs) are also termed premature ventricular beats (PVBs) or ventricular premature contractions (VPCs).

Etiology

An irritable focus in the ventricle initiates a contraction before the normally expected beat. The irritability may be due to acute myocardial infarction (most common), atherosclerotic heart disease (ASHD), CHF, drug toxicity, hypoxia, electrolytes, acidosis, or bradycardia (Fig. 11–16).

Identifying Characteristics

The rate is variable. Rhythm is irregular because of the premature beat. P waves are present but frequently not visible. P waves are most commonly lost in the QRS complex of the PVC. However, they may be slightly before or after the PVC. The PR interval is not present, since the atrial impulse does not conduct the PVC. The QRS complex is wide and bizarre, exceeding 0.12 sec and frequently being greater than 0.14 sec. It usually has a compensatory pause that is equal to two PP distances following the PVC.

Risk

The danger of a PVC is the possibility of increasing myocardial irritability leading to an increasing frequency of PVCs. With an increased occurrence of PVCs, ventricular tachycardia and/or ventricular fibrillation may occur. There is an increased potential for problems when any of the following occur:

1. PVCs occur from more than one focus (multiform PVCs).
2. PVCs occur more often than 6/min, including rhythms such as bigeminy (every other beat is a PVC), or short runs of PVCs occur frequently (two to three sequential PVCs) every few beats.
3. There are variable coupling intervals (the period between the beginning of a normal QRS and the beginning of the QRS of the PVC).
4. The PVC occurs on the T wave of the preceding complex (described as the R-on-T phenomenon). If the PVC occurs on the T wave, it may precipitate ventricular fibrillation.

Treatment

Lidocaine bolus followed by a lidocaine drip is the treatment of choice. (*Note:* If a lidocaine bolus has been given and 10–15 min have elapsed, another bolus must be administered before the drip is hung to establish and maintain therapeutic blood levels of the drug.) If hypokalemia is present, potassium may terminate the PVCs. If lidocaine is an unsuccessful treatment, procainamide or bretylium may be tried.

Chronic PVC control is usually with oral preparations, such as tocainide or mexilitine. Many

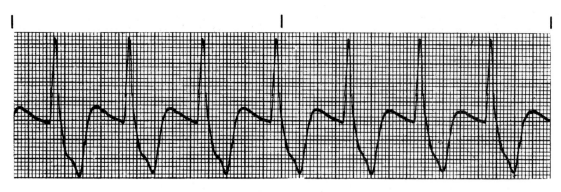

Figure 11–15. Accelerated idioventricular rhythm.

agents are available for the control of chronic PVCs. If PVCs are not controlled by conventional therapies, amniodorone may be required. Amniodorone is usually used as an end-stage treatment because of the multiple side effects associated with this agent. However, amniodorone is increasingly used since, unlike many other antidysrhythics, it has not been shown to have a proarrhythmic effect. In the past few years, a trend toward tolerating PVCs, especially in the absence of acute ischemia, is developing.

Nursing Intervention

Document the dysrhythmia with a rhythm strip. Differentiate the PVC from an atrial premature contraction (APC) with aberrant conduction. Monitor the patient closely for increasing frequency of PVCs or the development of multiform PVCs. Bolus with lidocaine or another antidysrhythmic agent and document the effect. Prepare a continuous drip to maintain control over the PVC frequency. Notify the physician. Observe the patient and monitor closely for ventricular tachycardia and ventricular fibrillation.

Differentiating APCs with Aberrant Conduction from PVCs

Atrial premature contractions with abnormal (aberrant) conduction can mimic PVCs. Criteria that help different APCs with aberrant conduction from PVCs have been described in both medical and nursing research articles. Table 11–2 provides the criteria necessary to aid differentiation. The key to identifying an aberrantly conducted APC centers around two features. First, identify any characteristics of an APC that are different from those of a PVC. For example, in Fig. 11–17, note the P wave on the downstroke of the T wave. This is suggestive of an APC. Second, note the shape of the QRS complex. The morphology or appearance of the QRS complex is a key factor in differentiating APCs with aberrancy from PVCs. Table 11–2 provides clues to QRS complex appearances in the two dysrhythmias. The CCRN exam frequently has a question, and sometimes a rhythm strip, on differentiating between the two, so it is wise to be familiar with the differences.

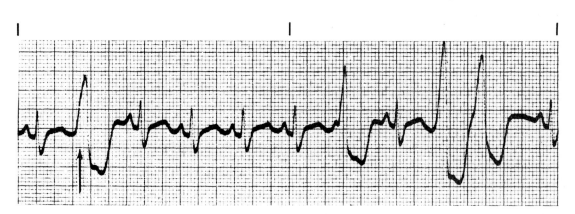

Figure 11–16. Premature ventricular contraction (PVC, PVB, or VPC).

TABLE 11–2. DIFFERENTIATING APCs WITH ABERRANT CONDUCTION FROM PVCs

Criteria for PVCs	Criteria for APCs
Extreme right axis	rSR′ in V₁
Rr′ in V₁	Bi- or triphasic QRS
rS in V₆	Normal axis
Precordial concordancy (all V leads show same axis pattern, i.e., upright or inverted)	
Initial R wave >.03 sec	
Beginning of R to nadir (lowest point) of S wave >.10 sec	

Ventricular Tachycardia

Etiology

Advanced irritability of the ventricles allows a ventricular focus to become the heart's pacemaker. The myocardial irritability may be due to ASHD, CHF, acute myocardial infarction, electrolyte imbalance, hypoxia, acidosis, or occasionally drugs (Fig. 11–18).

Identifying Characteristics

The rate is greater than 100, often 120–220 beats/min. The rhythm is regular or only slightly irregular. P waves are usually not discernible, although it is important to try to identify them. If P waves are present, they will not be related to the QRS complex (AV dissociation exists). No measurable PR interval exists. The QRS complex is wide and bizarre, resembling essentially a salvo (or burst) of premature ventricular contractions. A ventricular focus initiates ventricular depolarization.

Risk

The risk with ventricular tachycardia is the potential to develop dangerous or lethal reductions in cardiac output.

Treatment

According to the American Heart Association (AHA), several types of ventricular tachycardia exist. Treatment is dependent on the type of ventricular tachycardia. The types of ventricular tachycardia and treatments are listed in Table 11–3.

Nursing Intervention

Document this dysrhythmia with a rhythm strip. If the patient is unconscious, immediate defibrillation and institution of cardiac arrest procedures are essential.

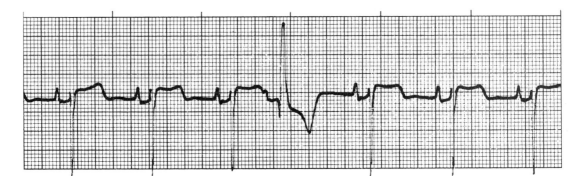

Figure 11–17. Aberrantly conducted APC.

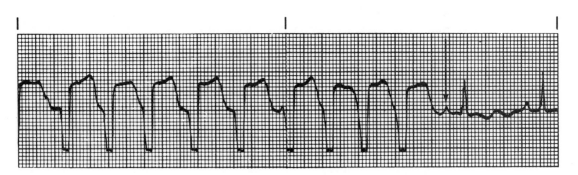

Figure 11–18. Ventricular tachycardia terminating spontaneously.

TABLE 11–3. VENTRICULAR TACHYCARDIA CATEGORIES AND TREATMENT

Characteristics	Treatment
No symptoms	Lidocaine Pronestyl Bretylium
Mild symptoms (chest pain, shortness of breath)	Synchronized Cardioversion, beginning at 50 joules and progressing to 360 joules
Serious symptoms (pulmonary edema, hypotension)	Defibrillation, beginning at 50 joules and progressing to 360 joules
No pulse	Treat as ventricular fibrillation

Ventricular Fibrillation

Etiology

Due to extensive ventricular irritability, ventricular fibers fail to depolarize in sequence; instead, they depolarize individually, creating an uncoordinated series of muscle depolarization. No substantial cardiac output is generated. Ventricular fibrillation may occur after an acute myocardial infarction. It may, however, occur as a result of ASHD, CHF, digitalis or other drug toxicity and electrolyte imbalance (Fig. 11–19).

Identifying Characteristics

There is no identifiable rate. The rhythm is irregular and immeasurable. P waves are replaced by undulating waves as the baseline. The PR interval is nonexistent or immeasurable. The QRS complex is an undulating, asymmetrical line.

Risk

The development of neurodynamic collapse may occur within seconds, followed by death within 4 to 8 minutes.

Treatment

Immediate defibrillation is the only possible means of establishing a viable cardiac rhythm. The AHA has recommended a series of actions to occur when ventricular fibrillation occurs. Essentially, these actions are as follows:

1. Defibrillate initially at 200 joules. If unsuccessful (determined by assessing for the return of a pulse), repeat the defibrillation at 300 joules. If still unsuccessful, repeat at 360 joules.
2. If initial defibrillations are unsuccessful, begin cardiopulmonary resuscitation (CPR) and establish artificial airway and venous access.
3. Administer epinephrine (1 mg). Epinephrine can be repeated every five minutes.
4. Defibrillate at 360 joules.
5. If unsuccessful, restart CPR and give lidocaine (1 mg/kg). Lidocaine can be repeated up to a total of 3 mg/kg, although usually the repeat doses are at 0.5 mg/kg.
6. Defibrillate at 360 joules.
7. If unsuccessful, restart CPR and consider bretylium (5 mg/kg). Bretylium can be given to a total dose of 30 mg/kg.
8. Defibrillate at 360 joules.

During the sequence, sodium bicarbonate can be considered to correct an acidosis. If the rhythm terminates, start a drip of whichever drug (lidocaine or bretylium) was likely responsible for aiding in the termination of the rhythm.

Nursing Intervention

Document the dysrhythmia with a rhythm strip and keep the monitor recorder running throughout the dysrhythmia. Initiate cardiac arrest procedures and follow the above guidelines.

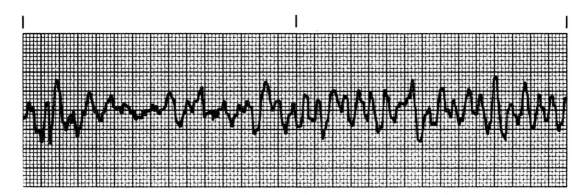

Figure 11–19. Ventricular fibrillation.

Cardiomyopathies and Pericarditis

EDITORS' NOTE

It is somewhat disproportionate to have a whole chapter on cardiomyopathies when the CCRN exam will not have more than a few questions on this topic. This chapter is intentionally short, with an emphasis on practical information which will be seen both in practice and on the exam. Much of the information in this chapter is also found in the discussion of congestive heart failure.

CARDIOMYOPATHIES

Clinical Presentation

Cardiomyopathy has been in the past roughly defined as heart muscle disease of unknown etiology. However, that is not exactly true since the origins of some types, such as ischemic cardiomyopathy, are known. Different potential origins of cardiomyopathies are listed in Table 12–1. Regardless of the origin, the disease tends to involve most of the muscle of the heart, although different parts of the heart might be more affected than others. This presents a clinical picture whereby the cardiomyopathy can appear differently in different patients. One patient might exhibit more left-sided dysfunction, while another might exhibit right-sided dysfunction. Some patients might have systolic ventricular failure, others diastolic dysfunction. The most common presentation appears to be a combination of the above. All cardiomyopathies will involve increased ventricular pressures by the time they present with symptoms.

There are three common presentations of cardiomyopathy, dilated, hypertrophic, and constrictive

(Fig. 12–1). The most common is dilated cardiomyopathy. This type of cardiomyopathy presents with symptoms resembling congestive heart failure (CHF). The patient will have a decreased stroke volume and ejection fraction, and symptoms of pulmonary congestion. Left ventricular (LV) volumes are increased. Eventually, hypotension will occur with death resulting from severe LV failure. Dilated cardiomyopathy presents with a highly compliant ventricle. This usually means that higher ventricular filling pressures (pulmonary capillary wedge pressure, PCWP = 20 mm Hg) can be tolerated relatively easily. Fluid administration of this PCWP can be employed without a major increase in extravascular lung water. However, the key parameter to monitor is stroke volume (and ideally, ejection fraction).

Hypertrophic cardiomyopathy is more of a diastolic dysfunction as a result of the inability of the heart to relax during diastole. Clinical symptoms include pulmonary congestion but close to normal stroke volume and ejection fraction, at least until end stages.

Constrictive cardiomyopathy presents with a very noncompliant ventricular muscle, leading to presentations of CHF. Ventricular volumes are decreased, although stroke volume and ejection fraction can be maintained at near normal levels.

Diagnosis

The only clear diagnostic technique is the use of endomyocardial biopsy. The prognosis for all cardiomyopathy is poor. No curative measures currently exist.

Treatment

Dilated cardiomyopathy is usually treated similarly to CHF. Inotropic agents (dobutamine in acute cases,

TABLE 12–1. POSSIBLE CAUSES OF CARDIOMYOPATHY

Dilated	Idiopathic (unknown)
	Inflammatory/infectious
	Autoimmune disease
	Toxic (drugs, alcohol)
	Hereditary
	Ischemic
	Metabolic (uremia, vitamin deficiency)
	Endocrine (thyroid)
Constrictive	Idiopathic
	Interstitial disease (sarcoidosis)
	Eospinophilic heart disease
	Radiation
	Drug toxicity
Hypertrophic	Idiopathic
	Systemic hypertension

digoxin in chronic cases), diuretics, vasodilators, and beta blockers are commonly used. Aggressive measures such as cardiomyoplasty and mechanical support devices may be used until heart transplantation is possible.

Treatment of constrictive cardiomyopathy is difficult. The focus is generally on diuretics and afterload reducers in an attempt to improve diastolic dysfunction. While this might help temporarily, eventually systemic hypotension results with a worsening of clinical symptoms. Treatments tend to be supportive, although if a specific condition is present, such as eosinophilic cardiomyopathy, then cytotoxic agents (hydroxyurea) or steroids might be used.

In hypertrophic cardiomyopathy the focus is on reducing afterload, particularly with beta blockers. Diuretics and other afterload reducers, such as calcium channel blockers, might be used. If atrial dysrhythmias (such as atrial fibrillation) develop, electrotherapy (cardioversion) or drugs for supraventricular tachycardia would be employed.

PERICARDITIS

Etiology

Pericarditis may be present or may develop in essentially any disease process. It may be due to a virus or bacteria (most common), have a metabolic cause, such as seen in uremia, or be due to an unknown cause. It may be secondary to systemic disease or myocardial trauma, or it may follow acute myocardial infarction.

Clinical Presentation

Symptoms vary with the etiology of the pericarditis. Most commonly, pain is present. The pain may mimic an acute myocardial infarction (MI), angina, or pleurisy. Pain usually increases with deep respiration and when the patient is lying supine. Sitting up and leaning forward usually diminishes the pain. Fever is commonly present because of the infectious or inflammation process. Pericardial friction rub may be present for only a few days (post-MI) or prolonged for many days (uremia). The pericardial friction rub is a scratchy, superficial sound with three components best heard at the lower left sternum. Classical ECG changes are ST segment elevation in all leads except avR.

Complications

Complications of pericarditis include dysrhythmias, tamponade, and restriction of ventricular contraction. Each complication must be treated promptly. Hemodynamic monitoring with a pulmonary artery catheter is useful in early detection of tamponade. Equalization of pressures in the heart, particularly the central venous pressure (CVP) and the PCWP, may signal the presence of tamponade. Auscultation of heart sounds is essential on a regular and frequent schedule, with the clinician attempting to identify whether a muffling of the heart sounds has occurred.

Treatment

Pain relief is essential to promote normal and adequate ventilation. Anti-inflammatory and steroid therapies may be tried. Treatment of the underlying cause is imperative. Antipyretic agents will control the fever if the patient is uncomfortable. Pericardiocentesis or a pericardial window may be performed if the possibility of developing a tamponade is present. Anticoagulants are contraindicated in order to avoid an increase in pericardial fluid.

Nursing Intervention

Perform continuous ECG monitoring for signs of dysrhythmias that may indicate the early development of cardiac tamponade. The most dangerous dysrhythmia is electromechanical dissociation (an ECG pattern is present but there is no pulse). Monitoring with a pulmonary artery catheter is more sensitive to early changes. The standard nursing interventions involved with pulmonary artery monitoring are employed in these instances. The nurse should be prepared to assist with an emergency pericardiocentesis if it becomes warranted. Especially close auscultation of cardiac sounds is imperative for

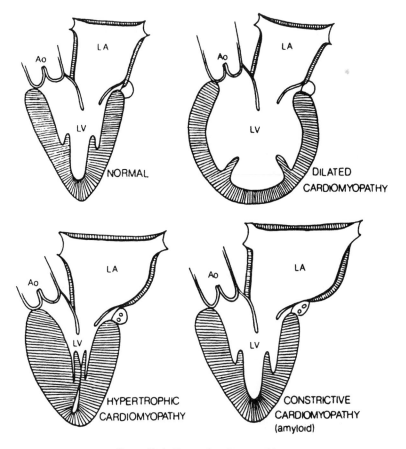

Figure 12–1. Types of cardiomyopathies.

early intervention. Medications to relieve pain and fever are administered as ordered.

Arterial blood gases or pulse oximetry should be monitored at regular intervals to determine ventilatory status and to allow early intervention if hypoxemia develops. Emotional support of the patient and explanations of the close monitoring will help to alleviate some of the patient's anxiety.

Cardiac Tamponade

If fluid accumulates in the pericardial sac, the potential exists for the development of cardiac tamponade. Cardiac tamponade will cause a constrictive effect on the heart, producing a condition initially like diastolic dysfunction (the heart cannot relax and fill with blood). This is particularly aggravated on inspiration, where increased right ventricular volume (due to inspiration) increases the pericardial pressure. This limits LV expansion and produces a drop in blood pressure during inspiration. The term pulsus paradoxus, where the systolic blood pressure decreases by about 20 mm Hg, is commonly seen with cardiac tamponade. Other clinical features include an equalization of left and right filling pressures (the CVP and PCWP are about the same) and pulmonary and venous engorgement.

Treatment involves treating the underlying cause of the fluid or blood in the pericardial sac. Emergent treatment might involve pericardiocentesis.

Treatment of Cardiac, Valvular, and Vascular Insufficiency, and Trauma

EDITORS' NOTE

Cardiovascular surgery has assumed a greater role in critical care over the past decade, and the CCRN exam reflects this trend. Expect several questions on topics of cardiovascular surgery, including a few (usually only one or two) on cardiac transplantation. Use this section in conjunction with the preceding chapters in order to be able to apply hemodynamic analysis to the concept of cardiovascular surgery. This will help in understanding the assessment of and need for surgical treatment of cardiovascular disorders.

CARDIAC, VALVULAR, AND VASCULAR SURGERY

Cardiovascular surgery in the critical care environment can include many procedures, although the key surgical interventions generally center around cardiac or vascular circulation problems. The cardiac disturbances that require emergency surgery include acute coronary artery obstruction, ventricular septal rupture, pericardial tamponade, and papillary muscle rupture. Other than acute coronary artery obstruction, the problems present with symptoms similar to those of cardiogenic shock and will not be discussed here. While this section will not specifically address emergent problems except for the acute obstructed artery, the principles discussed cover most essential information related to cardiovascular surgery. This section does not address all possible

surgical interventions but rather focuses on the common major cardiac and vascular surgeries of coronary artery bypass grafting (CABG), vascular aneurysm, and occlusive disease interventions. An introduction to the principles of cardiac transplantation will round out this section.

Knowledge of these common problems and the associated nursing care will prepare you for most CCRN questions on this content area, including the emergent surgical procedures. With the greater emphasis on the cardiovascular component of the CCRN exam, understanding cardiovascular surgical concepts has increased in importance.

Coronary Artery Bypass Grafting

Coronary artery bypass grafting (CABG) is the technique of using blood vessels obtained from another part of the body to replace obstructed coronary arteries. The internal mammary artery is generally used because of its long-term patency rates. The saphenous vein is generally harvested because the majority of patients requiring surgical revascularization need three or more bypass grafts. Other alternative conduits include the free radial artery, gastroepiploic artery, and inferior epigastric artery. Nursing care postoperatively differs somewhat for the different types of grafts; with saphenous vein removal, for example, one must care for the wound created by removal of the graft. Otherwise, postoperative care does not markedly change.

Determination of the Need for CABG
Indications for surgical revascularization continue to be revised as the roles of less invasive forms of

treatment are refined. Percutaneous transluminal coronary angioplasty (PTCA) and CABG are the two major revascularization therapies. General criteria for invasive revascularization are presented in Table 13–1.

CABG remains the treatment of choice in patients with triple vessel disease with left ventricular dysfunction or complex lesions and those with greater than 75% left main coronary artery stenosis. Other considerations include age, general health status, associated cardiac disease and co-morbid conditions. If there are multiple obstructions in a single artery, making bypass difficult, surgery is generally not indicated or helpful. Pain relief from bypass surgery is individualized, since bypass surgery is effective primarily if blood flow to viable cardiac muscle is reestablished:

Indications for emergency operation are as follows:

1. Complications of PTCA.
2. Ischemia that is uncontrolled by medical therapy.
3. Evolving myocardial infarction (MI).

The emergent CABG patient has either unstable hemodynamics (hypotension), unremitting chest pain despite maximal medical treatment, or the potential to become unstable (subjective assessment). Elective surgeries are utilized for those patients with hemodynamic stability and symptoms partially controlled through medical therapy. Unfortunately, surgical revascularization is not a curative therapy. Some patients require reoperation because of coronary artery disease progression or loss of graft patency. Patients undergoing reoperation have at least double the operative risk because the average age is higher and the atherosclerotic disease is more advanced. Patients undergoing reoperation tend to be more challenging to care for because of these considerations.

TABLE 13–1. INDICATIONS FOR INVASIVE REVASCULARIZATION PROCEDURES

- Stable angina refractory to medical therapy and interfering with the patient's ability to function at an acceptable level of activity.
- Exercise-induced hypotension or ventricular dysrhythmias secondary to myocardial ischemia
- Left ventricular dysfunction and clinical evidence of congestive heart failure
- Unstable angina
- Acute myocardial ischemia or infarction

Surgical Procedure

The surgical techniques utilized during CABG are unlikely to be covered on the CCRN exam. However, this section contains information that provides a useful background on the surgical procedure.

During CABG, several surgical techniques are employed to improve success rates. The patient is typically cooled to near 28–30°C (to reduce oxygen demands) and is placed on cardiopulmonary bypass (CPB). CPB is a technique for diverting blood from the heart during surgery while simultaneously oxygenating the blood and removing carbon dioxide. During CPB, three maneuvers help achieve safe and successful extracorporeal oxygenation: hemodilution, hypothermia, and anticoagulation. While these techniques help reduce complications, they also form the basis for many of the postoperative observations by the critical care nurse.

Physiologic consequences of CPB include the following:

1. Damage to blood elements (i.e., platelets, red blood cells, white blood cells, and plasma proteins).
2. Incorporation of abnormal substances into the blood (i.e., bubbles, fibrin particles, and platelet aggregates).
3. Systemic inflammatory response which results in an increased capillary permeability and fluid in the interstitial space.
4. An initial decrease in systemic vascular resistance, then a progressive increase as hypothermia is induced.
5. An increase in circulating catecholamines.
6. An increase in venous tone.

As fluid leaks from the blood vessels, the nurse should be alert for the need to give volume (either crystalloid or colloid) to maintain fluid status. Patients may gain several pounds following CPB due to the loss of vascular volume into the interstitial space. Careful observation of urine output to assess vascular volume is helpful. Impaired gas exchange as manifested by low arterial oxygen pressure/saturation (PaO_2/SaO_2) levels also indicates excess capillary leaking. Improved blood gases can indicate clearing of third space volume.

Postoperative bleeding is usually not due to CPB. Measurement of the partial thromboplastin time will best detect an excessive heparin effect from CPB. Protamine sulfate is given to reverse heparin-induced anticoagulation. Protamine sulfate can cause a severe adverse reaction accompanied by profound vasodilation and hypotension.

Postoperative Measures

The primary postoperative assessments following CABG involve hemodynamic monitoring, pain relief, dysrhythmia control, and recovery from surgical techniques such as CPB. Hemodynamic monitoring centers on maintaining adequate blood pressure, cardiac indices (greater than 2.2 L/min/m^2), and tissue oxygenation (SvO$_2$ above 0.60). Acceptable blood pressure and cardiac index are achieved through providing sufficient preload (assessed via central venous pressure (CVP) and/or pulmonary capillary wedge pressure (PCWP) monitoring), afterload reduction, and the use of inotropes to enhance contractility and maintain normal stroke volumes. As the patient warms postoperative, vasopressors may initially need to be used to maintain blood pressure. A temporary external pacemaker, antidysrhythmic agents, and sedatives may also be employed to optimize hemodynamic status.

More aggressive measures to maintain cardiac output may be required. This would include the use of artificial devices for mechanical support. Devices that may be utilized include an intraaortic balloon pump (IABP); ventricular assist devices (VADs) for right, left, or biventricular support; extracorporeal membrane oxygenator (ECMO); and CPB-portable system. However, few if any questions on the CCRN exam cover these aggressive measures at this time.

Problems encountered in the early postoperative period include the following:

1. Bleeding: either from a surgical site or due to a coagulopathy. This may result in cardiac tamponade. Postoperative blood loss should not exceed 300 mL/hr in the first several hours. After this time period, bleeding should be less than 150–200 mL/hr. The average blood loss is 1L total. The physician should be notified when blood loss is excessive. Autotransfusion is typically employed to aid in the replacement of normal blood loss. Autotransfusion is the reinfusion of shed mediastinal blood. In most centers all mediastinal blood shed is filtered and returned to the patient.
2. Low cardiac output syndrome: where the cardiac index is less than 2.0 L/min/m^2. Postoperative causes of low cardiac index include hypovolemia, elevated systemic vascular resistance (SVR), myocardial dysfunction, cardiac tamponade, and dysrhythmias.
3. Profound hypotension.
4. Hypertension.
5. Electrolyte imbalances (primarily hypokalemia).
6. Dysrhythmias (primarily PVCs, atrial fibrillation, atrial flutter).
7. Cardiac arrest.

Monitoring of temperatures is typically indicated by pulmonary artery or rectal (or bladder) temperature probes. The patient will attempt to rewarm through shivering; although this reflex is effective, the increase in oxygen consumption is undesirable. The nurse can aid in rewarming the patient through external methods (blankets, radiant lights) and internal methods (warmed blood, warmed inspired gases). Some institutions advocate the administration of paralytic agents to avoid the muscle activity associated with shivering. Avoidance of marked shivering is one key goal in the rewarming therapy.

During rewarming, the patient appears to be hypovolemic as vasodilation occurs. Volume replacement and vasopressors may be required to initially combat the decrease in PCWP and CVP, and less of SVR.

The nurse needs to maintain pain reduction while simultaneously allowing for recovery of ventilatory function. Aggressive pulmonary toilet via suctioning initially and then encouraging coughing will aid in reducing pulmonary complications. The nurse's support in pain reduction and the sensitivity shown for the patient's adjustment to temporary dependence on nursing will aid adaptation to the immediate postoperative recovery.

Dysrhythmia control centers on two factors. First, any metabolic disturbance that may precipitate either atrial or ventricular dysrhythmias should be corrected. For example, potassium (K$^+$) levels should be monitored when dysrhythmias, particularly ventricular ectopy (premature ventricular contractions, PVCs), exist. Second, pharmacological or electrical therapy can be utilized to control dysrhythmias. Pharmacological treatments are dictated by the type of dysrhythmia. For example, atrial tachycardias are treated with agents such as beta blockers (esmolol), calcium channel blockers (verapamil, diltiazem), adenosine, or a combination of these agents. Electrical cardioversion may also be used. Ventricular tachycardias and PVCs are treated with lidocaine, procainamide, or bretylium.

Electrical therapy is usually performed through epicardial pacing wires placed on the right atrium and ventricle near the end of the CABG procedure. These pacing wires can be used postoperatively to manage both supraventricular tachycardias and bradycardias. Postoperative bradycardia is the most common indication for use of the pacing wires. Atrial (for bradycardia) or atrioventricular (AV) sequential (for AV block) pacing is preferable to ventricular pacing, because atrial kick accounts for 15–30% of cardiac output. Certain dysrhythmias (paroxysmal atrial tachycardia, atrial flutter) may be treated with rapid overdrive pacing. A wide variety of external temporary pacemakers are available.

Complications of Cardiac Surgery

Potential complications of cardiac surgery include hemorrhage, cardiac tamponade, MI, ventricular dysfunction, dysrhythmias, and death. In addition, patients may be predisposed to problems with other organ systems (i.e., neural, pulmonary, renal).

Cardiac tamponade is one of the most challenging complications to manage in the postoperative period. Cardiac tamponade describes a condition in which the heart is compressed by blood that has accumulated in the pericardial space or mediastinum. The heart is unable to fill adequately causing cardiac output and blood pressure to fall. The usual signs of tamponade are enlargement of the cardiac silhouette on roentgenography, equalization of right and left heart filling pressures (CVP, PAD), pulsus paradoxus, and acute hypotension. Typically, patients with initially heavy bleeding from chest tubes suddenly stop bleeding and become hypotensive. Temporary measures to support cardiac function include volume administration and inotropic support. Emergent treatment involves reopening of the sternal incision in the ICU and an immediate return to the operating room.

Cardiac Transplantation

Heart transplantation is generally not covered on the CCRN exam. Nonetheless, transplantation may be an option for patients with cardiomyopathy, and you should be familiar with the procedure.

In patients with cardiomyopathies or reduced cardiac function from coronary artery disease, CABG will not improve cardiac performance. Replacement of the heart is indicated in patients with end-stage heart disease untreatable by medical or CABG intervention. Once identified as a candidate for transplantation and no contraindications to the transplant are present (Table 13–2), the patient is categorized as to severity. The patient typically has less than 1 year of expected survival without transplantation. The time between being placed on the

TABLE 13–2. ELIGIBILITY CRITERIA FOR CARDIAC TRANSPLANTATION

1. End-stage, ischemic, valvular, or congenital heart disease with maximal medical therapy, not amenable to conventional or high-risk surgery.
2. NYHA functional class III–IV congestive heart failure with maximal medical therapy.
3. Prognosis for 1 year survival <75%.
4. Age generally younger than 65 years.
5. Psychologically stable, compliant, reliable. Patient should be able to understand the procedure and risks involved.
6. Strong family support system.
7. Able to adhere to complex medical regimen.
8. Absence of the following contraindicating factors:
     Systemic disease or infection
     Serious, irreversible impairment of hepatic, renal, or pulmonary functions
     Recent cerebrovascular accident or neurologic deficits
     Recent pulmonary embolization or infarction
     Peptic ulcer disease
     Active substance abuse
     Pulmonary vascular resistance greater than 6 Wood units
     Psychological instability
     Malignancy
9. Relative contraindications:
     Advanced peripheral atherosclerosis
     Diabetes mellitus

list and undergoing transplantation is highly variable and can serve as a major source of anxiety to the potential recipient.

The success rate for transplantation is very good, with 1-year survival for heart transplantation at 76%, and thereafter there is approximately a 4% mortality per year over the subsequent 11 years. However, the shortage of donors means that not all patients who might benefit from transplantation actually undergo the procedure.

The surgical procedure has been improved since the time of the first transplantation in 1966, but the prime difference has been in the area of immunosuppression. Suppression of rejection through such agents as cyclosporine, azathioprine, and corticosteroids has been the major factor in improving outcome following transplantation.

Postoperative care is similar to that for CABG surgery with the exception of medications for immunosuppression. The electrocardiogram (ECG) has two sinus nodes initially (due to the retention of the recipient sinus node), and the recipient sinus node gives P waves unrelated to the QRS complex. Since the transplanted heart has no innervation from the autonomic nervous system, normal cardiac responses to various reflexes do not occur. In addition, the patient will feel no angina-like pain. Because of the denervation, sympathetic stimulants such as isoproterenol may be necessary to increase heart rate and support cardiac function until the ventricle adjusts to the absense of autonomic innervation.

Valvular Heart Disease

The cardiac valves provide for a unidirectional forward flow of blood through the heart. Dysfunctional cardiac valves are classified as stenotic or incompetent. When a cardiac valve restricts the forward flow of blood, it is referred to as stenotic. If the cardiac valve does not close competently, thereby allowing backward flow of blood, it is known as an incompetent (regurgitant, or insufficient) valve.

Valves that are stenotic cause an elevated afterload, subsequently resulting in hypertrophy of the atrium or the ventricle, which is contracting against the increased pressure load. Regurgitant valves allow blood to flow back into the preceding heart chamber, thus causing volume overload and dilation of the chamber.

The primary cause of acquired valvular heart disease is rheumatic fever. Other causes of valvular heart disease include infective endocarditis, degenerative changes of the tissue, trauma, papillary muscle rupture from myocardial infarction, systemic diseases, and others. The aortic valve and the mitral valve are more commonly affected by acquired valvular heart disease than the tricuspid or pulmonic valves.

Mitral insufficiency allows blood to be ejected back into the left atrium. The patient presents with dyspnea, orthopnea, paroxysmal nocturnal dyspnea, elevated PCWP, pulmonary hypertension, decreased cardiac output, crackles, holosystolic murmur heard best at the apex, S_3, atrial fibrillation, and signs of right heart failure. The progression of mitral insufficiency is slow and patients may remain asymptomatic for years. Postoperative care of patients requiring valvular surgery is similar to the general care of the cardiac surgery patient.

Mitral stenosis is most commonly due to rheumatic fever. The symptoms are produced as the size of the opening decreases. As the opening is reduced, symptoms that develop include dyspnea on exertion, progressive fatigue, cough, hemoptysis, right heart failure, elevated PCWP, elevated right ventricular pressures, and atrial fibrillation. Medical therapy for mitral stenosis includes treatment for pulmonary edema and anticoagulants for prophylaxis of embolization. However, the definitive treatment for mitral stenosis is surgical intervention.

Aortic insufficiency results in left ventricular (LV) overload causing dilation and hypertrophy of the left ventricle. The presentation of aortic insufficiency includes fatigue, dyspnea, paroxysmal nocturnal dyspnea, orthopnea, angina, widened pulse pressure, S_3, systolic murmur heard best in aortic area and Erb's point, sinus tachycardia, and elevated PCWP. Symptoms of heart failure, hypertension, and dysrhythmias are medically managed.

Aortic stenosis causes an obstruction of the blood from the left ventricle to the systemic circulation during systole. Symptoms of aortic stenosis include syncope, fatigue, palpitations, and angina. As the disease valve continues to narrow, symptoms of left heart failure develop. Surgical repair is the treatment of choice for patients with aortic disease. However, medical therapy is needed for angina, heart failure, and dysrhythmias.

Vascular Surgery

The two most common problems requiring vascular surgery are aneurysms and occlusions. Aneurysms are more problematic when they occur in major arteries. Occlusions are problematic when they occur in major arteries or veins.

Aortic Aneurysms

The two common types of aortic aneurysms are thoracic and abdominal. Abdominal aneurysms are more common (65% of aneurysms) than thoracic aneurysms. The aneurysm can typically take on one of two patterns: a weakness and bulging of the entire vessel wall, or a weakness within the vessel wall (intimal tear or dissection). It is estimated that 5% of individuals over the age of 60 have an abdominal aortic aneurysm (AAA).

Aortic Dissection

Aortic dissection is potentially life threatening because of rapid progression of shock, loss of vascular volume, potential bleeding into the pericardial sac (tamponade resulting), and disruption of the aortic valve with resultant LV failure. Ascending aortic involvement is more difficult to surgically correct than descending aortic dissecting aneurysms because of the proximity of the major cardiac structures.

The origin of aortic dissection is usually hypertension. The presentation is one of hypertension with severe unremitting chest and or abdominal pain frequently radiating to the back. Immediate surgical treatment is necessary. Medical management with antihypertensives can take place but may be unsuccessful.

Abdominal Aneurysms

Abdominal aneurysms may occasionally be identified by noting a palpable mass on physical exam. Symptoms may include abdominal or back pain with tenderness on palpation.

Diagnosis of Aneurysms

The use of computerized tomography (CT) and magnetic resonance imaging (MRI) to identify abdominal and thoracic vascular structures is common practice. Routine chest and abdominal x-rays and ultrasound may detect the aneurysm, although the detail is not as great as with CT or MRI. Angiography is a good test to demarcate the boundaries of the blood vessels.

Treatment of Aneurysms

Replacement of the aneurysm with a graft is the most common surgical intervention. Figure 13–1 contains an example of the surgical replacement technique. The closer the aneurysm is to the heart, the more difficult the surgery will be. Thoracic aneurysms of the descending aorta and abdominal aneurysms offer the surgeon a better operative field and reduce postoperative complications.

Currently investigation of endovascular surgical grafting techniques are being undertaken. If effective this will eliminate the need for cross-clamping the aorta and therefore decrease most of the complications of major aortic surgery.

Postoperative Considerations

The most serious complication following aortic surgery is MI, accounting for almost half of the postoperative mortality from aortic surgery. Monitoring cardiovascular performance such as cardiac index, stroke index or volume, PCWP, CVP, ST segments, and ECG rhythms is helpful in assessing cardiac performance.

The second most common complication is bleeding, which results from injury or from coagulopathies. The nurse must be aware of symptoms of hypovolemia (Chapter 10) indicating a potential bleed. The presence of a strong pulse on palpation of the femoral artery gives an indication of adequate patency of the aorta.

Renal failure, the third complication, is especially great in patients with pre-existing kidney disease. Acute renal failure is usually caused by periods of prolonged ischemia either from extended aortic cross-clamping above the renal arteries, hypotensive episodes before, during, or after surgery, and or atheroembolization of the renal arteries. Renal func-

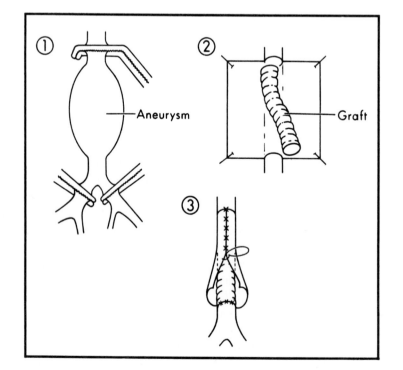

Figure 13–1. Aneurysm graft technique.

tion is assessed through measurement urine volume, intake and output, and serum and urine creatinine and electrolytes.

Acute limb ischemia is most commonly the result of atheroembolism and can occur in one or both legs. Significant cutaneous ischemia may occur despite maintenance of palpable pedal pulses (blue toe syndrome or trash foot). Assessment of pulses, skin color, temperature, movement, and sensation should be completed hourly. Pain in an extremity can be a significant indicator of acute ischemia.

Ruptured Abdominal Aortic Aneurysms

At least 50 percent of patients who experience ruptured abdominal aortic aneurysms (AAA) die before reaching the hospitals. Although the risk of rupture correlates with aneurysm size, even small aortic aneurysms can rupture. Symptoms most commonly associated with a ruptured AAA are abdominal and back pain, tender abdominal mass, hypotension, and/or shock. These symptoms occur in 50% or less of patients. The location of pain is dependent on the location of the retroperitoneal hematoma.

Mortality with a ruptured AAA ranges from 15 to 88%, and is most commonly the result of a delay in operating. The team needs to be prepared for massive infusion of fluid and blood products perioperatively. The same complications exist with the ruptured AAA as with elective AAA repair, but they occur with greater frequency. Patients with ruptured AAA repair have a 50% chance of renal failure and a 20% chance for a myocardial infarction. The patient usually has a longer ventilator course, and is more prone to colon ischemia than with elective AAA repair.

Bowel and spinal cord ischemias are less common complications but when they occur have high incidences of morbidity and mortality. Respiratory complications may be avoided through routine postoperative therapy, i.e., incentive spirometry, early ambulation and, if necessary, postural drainage and percussion.

Occlusive Disorders

Obstruction of arterial or venous flow due to atherosclerosis is the most common cardiovascular disturbance. Obstruction can occur anywhere along the major arterial tree, although in critical care settings, aortofemoral obstructions are most likely to bring the patient to the ICU setting.

Obstruction due to arterial flow usually results in pain on exercise. Lower-extremity obstruction is more common than upper-extremity obstruction. Pain in the legs upon activity due to obstruction is called intermittent claudication. Arterial obstructions are potentially more dangerous because of the loss of oxygen and substrates necessary for energy generation. Venous obstructions tend to be more chronic and are less likely to be seen in the critical care settings.

Clinical indications of decreased arterial blood flow include diminished pulses, loss of temperature (cool skin), change in color (cyanosis reflects venous obstruction, pallor reflects arterial obstruction), and diminished sensation. If the obstruction is sudden, severe pain distal to the obstruction is a common symptom.

Assessment of the need for surgery generally includes Doppler ultrasound studies and possibly abdominal aortic ultrasound and CT exams. Surgery is indicated when the patient has symptoms severe enough to restrict activities of daily living.

Surgical Intervention

The optimal surgical method to relieve obstruction to blood flow is dependent on the location of the obstruction. Figure 13–2 illustrates the most common types of surgical procedures to bypass obstructions of the aorta and femoral arteries.

Endovascular therapies (balloon angioplasties, atherectomy, and laser angioplasties) have not proven to be effective in peripherral vascular disease.

Postoperative Considerations

Assessment of blood flow is an important nursing measure both pre- and postoperatively. Blood flow assessment includes pulse quality, capillary refill, and sensation. Pulse presence does not necessarily mean that the graft has good patency. Doppler assessment is a better parameter to measure flow than is palpation.

Loss of flow following surgery can be due to failure of the bypass graft or obstruction as a result of clot formation. In the case of clot formation, the danger for potential embolization exists. In arterial surgery, the emboli will obstruct a site beyond the site of surgery and may result in loss of a portion of the extremity involved. If obstruction is on the venous side, the emboli will result in pulmonary embolization. Symptoms of pulmonary emboli are chest pain, shortness of breath, decreased PaO_2/SaO_2, and elevation of pulmonary artery pressures.

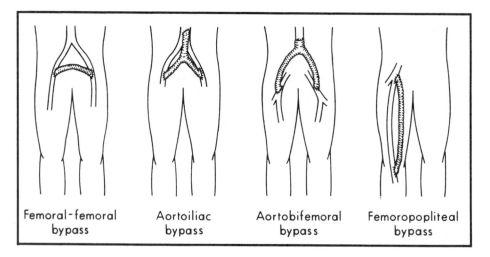

Femoral-femoral bypass   Aortoiliac bypass   Aortobifemoral bypass   Femoropopliteal bypass

Figure 13–2. Femoral vascular bypass techniques.

CARDIAC TRAUMA

EDITORS' NOTE

Expect two to four questions that cover cardiac trauma on the exam. This section, in conjunction with the previous sections, will enable the clinician to understand the hemodynamic effects of cardiovascular trauma.

Cardiac injuries can be some of the most life-threatening trauma injuries and are second in mortality only to neurological injuries. Most are the result of motor vehicle crashes, and are therefore the result of blunt trauma. There is an increasing number of chest injuries due to gunshot wounds and stabbings. Injury to the heart and or great vessels causing disruption of the structures can reduce circulating blood volume, and lead to hypovolemia and shock. Direct trauma to the heart muscle, as in myocardial contusion, can lead to a decrease in myocardial contraction, resulting in low cardiac output.

Cardiac Contusion

Cardiac contusion is the most common blunt injury to the heart. It is only rarely fatal. Suspect myocardial contusion if the patient has anterior chest wall trauma, and/or fractures of the sternum or ribs. Signs and symptoms are the same as for myocardial ischemia and/or infarction. Specific treatment is to monitor cardiac status with daily ECGs, since some ST- and T-wave changes may not become apparent for up to 48 hr. Dysrhythmias are the greatest con-

cern and are treated with standard antidysrhythmic agents as needed. Isoenzyme level elevations, specifically creatine phosphokinase-MB band and troponin I, are perhaps the most accurate indicators of myocardial injury. Two-dimensional echocardiography and/or multigated angiography may be useful in determining abnormalities in ventricular wall movement and ejection fraction. Severe visceral injury may result in delayed cardiac rupture, ventricular septal defect, and ventricular aneurysm, all of which would receive conventional treatment. Symptoms include angina-like chest pain, unexplained tachycardia, and after some time elapse, a pericardial friction rub.

Cardiac Rupture

This is a blunt trauma injury and is the most common cause of death. In sequence of frequency of rupture, it is right ventricle, left ventricle, right atrium, and left atrium. There is no treatment for cardiac rupture other than surgical intervention.

Valvular Injury

This is a blunt trauma injury. The aortic valve is the most commonly injured valve. Signs and symptoms are valve regurgitation and congestive heart failure. Specific treatment could include valve replacement or the normal medical treatment for congestive heart failure.

Cardiac Tamponade

This may result from blunt or penetrating trauma to the pericardium and/or the heart. Blood gets into the pericardial sac but cannot get out. As more blood enters the sac, more pressure is placed against the heart, which inhibits or compromises ventricular filling (Fig. 13–3). A subsequent decrease in stroke volume leads to a decrease in cardiac output.

Cardiac tamponade presents with hypotension, muffled or distant heart sounds, and distended neck veins. Additional clues are a falling systolic blood pressure, narrow pulse pressure, pulsus paradoxus (more than a 20 mm Hg drop in systolic blood pressure during inspiration), elevated central venous pressure, and various degrees of shock. In a trauma patient the classic symptoms may be obscured by hypovolemic shock.

Treatment and Nursing Intervention

The objective of treatment is to confirm the diagnosis and relieve the tamponade. This is best accomplished by a pericardiocentesis. Anesthesia is achieved with xylocaine. The patient is placed supine with the head elevated at a 45° angle. A 16- or 18-gauge, 6-inch or longer, over-the-needle catheter is attached to a 60-ml syringe. The needle is inserted at a 45° angle, lateral to the left side of the xiphoid, 1 to 2 cm inferior to the left of the xiphochondral junction (Fig. 13–4). Blood is aspirated during introduction of the needle. Usually some immediate improvement in cardiac performance is noted upon

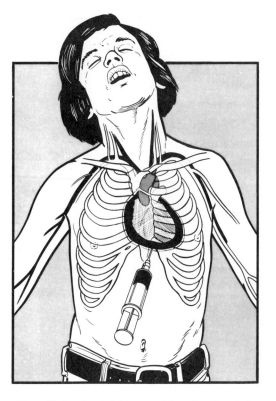

Figure 13–4. Paraxiphoid approach to pericardiocentesis.

aspiration of fluid from the pericardial sac. Pericardial blood should not clot. Rapid clotting of pericardial blood can mean the heart has been entered by the pericardial needle. The underlying cause for the tamponade must be determined. If pericardiocentesis does not relieve the tamponade, thoracotomy for direct repair of the pericardial wound is indicated.

Aortic Rupture

Aortic rupture is the result of blunt trauma deceleration injury. Although most patients die immediately, 10 to 20% survive to reach a hospital when a tamponade occurs around the rupture. This allows some blood to leave the left ventricle and pass beyond the distal end of the rupture.

Aortic rupture is diagnosed by aortogram. Roentgenography may reveal a widened mediastinum, which is suggestive of aortic rupture. The aortogram will identify the area of rupture. Figure 13–5 identifies the most common sites of aortic rupture.

Symptoms may include an increased blood pressure and pulse in the upper extremities, a decreased blood pressure and pulse in the lower

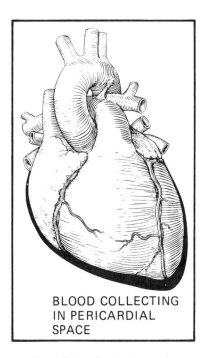

BLOOD COLLECTING IN PERICARDIAL SPACE

Figure 13–3. Cardiac tamponade.

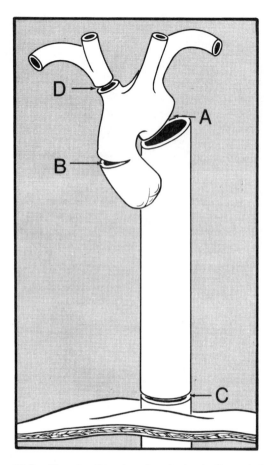

Figure 13–5.   Sites of aortic rupture. A, arch of aorta; B, area just above aortic valve; C, end of thoracic aorta; D, subclavian vein. The aortic arch is the most common site; the subclavian vein is the least common.

extremities, and the X-ray picture of a widened mediastinum. Shortness of breath, weakness, chest or back pain, and varied abnormalities involving the lower extremities may be present.

Treatment and Nursing Intervention

Treatment consists of thoracotomy to repair the rupture. If the thoractomy cannot be performed immediately, the patient is medically treated as a patient with dissecting aortic aneurysm until surgery.

Nursing interventions include monitoring the respiratory, cardiovascular, neurologic, and renal systems, since these suffer first due to the decreased blood flow. Sodium nitroprusside is usually administered until the patient can be taken to surgery. Nursing care of the patient on ventilatory support and in need of close monitoring before and after surgery applies to the patient with a ruptured aorta.

CARDIOVASCULAR BIBLIOGRAPHY

Ahrens, T.S., & Taylor, L. (1992). *Hemodynamic Waveform Analysis.* Philadelphia: W.B. Saunders.

Anderson, L.A. (1994). An update on the cause of abdominal aortic aneurysms. *J Vasc Nurs, 12*(4), 95–100.

Appel-Hardin, S. (1992). The role of the critical care nurse in noninvasive temporary pacing. *Crit Care Nurse, 12,* 10–19.

Baumgartner, W.A., Owens, S.G., Cameron, D.E., & Reitz, B.A. *The Johns Hopkins Manual of Cardiac Surgical Care.* St. Louis: C.V. Mosby, 1994.

Benedict, C.R., Mueller, S., Anderson, H.V., & Willerson, J.T. (1992). Thrombolytic therapy: A state of the art review. *Hosp Pract, 27,* 61–72.

DeAngelis, R. (1991). The cardiovascular system. In *Core Curriculum for Critical Care Nursing,* 4 ed. Ed. Alspach, J.G. Philadelphia: W.B. Saunders, 132–314.

Dracup K. (1995). *Meltzer's Intensive Coronary Care: A Manual for Nurses,* 5 ed. Stamford, CT: Appleton & Lange.

Emergency Nurses Association (1995). *Trauma Nursing Core Course,* 4 ed.

Finkelmeier, B.A. (1995). Diagnostic evaluation of cardiac disease. In *Cardiothoracic Surgical Nursing.* Philadelphia: J.B. Lippincott.

Hatswell, E.M. (1994). Abdominal aortic aneurysm surgery, Part I: An overview and discussion of immediate perioperative complications. *Heart Lung, 23*(3), 228–239.

Hatswell, E.M. (1994). Abdominal Aortic Aneurysm Surgery, Part II: Major complications and nursing implications. *Heart Lung, 23*(4), 337–341.

Hosenpud, J.D., Novick, R.J., Breen, T.J., Keck, B., & Daily, P. (1995). The registry of the International Society for Heart and Lung Transplantation: Twelfth official report—1995. *J Heart Lung Transplant, 14*(5), 805–815.

Hurn, P.D., & Hartsock, R.L. (1994). Thoracic Injuries. In *Trauma Nursing from Resuscitation through Rehabilitation.* Ed. Cardona, V.D. Philadelphia: W.B. Saunders.

Ide, B. (1995). Bedside electrocardiographic assessment. *J Cardiovasc Nurs, 9,* 10–23.

Joint National Committee on Detection, Evaluation and Treatment of High Blood Pressure. (1984). The 1984 Report of the Joint National Committee. *Arch Intern Med, 144,* 1045.

Kennedy, G., issue ed. (1996). Advanced heart failure. Reigel, B., & Vitello-Cicciu, J.M., journal eds. *J Cardiovasc Nurs, 10*(2).

Kinney, M.R., Packa, D.R., Andreoli, K.G., & Zipes, D.P. (1991). *Comprehensive Cardiac Care,* 7 ed. St. Louis: C.V. Mosby.

LeDoux, D. (1995). *12 Lead ECG Interpretation: A Self-Teaching Manual.* St. Louis: McGraw-Hill.

Lefor, N., Cardello, F.P., & Felicetta, J.V. (1992). Recognizing and treating Torsade de Pointes. *Crit Care Nurse, 12,* 20–29.

McGriffin, D.C., Kirklin, J.K. (1995). Cardiopulmonary bypass for cardiac surgery. In *Surgery of the Chest*, 6 ed. Ed. Sabison, D.C., Jr., & Spencer, F.C. Philadelphia: W.B. Saunders.

Mullholland, G.C., & Brewer, B.B. (1990). *Improving Your Skills in 12-Lead ECG Interpretation.* Baltimore: Williams & Wilkins.

Norman, A.E. (1992). *12 Lead ECG Interpretation: A Self-Teaching Manual.* St. Louis: McGraw-Hill.

Notterman, D.A. (1991). Inotropic agents. Catecholamines, digoxin, amrinone. *Crit Care Clin, 7,* 583–613.

Perler, B. (1995). Ruptured Abdominal Aortic Aneurysm. In *Current Surgical Therapy.* Ed. Cameron, J.L. St. Louis: C.V. Mosby.

Prolux, R., Guidetti, K., Bagg, A.M., & Marchette, L. (1992). Detection of right ventricular myocardial infarction in patients with inferior wall myocardial infarction. *Crit Care Nurse, 12,* 50–59.

Schlant, R.C., & Sonnenblick, E.H. (1994). Pathophysiology of heart failure. In *Hurst's The Heart,* 8 ed. Ed. Schlant, R.C., Alexander, R.W., O'Rourke, R.A., Roberts, R., & Sonnenblick, E.H., McGraw-Hill: New York.

Smith, T.W., & Kelly, R.A. (1992). Therapeutic strategies for CHF in the 1990s. *Hosp Pract 26,* 127–150.

Stier, F. (1992). Antidysrhythmic agents. *AACN Clin Issues Crit Care, 3,* 483–493.

Sweetwood, H.M. (1983). *Clinical Electrocardiography for Nurses.* Rockville, MD: Aspen.

Warbinek, E., & Wyness, M.A. (1994). Caring for patients with complications after elective abdominal aortic aneurysm surgery: A case study. *J Vasc Nurs, 12*(3), 73–79.

Williams, G.M. (1995). Ruptured abdominal aortic aneurysm. *Current Surgical Therapy.* Ed. Cameron, J.L. St. Louis: C.V. Mosby.

Cardiovascular Practice Exam

Questions 1 and 2 are based on the following scenario:

A 69-year-old male is admitted to the unit with the diagnosis of acute inferior wall MI (myocardial infarction). He has a history of peripheral vascular disease and COPD (chronic obstructive pulmonary disease). During your shift he begins to complain of shortness of breath. His 12-lead ECG shows ST-segment depression in leads V1–V4. He has dependent crackles in his posterior lobes along with expiratory wheezing. His pulse oximeter is reading 0.95 on 2 L/min per nasal cannula. He has the following laboratory data:

pH	7.37
$PaCO_2$	52
PaO_2	69
HCO_3	33
CPK	33
CPK-MB	4
troponin I	0.5

He has an S_3 (gallop) and a II/VI systolic murmur. The following hemodynamic information is available:

blood pressure	104/60
pulse	114
cardiac index	2.0
cardiac output	4.4
arterial pressure	40/24
PCWP	22
CVP	11

1. Based on this information, what is likely happening?
   (A) exacerbation of the COPD
   (B) development of congestive heart failure
   (C) development of inferior MI
   (D) development of pericardial tamponade

2. Based on the above information, what would be the best treatment to improve the symptoms?
   (A) oxygen therapy
   (B) dopamine
   (C) nicardipine
   (D) dobutamine

3. A 76-year-old female is in the unit with the diagnosis of CHF (congestive heart failure). The physician inserts a pulmonary artery catheter to aid in assessment of therapeutic interventions. One of the therapies she selects is dobutamine. With the addition of dobutamine to the treatment regimen, which parameters would you expect to see change if the therapy is successful?
   (A) increase in stroke volume
   (B) increase in wedge pressure
   (C) increase in systemic vascular resistance
   (D) decrease in mean arterial pressure

Questions 4 and 5 are based on the following scenario:

A 71-year-old male is admitted to the unit with shortness of breath, orthopnea, and progressive reduction in exercise tolerance. He states he has "not ever been to a doctor." His lung sounds demonstrate crackles in most of his posterior lobes. A pulse oximeter indicates a value of 0.89. A pulmonary artery catheter is placed to help identify the origin of the shortness of breath. The following data are available:

blood pressure	118/70
pulse	110
respiratory rate	28
temperature	37.1
cardiac index	2.2
stroke index	20
arterial pressure	36/22
PCWP	20
CVP	6

4. Based on the above information, what condition is likely developing?
   (A) noncardiogenic pulmonary edema
   (B) primary pulmonary hypertension
   (C) sepsis
   (D) left ventricular failure

5. What therapy would most likely improve his symptoms?
   (A) oxygen therapy
   (B) phenylephrine
   (C) furosemide
   (D) gentamycin

6. What is the approximate normal right atrial CVP (central venous pressure) value?
   (A) 2 to 6 mm Hg
   (B) 5 to 10 mm Hg
   (C) 8 to 12 mm Hg
   (D) 12 to 18 mm Hg

7. Which of the following is the outermost lining of the heart?
   (A) endocardium
   (B) myocardium
   (C) transcardium
   (D) pericardium

8. Which of the following statements regarding the coronary sinus is correct?
   (A) It provides arterial blood flow to the lateral left ventricular wall.
   (B) It provides arterial blood flow to the sinus node.
   (C) It is the main venous drainage vessel of the heart.
   (D) It stimulates secretion of the atrial naturietic factor.

9. Left atrial pressure approximates which pressure?
   (A) pulmonary mean pressure
   (B) left ventricular end diastolic pressure
   (C) right atrial pressure
   (D) CVP (central venous pressure)

10. Of the following four factors, three determine stroke volume. Identify the factor that does NOT affect stroke volume.
    (A) preload
    (B) afterload
    (C) contractility
    (D) mean arterial pressure

11. Which of the following are atrioventricular valves?
    (A) mitral and tricuspid
    (B) pulmonic and aortic
    (C) mitral and aortic
    (D) tricuspid and pulmonic

12. The A wave on the CVP (central venous pressure) and PCWP (pulmonary capillary wedge pressure) tracing represents which physical event?
    (A) ventricular filling
    (B) atrial contraction
    (C) atrial filling
    (D) tricuspid and mitral valve movement

13. The C wave on the CVP (central venous pressure) and PCWP (pulmonary capillary wedge pressure) tracing occurs due to which anatomic event?
    (A) pulmonic and tricuspid valve closure
    (B) aortic and mitral valve opening
    (C) mitral and tricuspid valve closure
    (D) mitral and tricuspid valve opening

14. What is the normal right ventricular end diastolic pressure?
    (A) 2 to 6 mm Hg
    (B) 5 to 10 mm Hg
    (C) 10 to 15 mm Hg
    (D) >20 mm Hg

15. Which of the following is an estimate of right ventricular preload?
    (A) pulmonary capillary wedge pressure
    (B) central venous pressure
    (C) pulmonary artery mean pressure
    (D) coronary sinus pressure

16. Afterload is estimated by which parameter?
    (A) CVP (central venous pressure)
    (B) PCWP (pulmonary capillary wedge pressure)
    (C) stroke volume
    (D) SVR (systemic vascular resistance)

17. Which hemodynamic waves are produced by the atria?
    (A) A, C, and V waves
    (B) arterial systolic waves
    (C) augmented diastolic waves
    (D) X, Y, and Z waves

18. Left ventricular (LV) failure alone presents with all but one of the following signs. Select the INCORRECT sign.
    (A) increased CVP (central venous pressure)
    (B) increased PCWP (pulmonary capillary wedge pressure)
    (C) increased LV end diastolic pressure
    (D) increased pulmonary mean arterial pressure

19. Two circumstances may produce a systolic murmur. One exists when backward flow of blood (regurgitant flow) occurs through a valve that is normally closed during systole. The second exists when blood has difficulty getting past a valve (stenosis) that is normally easily opened. Which two situations may produce a systolic murmur?
(A) aortic stenosis and mitral regurgitation
(B) pulmonic regurgitation and tricuspid stenosis
(C) aortic and tricuspid stenosis
(D) pulmonic and mitral regurgitation

20. Which part of the ECG (electrocardiogram) correlates to a diastolic murmur?
(A) PR interval
(B) QRS complex
(C) ST segment
(D) post-T wave

21. The PCWP (pulmonary capillary wedge pressure) is used to estimate which of the following pressures?
(A) left atrial pressure and left ventricular end diastolic pressure
(B) right atrial pressure and right ventricular end diastolic pressure
(C) central venous and pulmonary arterial pressures
(D) mean pulmonary artery and right ventricular peak pressures

22. Pericardial tamponade presents with all but one of the following symptoms. Identify the symptom NOT associated with pericardial tamponade.
(A) equalization of left and right atrial pressures [CVP (central venous pressure) and PCWP (pulmonary capillary wedge pressure)]
(B) left ventricular failure without right ventricular involvement
(C) hypotension
(D) distended neck veins

23. Left ventricular (LV) preload is estimated from all of the following pressures but one. Identify the one pressure that does NOT permit one to estimate left ventricular preload.
(A) CVP (central venous pressure)
(B) PCWP (pulmonary capillary wedge pressure)
(C) left atrial pressure
(D) LV end diastolic pressure

24. Right ventricular failure is manifested by which of the following signs?

(A) increased CVP (central venous pressure)
(B) increased PCWP (pulmonary capillary wedge pressure)
(C) decreased pulmonary artery pressure
(D) increased systemic arterial pressure

Questions 25 and 26 refer to the following scenario:

A 62-year-old male is admitted to your unit with the diagnosis of acute subendocardial infarction. He presently has no chest pain and vital signs are normal. As you are talking with him, he complains of sudden, severe shortness of breath. His blood pressure is 80/50, pulse 118, respiratory rate 34. Heart sounds are easily heard but he has a new systolic murmur, grade V/VI. Hemodynamic data indicate the following:

pulmonary arterial pressure	38/25
PCWP	24
CVP	7
cardiac output	3.2
cardiac index	1.7

25. Based on the preceding information, which condition is likely to be developing?
(A) pericardial tamponade
(B) mitral valve rupture
(C) ventricular wall rupture
(D) aortic valve rupture

26. Which treatment would be indicated for this condition?
(A) immediate surgery
(B) dopamine nitroprusside
(C) fluid challenges
(D) thrombolytic therapy

27. Dysfunction of the papillary muscle producing mitral regurgitation would be seen in which part of the left atrial PCWP (pulmonary capillary wedge pressure) tracing?
(A) giant A waves
(B) absent A waves
(C) giant C waves
(D) giant V waves

28. Phase 0 of cellular impulse transmission refers to which phase of electrical action?
(A) depolarization
(B) early repolarization
(C) end repolarization
(D) myocardial relaxation

29. Spontaneous diastolic depolarization occurs during which phase of the cardiac action potential?

(Answers cont'd.)

(A) phase 0
(B) phase 1
(C) phase 3
(D) phase 4

30. Which electrolyte is responsible for initial depolarization?
(A) sodium
(B) potassium
(C) chloride
(D) calcium

31. Which cation activates the second (slow channel) inward flow of ions during cardiac depolarization?
(A) sodium
(B) potassium
(C) chloride
(D) calcium

32. Which ion leaves the cell during depolarization to counter the inward flow of sodium?
(A) phosphate
(B) potassium
(C) chloride
(D) calcium

33. Which of the following cardiac chambers contains deoxygenated blood?
(A) right ventricle
(B) left ventricle
(C) pulmonary veins
(D) left atrium

34. Where is the SA (sinoatrial) node located?
(A) right atrium
(B) left atrium
(C) right ventricle
(D) superior vena cava

35. Which component of blood pressure regulation has the strongest effect on controlling the blood pressure?
(A) stroke volume
(B) cardiac output
(C) systemic vascular resistance
(D) mean arterial pressure

36. Which of the following corresponds most closely to the normal ejection fraction?
(A) 10 to 20%
(B) 25 to 35%
(C) 40 to 50%
(D) >60%

37. Starling's law refers to which of the following relationships?

(A) As fluid fills the lungs, gas exchange decreases.
(B) As coronary blood flow increases, preload falls.
(C) As afterload increases, stroke volume improves.
(D) As muscle stretches, contraction strength increases.

38. Normally, at approximately which PCWP (pulmonary capillary wedge pressure) does lung water begin to accumulate?
(A) 8 to 12 mm Hg
(B) 12 to 18 mm Hg
(C) >18 mm Hg
(D) PCWP pressure does not correlate with lung water

39. Which of the following is the most common reason for the PCWP (pulmonary capillary wedge pressure) and CVP (central venous pressure) to increase?
(A) left and right ventricular failure
(B) excess blood volume
(C) right ventricular failure
(D) pulmonary hypertension

40. Reduction of myocardial oxygen consumption is best achieved through which of the following changes?
(A) reducing afterload
(B) reducing preload
(C) increasing contractility
(D) increasing preload

41. Which neurological structure or system has the strongest effect on regulating the heart rate?
(A) sympathetic nervous system
(B) parasympathetic nervous system
(C) adrenergic system
(D) cerebellum

42. Which of the following could produce giant A waves?
(A) aortic stenosis
(B) mitral regurgitation
(C) mitral stenosis
(D) hypovolemia

43. Posterior hemiblock is seen when which conduction defect occurs?
(A) obstruction of the left main bundle branch
(B) obstruction of the right main bundle branch
(C) blockage of the posterior portion of the right bundle
(D) blockage of the posterior portion of the left bundle

44. What is the preferred first treatment for ventricular fibrillation?
    (A) CPR (cardiopulmonary resuscitation)
    (B) lidocaine, 1 mg/kg
    (C) synchronized cardioversion, 50 to 100 joules
    (D) defibrillation, 200 to 300 joules

45. Which of the the following leads are used in the diagnosis of an inferior MI (myocardial infarction)?
    (A) V_1, V_2, V_3, V_4
    (B) I, aVL
    (C) V_5, V_6
    (D) II, III, aVF

46. Which of the following leads are used in the diagnosis of an anterior MI (myocardial infarction)?
    (A) V_1, V_2, V_3, V_4
    (B) I, aVL
    (C) V_5, V_6
    (D) II, III, aVF

47. Which of the following leads are used in the diagnosis of a lateral MI (myocardial infarction)?
    (A) V_1, V_2, V_3, V_4
    (B) I, aVL, V_5, V_6
    (C) V_{2R}, V_{3R}, V_{4R}
    (D) II, III, aVF

48. Which of the following leads are used in the diagnosis of a right ventricular MI (myocardial infarction)?
    (A) V_1, V_2, V_3, V_4
    (B) I, aVL, V_5, V_6
    (C) aVR, aVL, aVF
    (D) V_1, V_2, V_{4R}, V_{6R}

49. An atrial premature beat with aberrant conduction usually has which of the following characteristics?
    (A) left bundle branch block
    (B) left anterior hemiblock
    (C) right bundle branch block
    (D) posterior hemiblock

50. Interpret the following ECG rhythm strip. Sinus rhythm with: *See art below.*
    (A) left ventricular PVC (premature ventricular contraction)
    (B) APC (atrial premature contraction) with aberrant conduction
    (C) right ventricular PVC
    (D) interpolated PVC

51. Interpret the following ECG rhythm strip. *See art below.*
    (A) sinus tachycardia
    (B) atrial tachycardia

(Answers cont'd.)

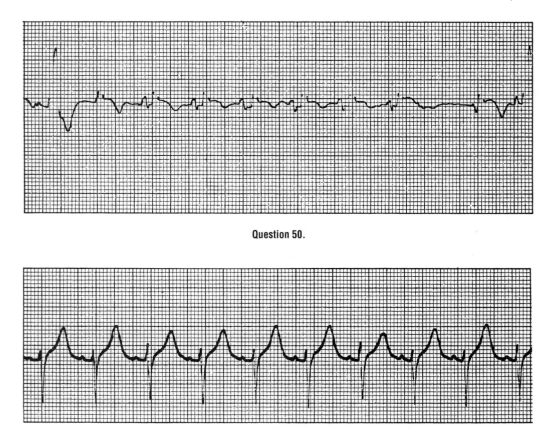

Question 50.

Question 51.

(C) atrial flutter
(D) atrial fibrillation

52. Interpret the following ECG rhythm strip. *See art below.*
(A) sinus tachycardia
(B) atrial tachycardia
(C) atrial flutter
(D) atrial fibrillation

53. Interpret the following ECG rhythm strip. *See art below.*

(A) sinus tachycardia
(B) atrial tachycardia
(C) atrial flutter
(D) atrial fibrillation

54. Interpret the following ECG rhythm strip. *See art below.*
(A) sinus tachycardia
(B) atrial tachycardia
(C) atrial flutter
(D) atrial fibrillation

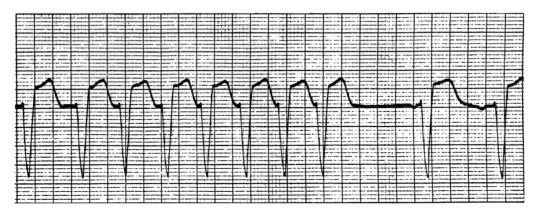

Question 52.

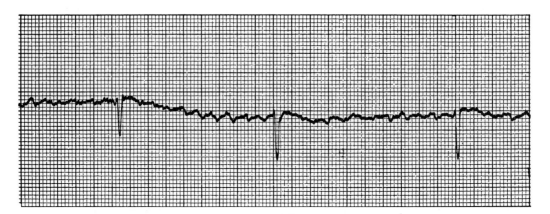

Question 53.

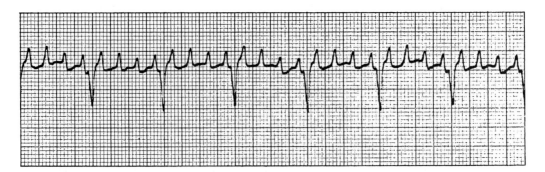

Question 54.

55. Interpret the following ECG rhythm strip. *See art below.*
    (A) first-degree block
    (B) second-degree block, type I
    (C) second-degree block, type II
    (D) third-degree block

56. Interpret the following ECG rhythm strip. *See art below.*

    (A) first-degree block
    (B) second-degree block, type I
    (C) second-degree block, type II
    (D) third-degree block

57. Interpret the following ECG rhythm strip. *See art below.*
    (A) first-degree block
    (B) second-degree block, type I

(Answers cont'd.)

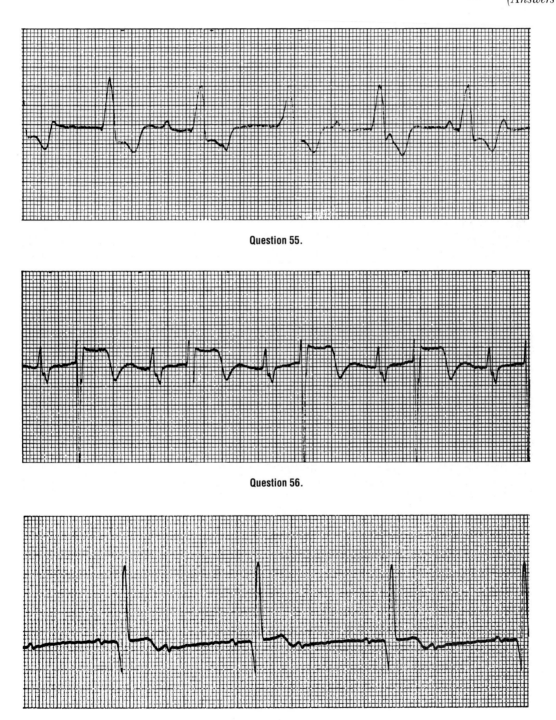

Question 55.

Question 56.

Question 57.

(C) second-degree block, type II

(D) third-degree block

58. Interpret the following ECG rhythm strip. *See art below.*
    (A) first-degree block
    (B) second-degree block, type I
    (C) second-degree block, type II
    (D) third-degree block

59. Interpret the following ECG rhythm strip. *See art below.*

(A) multiform PVC (premature ventricular contraction)

(B) ventricular tachycardia

(C) ventricular fibrillation

(D) SVT with abberancy

60. Interpret the following ECG rhythm strip. Atrial fibrillation with: *See art below.*
    (A) multiform PVC (premature ventricular contraction)
    (B) ventricular tachycardia

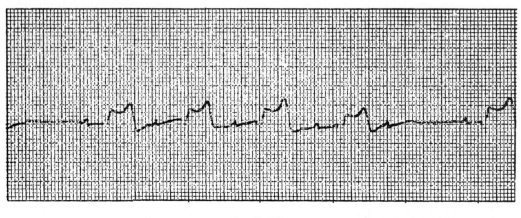

Question 58.

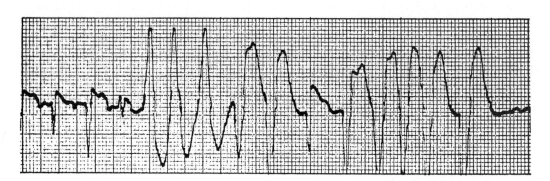

Question 59.

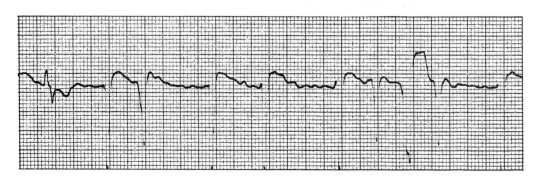

Question 60.

(C) ventricular fibrillation
(D) torsade de pointes

61. Interpret the following ECG rhythm strip. *See art below.*
    (A) multiform PVC (premature ventricular contraction)
    (B) ventricular tachycardia
    (C) ventricular fibrillation
    (D) torsade de pointes

62. APCs (atrial premature contractions) with abberant conduction can be differentiated from PVCs (premature ventricular contractions) by noting ECG changes. All of the following but one are associated with PVCs rather than APCs. Identify the one associated with APCs.
    (A) taller left peak (Rr') in V_1
    (B) right bundle branch block
    (C) marked left axis deviation
    (D) rS pattern in V_6

63. Which of the following corresponds most closely to the definition of precordial concordancy?
    (A) rsR' in V_1 to V_4
    (B) all QRS complexes have the same axis in V_1 to V_6
    (C) all T waves are inverted in V_1 to V_6
    (D) left axis deviation in I and aVF

64. Inferior MIs (myocardial infarctions) produce conduction defects different from those seen in anterior MIs. Which type of dysrhythmia is more likely to occur in inferior than anterior MIs?
    (A) second-degree type I
    (B) second-degree type II
    (C) multiform PVCs (premature ventricular contractions)
    (D) APCs (atrial premature contractions) with aberrancy

65. Anterior hemiblock is manifested by which of the following 12-lead ECG patterns?

(A) left axis deviation greater than −30°
(B) right axis deviation greater than +90°
(C) Q wave in V_1 to V_3
(D) large R wave in I and aVL

66. Posterior hemiblock is manifested by which of the following 12-lead ECG patterns?
    (A) left axis deviation greater than −30°
    (B) right axis deviation greater than +90°
    (C) Q wave in V_1 to V_3
    (D) large R wave in I and aVL

67. Left ventricular hypertrophy is manifested by which of the following ECG changes?
    (A) left anterior hemiblock patterns
    (B) left bundle branch block patterns
    (C) S wave in V_1 and R wave in V_5 totaling more than 35 mm
    (D) R wave in III and S wave in aVL totaling greater than 30 mm

68. Right ventricular hypertrophy is manifested by which of the following ECG changes?
    (A) right anterior hemiblock patterns
    (B) right bundle branch block patterns
    (C) S wave in V_1 and R wave in V_5 totaling more than 35 mm
    (D) R:S ratio greater than 1:1 in V_1

69. Which of the following is NOT an example of atrioventricular (AV) dissociation?
    (A) ventricular tachycardia
    (B) third-degree heart block
    (C) first-degree heart block
    (D) atrial tachycardia with 2:1 block

70. What is the initial treatment of sinus tachycardia?
    (A) verapamil
    (B) initially try carotid massage, then give digoxin
    (C) esmolol or propranolol
    (D) There is no primary treatment; find the source of the tachycardia.

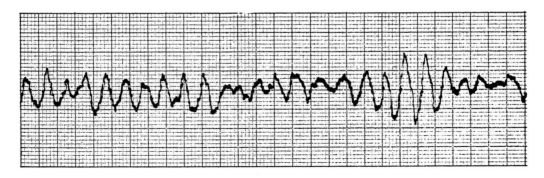

Question 61.

71. Which of the physical treatments listed below is NOT a form of parasympathetic stimulation for atrial tachycardia?
    (A) carotid massage
    (B) pressure on the eyeball
    (C) Valsalva manuever
    (D) hepatojugular reflux

Questions 72 and 73 refer to the following scenario:

A 65-year-old male is admitted to your unit with chest pain. The chest pain developed 2 hr ago at home. The pain went away for a while while he rested but then returned. Currently, he has substernal chest pain radiating to the left arm and chin. The pain is the same regardless of position. No change in the pain occurs during inspiration. Vital signs are as follows: blood pressure 132/86, pulse 96, respiratory rate 25. His 12-lead ECG shows depressed ST segments in the inferior leads. Small Q waves, less than one-third the height of the R wave, are present in the inferior leads.

72. Based on the preceding information, which condition is likely to be developing?
    (A) angina
    (B) acute myocardial infarction
    (C) pericarditis
    (D) pericardial tamponade

73. What would be the most likely treatment for the condition?
    (A) nitrates and beta blockers
    (B) thrombolytic therapy
    (C) pericardiocentesis
    (D) aspirin and analgesics

Questions 74 and 75 refer to the following scenario:

A 72-year-old male is admitted to your unit with the diagnosis of anterior MI (myocardial infarction). During your shift, you notice that he has developed a 2:1 heart block and a constant PR interval, with a ventricular response rate of 42. His blood pressure is 84/50.

74. Based on the preceding information and considering the type of MI (myocardial infarction), which type of heart block is likely?
    (A) first-degree
    (B) second-degree type I
    (C) second-degree type II
    (D) third-degree

75. Which treatment is likely to be most effective in stabilizing this rhythm?
    (A) pacemaker
    (B) calcium chloride
    (C) dopamine
    (D) epinephrine

76. For what does the first letter in VVI stand?
    (A) ventricular paced
    (B) ventricular sensed
    (C) ventricular inhibited
    (D) ventricular programmed

77. For what does the second letter in VVI stand?
    (A) ventricular paced
    (B) ventricular sensed
    (C) ventricular inhibited
    (D) ventricular programmed

78. In the following rhythm strip, identify the pacemaker operational state. *See art below.*
    (A) capturing properly at 1:1
    (B) failing to sense
    (C) failing to capture
    (D) producing pacemaker-generated ventricular ectopic beats

79. Which of the following is an advantage of a transcutaneous pacemaker?
    (A) It is easy to apply.
    (B) It requires lower electrical stimulation to capture the heart rate.

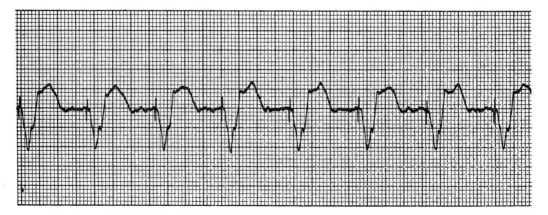

Question 78.

(C) It requires peripheral intravenous access.

(D) Electrical stimulation is not perceived by the patient.

Questions 80 and 81 refer to the following scenario:

A 45-year-old male is admitted to the unit with the diagnosis of inferior MI (myocardial infarction). Currently, he has no chest pain or shortness of breath. Two hours after admission, he develops a bradycardia of 50 beats/min with a blood pressure of 86/54. He also develops uniform PVCs (premature ventricular contractions) at the rate of 10/min.

80. Based on the diagnosis of inferior MI (myocardial infarction), how long will the bradycardia last?
    (A) It usually will be permanent and symptomatic.
    (B) It usually will be transient and possibly symptomatic.
    (C) Bradycardias are so uncommon with inferior MIs that some degree of CHF (congestive heart failure) must be present and the bradycardia will exist until the CHF is resolved.
    (D) It usually will be permanent but asymptomatic.

81. Treatment for this dysrhythmia would most likely include which medication?
    (A) lidocaine
    (B) dopamine
    (C) atropine
    (D) diltiazen

82. What is the inherent rate of the AV (atrioventricular) node area?
    (A) 20 to 40
    (B) 40 to 60
    (C) 60 to 80
    (D) The AV node area has no inherent rate.

83. Anterior MIs (myocardial infarctions) produce conduction defects different from those seen in inferior MIs. Which type of dysrhythmia is more likely to occur in anterior than inferior MIs?
    (A) APCs (atrial premature contractions) with aberrancy
    (B) second-degree type I
    (C) second-degree type II
    (D) multiform PVCs (premature ventricular contractions)

84. Passage of the electrical impulse through the AV (atrioventricular) node is represented by which ECG complex?
    (A) PR interval
    (B) QRS complex
    (C) ST segment
    (D) T wave

85. Atrial tachycardia is initially treated with which pharmacological agent?
    (A) atropine or isoproterenol
    (B) diltiazem or adenosine
    (C) digitalis or pronestyl
    (D) propranolol or metaprolal

Questions 86 and 87 refer to the following scenario:

A 66-year-old female is admitted to your unit with the diagnosis of anterolateral MI (myocardial infarction). She has no complaints of chest pain or discomfort. While you are interviewing her, she goes into the rhythm displayed below. You ask her how she feels and she replies "I feel fine. You look worried though. Is something wrong?" Her blood pressure is 118/78.

86. What is your interpretation of the dysrhythmia?
    See art below.
    (A) accelerated idioventricular rhythm
    (B) aberrantly conducted APCs (atrial premature contractions)

(Answers cont'd.)

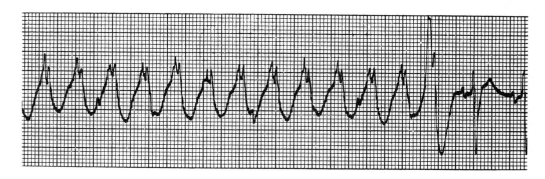

Question 86.

(C) artifact

(D) ventricular tachycardia

87. What would be the treatment for this rhythm?
    (A) observation; no treatment necessary
    (B) lidocaine
    (C) synchronized defibrillation at 50 joules
    (D) unsynchronized defibrillation at 200 joules

88. A junctional rhythm has all of the following characteristics but one. Which of the following characteristics is NOT indicative of a junctional rhythm?
    (A) normal QRS complex
    (B) wide QRS complex
    (C) heart rate between 40 and 60 beats/min
    (D) absent P waves

89. Which lead is most likely to detect aberrantly conducted APCs (atrial premature contractions)?
    (A) lead II
    (B) lead III
    (C) lead aVF
    (D) V_1 lead

90. Of the following findings, all but one indicate an increased seriousness of PVCs (premature ventricular contractions). Select the factor that does NOT increase the seriousness of PVCs.
    (A) uniform appearance
    (B) multiform complexes
    (C) PVC on T wave (R on T phenomenon)
    (D) frequency greater than 10/min

91. APCs (atrial premature contractions) with aberrant conduction can be differentiated from PVCs (premature ventricular contractions) by noting ECG changes. All of the following findings but one are associated with APCs rather than PVCs. Identify the one associated with PVCs.
    (A) second R wave larger than the first in V_1
    (B) right bundle branch block
    (C) right axis deviation
    (D) A-V dissociation

92. Which of the following isoenzymes is most diagnostic in identifying MI (myocardial infarction)?
    (A) CPK (creatine phosphokinase)—MB band
    (B) CPK—MM band
    (C) CPK—BB band
    (D) LDH (lactic acid dehydrogenase)—1

Questions 93 and 94 refer to the following scenario:

A 51-year-old male is admitted to your unit with the symptoms of crushing chest pain, unrelieved by nitrates or rest. He has 3-mm elevated ST segments in V_1 through V_4, with ST depression in II, III, and aVF. His blood pressure is 94/64, pulse 110, and respiratory rate 32.

93. Based on the preceding information, which type of MI (myocardial infarction) would most likely be represented by the ECG changes?
    (A) anterior
    (B) inferior
    (C) lateral
    (D) posterior

94. Is ECG confirmation of an MI (myocardial infarction) present in this patient?
    (A) no, due to the absence of Q waves
    (B) no, due to ST depression in the inferior leads
    (C) yes, due to ST segment elevation in V_1 through V_4
    (D) yes, due to absence of lateral ECG changes

95. Which type of MI (myocardial infarction) has the highest mortality rate?
    (A) anterior
    (B) inferior
    (C) lateral
    (D) posterior

96. Unstable angina is characterized by all of the following features but one. Which feature does NOT characterize unstable angina?
    (A) increasing frequency of chest pain
    (B) chest pain at rest
    (C) increasing severity of symptoms
    (D) Q wave formation

97. The LDH (lactate dehydrogenase) "flip," after which LDH-1 exceeds LDH-2, is potentially useful in which situation?
    (A) differentiating angina from MI (myocardial infarction)
    (B) identifying MIs in patients who present after CPK (creatine phosphokinase) levels have returned to normal
    (C) verifying the presence of Prinzmetal's angina
    (D) differentiates anterior from inferior MIs

Questions 98 through 100 refer to the following scenario:

A 65-year-old female is admitted to the unit with chest pain. Physically, she has no shortness of breath or orthopnea, some noticeable jugular venous distension, and clear breath sounds. Her ECG shows large R waves in V_1 and V_2.

Hemodynamic studies reveal the following:

blood pressure	102/72
pulse	105
pulmonary arterial pressure	30/16
PCWP	13
CVP	16
cardiac output	4.6
cardiac index	2.4

98. Which condition is likely to be present based on the preceding information?
    (A) right ventricular hypertrophy
    (B) right ventricular infarction
    (C) left ventricular infarction
    (D) pericardial tamponade

99. What other leads may be useful in establishing a diagnosis in this patient?
    (A) MCL_1
    (B) MCL_5
    (C) aVR
    (D) V_{4R} and V_{6R}

100. Hemodynamic support would most likely include which of the following strategies:
     (A) fluids to keep the CVP (central venous pressure) elevated
     (B) diuretics to reduce the CVP
     (C) dopamine to increase the blood pressure
     (D) nitroglycerine to reduce the preload

101. Which type of medication is common in the treatment of unstable angina?
     (A) diuretics
     (B) vasodilators
     (C) beta blockers
     (D) sympathetic stimulants

Questions 102 and 103 refer to the following scenario:

A 59-year-old male is admitted to your unit with the diagnosis "rule out myocardial infarction." He stated 1 hr ago that he was at work when he felt severe chest pain, became cool and clammy, and felt nauseated. He came immediately to the hospital. The ECG indicates ST segment elevation in leads II, III, and aVF. ST-segment depression exists in V_1 through V_6. He has not responded to nitrates in the emergency room or the ICU. His vital signs are as follows:

blood pressure	98/68
pulse	107
respiratory rate	32

102. Which type of MI (myocardial infarction) is represented on the ECG changes?
     (A) anterior
     (B) inferior
     (C) lateral
     (D) posterior

103. Based on the preceding description, which initial treatment is indicated?
     (A) dobutamine
     (B) thrombolytic therapy
     (C) CABG (coronary artery bypass graft)
     (D) angioplasty

104. Thrombolytic therapy is commonly associated with complications. Which of the following is NOT a complication of thrombolytic therapy?
     (A) bradycardias
     (B) bleeding from venipuncture sites
     (C) ventricular ectopy
     (D) extension of the MI (myocardial infarction) due to embolic phenomena

105. Which of the following is an indication for angioplasty?
     (A) proximal stenosis of a coronary artery
     (B) distal stenosis of a coronary artery
     (C) multiple obstructions in coronary arteries
     (D) no prior episodes of angina

106. A patient who has failed to derive benefit from a medication regimen for unstable angina may benefit in reduction of pain from which treatment?
     (A) valvuloplasty
     (B) thrombolytic therapy
     (C) beta blockade
     (D) CABG (coronary artery bypass graft)

107. Indications for thrombolytic therapy (with optimal prognosis) include which of the following?
     (A) onset of pain less than 8 hr
     (B) onset of pain less than 4 hr
     (C) no prior MI (myocardial infarction)
     (D) ST-segment depression in two consecutive leads

108. Dopamine is used with caution in patients with MI (myocardial infarction) for which reason?
     (A) its potential for increasing myocardial oxygen consumption
     (B) because it has no inotropic component
     (C) because it may cause reflex bradydysrhythmias
     (D) due to the increase in the fibrillation threshold

109. Which of the following medications is an example of an agent that is expected to reduce directly myocardial oxygen consumption?
    (A) labetalol
    (B) dobutamine
    (C) dopamine
    (D) furosemide

110. Assuming vascular volume is adequate, which medication would have the strongest effect on raising the blood pressure in a hypotensive patient?
    (A) norepinephrine (Levophed)
    (B) dobutamine (Dobutrex)
    (C) epinephrine (Adrenalin)
    (D) esmolol (Brevibloc)

111. What is the stroke volume in a patient who has a cardiac output of 5.2 L/min and a heart rate of 80 beats/min?
    (A) 11 ml
    (B) 52 ml
    (C) 65 ml
    (D) 101 ml

112. Pulsus paradoxus is utilized to identify which one of the following conditions?
    (A) cardiac tamponade
    (B) myocardial infarction
    (C) respiratory failure
    (D) ruptured papillary muscle

113. Orthostatic hypotension results from which of the following conditions?
    (A) left ventricular failure
    (B) pulmonary hypertension
    (C) hypovolemia
    (D) portal hypertension

114. Orthostatic hypotension is manifested by which of the following clinical symptoms following a change from lying down to sitting up?
    (A) a systolic blood pressure fall of more than 25 mm Hg and a decrease in diastolic blood pressure of more than 10 mm Hg
    (B) systolic blood pressure is unchanged while a decrease in diastolic blood pressure of more than 10 mm Hg occurs
    (C) a decrease in systolic blood pressure while diastolic blood pressure slightly increases
    (D) an increase in systolic blood pressure while diastolic blood pressure falls

115. Measurement of orthostatic hypotension occurs during measurement of blood pressure with position changes. Select the position change by means of which orthostatic hypotension should be measured.
    (A) move from upright to supine
    (B) move from sitting to standing
    (C) move from supine to upright
    (D) turn from left side to right

116. Which medication has the strongest effect (assuming normovolemia) in elevating the blood pressure?
    (A) dobutamine (Dobutrex)
    (B) isoproterenol (Isuprel)
    (C) esmolol (Brevibloc)
    (D) dopamine (Intropin)

117. Furosemide (Lasix) is considered to affect primarily which component of stroke volume?
    (A) preload
    (B) afterload
    (C) contractility
    (D) aortic distensibility

118. Which medication promotes the largest increase in myocardial oxygen consumption (MVO_2)?
    (A) nitroglycerine
    (B) nitroprusside
    (C) dobutamine
    (D) dopamine

119. Vasodilator drugs have which of the following effects on hemodynamics?
    (A) decreased SVR (systemic vascular resistance), increased PCWP (pulmonary capillary wedge pressure), decreased cardiac output
    (B) increased SVR, decreased PCWP, decreased cardiac output
    (C) increased CVP (central venous pressure), increased SVR, increased cardiac output
    (D) decreased CVP, decreased PCWP, increased cardiac output

120. Physical signs associated with CHF (congestive heart failure) include all but one of the following. Identify the one sign that is NOT associated with CHF.
    (A) dependent crackles
    (B) S_3 heart sound
    (C) dependent edema
    (D) Kussmaul respiration

Questions 121 and 122 refer to the following scenario:

A 72-year-old male is admitted with the diagnosis of CHF (congestive heart failure). He complains of shortness of breath but does not complain of chest pain. He has bibasilar crackles and distended neck veins. His vital signs are blood pressure 112/82, pulse 110, respiratory rate 29. Pulmonary artery catheter readings reveal the following:

arterial pressure	38/23
PCWF	22
CVP	15
cardiac output	3.6
cardiac index	2.1

121. Based on the preceding data, which condition does this patient exhibit?
(A) left ventricular failure alone
(B) right ventricular failure alone
(C) biventricular failure
(D) chronic obstructive pulmonary disease

122. All of the following medications would be used to treat the condition but one. Identify the medication that would NOT be used for this patient.
(A) low-dose dobutamine
(B) nitroglycerine
(C) furosemide
(D) high-dose dopamine

Questions 123 and 124 refer to the following scenario:

A 68-year-old female is admitted to your unit complaining of fatigue, shortness of breath, and "swollen feet." She has the following vital signs: blood pressure 188/106, pulse 108, respiratory rate 30. Pulmonary artery catheter readings reveal the following information:

arterial pressure	42/25
PCWP	21
CVP	17
cardiac output	3.3
cardiac index	1.9

123. If a vasodilator were to be used in this patient, which would be the optimal agent to employ?
(A) nitroglycerine (Nitrostat)
(B) phenylephrine (Neo-Synephrine)
(C) diazoxide (Hyperstat)
(D) nitroprusside (Nipride)

124. What would be the reason she has shortness of breath and fatigue?
(A) biventricular failure
(B) underlying chronic lung disease

(C) right ventricular failure
(D) pulmonary hypertension

Questions 125 and 126 refer to the following scenario:

A 75-year-old female is admitted to your unit from the emergency room with severe shortness of breath and orthopnea. She is very anxious and restless. She has a history of CHF (congestive heart failure) and was fine until this morning, when the respiratory difficulties started and became progressively worse. Her ECG shows nonspecific ST changes. Breath sounds reveal crackles throughout her lungs. Her blood pressure is 82/56, pulse 118, respiratory rate 38.

125. Based on these symptoms, which condition is probably developing?
(A) right ventricular failure
(B) pulmonary edema
(C) myocardial infarction
(D) pulmonary emboli

126. Which of the following would probably NOT be used in the treatment of this patient?
(A) dopamine
(B) nitroprusside
(C) dobutamine
(D) furosemide

127. If the physician ordered nitroprusside and dobutamine in a patient with CHF (congestive heart failure), what is the goal of this type of medication regimen?
(A) reduced preload and improved contractility
(B) increased preload and reduced afterload
(C) reduced afterload and reduced contractility
(D) reduced afterload and improved contractility

128. The use of furosemide (Lasix) and morphine in pulmonary edema is designed to improve myocardial function by which action?
(A) reduce preload and myocardial oxygen consumption
(B) reduce afterload and myocardial oxygen consumption
(C) increase preload and improve contractility
(D) improve contractility while increasing afterload

129. Which of the following medications is NOT a positive inotrope?
(A) dopamine
(B) dobutamine

(Answers cont'd.)

(C) amrinone
(D) nitroprusside

130. Which of the following medications is a beta blocker?
(A) esmolol
(B) nifedipine
(C) mexiletine
(D) captropril

131. Vasodilation may help reduce myocardial oxygen consumption in the failing left ventricle. Which of the following medications produce(s) vasodilation that could be useful in the treatment of congestive heart failure?
   I. nitroprusside (Nipride)
  II. phenylephrine (Neo-Synephrine)
 III. nifedipine (Procardia)
      (A) I
      (B) II and III
      (C) II
      (D) I and III

132. Which of the following is NOT a calcium channel blocker?
(A) nifedipine
(B) diltiazem
(C) verapamil
(D) diazoxide

133. Pericarditis presents on the 12-lead ECG with which of the following changes?
(A) Q waves in precordial leads
(B) left axis deviation
(C) generalized elevation of ST segments
(D) depression of ST segments

134. Which of the following is NOT a symptom of pericarditis?
(A) fever
(B) increased pain on left lateral position
(C) pericardial friction rub
(D) chest pain unchanged with respiration

135. Early stages of hypovolemic or cardiogenic shock may exhibit normal blood pressure due to which of the following compensating mechanisms?
(A) increased SVR (systemic vascular resistance)
(B) increased preload
(C) decreased afterload
(D) increased stroke volume

136. Where should inflation of the balloon in an IABP (intra-aortic balloon pump assist) occur?
(A) near the T wave on the ECG
(B) at end diastole

(C) at end systole
(D) near the dicrotic notch

137. Which of the following is one danger of abdominal aortic aneurysm repair?
(A) obstruction of renal blood flow
(B) interference with coronary diastolic filling
(C) creation of pulmonary emboli
(D) pericardial tamponade

138. Deflation of the balloon in an IABP (intra-aortic balloon pump assist) should occur at what point?
(A) near the T wave on the ECG
(B) before the QRS complex
(C) at end systole
(D) near the dicrotic notch

139. Hypovolemic shock differs from cardiogenic shock by exhibiting which one of the following hemodynamic changes?
(A) high preload
(B) low preload
(C) high SVR (systemic vascular resistance)
(D) low stroke volume

140. Which of the following agents would most reliably raise the blood pressure in cardiogenic shock?
(A) dopamine
(B) dobutamine
(C) fluid bolus
(D) nitroprusside

141. Which of the following are two benefits of an IABP (intra-aortic balloon pump) assist?
(A) decreased preload and increased afterload
(B) increased contractility and afterload
(C) decreased afterload and increased coronary artery filling
(D) increased coronary filling and increased preload

142. Which physical maneuver is most likely to result in improved blood pressure?
(A) placing the patient in the Trendelenburg (head-down) position
(B) sitting the patient in a semiupright position
(C) placing the patient in a prone position
(D) placing the patient in a supine position and elevating the legs

143. Which of the following is NOT a cause of hypovolemic shock?
(A) pulmonary capillary leak syndrome
(B) cardiogenic shock

(C) postoperative bleeding

(D) fracture of a long bone

144. Cardiogenic shock is characterized by which of the following parameters?
    I. cardiac index less than 2.2 L/min/m^2
    II. PCWP (pulmonary capillary wedge pressure) greater than 22 mm Hg
    III. CVP (central venous pressure) between 5 and 10 mm Hg
    (A) I only
    (B) I and II
    (C) II and III
    (D) III only

Questions 145 and 146 refer to the following scenario:

At 1600, a 67-year-old female is admitted to your unit from the emergency room with hypotension. Her husband states that she had complained of shortness of breath earlier in the day and since noon he has not been able to awaken her. She is currently unresponsive except to painful stimuli. Her blood pressure is 78/50, pulse 118. A pulmonary artery catheter is inserted and gives the following information:

arterial pressure	44/26
PCWP	25
CVP	15
cardiac output	3.7
cardiac index	1.6
$S_{\bar{v}}O_2$	0.40

145. Based on the preceding information, which condition is developing?
    (A) cardiogenic shock
    (B) hypovolemic shock
    (C) right ventricular failure with pulmonary hypertension
    (D) sepsis with a low SVR (systemic vascular resistance)

146. Which treatment should be initiated for this patient?
    (A) fluid bolus
    (B) dobutamine and dopamine
    (C) Furosemide and nitroprusside
    (D) epinephrine and furosemide

Questions 147 and 148 refer to the following scenario:

A 58-year-old male is admitted to your unit with hypotension and the diagnosis "rule out myocardial infarction." He has a blood pressure of 82/52, pulse

122. During physical assessment, he exhibits marked orthopnea, extreme anxiety, and crackles throughout his lungs but more prominent posteriorly. He is to have a pulmonary artery catheter inserted in the next hour.

147. Based on these symptoms, what would you expect the hemodynamic data from the pulmonary artery catheter to reveal?
    (A) PCWP < 10, CI (cardiac index) < 2 L/m^2
    (B) PCWP > 22, CI < 2 L/m^2
    (C) CVP > 15, CI > 4 L/m^2
    (D) SVR (systemic cardiac resistance) > 2000 dynes/sec·cm, CI > 4 L/m^2

148. What treatment would be most effective initially for this patient?
    (A) high-dose dopamine and nitroprusside
    (B) furosemide and dobutamine
    (C) dobutamine and epinephrine
    (D) digitalis and furosemide

149. Vasoconstriction can increase the blood pressure while also increasing myocardial oxygen consumption. Which of the following drugs could be expected to produce vasoconstriction and thereby raise the blood pressure and increase MVo$_2$ (myocardial oxygen consumption)?
    I. dopamine
    II. dobutamine
    III. norepinephrine
    (A) I and II
    (B) I and III
    (C) II and III
    (D) I, II, and III

Questions 150 and 151 refer to the following scenario:

A 57-year-old male is admitted to your unit postoperatively for repair of a fractured femur and a splenectomy after a motor vehicle accident. Four hours postoperatively, his level of consciousness begins to decrease. Vital signs are as follows: blood pressure 88/58, pulse 113, respiratory rate 28. His skin is cool and clammy. He has no complaints of shortness of breath; breath sounds are clear. His pulmonary artery catheter provides the following data:

arterial pressure	21/7
PCWP	4
CVP	2
cardiac output	3.6
cardiac index	1.7

150. Based on the preceding information, which condition appears to be developing?

(Answers cont'd.)

(A) left ventricular failure
(B) right ventricular failure
(C) cardiogenic shock
(D) hypovolemic shock

151. In a patient with acute blood loss, which of the following would most reliably increase the vascular volume?
(A) NS (normal saline)
(B) LR (lactated Ringer's)
(C) hetastarch (Hespan)
(D) 5% dextrose in water (D_5W)

152. Sympathetic stimulants, such as dopamine, are not indicated in hypovolemia until the blood volume has been corrected. Which of the following is the best explanation for this approach?
(A) Massive sympathetic stimulation is already present and cannot reach effectiveness without adequate fluid volume.
(B) Sympathetic stimulation only works when vasodilation is the primary problem.
(C) Sympathetic stimulation cannot occur until vascular baroreceptors have been inactivated.
(D) Dopamine is indicated in hypovolemia before fluid replacement.

Questions 153 to 155 refer to the following scenario:

A 71-year-old female is in your unit following colon resection. Because of an episode of hypotension in the operating room, a pulmonary artery catheter was inserted. On postoperative day 1, her morning hematocrit was 35, hemoglobin 11.5. Her afternoon hematocrit is 27, hemoglobin 9. She has no complaints of pain that differ from those reported in the morning. The following are the pulmonary artery catheter readings from the morning and afternoon. She has received one liter of normal saline over the past 12 hr. The house officer is not concerned over the change, attributing the change to dilutional factors.

	MORNING	AFTERNOON
blood pressure	98/58	94/56
pulse	102	115
pulmonary arterial pressure	24/12	20/8
PCWP	10	5
CVP	4	3
cardiac output	3.9	3.7
cardiac index	2.5	2.4

153. Based on the preceding information, which condition is developing?
(A) The data support dilutional reasons for the drop in hematocrit and hemoglobin.

(B) hypovolemia
(C) left ventricular failure
(D) pericardial tamponade

154. Which parameters best separate dilutional from actual decreases in the hematocrit and hemoglobin?
(A) heart rate, cardiac output, and SVR (systemic vascular resistance)
(B) stroke volume, heart rate and PCWP (pulmonary capillary wedge pressure)
(C) PCWP and cardiac output
(D) blood pressure and CVP (central venous pressure)

155. Why would the cardiac output not change substantially if the patient was developing hypovolemia?
(A) The stroke volume increased to offset the loss of blood volume.
(B) The PCWP (pulmonary capillary wedge pressure) decrease reduced myocardial oxygen consumption and improved contractility.
(C) The heart rate increased to offset the loss of blood volume.
(D) The mean arterial pressure increased to offset the loss of blood volume.

156. Which of the following is NOT an indication for a CABG (coronary artery bypass graft)?
(A) unstable angina
(B) 90% narrowing of LAD (left anterior descending) coronary artery
(C) distal stenosis of LAD coronary artery
(D) multiple vessel stenosis

157. Which of the following is a common sign in cardiac tamponade?
(A) decreased PCWP (pulmonary capillary wedge pressure)
(B) increased diastolic blood pressure
(C) pulsus paradoxus
(D) ejection fraction > 75%

158. Which blood vessel is commonly used as the graft vessel in a CABG (coronary artery bypass graft)?
(A) femoral vein
(B) axillary artery
(C) a coronary artery that is unobstructed
(D) internal mammary artery

159. Nursing care of the patient following cardiopulmonary bypass surgery includes observation of all of the following measures but one. Which

of the following is NOT a postoperative measure for the nurse to assess?
(A) body temperature
(B) pulmonary gas exchange
(C) PT (prothrombin time)
(D) PCWP (pulmonary capillary wedge pressure) and CVP (central venous pressure)

160. Which of the following is the best method to treat cardiomyopathy?
(A) heart transplantation
(B) CABG (coronary artery bypass graft)
(C) IABP (intraaortic balloon pump) assist
(D) coronary angioplasty

161. Approximately what percent of heart transplant recipients are alive after five years?
(A) <25%
(B) 25 to 50%
(C) 50 to 75%
(D) If they survive the first year, 100% survival at 5 years

162. What is the most common type of aortic aneurysm?
(A) ascending thoracic
(B) descending thoracic
(C) abdominal
(D) aortic arch

163. Dissecting aneurysms present with several symptoms. Which of the following is NOT a symptom of a dissecting aortic aneurysm?
(A) gastrointestinal bleeding
(B) severe abdominal pain
(C) pain radiating to the back
(D) palpable abdominal mass

164. Dissection of an artery occurs because of which type of injury to the blood vessel?
(A) intimal tear
(B) weakness of the entire vessel wall
(C) severance of the arterial wall
(D) bleeding into an already formed aneurysm

165. Which of the following is the most common complication causing death following aortic surgery?
(A) stress ulcers
(B) ATN (acute tubular necrosis)
(C) bleeding
(D) MI (myocardial infarction)

166. All of the following but one are symptoms of obstructed arterial flow. Select the one that represents venous, NOT arterial, obstruction.
(A) pallor of the skin
(B) cyanosis of the skin

(C) intermittent claudication
(D) decreased pulses

167. Which of the following is a common sign of acute arterial obstruction?
(A) pain distal to the obstruction
(B) edema distal to the obstruction
(C) cyanosis distal to the obstruction
(D) warm skin proximal to the obstruction

168. Deep venous thrombosis can potentially release emboli. Which of the following could result from the emboli of a deep venous thrombosis?
(A) loss of dorsalis pedal pulse
(B) loss of pulses in the femoral artery
(C) superior vena caval syndrome
(D) pulmonary emboli

169. Which of the following is NOT a parameter commonly measured in a patient after a CABG (coronary artery bypass graft)?
(A) temperature
(B) PCWP (pulmonary capillary wedge pressure)
(C) cardiac output
(D) ejection fraction

Questions 170 and 171 refer to the following scenario:

A 57-year-old male is admitted to your unit following a CABG (coronary artery bypass graft). At 0400 he is alert and oriented and is extubated without difficulty. At 0500, he is lethargic despite not receiving analgesics. He has a mediastinal chest tube that has drained 500 ml in the last hour. Pulmonary artery catheter and blood gas information are listed below:

	0400	0500
blood pressure	100/70	100/66
pulse	100	110
PCWP	15	10
CVP	10	7
cardiac output	4.3	4.0
cardiac index	2.5	2.4
PaO_2	82	77
SaO_2	0.96	0.95
FiO_2	0.40	0.40
$PaCO_2$	37	39
pH	7.37	7.35
HCO_3^-	24	23

170. Based on the preceding information, the patient is probably developing which of the following?
(A) tension pneumothorax
(B) mediastinal bleeding

(Answers cont'd.)

(C) adult respiratory distress syndrome
(D) CHF (congestive heart failure)

171. Which treatment would be optimal for the patient at this time?
(A) initiation of dobutamine
(B) addition of epinephrine
(C) autotransfusion
(D) added pleural and mediastinal chest tubes

Questions 172 through 174 refer to the following scenario:

A 62-year-old male is admitted to your unit postoperatively following abdominal aortic aneurysm repair. Four hours after returning from the operating room, he begins to complain of chest pain and shortness of breath. Breath sounds are equal with inspiratory crackles noted posteriorly. Heart sounds indicate a clear S_1, S_2, and S_3.

172. On the basis of this information, the patient is most likely developing which of the following?
(A) MI (myocardial infarction)
(B) pulmonary emboli
(C) tension pneumothorax
(D) dissecting thoracic aneurysm

Before answering questions 173 and 174, please read the following additional information:

Based on the development of chest pain, the patient has a pulmonary artery catheter inserted and blood gases are obtained. Analysis of this formation discloses the following:

blood pressure	96/64
pulse	112
arterial pressure	34/20
PCWP	19
CVP	11
cardiac output	3.8
cardiac index	2.2
PaO_2	68
SaO_2	0.92
FiO_2	0.40
$PaCO_2$	35
pH	7.40
HCO_3^-	25

173. Based on the preceding information, which condition is most likely to be developing?
(A) MI (myocardial infarction)
(B) pulmonary emboli
(C) tension pneumothorax
(D) dissecting thoracic aneurysm

174. Treatment to support these hemodynamics would most likely include which of the following?
(A) fluid bolus
(B) dobutamine
(C) dopamine
(D) nitroprusside

Questions 175 through 177 refer to the following scenario:

A 68-year-old female is admitted to your unit after a CABG (coronary artery bypass graft). Eight hours following surgery, she is extubated and experiencing only mild chest discomfort. Over the next hour, she begins to complain of vaguely increasing discomfort. Her pleural tube is bubbling in the water seal chamber. No drainage is present from the mediastinal tube. Her blood pressure fluctuates with respiration, decreasing by 20 mm Hg during inspiration. Her lung sounds are clear; heart sounds are normal but distant.

175. Based on the preceding information, which condition is most likely to be developing?
(A) tension pneumothorax
(B) pneumomediastinum
(C) left ventricular failure
(D) pericardial tamponade

Before answering question 176, please read the following additional information:

A pulmonary artery catheter reveals the following information:

blood pressure	92/58
pulse	115
arterial pressure	36/22
PCWP	18
CVP	18
cardiac output	3.2
cardiac index	1.9

176. With the added information, does your interpretation of the situation change? Which condition is developing in this patient?
(A) tension pneumothorax
(B) dissecting aortic aneurysm
(C) pulmonary emboli
(D) cardiac tamponade

177. Which treatment would be indicated in this patient?
(A) pleural chest tube insertion
(B) insertion of a new mediastinal tube
(C) dopamine
(D) reintubation and placing the patient on positive pressure ventilation

178. Interpret the following 12-lead ECG. *See art below.*
- **(A)** anterior hemiblock
- **(B)** posterior hemiblock
- **(C)** right bundle branch block
- **(D)** left bundle branch block

179. Interpret the following 12-lead ECG. *See art below.*
- **(A)** anterior MI (myocardial infarction)
- **(B)** inferior MI
- **(C)** posterior MI
- **(D)** lateral MI

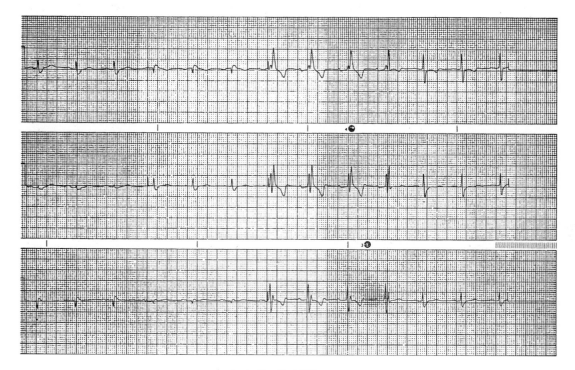

Question 178.

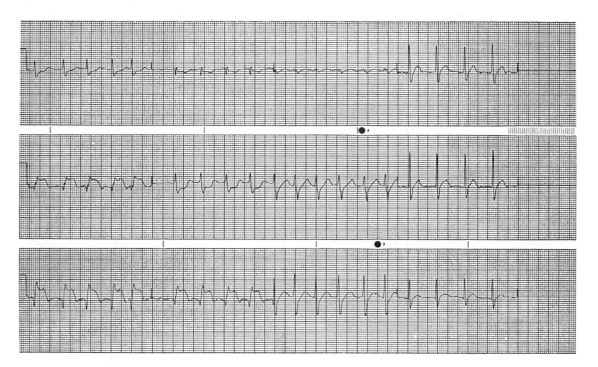

Question 179.

180. Interpret the following 12-lead ECG. *See art below.*
  (A) anterior MI (myocardial infarction)
  (B) inferior-lateral MI
  (C) posterior MI
  (D) lateral MI

181. In the following ECG, identify the major electrocardiographic abnormality. *See art below.*
  (A) inferior ischemia
  (B) left ventricular hypertrophy
  (C) right ventricular hypertrophy
  (D) anterior ischemia

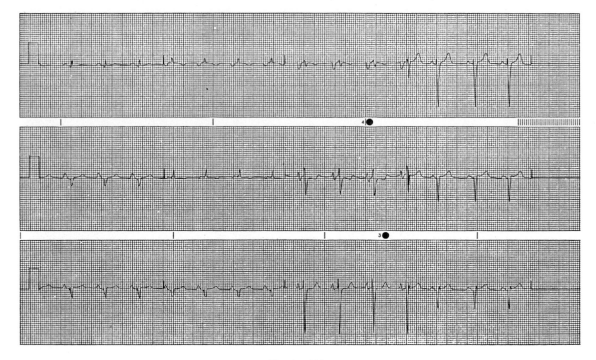

Question 180.

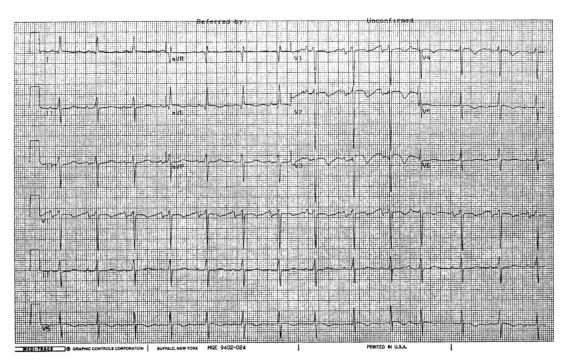

Question 181.

182. Interpret the following 12-lead ECG. *See art below.*
- **(A)** anterior MI (myocardial infarction)
- **(B)** new inferior MI
- **(C)** posterior MI
- **(D)** anterior and old inferior MI

183. In the following ECG, identify the major electro-cardiographic abnormality. *See art below.*
- **(A)** inferior ischemia
- **(B)** left ventricular hypertrophy
- **(C)** right ventricular hypertrophy
- **(D)** anterior ischemia

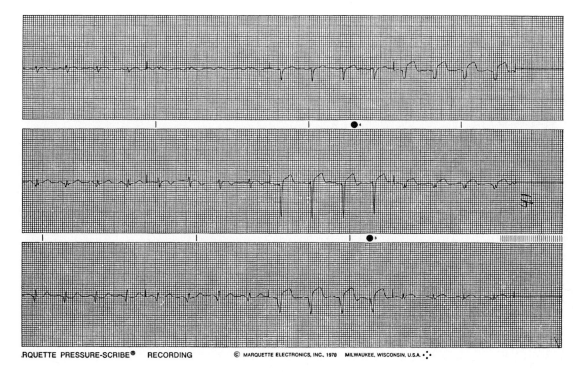

Question 182.

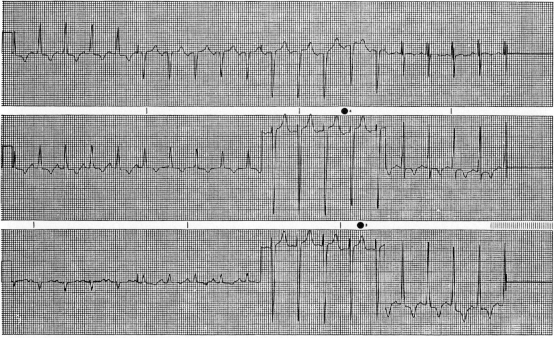

Question 183.

184. Interpret the following 12-lead ECG. *See art below.*
(A) anterior hemiblock
(B) posterior hemiblock
(C) right bundle branch block
(D) left bundle branch block

185. Interpret the following 12-lead ECG. *See art below.*
(A) anterior hemiblock
(B) posterior hemiblock
(C) right bundle branch block
(D) left bundle branch block

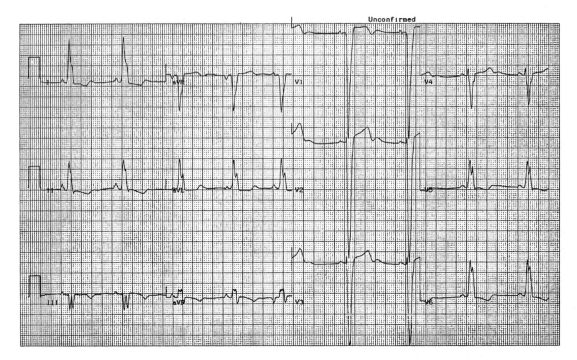

Question 184.

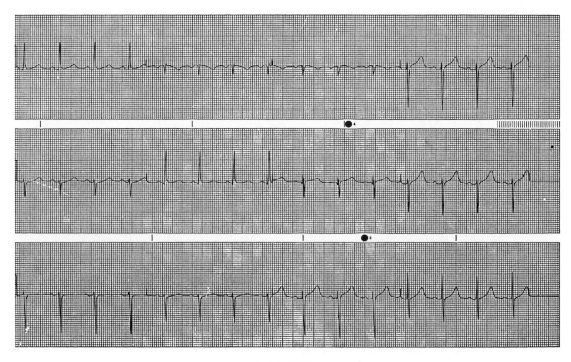

Question 185.

186. Which abnormality is present in the following ECG? *See art below.*
(A) left ventricular ectopy
(B) pericarditis
(C) left axis deviation
(D) right axis deviation

187. In the following ECG, identify the major electrocardiographic abnormality. *See art below.*
(A) inferior ischemia
(B) left ventricular hypertrophy
(C) right ventricular hypertrophy
(D) anteriolateral ischemia with RBBB (right bundle branch block)

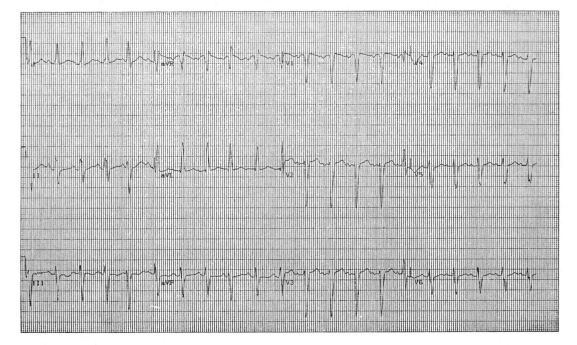

Question 186.

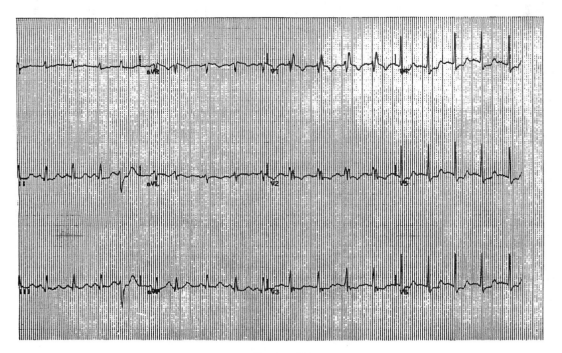

Question 187.

188. Interpret the following 12-lead ECG. *See art below.*
 (A) anterior hemiblock
 (B) atrial tachycardia with aberrancy
 (C) ventricular tachycardia
 (D) left bundle branch block

189. In the following ECG, identify the major electrocardiographic abnormality. *See art below.*
 (A) left bundle branch
 (B) left bundle branch block
 (C) right ventricular hypertrophy
 (D) anterior ischemia

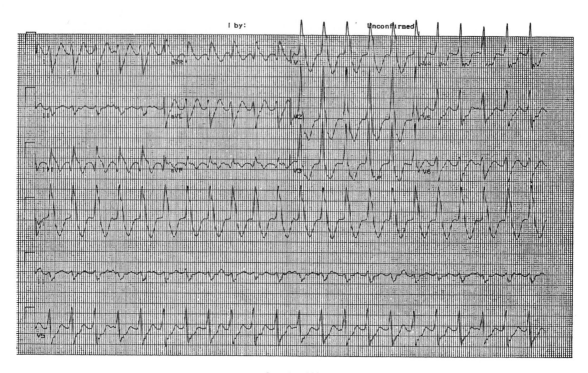

Question 188.

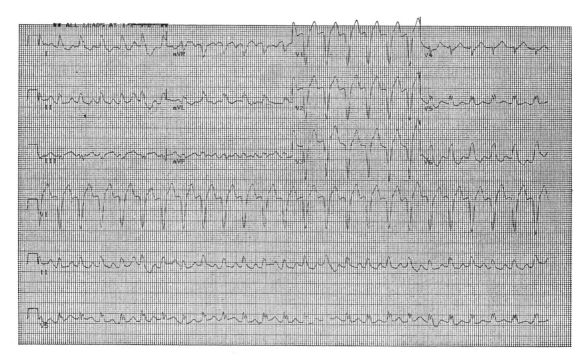

Question 189.

190. In a patient admitted with the diagnosis of cardiac contusion, which physical sign would correlate best with this diagnosis?

(A) distended neck veins
(B) tachycardia disproportionate to injury
(C) shortness of breath
(D) ecchymotic area over the entire sternum

Cardiovascular Practice Exam

1. _____
2. _____
3. _____
4. _____
5. _____
6. _____
7. _____
8. _____
9. _____
10. _____
11. _____
12. _____
13. _____
14. _____
15. _____
16. _____
17. _____
18. _____
19. _____
20. _____
21. _____
22. _____
23. _____
24. _____
25. _____
26. _____
27. _____

28. _____
29. _____
30. _____
31. _____
32. _____
33. _____
34. _____
35. _____
36. _____
37. _____
38. _____
39. _____
40. _____
41. _____
42. _____
43. _____
44. _____
45. _____
46. _____
47. _____
48. _____
49. _____
50. _____
51. _____
52. _____
53. _____
54. _____

55. _____
56. _____
57. _____
58. _____
59. _____
60. _____
61. _____
62. _____
63. _____
64. _____
65. _____
66. _____
67. _____
68. _____
69. _____
70. _____
71. _____
72. _____
73. _____
74. _____
75. _____
76. _____
77. _____
78. _____
79. _____
80. _____
81. _____

82. _____
83. _____
84. _____
85. _____
86. _____
87. _____
88. _____
89. _____
90. _____
91. _____
92. _____
93. _____
94. _____
95. _____
96. _____
97. _____
98. _____
99. _____
100. _____
101. _____
102. _____
103. _____
104. _____
105. _____
106. _____
107. _____
108. _____

109. _____	130. _____	151. _____	171. _____
110. _____	131. _____	152. _____	172. _____
111. _____	132. _____	153. _____	173. _____
112. _____	133. _____	154. _____	174. _____
113. _____	134. _____	155. _____	175. _____
114. _____	135. _____	156. _____	176. _____
115. _____	136. _____	157. _____	177. _____
116. _____	137. _____	158. _____	178. _____
117. _____	138. _____	159. _____	179. _____
118. _____	139. _____	160. _____	180. _____
119. _____	140. _____	161. _____	181. _____
120. _____	141. _____	162. _____	182. _____
121. _____	142. _____	163. _____	183. _____
122. _____	143. _____	164. _____	184. _____
123. _____	144. _____	165. _____	185. _____
124. _____	145. _____	166. _____	186. _____
125. _____	146. _____	167. _____	187. _____
126. _____	147. _____	168. _____	188. _____
127. _____	148. _____	169. _____	189. _____
128. _____	149. _____	170. _____	190. _____
129. _____	150. _____		

1.	B	p 52	28.	A	p 8	55.	D	p 74	82.	B	p 60
2.	D	p 19	29.	D	p 12	56.	A	p 72	83.	C	p 68
3.	A	p 19	30.	A	p 8	57.	C	p 73	84.	A	p 30
4.	D	p 51–52	31.	D	p 8	58.	B	p 73	85.	B	p 99
5.	C	p 20–21	32.	B	p 8	59.	B	p 108	86.	D	p 108
6.	A	p 51	33.	A	p 9	60.	A	p 108	87.	B	p 109
7.	D	p. 4	34.	A	p 12	61.	C	p 109	88.	B	p 103
8.	C	p 13	35.	C	p 23	62.	B	p 108	89.	D	p 27
9.	B	p 52	36.	D	p 47	63.	B	p 108	90.	A	p 106
10.	D	p 48	37.	D	p 48	64.	A	p 68	91.	D	p 108
11.	A	p 9–10	38.	C	p 48	65.	A	p 76	92.	A	p 66, 68
12.	B	p 54–55	39.	A	p 50–52	66.	B	p 76	93.	A	p 66
13.	C	p 15	421	A	p 21	67.	C	p 42–45	94.	A	p 66
14.	A	p 51	41.	B	p 95	68.	D	p 42–45	95.	A	p 68
15.	B	p 51	42.	C	p 54	69.	C	p 75	96.	D	p 65–66
16.	D	p 52	43.	D	p 75	70.	D	p 97	97.	B	p 67
17.	A	p 54–55	44.	D	p 109	71.	D	p 99	98.	B	p 68
18.	A	p 83	45.	D	p 66	72.	A	p 65	99.	D	p 68
19.	A	p 11	46.	A	p 66	73.	A	p 65	100.	A	p 68
20.	D	p 11	47.	B	p 66	74.	C	p 67	101.	C	p 65
21.	A	p 52	48.	D	p 66	75.	A	p 73	102.	B	p 66
22.	B	p 123	49.	C	p 107–108	76.	A	p 77–78	103.	B	p 68
23.	A	p 51, 52	50.	B	p 107–108	77.	B	p 77–78	104.	D	p 68–69
24.	A	p 51, 83	51.	A	p 97	78.	A	p 78	105.	A	p 69
25.	B	p 11	52.	B	p 99	79.	A	p 77	106.	D	p 65
26.	A	p 70	53.	D	p 102	80.	B	p 68	107.	B	p 68–69
27.	D	p 54	54.	C	p 101–102	81.	C	p 73	108.	A	p 19

109. A _p 49_	130. A _p 22_	151. C _p 93, 94_	171. C _p 117_
110. A _p 23_	131. D _p 20–21_	152. A _p 48, 91_	172. A _p 120_
111. C _p 47–48_	132. D _p 22_	153. B _p 52, 91_	173. A _p 52, 120_
112. A _p 113_	133. C _p 112_	154. B _p 52, 91_	174. B _p 19_
113. C _p 93_	134. D _p 112_	155. C _p 52, 91_	175. D _p 113_
114. A _p 93_	135. A _p 91_	156. C _p 116_	176. D _p 113_
115. C _p 93_	136. D _p 89_	157. C _p 123_	177. B _p 113_
116. D _p 23_	137. A _p 120_	158. D _p 115_	178. C _p 76_
117. A _p 20_	138. B _p 89_	159. C _p 117_	179. B _p 66_
118. D _p 23_	139. B _p. 88_	160. A _p 112_	180. B _p 66_
119. D _p 21_	140. A _p 88_	161. C _p 118_	181. D _p. 33–35_
120. D _p 83_	141. C _p 89_	162. C _p 119_	182. D _p 66_
121. C _p 83_	142. D _p 94_	163. A _p 119_	183. B _p 42–45_
122. D _p 83–84_	143. B _p 92_	164. A _p 119_	184. D _p 41, 66_
123. A _p 21_	144. B _p 48, 88_	165. D _p 120_	185. A _p 42, 66_
124. A _p 83_	145. A _p 48, 88_	166. B _p 121_	186. C _p 35–39_
125. B _p 84_	146. B _p 88_	167. A _p 121_	187. D _p 66, 76_
126. B _p 84_	147. B _p 48, 88_	168. D _p 121_	188. C _p 66_
127. D _p 19–21_	148. B _p 88_	169. D _p 117_	189. A _p 66_
128. A _p 20_	149. B _p 23_	170. B _p 117_	190. B _p 121_
129. D _p 19_	150. D _p 52–92_		

II

PULMONARY

Pamela Becker Weilitz

Pulmonary Anatomy and Physiology

EDITORS' NOTE

The CCRN exam will have a few questions that are directly related to the anatomy of the pulmonary system. However, as you read this chapter, concentrate on understanding the major pulmonary features rather than minute details. For example, the CCRN exam is not likely to ask what the larynx is composed of (e.g., cartilage), but it may give a clinical scenario involving right mainstem intubation secondary to the anatomy of the tracheobronchial tree that facilitates right mainstem entry by an endotracheal tube. Try to understand the anatomy as it relates to clinical application rather than memorizing details of anatomy.

Understanding concepts in pulmonary physiology is crucial to applying the clinical concepts necessary in the CCRN exam section on pulmonary critical care. While much of this chapter is explanatory and somewhat theoretical, it is important to be familiar with most of the concepts presented. As you read this chapter, focus on understanding key principles rather than on minute details. This is a long chapter, and it may be useful to read it in sections in order to improve understanding of the key concepts. You can expect the CCRN exam to have several questions addressing major concepts in pulmonary physiology, so be familiar with the information in this chapter.

The major function of the pulmonary system is the exchange of oxygen and carbon dioxide in the body. The pulmonary anatomy includes the thoracic cage, the muscles of the chest, the upper airway, and the lower airway. Pulmonary physiology is the key to understanding pulmonary disturbances and includes gas exchange principles and analysis of blood gases.

THE THORACIC CAGE

The thoracic cage (Fig. 14–1) is the bony frame of the chest. The thorax is shaped like an inverted cone with the apex about 2.5 cm above the clavicles. The clavicles and first ribs form the protective barrier of the superior portion of the thoracic cage. The diaphragm is the inferior portion of the thoracic cage.

The sternum makes up the anterior portion of the thoracic cage and is actually three connected flat bones: the manubrium, the body, and the xiphoid process. Seven pairs of ribs attach to the sternum, called the "true ribs." The remaining five ribs form the anterior portion of the thoracic cage. Each rib is attached to the rib above it by intercostal muscles and cartilage. The posterior thoracic cage is formed by the vertebrae and 12 pairs of ribs attached to the vertebrae. The ribs are C-shaped and serve as the bony protective sides of the thoracic cage (Fig. 14–2).

MUSCLES OF RESPIRATION

The diaphragm is the major muscle of respiration. On inspiration, the diaphragm contracts (Fig. 14–3), lengthening the chest cavity. The external intercostal muscles contract to raise the ribs, enlarging the diameter of the chest. On expiration, the diaphragm relaxes, becoming dome shaped, decreasing the size of the thorax (Fig. 14–3).

Expiration is passive, accomplished by relaxation of the diaphragm and external intercostal muscles, and the lungs' normal tendency to collapse. Relaxation of the musculature is the major mechanism for exhalation.

The intercostal muscles are composed of two layers: the internal and external intercostals. Changes in the chest muscles alter normal thoracic pressures,

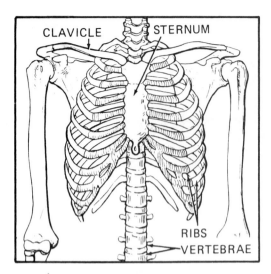

Figure 14–1. The thoracic cage.

affecting ventilation. The internal intercostal muscles pull the ribs down and inward. They are used for forceful expiration, coughing, and sneezing, and in other stressful states and exertional activities. The intercostal muscles may facilitate a smooth transition from inspiration to expiration.

In pulmonary distress and/or disease, accessory muscles are used to facilitate inspiration. The accessory muscles of respiration include the scalene, sternocleidomastoid, trapezius, and pectoralis muscles.

THE MEDIASTINUM

The lung parenchyma and the mediastinum are contained within the bony thoracic cage. The mediastinum is a space midline in the chest and contains the heart, great vessels, trachea, major bronchi, esophagus, thymus gland, lymphatics, and various nerves (Fig. 14–4).

THE PLEURA

Each lung lies free in its own pleural cavity except at its single point of attachment, the hilum (Fig. 14–4). The pleural covering of each lung is composed of two layers. The visceral layer is contiguous with the lung and does not have sensory (pain) nerve fibers. The parietal layer is the outer pleural layer that lines the inside of the thoracic cage and contains sensory nerve fibers. The two pleural layers are separated by a small amount of pleural fluid that allows the two surfaces to slide easily over each other during inspiration and expiration. If the pleura

become inflamed, movement is restricted and the irritation results in pleuritic pain. The diaphragm is the inferior border for each pleural space; the chest wall the lateral border, and the mediastinum the medial border.

THE LUNG

Each lung is made up of lobes. There are three lobes on the right and two on the left. Each lobe of the lung is separated from the adjacent lobe by fissures. The left lung also has an upper and lower division of its superior lobe, separated by a fissure. This fissure is called the lingula. The area of the lingula is equal to or smaller than the middle lobe of the right lung. Each lobe is further divided into segments; 10 in the right lung and 8 in the left lung (Fig. 14–5).

THE UPPER AIRWAY

The upper airway consists of the mouth, nose and oral pharynx, and larynx. The larynx functions in part as a transitional structure between the upper and lower airways. The purpose of the upper airway is to warm, humidify, and filter the inspired air. This is essential to protect the lower airway and alveoli.

The entire upper airway is lined with a mucous membrane that moisturizes and warms the inspired air by means of the vast blood supply and thick layer of watery mucus produced by serous glands and the thick, tenacious mucus produced by the epithelial goblet cells. The ciliated portions of the upper

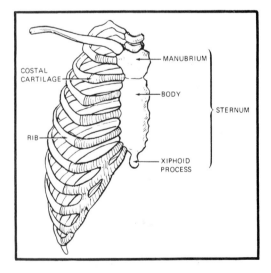

Figure 14–2. The sternum.

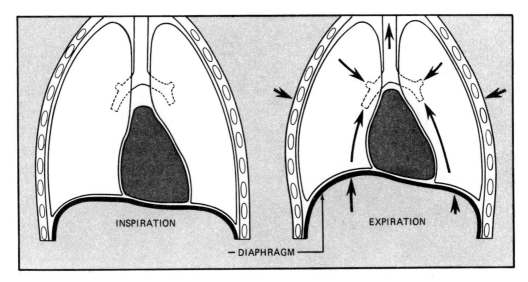

Figure 14–3. The diaphragm on inspiration and expiration.

airway filter pollutants, irritants, and fine particles (1–4 μm in size). Particles come in contact with the respiratory mucosa and are trapped. They are carried to the pharynx by the mucous blanket, where they are swallowed.

The Nose

Air normally enters the respiratory system through the nose. The nose has skeletal rigidity, which maintains patency during inspiration. The first two-thirds of the nose are cartilaginous, and the last one-third bony. The cartilaginous septum, straight at birth, frequently becomes deviated during life and may obstruct air flow. The nasal septum divides the nose into two fossae; the lateral borders are the alae. The openings between the alae and the nasal septum are the nostrils or the nares. The nose has a small inlet and a large outlet, allowing inspired air to have maximum contact with the upper airway mucosa. By sniffing through the nose, inhaled air is directed toward the superior turbinates and olfactory bulb (Fig. 14–6).

The first one-third of the nose is lined with nonciliated, squamous epithelium. The remaining two-thirds of the nose are lined with ciliated, pseudostratified epithelium. Coarse particles larger than 4 μm are entrapped by nasal hairs. The nasopharynx is lined with ciliated, pseudostratified epithelium.

The Pharynx

The main function of the pharynx is to collect incoming air from the mouth and nose and project it downward to the trachea. The pharynx is subdivided into the nasopharynx, the oropharynx, and the laryngopharynx (Fig. 14–6). The nasopharynx is the space behind the oral and nasal cavities and above the soft palate; it contains the orifices of the eustachian tubes. The pharyngeal tonsils (adenoids), an important defense mechanism of the pulmonary system, are located in the superior nasopharynx.

The oropharynx is the area from the soft palate to the base of the tongue. It receives air from the mouth and nose, and food from the mouth. The faucial tonsils are located at the anterolateral borders of the oropharynx.

The laryngopharynx is the lower portion of the pharynx, extending from the base of the tongue to the opening of the esophagus. The laryngopharynx

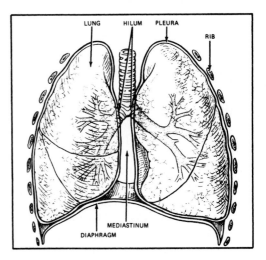

Figure 14–4. The mediastinum and hilum.

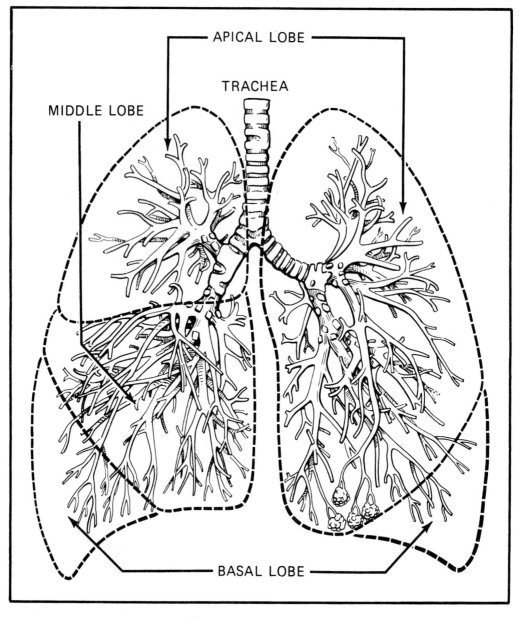

Figure 14–5. Lobes of the lung.

contains muscles within its wall, the pharyngeal constrictors, that aid in the mechanism of swallowing.

The Larynx

The larynx lies in the anterior portion of the neck, extending from cervical vertebrae through (C4–6), and connecting the upper and lower airway. It aids in speech, and is an essential part of the mechanism of coughing. The larynx is composed of cartilage, connected by membranes, and muscle. The laryngeal mucosa is stratified, squamous epithelium above the vocal cords and pseudostratified, columnar epithelium below.

The glottis is the opening into the larynx. The epiglottis, a flexible cartilage attached to the thyroid cartilage, helps prevent foreign material from entering airway by covering the glottis during swallowing. In the adult, the thyroid cartilage (Fig. 14–7) is the narrowest part of the air passage of the larynx. As muscles in the larynx contract, the vocal cords change shape and vibrate. This vibrating of the vocal cords produces sound.

The cricoid cartilage is a complete ring located just below the thyroid cartilage, where the vocal cords are located. The cricothyroid membrane is an avascular structure that connects the thyroid cartilage and cricoid cartilages. It is through this mem-

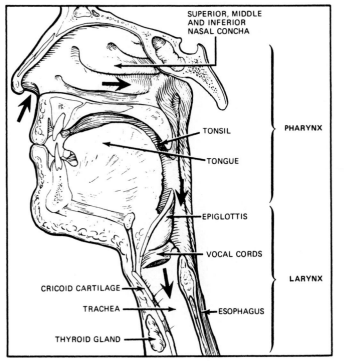

Figure 14–6. The upper airway, pharynx, and larynx.

brane that an airway may be established in an emergency. The posterior wall of the larynx and the vocal cords will not be injured.

LUNG DEFENSE MECHANISMS

The mucociliary escalator is the primary protective mechanism for the entire respiratory system. The entire respiratory tree is lined with varying types of epithelial cells. The airway is lined with cilia, which

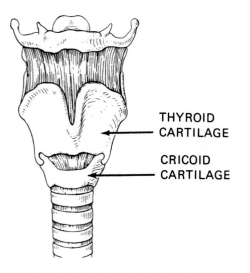

Figure 14–7. The thyroid-cricoid cartilages.

are fine, hairlike filaments projecting into the airway lumen. Goblet cells in the epithelium produce watery and thick mucous that covers the inside of the airway lumen. The mucous lining is called the mucous blanket. Various mechanisms move the mucous blanket to the pharynx, where it will be swallowed, to the larynx, where coughing will expel it, and to the nose, where it will be expelled by blowing and sneezing. Cilia lining the larger airways will help to move the mucous blanket up the respiratory tract by the cilia's continuous undulating movement, referred to as the mucociliary escalator (Fig. 14–8).

The sneeze reflex is a reaction to irritation in the nose. The cough reflex is a reaction to irritation in the upper airway distal to the nose. Both processes are complex mechanisms that require the integration of increased intrathoracic pressure, complete and tight closure of the epiglottis and vocal cords, and strong contraction of the abdominal musculature, diaphragm, and intercostal muscles.

THE LOWER AIRWAY

The lower airway consists of two divisions, the tracheobronchial tree and the lung parenchyma. The tracheobronchial tree is a system of progressively narrower conducting tubes providing air passage to the alveoli. The trachea divides into the right and left

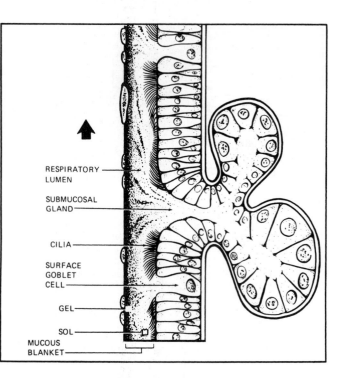

Figure 14–8. The mucociliary escalator.

main-stem bronchi. Further subdivisions include the bronchi, bronchioles, terminal bronchioles, and alveoli.

Trachea

The trachea extends from approximately C6 to the carina, the point of bifurcation of the right and left main-stem bronchi. It is composed of C-shaped cartilaginous rings with a posterior muscle that is membranous and friable. This muscle relaxes on inspiration, increasing the tracheal diameter. On exhalation, the muscle contracts, decreasing the tracheal diameter. Occasionally, the muscle relaxes and

bows in on exhalation, decreasing the effectiveness of the mucociliary stream in clearing secretions from the lungs (Fig. 14–9).

The trachea divides into the right and left mainstem bronchi at the carina, located at the angle of Louis at the sternomanibrial junction, about the second intracostal space. The right mainstem bronchus comes off the trachea in almost a straight line while the left mainstem bronchus comes off the trachea at an angle of approximately 40°. The right mainstem bronchus is wider in diameter than the left. Foreign matter tends to lodge in the right mainstem bronchus because of its size and the angle it takes off the trachea (Fig. 14–10).

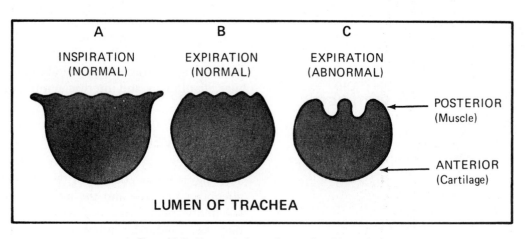

Figure 14–9. Movement of posterior muscles of the trachea.

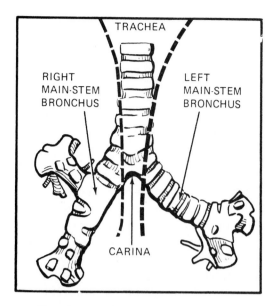

Figure 14–10. Right and left main-stem bronchi.

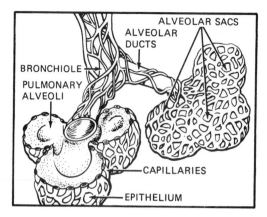

Figure 14–11. Terminal bronchiole and alveolar sac.

The right and left mainstem bronchi separate into 22 divisions before the terminal respiratory bronchioles. These divisions are cartilaginous; the terminal respiratory bronchioles are small tubes without cartilage. Only smooth muscle surrounds the respiratory epithelium. Contraction of this smooth muscle results in bronchospasm.

The respiratory bronchioles branch into alveolar ducts, and then into the alveoli which make up the lung parenchyma. The alveoli and alveolar ducts have common walls, termed septae, which play an important role in the elastic recoil of the lung. The septal wall is composed of smooth muscle that contracts to narrow the alveolar duct lumen.

Alveolar Sacs and Cells

The terminal end of the tracheobronchial tree is the alveolar sacs. The alveolar sacs are dead-end structures, preventing ambient air from going further. The sacs are made up of 15–20 alveoli, sharing a common wall with adjacent sacs (Fig. 14–11).

The 200 to 600 million alveoli in the normal lung comprise an average total surface area of 40–100 m^2, approximately the size of a football field. The surface area is directly related to body length and decreases by about 5% per decade.

Alveolar sacs are lined with epithelium, composed of three types of cells. Type I cells are characterized by cytoplasmic extensions and are the cells that make up most of the lung. Type II alveolar cells are found where one extension interfaces with another and are active metabolic cells that contain organelles to synthesize surfactant. Type III alveolar cells are phagocytes that arise from bone marrow or may arise from type II cells.

Pulmonary Surfactant

Alveolar epithelium is lined with a phospholipid protein fluid called surfactant. The phospholipid is insoluble but highly permeable to all gases. The function of surfactant is to reduce the surface tension in the alveoli. Two pathologic states that are complicated by insufficient or absent surfactant are (1) hyaline membrane disease and (2) adult respiratory distress syndrome (ARDS).

Surfactant functions by forming a thin, monomolecular layer at the interface of the air and fluid in the alveoli. Without surfactant an air–fluid interface would produce surface tension that would collapse the small alveoli. By preventing the development of the air–fluid interface, surfactant decreases the surface tension in the alveoli. Surfactant provides stability to smaller alveoli that have a greater pressure and tend to collapse. Without the proper amount of surfactant, there is a filtration of fluid from the alveolar wall capillaries into the alveoli, leading to development of pulmonary edema and/or ARDS.

The alveoli are where gas exchange occurs. Oxygen diffuses across the alveolar epithelium, the basement membrane, and the small interstitial space, and through the capillary membrane, the plasma fluid, and the erythrocyte membrane. At this point, the capillary is so small the erythrocytes must line up in a single column to move through the capillary. Oxygen diffuses rapidly through the erythrocyte membrane and attaches to the hemoglobin molecule of the erythrocyte. Carbon dioxide molecules diffuse across the alveolar capillary membrane in the opposite direction at a rate 20 times faster than oxygen. The capillary endothelium is very sensitive and is easily damaged by endotoxins, oxygen, or other noxious substances.

PULMONARY CIRCULATION

The lung receives deoxygenated blood from the right side of the heart via the pulmonary artery. The oxygenated blood is returned to the left side of the heart via the pulmonary vein, where it is pumped from the left ventricle through the cardiovascular system.

The lungs' arterial system follows the bronchial tree, bifurcating at each bronchial division, following close to the bronchus and its subdivisions. As the bronchioles become smaller some arteries fail to bifurcate and nearby arteries send out branches from their stem to provide oxygenated blood to the central part of the alveolar tissue (Fig. 14–12).

Venous blood flows through the capillaries and venules to the periphery of the alveoli and then re-enters the venous circulation to be directed back to the right atrium.

The total volume and rate of pulmonary blood circulation is about 5 L/min. Blood flow is greatest to the dependent portions of the lung, because of gravity. Thus, in an erect person, the apex of the lung will have the least circulating blood volume. When the person is lying down, the anterior lung surfaces will have the least circulating blood volume.

The erythrocyte completes the pulmonary circulation very rapidly (within 0.75 sec at rest). This rapid circulation helps maintain adequate perfusion. The total volume of blood in the pulmonary arteries, veins, and capillaries is about 500 to 750 ml in the average adult male or about 10–15% of the total blood volume, serving as a reservoir in times of increased cardiac output.

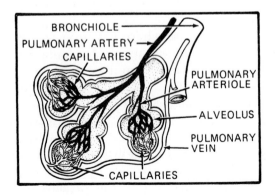

Figure 14–12. Blood flow in the parenchyma.

CONTROL OF VENTILATION

Three major factors control ventilation: neural, central chemical, and peripheral chemical control mechanisms.

Neural Control

The respiratory center is in the medullary portion of the brain stem. Neurons initiate impulses that result in inspiration. An increase in the rate of impulses results in an increase in respiratory rate; an increase in the strength increases tidal volume.

Normally, chemical factors keep the inspiratory and the expiratory centers in balance, resulting in normal ventilatory patterns. The inspiratory center is in the dorsal aspect of the medulla oblongata, in close association to the vagus nerve and the glossopharyngeal nerves. There appears to be an inherent automaticity in the electrical impulse release for inspiration. The apneustic center, in the pons, acts to prevent the interruption of these inspiratory impulses.

If the apneustic center takes control over the normally balanced ventilation pattern, apneustic breathing occurs, consisting of slight pauses following some expirations in an otherwise normal breathing pattern.

Expiration control is in the pneumotaxic center located in the upper pons. The neurons located there transmit impulses to limit inspiration. When the pneumotaxic center controls ventilation, there is irregular, deep, and shallow breathing with randomly spaced periods of varying lengths of apnea.

The walls of the pulmonary bronchi and bronchioles have stretch receptors that interact with the vagus nerve in what is known as the Hering–Breuer reflex. When they become overstretched, there is a feedback mechanism to the inspiratory center to prevent hyperinflation of the lungs.

Central Chemical Control

Cerebrospinal fluid (CSF) pH is the primary control of respiratory center stimulation. A change in the CSF hydrogen ion concentration occurs very quickly in relation to arterial carbon dioxide pressure $Paco_2$, resulting in the appropriate change in stimulation of the neural respiratory center. Acidosis, a rise in CSF hydrogen ion concentration, increases stimulation to respiratory centers. Alkalosis, a drop in CSF hydrogen ion concentration, decreases stimulation to neural respiratory centers.

Pa_{CO_2} is the normal neurochemical control of the respiratory cycle because of its effect on the CSF pH. A rise in CSF hydrogen ion concentration will first increase respiratory depth and then the respiratory rate.

Peripheral Chemical Control

Chemoreceptors are located at the bifurcation of the internal and external carotid arteries, carotid bodies, and aortic bodies at the aortic arch. These highly vascular, neural bodies are stimulated by any decrease in oxygen supply, such as decreased blood flow, decreased hemoglobin, increased pH, or increased Pa_{CO_2}. Stimulation of the carotid and/or aortic bodies will increase cerebral cortex activity, resulting in tachycardia, hypertension, increased respiratory rate, tidal volume, pulmonary resistance, bronchial smooth muscle tone, and adrenal gland secretions.

Factors Affecting Ventilation

Certain drugs depress the respiratory center by decreasing alveolar ventilation or blocking the central respiratory center. Decreased alveolar ventilation is characterized by shallow respirations and a respiratory rate less than 12 breaths/min.

Chronic respiratory disease may alter normal respiratory patterns. Patients with chronic CO_2 retention have a constantly elevated Pa_{CO_2}, decreasing the peripheral chemoreceptors' sensitivity to changes in hydrogen ion concentration. A decrease in arterial oxygen pressure (Pa_{O_2}) levels stimulates ventilation. High-flow oxygen therapy may result in apnea, suppressing the hypoxic drive mechanism.

PROCESS OF RESPIRATION

The process of respiration has four phases. Phase I is ventilation, the movement of ambient air into and out of the lungs. Phase II is the diffusion of oxygen and carbon dioxide in the alveoli. Phase III is the delivery of oxygen and removal of carbon dioxide from the cells. Phase IV is the regulation of ventilation.

Phase I—Ventilation

Normal barometric pressure at sea level is 760 mm Hg. For the average, healthy person at rest, the intrapleural pressure is slightly subatmospheric at 755 mm Hg. If the pressures were equal, there would be no flow of air into or out of the lung.

As inspiration begins, the thoracic cage increases in size, producing a negative intrapleural pressure, compared to the atmosphere, resulting in air flow into the lungs. If one considers atmospheric pressure to be zero (0), then resting intrapleural pressure is –5 and inspiratory intrapleural pressure is –10. As inspiratory muscle activity ends, the normal elastic recoil of the lung decreases thoracic cage size and gas flows out of the lung.

Lung Pressures

The pulmonary system is a low-pressure system. This low-pressure system allows the capillaries to distend easily to accommodate increased volumes from the systemic circulatory system in times of distress and/or exertion. The distensibility helps regulate resistance to blood flow through the pulmonary system. In the normal disease-free lung, the average pulmonary artery systolic pressure is 15–30 mm Hg and the average diastolic pressure is 5–15 mm Hg. The pressure necessary to move blood from the right heart to the left heart is the left atrial pressure, or the pulmonary capillary wedge pressure (PCWP). The normal left atrial and PCWP is 8–12 mm Hg. The mean pulmonary artery pressure must always be higher than the left atrial pressure in order to move blood from the right heart through the lungs to the left atrium.

Compliance

Compliance is a measure of the distensibility of the lungs and thorax. Compliance is expressed as change in volume (V) for a change in the intra-alveolar pressure (P). Greater compliance means there is a larger volume change in the lung for each pressure change. Reduced compliance means there is less volume change in the lung for each pressure change. In other words, the more pressure needed to change the volume in the lung, the less compliance.

Any disease that stiffens the lungs will decrease compliance. Diseases that increase congestion in the lungs, such as atelectasis, pneumonia, or pulmonary edema, result in decreased lung compliance and decreased gas exchange. Space-occupying neoplasms, infections, or increased extravascular lung water decrease lung compliance (Table 14–1).

Any condition that limits the ability of the bony thorax to expand will also decrease lung compliance. An example of a restrictive cause of decreased compliance is third-trimester pregnancy. During the third trimester of pregnancy abdominal contents are displaced upward, preventing the diaphragm from descending fully, decreasing the extent of chest wall

TABLE 14–1. CAUSES OF DECREASED LUNG COMPLIANCE

Intrathoracic	Extrathoracic
Atelectasis	Flail chest
Pneumonia	Barrel chest
Pleural effusion	Pectus excavatum
Empyema	Pectus carinatum
Lung abscess	Kyphosis
Bronchospasm	Scoliosis
Pulmonary edema	Kyphoscoliosis
Bronchitis	
Asthma	
Emphysema	
Adult respiratory distress syndrome (ARDS)	
Tension pneumothorax	

expansion. Obesity and abdominal distention also prevent full movement of the diaphragm. The obese patient has a decreased lung compliance as a result of the excess weight on the upper torso. The intercostal muscles cannot function efficiently as they attempt to lift the weight. Postoperative binders and chest splints decrease lung compliance over large segments of the thorax by limiting the expansion of the thorax.

There are two types of compliance, static and dynamic. Static compliance (Cst) is the change in lung volume per unit airway pressure change when the lungs are motionless. Static compliance can be measured only when there is no flow of gases, at the end of inspiration or expiration. Normally it is about 100 ml of pressure per centimeter of water pressure (cm H_2O). Static compliance measurements are a reliable index of lung compliance when no airway disease is present, as the presence of airway disease alters the rate of gas flow from the mouth to the alveoli, resulting in inaccurate values. If airway disease is present, most of the resistance to air flow will be in the medium size bronchi.

Dynamic compliance (Cdyn) can be easily tested in the clinical area. To get an estimate of the dynamic compliance for the patient on mechanical ventilation, divide the tidal volume (VT) by the peak airway pressure (PAP). Normal dynamic compliance is about 35–55 ml/cm H_2O.

Airway resistance results from impediment of gas molecule flow by the walls of the airway or obstruction, changing the ratio of alveolar pressure against the rate of air flow. Airway resistance is increased by secretions, artificial airways, endotracheal tubes, bronchospasms, laryngeal or tracheal strictures, edema, emphysema, or space-occupying lesions. A measure of airway resistance can be made by comparing the static and dynamic compliance.

Elastic Recoil

Intra-alveolar septae are a major factor in the elastic recoil of the interstitial parenchyma. The thorax, pleura, and lung parenchyma have opposing elastic forces. The fluid lining the alveoli and the interstitial parenchymal try to collapse the lungs, while the thoracic cage and pleura try to expand the lungs. As long as the thoracic cage and pleura are patent, these elastic forces balance each other. If the integrity of the pleura is compromised, the parenchymal forces become greater, and the lung collapses.

Air Flow

There are three basic types of air flow within the lung airways, turbulent, transitional, and laminar. Turbulent air flow occurs in large chambers such as the nose and oral pharynx (Fig. 14–13). Transitional air flow occurs in large-to-medium airways at points of bifurcation and/or narrowing. As air flows down the tracheobronchial tree, it branches into smaller and smaller tubes creating transitional air flow (Figure 14–14). Laminar air flow occurs in thin, flat, continuous sheets. The outermost layer of air has minimal contact with the air passage walls, providing slight filtering in the small peripheral airways (Figure 14–15).

Lung Volumes

The total lung capacity (TLC) is the maximum amount of gas that the lungs can hold (Fig. 14–16). Normal is about 4000–7000 ml. The TLC is composed of four discrete lung volumes measured by spirometry: the inspiratory reserve volume, the tidal volume, the reserve volume, and the residual volume. This relationship is expressed by the equation TLC = IRV + VT + ERV + RV.

Inspiratory reserve volume (IRV) is the amount of reserve or extra gas that can be inhaled at the end of a normal inspiration. Normal IRV may be as much as 3000 ml.

Tidal volume (VT) is the amount of gas that is exhaled or inhaled during normal breathing. Normal VT is 5–10 ml/kg or about 350–600 ml in a young adult.

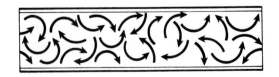

Figure 14–13. Turbulent air flow.

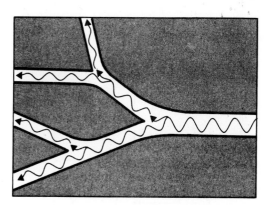

Figure 14–14. Transitional air flow.

Expiratory reserve volume (ERV) is the amount of gas that can be exhaled after a normal expiration. Normal ERV is about 1000–1500 ml.

Residual volume (RV) is the amount of gas that always remains in the lungs and cannot be exhaled.

There are four lung capacities which represent the combination of two or more lung volumes. The values listed for lung capacities are averages and will differ according to body size, weight, and age.

Vital capacity (VC) is the amount of gas that can be forcefully exhaled after a maximum inspiration (VC = VT + IRV + ERV) Normal is about 4000–5000 ml.

The inspiratory capacity (IC) is the amount of gas that can be inhaled after a normal exhalation (IC = VT + IRV). Normal is about 3500 ml.

The functional residual capacity (FRC), is the amount of air in the lungs after normal expiration (FRC = ERV + RV). Normal is about 2000–3000 ml.

These respiratory volumes and capacities can be used to establish a baseline and monitor the effectiveness of treatment modalities. Vital capacity, inspiratory force, and tidal volume are the most frequently measured parameters of respiratory muscle function.

Dead Space

Dead space (VD) is amount of inhaled gas that does not take part in gas exchange. Gas exchange only occurs in the terminal bronchioles and alveoli. There are two types of dead space, anatomical and physiological. Physiological dead space is the total amount of dead space in the lung. Anatomical dead space is estimated to be 150 ml or 1 ml/pound of ideal body weight (25–35% of VT). For a 500-cc tidal volume, approximately 350 ml reaches the alveoli.

The amount of inhaled air that reaches the alveoli and takes part in gas exchange is alveolar ventilation (VA). In a stable state, the arterial carbon dioxide is inversely related to alveolar ventilation, and indicates adequacy of gas exchange. VA is equal to VE (minute ventilation) − VD. VE is normally 5–10 LPM and is measured by multiplying VT × RR.

Phase II—Gas Diffusion

On inspiration, oxygen concentration or pressure is greater in the alveoli than the erythrocytes. The carbon dioxide concentration is greater in the erythrocytes than the alveoli. Therefore, the gas diffuses from the highest level of concentration toward the lower level of concentration.

The actual area of space the gases have to cross to diffuse is very thin, 0.2–0.5 µm. The alveoli and capillaries are so small and thin that under the microscope they look like a single sheet of blood. Instead, they are made up of six layers, the alveolus, alveolar membrane, interstitial space, capillary membrane, plasma, and the erythrocyte membrane. The gases must diffuse through these layers, known as the respiratory membrane, for gas exchange to take place. If the membrane becomes thickened, as in pulmonary edema or interstitial pulmonary fibrosis, the diffusion of gases is slowed. Another factor affecting diffusion through the respiratory membrane is the available surface area. If an area of the lung is filled with fluid or pus, its presence will cause gas diffusion to be slowed or stopped completely. In emphysema, the alveolar septae collapse, destroying the alveolar structure, and decreasing the surface area available for diffusion.

The specific composition of the alveolar, arterial, and venous compartments will directly affect the diffusibility of gases (Table 14–2).

OXYGEN TRANSPORT

Once oxygen has penetrated the erythrocyte membrane, it is carried through the systemic circulatory system to all body tissues. Oxygen is transported in only two possible forms in the body, either dissolved in plasma or combined with hemoglobin. The amount

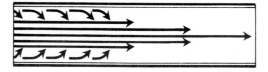

Figure 14–15. Laminar air flow.

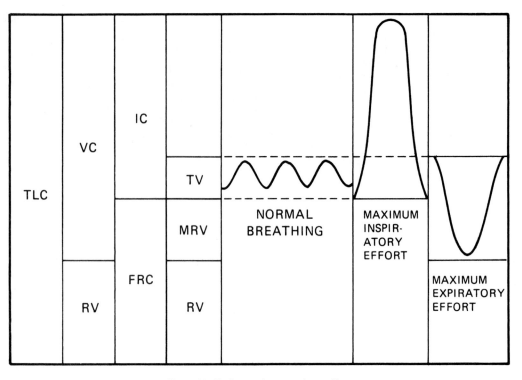

Figure 14–16. Lung volumes and capacities.

of oxygen dissolved in the plasma is very small and amounts to 0.003 ml 2/100 ml of blood, or 3% of the total body oxygen. PaO_2 measures dissolved oxygen. The remaining 97% of oxygen transported through the system's circulation in combination with hemoglobin (Hgb), oxyhemoglobin. A gram of hemoglobin combines with approximately 1.34 ml of oxygen. The transport of oxygen to body tissues is influenced most by cardiac output, hemoglobin concentration, and by oxygen–hemoglobin binding and releasing factors.

Cardiac output is usually 4–8 L/min. As the cardiac output varies, the quantity of blood oxygenated in the lungs also varies. In normal, healthy lungs, a slight decrease in cardiac output will not greatly alter oxygen content. A markedly decreased cardiac output will alter oxygen content, although the available blood will be maximally oxygenated. If hemoglobin is low, cardiac output will increase to help compensate and maintain an adequate oxygen content. The amount of oxygen transported per minute is determined by the cardiac output, even though there are other contributing factors.

Oxygen content (CaO_2) is the maximum potential amount of oxygen the blood can carry. It is expressed as milliliters of oxygen per 100 ml of blood. $CaO_2 = Hgb \times 1.34$ (cubic centimeters of oxygen) $\times SaO_2 + (PO_2 \times 0.0003)$. In calculating the oxygen content, the dissolved oxygen in plasma (PaO_2) is usually not included because of its small contribution. Oxygen content is equal to the actual amount of oxygen in both the plasma and the erythrocytes.

Oxygen saturation (SaO_2) is the ratio comparing the actual amount of oxygen that could be carried with the amount actually carried, expressed as a percentage.

Oxygen Capacity

Hemoglobin has a natural affinity for oxygen. Once the oxygen diffuses through the erythrocyte membrane, it readily attaches to the hemoglobin molecule. With a hemoglobin level of 15 g%, 100 ml of blood will have enough hemoglobin to carry 20 cc of oxygen. Hemoglobin cannot be oversaturated; 100% is the maximum under human physiological conditions.

TABLE 14–2. COMPOSITION OF PULMONARY GASES

Alveolar	Arterial	Venous	Atmospheric
$PH_2O = 47$	$PH_2O = 47$	$PH_2O = 47$	$PH_2O = 47$
$PACO_2 = 40$	$PaCO_2 = 40$	$PVCO_2 = 46$	$PICO_2 = 0$
$PAO_2 = 100-110$	$PaO_2 = 92$	$PVO_2 = 40$	$PIO_2 = 150$
$PAN_2 = 563$	$PaN_2 = 563$	$PVN_2 = 563$	$PIN_2 = 563$
			760 mm Hg

P, pressure or partial pressure; A, alveolar; O_2, oxygen; a, arterial; CO_2, carbon dioxide; V, venous; N_2, nitrogen; I, inspired; H_2O, water.

Oxygen Transport

Oxygen transport is the amount of oxygen delivered to the cells, expressed as milliliters of oxygen per minute. O_2 transport = CaO_2 × 10 × cardiac output, expressed in liters per minute. Normal oxygen transport is between 600 and 1000 ml/min or 10–12 cc/kg.

Oxygen content and oxygen transport are a more reliable index of oxygenation than the PaO_2 alone because the hemoglobin level and cardiac output are taken into consideration.

Oxygen Consumption (Vo₂)

Oxygen consumption is the amount of oxygen used per minute. Normal Vo_2 is approximately 3.5 ml/kg/min. A 70-kg person would use approximately 245 ml/min of oxygen at rest. Under normal circumstances, only 25–30% of the transported oxygen is used by the cells. If oxygen transport is 1000 ml/min and Vo_2 is 250 ml/min, 25% of the oxygen transported was used. The oxygen extraction rate is the difference between the oxygen transported and the oxygen consumed. As the oxygen extraction rate increases, cellular oxygenation is threatened. Rates over 40% require assessment of oxygen transport and consumption components.

Oxyhemoglobin Dissociation

Factors affecting oxygen–hemoglobin binding and releasing include temperature, pH, PCO_2, acidosis or alkalosis, and 2,3-diphosphoglycerate (2,3-DPG). The oxyhemoglobin curve is an S-shaped curve representing the nonlinear relationship of the PaO_2 and the SaO_2 (Fig. 14–17).

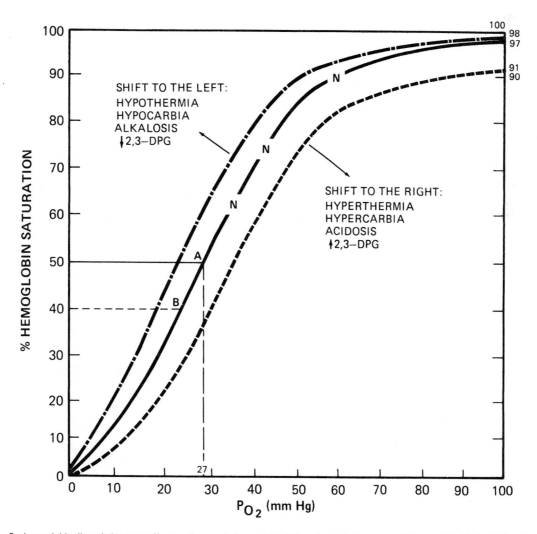

Figure 14–17. Oxyhemoglobin dissociation curve. N, normal curve; A, hemoglobin 50% saturated with oxygen; B, hemoglobin binds tightly with oxygen, preventing its release to the tissues, leading to hypoxia.

The amount of oxygen dissolved in the plasma, the PaO_2, provides the driving pressure that forces oxygen to combine with hemoglobin. The driving pressure of dissolved oxygen exists until the alveolar (PaO_2) and the arterial (PaO_2) pressures are almost equal. With the oxygen pressure gradient between the alveolus and the erythrocyte at equilibrium, the point of the normal curve is the upper right. In the healthy person, the oxygen tension is 95–97 mm Hg with a hemoglobin saturation (SaO_2) of about 97%.

There is a steep down-slope portion to the curve, indicating a move from the lungs into the systemic circulation. The SaO_2 and the PaO_2 are dropping because the hemoglobin is readily giving up oxygen to the tissue capillaries. As the hemoglobin moves through the body, the PaO_2 drops and hemoglobin loses its affinity for oxygen, readily releases it into the tissues. When SaO_2 drops to 50%, the P_{50}, the hemoglobin begins to give up to its oxygen much less readily. At the P_{50}, the partial pressure of arterial oxygen is about 27 mm Hg. The normal curve can be shifted to the right or to the left by many factors. A shift in either direction indicates a change from the normal SaO_2 and PaO_2.

A shift to the right occurs in acidosis, hypercarbia, increased carbon dioxide, and fever. A shift to the right means there is less oxygen in the blood. It also means oxygen is more readily given up to the tissues by the hemoglobin, preventing hypoxia. If shift persists, eventually the decreased oxygen content will not prevent tissue hypoxia.

A shift to the left occurs in alkalosis, hypocarbia, and hypothermia. In a shift to the left, hemoglobin binds oxygen much more tightly and releases less oxygen to the tissues. The arterial oxygen tension and hemoglobin saturation are only very slightly changed from the normal curve.

2,3-Diphosphoglycerate (2,3-DPG) is an important organic phosphate that will shift the normal curve to the right and left. 2,3-DPG is a phosphate-type enzyme that is present in erythrocytes. An increase of 2,3-DPG in the hemoglobin of erythrocytes shifts the curve to the right and facilitates release of oxygen in the tissues. A decrease of 2,3-DPG in the hemoglobin of erythrocytes shifts the curve to the left and hinders the release of oxygen into the tissues.

Causes of Hypoxemia

Normal pulmonary anatomy accounts for the 2–5% of the blood flowing through the lungs that does not come in contact with inspired air for gas exchange. Anatomic shunt occurs when there is adequate ventilation to the alveoli, but perfusion is absent or markedly decreased and blood does not have the chance to participate in gas exchange (Fig. 14–18). This can be due to an anatomic aberration of the circulatory system of the lungs, such as an anomaly in the pulmonary vasculature, which channels unoxygenated blood into the left atrium through the thebesian, pleural, and bronchial veins. The danger of these are a low PaO_2 (<60 mm Hg) can produce pulmonary hypertension, increased breathing, and low SaO_2 levels.

Decreased alveolar ventilation (VA) results in rising $PACO_2$, causing displacement of oxygen and lowering PaO_2. Hypoventilation-induced hypoxemia is easily treated with oxygen therapy; however, the decreased VA must be improved or respiratory failure will occur.

Intrapulmonary, or physiological, shunt is that portion of the pulmonary blood flow not exposed to functioning alveoli (Fig. 14–19). It provides a measure of efficiency of gas exchange in the lungs. Accumulated secretions, atelectasis, pulmonary edema, neoplasms, and foreign objects are only a few of many causes of obstruction.

Intrapulmonary shunts are also referred to as low ventilation/perfusion (V/Q) ratios. When alveolar ventilation is reduced without a subsequent reduction in perfusion, venous blood is not completely oxygenated. Normal venous oxygen levels are low (PvO_2 35–45 mm Hg and SvO_2 0.60–0.75), and more poorly oxygenated blood becomes mixed with oxygenated blood, resulting in hypoxemia (PaO_2 below 60 mm Hg). Intrapulmonary shunt is measured by shunt equations or estimated from oxygen

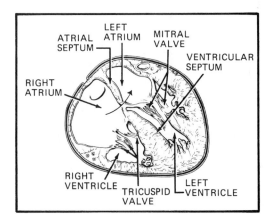

Figure 14–18. Anatomical shunt.

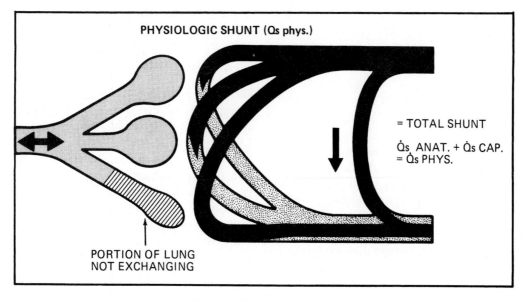

PHYSIOLOGIC SHUNT (Qs phys.)

= TOTAL SHUNT

$\dot{Q}s$ ANAT. + $\dot{Q}s$ CAP.
= $\dot{Q}s$ PHYS.

PORTION OF LUNG
NOT EXCHANGING

Figure 14–19. Physiological shunt.

tension indices, such as the PaO_2/FIO_2 ratio or a/A ratio. Normal PaO_2/FIO_2 ratio is >286. The lower it becomes, the worse the shunt.

CARBON DIOXIDE TRANSPORT

Carbon dioxide is a byproduct of metabolism. It is effectively eliminated only through respiration and is reflected in changes in $PaCO_2$ values. Carbon dioxide is transported in the blood in five different states: (1) dissolved in plasma; (2) as bicarbonate ion; (3) as carbonic acid; (4) in combination with hemoglobin; and (5) an extremely small amount as the carbonate ion.

Much like oxygen, only a very small amount of carbon dioxide is transported in the dissolved state, making up about 7% of the total carbon dioxide. The presence of carbon dioxide in a dissolved state creates a pressure gradient or driving force measured as carbon dioxide tension, or $PaCO_2$. The pressure gradient of the dissolved carbon dioxide at the tissue level continues until the blood reaches the pulmonary capillaries. Since no carbon dioxide is normally inhaled, the pressure gradient is almost completely one-sided, pushing carbon dioxide from the capillary into the alveoli.

The dissolved carbon dioxide in the blood reacts with water to form carbonic acid. The amount of carbon dioxide that diffuses into the erythrocyte comes into contact with carbonic anhydrase, an enzyme that is a strong catalyst enabling dissolved carbon dioxide to convert to carbonic acid rapidly.

About 70% of the body's carbon dioxide waste is handled by the lungs through exhalation. As soon as carbonic acid is formed, it is immediately broken down into hydrogen and bicarbonate ions through the process of dissociation. The hydrogen ions combine with hemoglobin, the bicarbonate ions diffuse into the plasma, and chloride ions diffuse into the erythrocytes to maintain homeostasis. Movement of the bicarbonate ion results in a chloride shift, allowing chloride to move into the erythrocytes. Since this is the body's most important way of transporting carbon dioxide, it is important to review the steps of the chemical reactions.

1. Carbon dioxide enters the erythrocyte and does two things:
   (A) combines with hemoglobin

   $$CO_2 + Hgb \rightarrow Hgb\,CO_2$$

   (B) combines with water

   $$CO_2 + H_2O$$
   carbon dioxide + water
   $$CA \longleftrightarrow H_2CO_3$$
   carbonic anhydrase $\longleftrightarrow$ carbonic acid

2. The carbonic acid of step B dissociates

   $$H_2CO_3 \longleftrightarrow HCO_3^- + H^+$$
   carbonic acid $\longleftrightarrow$ bicarbonate ion + hydrogen ion

3. Bicarbonate ion leaves the erythrocyte and enters the plasma, allowing the chloride ion to enter the erythrocyte (the chloride shift).

4. The hydrogen ion from step C binds with hemoglobin

$$H^+ + Hgb \longleftrightarrow HHgb$$

VENTILATION PHYSIOLOGY

The acid-base state in our bodies is kept within a very narrow range. An acid state that is not corrected will eventually result in a coma and then death. A base or alkalotic state that is not corrected will eventually result in convulsion, tetany or eventually death.

An acid is a chemical substance that dissociates into positive or negative electrically charged ions by and gives up a hydrogen (H^+) proton to the solution. The positive ion is a cation and the negative ion is an anion. A base is a substance that can and will accept a hydrogen proton while in solution. Water is the most common and abundant base in the body. The pH represents the hydrogen ion concentration and is an expression of the hydrogen ion concentration as a negative logarithm.

Two types of acids are formed in the body: volatile acids or nonvolatile (fixed) acids. These acids are formed by the metabolism of food and by anaerobic glycolysis.

Volatile acids are those acids that can form a gas, and because of an open system, can be eliminated in their gaseous form. All volatile acids can, therefore, be eliminated by the lungs. The main source of volatile acids is the body's metabolism of glucose and fat. Carbonic acid is the major volatile acid in the body. It is made by the combination of carbon dioxide and water: $CO_2 + H_2O \longleftrightarrow H_2CO_3$. The double-direction arrow indicates that the reaction readily moves in either direction.

Acids that cannot be converted into their gaseous form for elimination are termed nonvolatile or fixed acids. Nonvolatile acids are excreted mainly by the kidneys via the urine and in the stool. Nonvolatile acid sources are anaerobic glycolysis, amino acid metabolism, and phosphoprotein/phospholipid metabolism. The kidneys excrete these fixed acids, totaling about 50 mEq/day. Disease can also produce nonvolatile acids.

ACID-BASE BALANCE

When there is any disruption in the acid-base balance of the arterial blood toward acidosis, the body has three main defense mechanisms: buffering, increasing alveolar ventilation, and/or increasing

hydrogen ion elimination along with increasing bicarbonate reabsorption.

Buffering

Buffering is an immediate response to an acid-base disturbance which prevents changes in hydrogen ion concentration. Increasing alveolar ventilation begins in 1–2 min. As the hydrogen ion concentration builds up the lungs attempt to reduce the amount of hydrogen ions by increasing ventilation. The kidneys provide the strongest defense against acid-base disturbances by increasing hydrogen ion elimination and increasing bicarbonate ion reabsorption. Unfortunately, it takes from several hours to several days for the kidneys to rebalance the hydrogen ion concentration.

There are three major buffering systems: (1) the bicarbonate buffer system; (2) the phosphate buffer system; and (3) the protein buffer system. The bicarbonate buffer system is the most important system because the end products of the chemical buffer are regulated by both the kidneys and the lungs. The chemical reaction in this system is reversible and occurs extremely rapidly:

$$H^+ + HCO_3^- \longleftrightarrow H_2CO_33 \longleftrightarrow CO_2 + H^+.$$

If the buffering moves toward the left, the bicarbonate ion is the end product, regulated by the kidneys. If the buffering moves toward the right, the end product is carbon dioxide, regulated by the lungs. The pH can be shifted up or down by either or both the renal and/or the respiratory system.

The phosphate buffer system is similar to the bicarbonate system in function and buffers best at a slightly different pH than bicarbonate, mainly in the tubular fluids of the kidney. This system buffers strong acids (e.g., hydrochloric acid) and strong bases (e.g., sodium hydroxide) into weak acids and bases that have little effect upon the blood pH.

The protein buffer system is the most inexhaustible buffering system in the body. All the plasma proteins and intracellular proteins, such as hemoglobin, buffer and the supply of protein is infinite. Proteins buffer carbon dioxide quickly and bicarbonate ions over a period of several hours. The importance of this system is that it helps buffer the extracellular fluids through diffusion of carbon dioxide and bicarbonate ion.

Increasing Alveolar Ventilation

If the buffering system has not rectified an acid-base disturbance within minutes, the respiratory system will become active. Alveolar hyperventilation increases the rate of carbon dioxide excretion, compensating for a metabolic acidosis. Alveolar hypoventilation does the opposite, compensating for a metabolic alkalosis. As alveolar ventilation increases the $PaCO_2$ decreases. The decreased $PaCO_2$ results in a respiratory-induced alkalosis, forcing the hydrogen to combine with HCO_3^-. If alveolar ventilation decreases the $PaCO_2$ level increases, resulting in a respiratory acidosis, as a result of the increased availability of hydrogen.

Increasing Hydrogen Ion Elimination/ Bicarbonate Reabsorption

The final mechanism the body can utilize to alter acid-base disturbances is increasing hydrogen ion elimination and bicarbonate ion reabsorption. This defense mechanism involves both the lungs and the kidneys. The kidney function of acid-base disturbances reacts within a few hours of the disturbance; however, it is a slow-acting defense mechanism and may take several days to rebalance the acids and bases. The kidneys are able to excrete some hydrogen ions in relation to excretion of nonvolatile acids. This is a very small amount of hydrogen ion elimination since the lungs excrete the majority of the hydrogen ions. At the same time the kidneys reabsorb bicarbonate ions in the proximal tubule to equal the excessive number of hydrogen ions. As this reabsorption proceeds, carbon dioxide and water are formed:

$$H^+ + HCO_3^- \longleftrightarrow H_2CO_3^- \longleftrightarrow CO_2 + H_2O.$$

If this reabsorption is not adequate to restore acid-base balance, sodium and hydrogen ions will trade places to maintain electrical neutrality and the sodium bicarbonate return from the kidney tubules to the plasma. If this does not re-establish acid-base balance, the kidneys will conserve still more bicarbonate by substituting ammonium ions (NH_4) for bicarbonate ions. Assuming the acid-base disturbance continues, and all of the possible bicarbonate ions have been retained, hydrogen ions will reach the distal tubules and combine with phosphates. These phosphates will be excreted in the urine. Alterations in potassium and extracellular fluid volume are final efforts of the kidney to restore acid-base balance.

ACID-BASE DISTURBANCES

The pH expresses the driving pressure of acid-base balance. The pH is a negative logarithm of the hydrogen ion concentration of the blood. The smaller the value of the pH, the greater the concentration of hydrogen ions and the more acidic the solution. Conversely, the larger the value of the pH, the smaller the concentration of hydrogen ions and the less acidic the solution. The normal range of pH for arterial blood is 7.35–7.45.

Acidosis is an acid-base disturbance with a predominant quantity of acid. Acidemia is a state of increased hydrogen ions reflected in an arterial blood pH below 7.35. Alkalosis is an acid-base disturbance in which acids are insufficient in quantity or base is in excess. Acid insufficiency is more commonly a cause than is base excess. Alkalemia is a state of decreased hydrogen ions reflected in an arterial blood pH above 7.45.

There are only two ways by which the pH may be returned toward the normal 7.40 in acid-base disturbances: compensation or correction. Compensation occurs when the body attempts to respond to the acid-base abnormality. If the primary disturbance is respiratory, the kidneys will respond to shift the pH toward normal. If the primary disturbance is metabolic, the respiratory system will attempt to compensate for the alteration.

In respiratory acidosis, the lungs are responsible for the altered state. The kidneys will try to compensate by excreting more acid in the urine and increasing reabsorption of the bicarbonate ion. These two concurrent actions will move the pH nearly back to the normal value of 7.40. In respiratory alkalosis the kidneys will try to compensate by increasing the amount of bicarbonate excreted.

In metabolic acidosis the respiratory system is stimulated to increase alveolar ventilation. The hyperventilation increases the excretion of carbon dioxide as an acid waste product of metabolic processes. This is an effective and rapid way to decrease $PaCO_2$. The respiratory system can compensate in metabolic acidosis in just a few hours. In metabolic alkalosis the respiratory system will hypoventilate, retaining carbon dioxide and shifting the pH toward normal. The body cannot fully compensate for metabolic alkalosis. The hypoventilation necessary for compensation causes a decrease in the PaO_2. When the oxygen level becomes too low, the respiratory system will respond to the decreased oxygen by increasing ventilation. Although this compensation effort is rapid, it is not a complete compensation. The most significant fact about compensation as a defense mechanism in acid-base disturbance is that the body never overcompensates and will return the pH to near normal (7.40), but it never "overshoots the mark."

RESPIRATORY IMBALANCES

Respiratory Acidosis

The normal Pa_{CO_2} is 35–45 mm Hg. If the Pa_{CO_2} is elevated, over 45 mm Hg, and the pH decreased, below 7.35, respiratory acidosis is present and indicates acute or chronic hypoventilation. Respiratory acidosis indicates inadequate alveolar ventilation.

Any clinical condition that depresses the respiratory center in the medulla oblongata may precipitate hypoventilation and result in respiratory acidosis. These conditions include head trauma, oversedation, and general anesthesia. More rarely, neoplasms in the medulla oblongata or nearby areas with increasing intracranial mass, size, and pressure may cause a respiratory acidosis. Neuromuscular diseases, including myasthenia gravis, Guillain-Barré syndrome, multiple sclerosis, amyotrophic lateral sclerosis, and trauma to the cervical spinal cord, may cause hypoventilation and resultant respiratory acidosis. Inappropriate mechanical ventilation may cause respiratory acidosis. Too low a respiratory rate or tidal volume and too much dead space in the tubing may result in respiratory acidosis. Obstructive lung diseases may result in a degree of V/Q disturbance, increasing the risk for developing both acute and chronic carbon dioxide retention.

Respiratory acidosis can best be treated by improving ventilation. This includes nursing measures such as protecting the airway through positioning or use of artificial airways. The key to treatment is to find the cause of the respiratory depression and correct it. A respiratory acidosis only requires active treatment if the increase in Pa_{CO_2} results in a pH of about 7.25. The more alert the patient, the longer intubation and mechanical ventilation can be delayed. For the patient on mechanical ventilation, the respiratory rate is increased to decrease the Pa_{CO_2} and maintain effective ventilation, or the tidal volume may be increased.

Respiratory Alkalosis

When the the Pa_{CO_2} is decreased, below 35 mm Hg, and the pH is increased, above 7.45, respiratory alkalosis is present, indicating hyperventilation. Restrictive lung diseases are common pathological causes of respiratory alkalosis. Other causes of respiratory alkalosis include anxiety, nervousness, agitation, hyperventilation via mechanical ventilation, and excessive Ambu-bagging during a cardiopulmonary arrest.

A respiratory alkalosis is treated by finding the cause of the excessive breathing, such as anxiety, pain, fear, hypoxemic compensation for a metabolic acidosis, or CNS disturbance. Correcting the causative problem will correct the respiratory alkalosis. If the patient is on mechanical ventilation, decreasing the respiratory rate, decreasing the tidal volume, or adding additional tubing (dead space) may correct the imbalance. If the pH is greater than 7.55, more aggressive measures such as administration of acetazolamide (Diamox), ammonium chloride, hydrochloric acid, or potassium chloride (KCl) are used.

METABOLIC DISTURBANCES

Base Excess

The bicarbonate ion (HCO_3) and base excess are the parameters of the arterial blood gases used to identify nonrespiratory imbalances. Base excess is an easy guide to use in distinguishing metabolic acidosis from alkalosis. Base excess is the amount of base above the normal level, after adjusting the level for hemoglobin. The normal midpoint value is zero. If the base excess is above +2, there is an excess of metabolic base in the body fluids and a metabolic alkalosis exists. If the base excess is below –2, there is not enough metabolic base in the body fluids and a metabolic acidosis exists.

Metabolic Alkalosis

Metabolic alkalosis is a condition with an excess base. The three most common causes are diuretic therapy, excessive vomiting, and excessive ingestion of alkaline drugs. Any condition that increases metabolic processes beyond the ability of the body to eliminate or neutralize the waste products results in an increase in bicarbonate ions. These conditions cause a loss of hydrogen ions (diuretics), chloride ions (vomiting), and potassium ions (hyperaldosteronism) through the kidneys. The effect is increased bicarbonate ion reabsorption in the kidneys, which forces excretion of the hydrogen, chloride, and potassium ions in the urine. Loss of gastric secretions from vomiting or through nasogastric suctioning results in metabolic alkalosis. Excessive ingestion of alkaline drugs such as antacids and soda bicarbonate may lead to metabolic alkalosis. Less commonly, treatment with corticosteroids, hyperaldosteronism, and Cushing's syndrome may result in a metabolic alkalosis.

A metabolic alkalosis is corrected by finding and treating the underlying cause. Most cases of metabolic alkalosis are due to electrolyte disturbances, such as hypokalemia (low potassium) or hyperchloremia (high chloride). In severe disturbances where the pH is greater than 7.60, hydrochloric acid or ammonium chloride may be administered.

Metabolic Acidosis

Metabolic acidosis occurs in the body when there is an increase of any metabolic acid, except carbon dioxide. Although carbon dioxide is an acid end product of body metabolism, it is excreted by the lungs and therefore classified as a respiratory acidosis when elevated. Metabolic acidosis may occur with an excess loss of body alkali (bicarbonate ion), with certain medications, with retention of hydrogen ions, and in prolonged vomiting and diarrhea of small intestinal fluids.

Metabolic acidoses are classified in two major groups: those with an increase in unmeasurable anions, and those with no increase in unmeasurable anions. To calculate unmeasurable anions, add the serum chloride and the bicarbonate ion values, then subtract this sum from the serum sodium level. If the difference is greater than 15 mEq/L, there is an increase in unmeasurable anions known as the anion gap. No real anion gap exists since postive (cations) and negative (anions) ions must always be present in equal numbers. However, it appears as if the anion gap is present since only the major ions (sodium, chloride, and bicarbonate) are measured.

Common causes of metabolic acidosis with an increase in unmeasurable anions include (the specific anion is in parentheses) diabetes mellitus (ketone bodies), uremia (phosphates and sulfates), lactic acidosis (lactate), aspirin poisoning (salicy-late), methyl poisoning (formic acid), ethylene glycol poisoning (oxalic acid and formic acid), and paraldehyde poisoning.

There are several common causes of metabolic acidosis with no increase in unmeasurable anions. Diarrhea is probably the most common cause. Large amounts of bicarbonate ion are in the intestines and are washed out in the diarrhea. The more severe the diarrhea, the greater the likelihood of metabolic acidosis. A general guide for the possible development of metabolic acidosis with no increase in unmeasurable anion is the presence below the umbilicus of a drainage tube (except a Foley catheter) such as that for drainage of the pancreas or a ureterosigmoidostomy, and other drainage tubes.

Another cause is uremia. In severe renal failure, the kidneys cannot excrete the normal acids formed daily by the body. As the acids build up, uremia develops, resulting in an increase in unmeasurable anions.

Metabolic acidosis is the most difficult acid-base disturbance to correct. The high hydrogen ion concentration stimulates the body to attempt compensation by increasing both the depth and the rate of respiration. Compensation is not usually enough by itself. The electrolytes are often quite abnormal and complicate the correction of the acid-base disturbance. A metabolic acidosis is treated by correcting the cause of the acidosis. Correcting the underlying cause will reverse the metabolic acidosis. If the pH is less than 7.25, sodium bicarbonate ($NaHCO_3$) may be ordered in a dose of 1 mEq/kg. If given judiciously, bicarbonate will begin to return the pH toward normal while the underlying cause of the imbalance is identified and treated.

If tissue hypoxia is present, the lactate (normally <2 mmol) may increase. Lactate values greater than 4, when associated with a decreased pH, are warning signs of tissue hypoxia.

Diagnosis and Treatment of Pulmonary Disorders

The CCRN exam will have questions that are related to ventilatory and oxygenation failure. This chapter will familiarize you with the diagnostic techniques to recognize these disorders and the pharmacologic interventions used to treat them.

INVASIVE AND NONINVASIVE DIAGNOSTIC STUDIES

Diagnostic studies used in identifying respiratory alterations include physical assessment, arterial blood gases, pulmonary function tests, and chest radiography.

Physical Assessment

Assessment of the respiratory system includes inspection, palpation, percussion, and auscultation of the lungs.

Inspection

Inspect the patient for respiratory pattern, chest symmetry, clubbing of the fingers, and color.

There are five basic terms used to describe breathing patterns: eupnea, tachypnea, hyperpnea, bradypnea, and apnea.

- Eupnea: regular rhythm and a respiratory rate of 12–20 breaths per minute (Fig. 15–1).
- Tachypnea: increased respiratory rate above 24 breaths/min with normal depth of respiration.

- Hyperpnea: increased depth of respiration at a normal respiratory rate.
- Bradypnea: decreased respiratory rate less than 10 breaths/min with normal depth of respiration.
- Apnea: the absence of breathing (Fig. 15–2).

The four common patterns of respiration seen in critical care are (1) *central neurogenic hyperventilation* (Fig. 15–3)—regular, deep, and rapid respirations without periods of apnea; (2) *Cheyne–Stokes respiration* (Fig. 15–4)—a pattern in which respirations start from apnea, reach a maximum in depth and rate, and then fade back to apnea; (3) *Kussmaul breathing* (Fig. 15–5)—a tachypnea pattern of labored, deep breaths; and (4) *Biot respirations* (Fig. 15–6); regular, fast and shallow breaths with irregular, abrupt periods of apnea.

Central neurogenic hyperventilation is caused by neurogenic dysfunction. Cheyne–Stokes respirations are caused by alterations in acid-base status, an underlying metabolic problem, or neurocerebral insult. Kussmaul breathing is associated with metabolic acidosis and renal failure. Biot respiration is caused by central nervous system disorders; however this pattern may be found in some healthy patients.

Pneumotaxic breathing occurs when the pneumotaxic center takes over control of ventilation. The pattern is irregular, deep, and shallow breathing with random periods of apnea of varying lengths (Fig. 15–7).

Inspect the patient's color for signs of cyanosis. Peripheral cyanosis has little clinical value, and often is the result of peripheral vasoconstriction. When you assess oxygenation from the physical examination, look at the mucosa of the oral cavity and mouth for signs of central cyanosis.

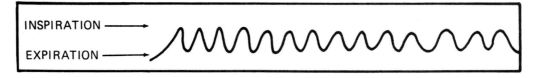

Figure 15-1. Spirometer pattern of normal ventilation.

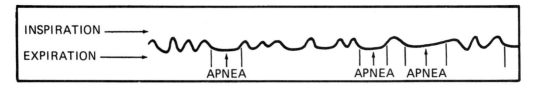

Figure 15-2. Spirometer pattern of apneustic breathing.

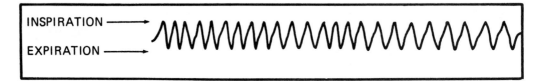

Figure 15-3. Spirometer pattern of central neurogenic hyperventilation.

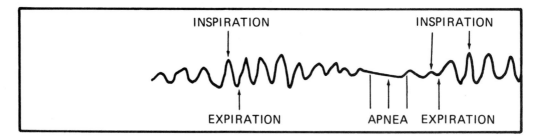

Figure 15-4. Spirometer pattern of Cheyne–Stokes breathing.

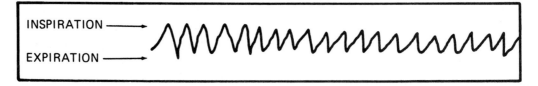

Figure 15-5. Spirometer pattern of Kussmaul breathing.

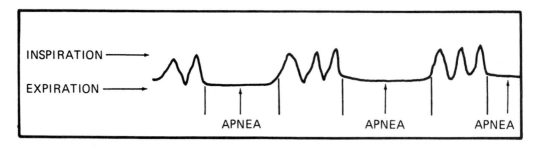

Figure 15-6. Spirometer pattern of Biot (cluster) breathing.

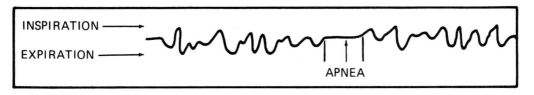

Figure 15–7. Spirometer pattern of pneumotaxic (ataxic) breathing.

Inspection for chest wall symmetry is important in diagnosing pneumothorax, and other processes that cause decreased or absent chest wall movement. Watch the patient breathe to determine if the accessory muscles of ventilation—the scalene, trapezius and sternocleidomastoid muscles—are being used. Their use suggests an increase in the work of breathing, often seen in patients with chronic obstructive pulmonary disease (COPD).

Clubbing of the digits indicates chronic oxygen deficit. The distal phalanges of the fingers become widened. This is most often seen in patients with cystic fibrosis, pulmonary hypertension, and end-stage COPD.

Palpation

Palpation of the chest wall can help further assess findings suggested by inspection. It is used to assess thoracic expansion, tactile and vocal fremitus, and subcutaneous emphysema.

Subcutaneous emphysema is assessed by the familiar crunching or popping that occurs on palpation. It occurs when a communication exists between the pleural space and subcutaneous tissue. By itself, it is not dangerous and does not require treatment.

Percussion

Percussion is the assessment of the lung by striking or tapping on the thorax. It can help to identify areas of consolidation, hyperresonance, and diaphragmatic excursion. A flat or dull sound over the lung indicates that an air-filled space has been replaced with fluid or tissue.

Auscultation

Lung sounds are frequently described in general terms regarding the quality of sound heard over each anatomic region. Tracheal and bronchial sounds reflect the airflow in the major airways. Bronchovesicular and vesicular sounds reflect the progression of airflow in more distal airways. The presence of bronchial sounds in the periphery or any place other than the bronchial area may reflect an abnormality. Any abnormal sound is referred to as an adventitious sound.

Crackles is the term used to describe the sounds heard during reopening of airways secondary to changes in forces surrounding the airways. The airways collapse primarily on expiration and their sounds can be heard throughout the lungs. Crackles can be due to pulmonary or cardiac origins. Differentiation of pulmonary crackles from those of cardiovascular origin is based on the fact that cardiac crackles are position dependent.

Wheezes are due to either partial or complete airway obstruction. Wheezes can be high- or low-pitched. The presence of a wheeze is assessed by identifying the location of the loudest wheeze and listening to the airflow distal to this point. The presence of airflow distal to the loudest wheeze location indicates airflow past the obstruction. If a wheeze disappears, either the obstruction is lessening or worsening. If airflow is more easily heard as the wheeze diminishes, then the lung is improving. If airflow diminishes, then the patient is worsening.

Lung sounds can be diminished by the presence of fluid or air between the lung and the stethoscope. For example, a pneumothorax or pleural effusion will diminish the intensity of lung sounds. On the other hand, consolidation of fluid in the lung itself will accentuate sound transmission. A pneumonia, for example, may accentuate the sound heard in the location of the pneumonia. A bronchial sound would be heard instead of the expected vesicular sound. Loss of airflow, such as with bronchoconstriction or obstruction, differs from consolidation in that reduction in airflow generally diminishes breath sounds. For example, atelectasis or airway obstruction will reduce the intensity of breath sounds. Identifying whether the source of the loss of breath sound is intrapulmonary (atelectasis, mucus plugs) or extrapulmonary (pneumothorax) is up to the clinician.

Interpreting Arterial Blood Gas Values

The identification of basic acid-base disturbances can be done by following a step-by-step procedure of analyzing arterial blood gas values (ABGs). The five important values used to interpret ABGs are shown in Table 15–1.

When the pH and the arterial carbon dioxide pressure ($Paco_2$) move in opposite directions, the primary cause of acid-base disturbance is respiratory. If the pH and the $Paco_2$ move in the same direction, the primary cause is metabolic.

Step 1: Look at the pH to identify the presence of acidosis or alkalosis.

- If it is 7.35–7.45, the pH is normal.
- If the pH is less than 7.35, an acidosis exists.
- If the pH is greater than 7.45, an alkalosis exists.

Step 2: Look at the $Paco_2$ to determine the primary disturbance.

- If the $Paco_2$ is between 35 and 45, a normal level exists. If the value is below 35, a respiratory alkalosis exists. If the value is above 45, a respiratory acidosis exist.
- If the $Paco_2$ moves in the same direction as the pH, the primary cause is metabolic.

Example 1:

pH = 7.25
$Paco_2$ = 26

Since the $Paco_2$ and pH moved in the same direction, the primary problem is a metabolic one. The pH is acidotic, therefore a metabolic acidosis exists. A respiratory alkalosis exists as well, as evidenced by the low $Paco_2$. The respiratory alkalosis is an attempt to compensate for the metabolic acidosis, but is unable to correct the acidosis.

Example 2:

pH = 7.24
$Paco_2$ = 59

Since the $Paco_2$ and pH moved in opposite directions, the primary problem is respiratory. As the $Paco_2$ is elevated and the pH is depressed, a pure respiratory acidosis exists.

TABLE 15–1. NORMAL ARTERIAL BLOOD GAS VALUES AT SEA LEVEL

	Range	Midpoint	Mixed Venous
ph	7.35–7.45	7.40	7.36–7.41
Po_2	80–100 mm Hg	93	35–40 mm Hg
Pco_2	35–45 mm Hg	40	41–51 mm Hg
Hco_3^-	22–26 mEq/L	24	22–26 mEq/L
So_2	95–100%	97%	70–75%
Base excess	+2	0	+2

Step 3: Look at the bicarbonate ion (HCO_3^-) value.

- If it is 22–26, consider it normal.
- If it is less than 22, a metabolic acidosis exists.
- If it is greater than 26, a metabolic alkalosis exists.

Example 3:

pH = 7.25
$Paco_2$ = 26
HCO_3^- = 17

A metabolic acidosis exists because the pH and $Paco_2$ moved in the same direction. The low HCO_3^- level confirms a metabolic acidosis.

	Example 1	Example 2	Example 3
pH	7.19	7.35	7.52
$Paco_2$	30	62	25
HCO_3^-	14	40	25

Practice ABG Interpretation

Example 1: Since the $Paco_2$ and pH moved in the same direction, the primary problem is metabolic. The pH and HCO_3^- confirm a metabolic acidosis. The low $Paco_2$, a respiratory alkalosis, is an attempt to correct for the metabolic acidosis. Since the pH is very low, this situation requires intervention to correct the metabolic acidosis.

Example 2: The $Paco_2$ is elevated, indicating a respiratory acidosis, but the pH is normal. The only way this could occur if a compensation had occurred to offset the acidosis. The high HCO_3^- confirms a metabolic alkalosis exists. The interpretation is respiratory acidosis compensated for by a metabolic alkalosis. Since the pH is normal, no acute danger exists in this patient.

Example 3: Since the $Paco_2$ and pH moved in opposite directions, the primary problem is respiratory. Because of the low $Paco_2$ and high pH, a respiratory alkalosis exists. No compensation has occurred, as evidenced by the normal HCO_3 level. In this case, a pure respiratory alkalosis exists.

The combination of an acidosis and an alkalosis is tolerated better by the body than two acidoses or alkaloses, as they tend to block compensation for each other, resulting in a severe acid-base and electrolyte disturbance.

Pulmonary Function Tests

Pulmonary function tests are used to evaluate the volumes and flow rate of the respiratory system with spirometry (Fig. 15–8).

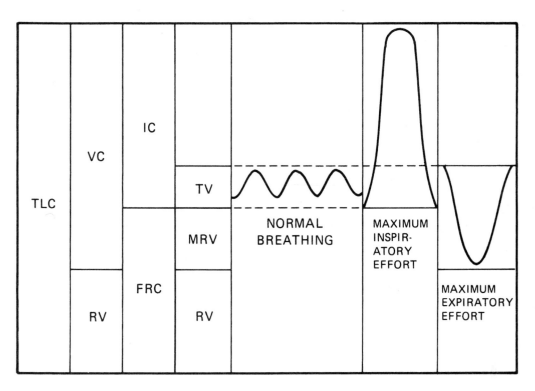

Figure 15–8. Lung volumes and capacities.

Measuring the flow of exhaled gas and the exhalation time helps distinguish between restrictive and obstructive lung diseases (Table 15–2). Forced vital capacity (FVC) measures the vital capacity that the patient can forcibly exhale and suggests the maximum volume of air available for airway clearance.

FEV_1 is the forced expiratory volume over 1 sec. The patient inhales as much as possible, holds his or her breath briefly, and then exhales as forcibly and quickly as possible. A decrease in the FEV_1 indicates obstruction to airflow.

Chest Radiography

The chest radiograph is used to evaluate the structures of the chest, the relationships between structures and the presence of air and fluid. The thoracic cage is made up of 12 ribs, 8 attached and 4 floating ribs inserted in the sternum at a 45° angle. The trachea is midline and tubular. The cardiac silhouette appears anteriorly, as a white solid structure in the left mediastinum. The normal heart width is less than one-half of the thorax.

Review of the chest film begins with the bony structures. Look for the presence of the ribs, and observe any notching or calcifications. Rib notching involves the third through the ninth ribs and is seldom seen in all the ribs of an individual patient. Rib notching has a number of causes (Table 15–3).

Determine that the major organs of the thorax are present, as well as their relationship to each other. Examine the cardiac silhouette for size and placement in the chest. The lungs are examined for expansion and any increased densities, such as that caused by fluid or masses.

Review the position of the hemidiaphragm. It is a rounded silhouette at the base of the thorax. The right side is slightly higher than the left. Flattening of the diaphragm is seen with chronic air-trapping, COPD, and asthma.

PULMONARY PHARMACOLOGY

Medications used in managing pulmonary disease include bronchodilators, corticosteroids, and anticholinergics.

TABLE 15–2. DIFFERENTIATING OBSTRUCTIVE AND RESTRICTIVE DISEASE

Parameter	Obstructive	Restrictive
Vital capacity	normal or ↓	↓
Functional residual capacity	↑	↓
Total lung capacity	↑	↓
Residual volume	↑	↓
FEV_1	↓	normal or ↓

TABLE 15–3. CAUSES OF RIB NOTCHING

Arterial
  High aortic obstruction
    Coarctation of the aorta
  Low aortic obstruction
    Aortic thrombosis
  Subclavian obstruction
    Arteritis
    Arteriosclerosis obliterans
  Pulmonary oligemia
    Tetralogy of Fallot
    Absent pulmonary artery
    Pulmonary valvular stenosis
    Pseudotruncus
    Emphysema
Venous
  Superior vena cava obstruction
Arteriovenous
  AV fistula of the chest wall
Neural
  Neurofibromatosis
Idiopathic
Normal

Bronchodilators

Bronchodilators are divided into classes: methylxanthines and sympathomimetics.

Methylxanthines

Theophylline (anhydrous) is an example of a methylxanthine. It is usually given orally, metabolized in the liver, and has a half-life of 3–6 hr. Its primary effect is bronchodilatation of the airways, although it also stabilizes mast cells and increases mucociliary clearance. The therapeutic range is 10–20 μg/ml. Aminophylline, a salt of theophylline, is administered parenterally, and rectally.

Side effects of theophyllines include tachycardia, tremor, nervousness, palpitations, dizziness, sweating, dysrhythmias, increased blood pressure, irritability, vomiting, nausea, headache, and restlessness.

Overdose of theophylline is critical, as there is no antidote. Early indicators of theophylline overdose include central nervous system changes, headache, confusion, gastrointestinal upset, palpitations, tachycardia, and tachypnea.

Sympathomimetics

Sympathomimetic bronchodilators are part of the class of adrenergic receptor agonists that stimulate alpha, beta-1 and beta-2 receptors, controlling smooth muscle activity, cardiac muscles and glands, and metabolic processes. The lungs contain beta-2 receptors. Stimulation results in relaxation of bronchial smooth muscle, decreased mucus secretion, increased mucociliary clearance and stabilization of the mast cell. Other beta-2 effects include dilatation of the major blood vessels, decreased blood pressure, and increased blood glucose levels.

Current therapy for bronchodilatation is the use of selective beta-2 agonists such as albuterol, terbutaline, and isoetharine. Sympathomimetics can be given parenterally, inhaled from metered-dose inhalers (MDIs), or nebulized.

Side effects of beta-2 agonists include stimulation of heart rate, contractility, and automaticity. They should be used with caution in patients with a history of tachycardia, dysrhythmias, ischemic heart disease, and uncontrolled hyperthyroidism. Tachycardia can be precipitated by vasodilatation and a fall in blood pressure. Patients with diabetes may have increased hyperglycemia. Pregnant women in the third trimester may have delayed or prolonged labor with the use of beta-2 agonists. Central nervous system side effects include anxiety, irritability, insomnia, and fine tremor.

Overdose of sympathomimetics can result in excessive cardiac stimulation. Carefully administered beta blockers can be used to counteract the overdose; however, be prepared for the resulting beta blockade in the lung.

Epinephrine, isoproterenol, and ephedrine all have beta adrenergic action. Epinephrine is the drug of choice for anaphylaxis because of its bronchodilating and cardiovascular effects. Subcutaneous epinephrine may be used to treat acute bronchospasm.

Isoproterenol is a pure beta adrenergic drug that can be injected or inhaled. Ephedrine is a weak bronchodilator that can be given orally. The use of isoproterenol and ephedrine as treatment for bronchospasm has been reduced dramatically with the newer drugs.

Corticosteroids

Corticosteroids are used to reduce inflammation and edema in the airway, stabilize mast cells, and restore bronchodilator response to sympathomimetics. Steroids can be given orally, parenterally, or nasally. Parenteral steroids, such as hydrocortisone, are used to treat severe bronchoconstriction. If prolonged therapy is needed, oral steroids such as prednisone may be used. Both parenteral and oral steroids have a systemic effect and can cause many side effects. These include edema, weight gain, hypernatremia, hypokalemia, hypertension, redistribution of body fat, osteoporosis, muscle weakness, and increased risk for peptic ulcer disease.

Dosage for hydrocortisone is 20–240 mg/day, depending on the severity of the presenting symptoms. Prednisone dosage is 5–60 mg/day. The tapering of prolonged systemic steroids is done gradually to avoid withdrawal symptoms from adrenal insufficiency. Even a few weeks of full-dose therapy can suppress the synthesis and release of cortisol into the bloodstream.

Inhaled steroids provide the same reduction of inflammation and edema of the lung without the major systemic effects. They are supplied in MDIs. The most common ones include beclomethasone dipropionate (Beclovent, Vanceril), flunisolide (Aerobid), and triamcinolone acetonide (Azmacort). Inhaled steroids are used in conjunction with bronchodilator therapy. The effect of inhaled steroids takes weeks to achieve; therefore, they are not used to treat acute bronchospasm and bronchoconstriction. The usual dose is 2 puffs qid or q6h. Azmacort has been shown to be effective in twice-daily dosing using 4–8 puffs each time.

The major side effect of inhaled steroids is infection with oral *Candida albicans*. Instructing the patient to rinse the mouth with water and expectorate after using the inhaler will prevent candidal development.

Mast Cell Stabilizers

Cromolyn (Intal) and nedocromil sodium (Tilade) are inhaled drugs used to stabilize the mast cells. They have no direct bronchodilator effect and are not used in acute situations. The drugs prevent the mast cells from releasing histamine and other mediators that lead to bronchoconstriction, edema, and inflammation of the airways. The dosage for cromolyn is 20 mg tid or qid. Tilade is given in doses of 4 mg qid. Twice-daily dosing has also been shown to be effective.

Anticholinergics

Anticholinergic drugs block the stimulation of cholinergic receptors by acetylcholine. Acetylcholine is a powerful bronchoconstrictor, stimulator of mucus production, and mast cell activator. Ipratropium (Atrovent) is an inhaled anticholinergic used as adjunctive therapy in chronic bronchitis and emphysema.

ADJUNCTIVE RESPIRATORY MONITORING

Adjunctive respiratory monitoring includes pulse oximetry, venous oximetry, and capnography (Table 15–4).

TABLE 15–4. NORMAL VALUES FOR PULSE OXIMETRY, VENOUS OXIMETRY, AND CAPNOGRAPHY

Parameter	Value	Significance
Pulse oximetry (SpO_2)	>92%	Normal
	<92%	Hypoxemia
Venous oximetry (SvO_2)	60–75%	Normal
	>75%	Decreased oxygen consumption
		Malposition of catheter
	<60%	Increased oxygen consumption or decreased oxygen delivery
Capnography ($PetCO_2$)	1–4 mm Hg <$PaCO_2$	Normal
	Widened gradient	V_A/Q mismatch

Oximetry

Pulse Oximetry

Pulse oximetry is a commonly used and excellent indicator of arterial oxygen saturation (SaO_2) values. It can decrease the need to obtain ABGs; however, it is recommended that ABGs be obtained initially to verify the accuracy of the pulse oximeter and to determine $PaCO_2$ levels. Pulse oximetry is most useful in trending saturations level during weaning from oxygen therapy or positive end expiratory pressure/continuous positive airway pressure levels. Spot checks or one-time pulse oximetry readings have little value and are not recommended.

Oximetry measures functional, not fractional, SaO_2. Therefore, the pulse oximetry reading is expected to be 2–4% higher than SaO_2 measured by an ABG.

Complications associated with the use of pulse oximetry are skin breakdown at the probe site and inaccurate readings due to venous stasis, low blood pressure (below 90 mm Hg systolic), and low perfusion states.

Venous Oximetry

Venous oximetry utilizes blood from the pulmonary artery to estimate overall oxygenation. The balance between oxygen transport and consumption is estimated by venous oxygen saturation (SvO_2) levels. As long as blood flow to the capillaries is relatively normal, SvO_2 levels provide relatively accurate reflections of cellular oxygenation. Normal SvO_2 values, between 0.60 and 0.75, indicate an adequate balance between oxygen delivery and consumption. If the

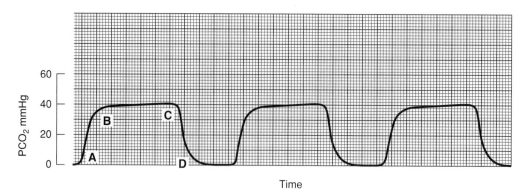

Figure 15–9. The normal capnogram. **(A)** Carbon dioxide concentration is zero, consists of gas from anatomic deadspace. **(B)** Alveolar plateau; minimal rise in carbon dioxide near end of exhalation. **(C)** End tidal carbon dioxide level (PetCO$_2$). **(D)** Inspiration, rapid fall in carbon dioxide.

SvO$_2$ falls less than 0.60, either oxygen transport has decreased or oxygen consumption has increased. While limitations exist with SvO$_2$ use, it remains one of the more valuable tools in the assessment of oxygenation. The SvO$_2$ levels will be higher, about 2%, than laboratory measured values, because it only measures oxyhemoglobin and reduced hemoglobin.

Complications associated with continuous SvO$_2$ monitoring include inadequate calibration of the monitor, infection from long-term catheter insertion, damage to the fiber optics in the catheter, and possible malposition of the catheter.

Capnography

Arterial carbon dioxide levels are the key to determining the adequacy of alveolar ventilation. Capnography is a noninvasive method to assess pulmonary function without sampling blood by analyzing exhaled carbon dioxide. The peak exhaled carbon dioxide value, end tidal carbon dioxide level (PetCO$_2$), is a close approx-imation of arterial carbon dioxide values. It is usually slightly lower than arterial values by 1–4 mm Hg and can be used to approximate PaCO$_2$.

When an increase in physiological deadspace exists, the PetCO$_2$ may not equal the PaCO$_2$. The clinician can monitor the PaCO$_2$–PetCO$_2$ gradient as an indicator of the severity of the pulmonary deadspace; the greater the gradient, the greater the deadspace. In patients with COPD the gradient may rise to 10–20 mm Hg as a result of the ventilation/perfusion mismatch.

A capnogram is a display of the PetCO$_2$ values or a recorded waveform of carbon dioxide concentration. Fast-speed capnograms are used for breath-to-breath analysis, while slow-speed capnograms are used for trending over time (Fig. 15–9).

Capnography is excellent at detecting tracheal intubations, since it will reflect a CO$_2$ waveform. Capnography is a standard for intubation in anesthesia.

Alternative Methods of Ventilatory Support

EDITOR'S NOTE

The CCRN exam will have questions that are related to ventilatory and oxygenation failure. This chapter will review the treatment for these conditions. It is important to understand the concepts of mechanical ventilation, positive end expiratory pressure/continuous positive airway pressure, and oxygen therapy.

OXYGEN THERAPY

Oxygen therapy is used to support oxygen transport while treating the underlying cause of oxygenation failure. There are two methods of delivering oxygen therapy, low- and high-flow systems (Table 16–1).

Low-Flow Oxygen Systems

Low-flow systems do not meet all inspiratory volume needs, requiring patients to entrain room air to meet their inspiratory needs. The advantage of a low-flow oxygen system is the ease of use. In a low-flow oxygen system, the fraction of inspired oxygen level (FIO_2) fluctuates with varying depths of inspiration. A shallow breath has a higher FIO_2 than a deep breath, even though the liter flow is the same, because less room air is entrained during inspiration. Low-flow systems provide FIO_2 levels between 24 and 44% with a nasal cannula or 40 and 60% with a simple face mask (Table 16–2). Rebreathing masks can provide higher levels of inspired oxygen; however they are not as reliable as high-flow systems.

Low-flow oxygen systems are useful in the less acutely ill patient or mouth-breathing patient. The oral inspiration of air draws nasal gases simultaneously into the lungs, allowing for effective oxygen therapy.

High-Flow Oxygen Systems

High-flow oxygen systems meet all inspiratory volume and flow requirements independent of inspiratory changes. High-flow systems are more difficult to apply, requiring face masks or ventilator circuits. High-flow oxygen systems provide stable FIO_2 levels, with oxygen concentrations 24–100% (Table 16–3). Critically ill patients with oxygenation disturbances will almost always require high-flow oxygen systems. Oxygen therapy should not be removed until a stable SpO_2 or $PaO_2/FIO_2 > 286$ is present.

Complications

As long as oxygen therapy generates an arterial oxygen pressure (PaO_2) level greater than 60 mm Hg or an arterial oxygen saturation (SaO_2) level greater than 0.90, no further increases in oxygen therapy should be instituted. Oxygen therapy is not without risk. An oxygen concentration in excess of 50% for more than 24 hr increases the potential for the development of oxygen toxicity and lung damage. Alveolar type II cells, responsible for producing surfactant, are impaired by high oxygen levels.

One of the factors promoting alveolar expansion is the presence of nitrogen, the most plentiful gas, making up approximately 79% of the barometric pressure. When 100% oxygen therapy is employed, nitrogen is completely displaced or washed out by

TABLE 16–1. LOW- AND HIGH-FLOW OXYGEN THERAPY

Low-Flow
Nasal cannula
Simple face masks
Rebreather masks
Non-rebreather masks

High-Flow
Venturi masks
Nebulizer-regulated FIo$_2$ systems
Ventilator circuits

TABLE 16–3. OXYGEN DELIVERY WITH THE VENTURI MASK SYSTEM

FIo$_2$ Desired	Liter Flow Required (L/min)	Air Entrainment Ratio	Liter Flow Delivered (L/min)
0.24	4	1:25	104
0.28	4	1:20	44
0.31	6	1:7	48
0.35	8	1:5	48
0.40	8	1:3	32
0.50	12	1:1.7	32

the oxygen, resulting in a PaO$_2$ of 400 to 600 mm Hg. If perfusion exceeds ventilation, all oxygen can be absorbed from the alveoli, resulting in atelectasis.

Continuous Positive Airway Pressure

Continuous positive airway pressure (CPAP) is positive airway pressure above atmospheric levels applied throughout the respiratory cycle for spontaneous breaths. CPAP stabilizes the airways during the expiratory phase. PaO$_2$ values can be increased if the functional residual capacity (FRC) can be increased and the time for gas exchange to occur is increased. CPAP increases FRC, improves distribution of ventilation, helps hold alveoli open, and opens smaller airways, improving oxygenation. CPAP added to T-piece weaning trials may help prevent microatelectasis and promote alveolar stability.

Positive End Expiratory Pressure

Positive end expiratory pressure (PEEP) is the application of a positive airway pressure at end exhalation while on mechanical ventilation. It improves oxygenation by the same mechanisms as CPAP. PEEP is effective in raising PaO$_2$ and SaO$_2$ levels by maintain-

TABLE 16–2. APPROXIMATE FIo2 WITH NASAL CANNULA AND FACE MASK

	Liter Flow (L/min)	Approximate FIo$_2$%
Nasal cannula	1	24
	2	28
	3	32
	4	36
	5	40
	6	44
Face mask	5–6	40
	6–7	50
	7–8	60

ing alveolar air flow during expiration. Airways have a tendency to collapse during expiration as a result of increasing pressures outside the airway.

Some clinicians believe in physiological PEEP, a concept which assumes some PEEP is present in all people because of resistance of the airways. Low levels of PEEP, such as 3–5 cm H$_2$O, may be ordered even in patients without oxygenation problems to simulate physiological PEEP.

Positive end expiratory pressure is indicated to help reduce FIO$_2$ levels or to elevate PaO$_2$/SaO$_2$ values when high FIO$_2$ levels are unsuccessful, to drive lung water back into the vascular system, or to reduce mediastinal bleeding postoperatively.

Optimal PEEP levels are achieved by the lowest level of PEEP needed to raise the PaO$_2$/SaO$_2$ levels, and do not result in cardiovascular compromise, such as decreased cardiac output, impeded right-heart filling, and tachycardia. The optimal PEEP level varies from patient to patient, although levels of PEEP higher than 20 cm H$_2$O are uncommon. Values between 9 and 15 cm H$_2$O are common in support of the patient with oxygenation problems.

Auto-PEEP

Auto-PEEP, also known as intrinsic PEEP, is the trapping of air in the alveoli, producing PEEP as the result of early airway closure or insufficient exhalation time. Patients at risk for the development of auto-PEEP include those with COPD or asthma, those greater than 60 years old with a history of cardiopulmonary disorders, or patients with increased minute ventilation (VE) of 20 L/min or more. It can be measured by obstructing the exhalation port of a ventilator immediately prior to an inspiratory effort.

Complications of auto-PEEP include increased work of breathing; barotrauma; hemodynamic compromise, such as decreased cardiac output and decreased venous return to the right heart; misinterpretation of pulmonary capillary wedge pressure

(PCWP) readings; increased intracranial pressure; decreased renal function; passive hepatic congestion; and increased intrapulmonary shunt.

Complications of PEEP and CPAP

Positive end expiratory pressure and CPAP have potential side effects related to the increased airway pressures. When PEEP or CPAP is applied, monitor the cardiac output must be carefully monitored. Cardiac output and stroke volume can fall as a result of the increased intrathoracic pressure. The increased intrathoracic pressure impedes venous blood return to the right heart, producing a pseudo-hypovolemia. If cardiac outputs are not available, the heart rate and systolic blood pressure are monitored. Increases in the heart rate and falls in systolic blood pressure may signal a reduction in cardiac output and stroke volume.

Barotrauma and pneumothorax are also complications of PEEP and CPAP. Lung sounds should be monitored and the thorax percussed for potential development of pneumothorax. Sustained peak airway pressures greater than 40 cm H_2O increase the risk for development of barotrauma.

ARTIFICIAL AIRWAYS

In order to use a ventilator, the patient must have an artificial airway, such as an endotracheal tube or a tracheostomy tube.

Endotracheal Tubes

Endotracheal tubes may be inserted nasally or orally. Intubation should be attempted only by trained and experienced clinicians. Immediately after intubation, all chest fields are auscultated to determine there are bilateral breath sounds. Chest roentgenography is important to ensure whether the tip of the endotracheal tube is about 1 inch (2–3 cm) above the carina.

Nasotracheal intubation is contraindicated in patients with increased ICP, head trauma, or chronic sinusitis. Disadvantages include the possibility of tissue necrosis, nosebleed, rupture of nasal polyps, and submucosal dissection. Increased mucus production as a result of the irritant properties of the tube increases the patient's susceptibility to infection, and stabilization of the tube is difficult if the patient is diaphoretic.

The advantages of orotracheal intubation are direct visualization and rapid intubation. Oral endotracheal tubes are repositioned to the opposite side of the mouth at least every 24 hr to prevent necrosis of the lips. Disadvantages of oral intubation include increased dryness of oral mucosa, increased mucus production, increased gagging, and increased susceptibility to infection.

Complications associated with intubation include laryngeal trauma, intubation of the right mainstem bronchus, and infection.

Tracheostomy

Tracheostomy, the formation of an opening into the trachea, may be performed if ventilatory support is expected to be long term. Tracheostomies bypass upper airway obstruction, decrease dead space, may help prevent aspiration, and may decrease the possibilities of necrosis and/or tracheoesophageal fistula formation. A sterile tracheostomy tube of the same size used in the patient is taped to the head of the bed for emergency replacement. An endotracheal tube of the same or smaller size is also acceptable for maintaining the airway in an emergency.

Suctioning

Maintaining patency of the airway can be facilitated through suctioning. Suctioning can be accomplished with a closed-system multiple-use catheter or the traditional single-use catheter.

Hyperoxygenation of the patient prior to suctioning reduces hypoxemia associated with suctioning. Patients who benefit from hyperventilation include those receiving an FIO_2 of 0.40 or higher, those who have demonstrated decreased SaO_2 with suctioning or cardiovascular compromise such as bradycardia or premature ventricular contractions (PVCs).

Suction pressures of less than 200 are generally adequate to remove secretions. Removing viscous, thick secretions is difficult even with adequate suction. The lack of benefit of instillation of saline in the endotracheal or tracheostomy tube has been well documented. Thinning of pulmonary secretions is accomplished by adequate fluid intake. Stimulating a cough is a very effective aid to secretion clearance.

Cuff Management

Most endotracheal tubes and tracheostomy tubes for initiation of mechanical ventilation have inflatable cuffs. The cuff provides a closed system with a seal and reduces aspiration of fluids into the lungs. Soft, low-pressure cuffs are preferred because they minimize tracheal necrosis and fistula development. Pressure is distributed over a large area, and only sufficient pressure to provide a seal is necessary. High-volume, low-pressure cuffs negate the need to deflate the cuff for a specified period of time each hour.

Policies vary from hospital to hospital regarding the measuring of cuff pressures. Generally, a minimal occlusive pressure is maintained at 25 cm H_2O or less, 20 mm Hg to prevent tracheal damage. If more pressure is required, the patient may need to have a large tube inserted. Cuff pressure is checked every 4–8 hr by using a blood pressure manometer, syringe and stopcock, or a pressure manometer specifically for measuring cuff pressures. This may be a shared responsibility with the respiratory care practitioner.

Deflation of the cuff is not recommended while mechanical ventilation is in place. During the weaning process, the patient may have periods of time off ventilation when the tracheostomy tube could be deflated. Before deflating the cuff, the patient should be suctioned carefully, especially orotracheally, to remove any secretions that may have accumulated on the top of the cuff. The patient must be monitored carefully for potential aspiration.

Complications

The major complication of a cuffed tube is obstruction from dried secretions (airway plugging). The increased mucus production stimulated by the foreign body puts the patient at increased risk for airway plugging. Maintaining adequate hydration and suctioning will help reduce the risk of plugging.

Endotracheal tubes can become displaced easily, leading to carinal rupture, unilateral lung ventilation, tension pneumothorax, and atelectasis. Signs of tube misplacement include diminished or absent lung sounds and little, if any, chest excursion on the contralateral side, expiratory wheezing, and sometimes uncontrollable coughing. Tension pneumothorax may occur in the lung that has become intubated—one of the most serious complications of ventilatory support. The only treatment is insertion of a chest tube to relieve the pressure and remove air. Without adequate treatment, tension pneumothorax can be rapidly fatal.

If a tracheostomy tube's position fluctuates with the patient's pulse, it is possible that the tube is rubbing against the innominate artery; in such a case the physician is notified immediately. Erosion of the artery usually results in exsanguination and death. A tracheostomy tube may become misplaced, causing subcutaneous and/or mediastinal emphysema or pneumothorax. Progressively deteriorating blood gases, poor air movement, and/or difficulty in suctioning should alert the clinician to a possible shift in the tracheostomy tube.

Tracheal dilatation, ischemia, and necrosis may occur because tracheostomy tubes and endotracheal tubes are round, whereas the trachea is oval. If ischemia and necrosis progress, a tracheoesophageal (TE) fistula may occur. If suspected, this can be easily tested by instilling methylene blue or cranberry juice into the mouth. If it is suctioned from the endotracheal tube or tracheostomy, a TE fistula may have developed. This may be minimized by the use of low-pressure cuffs.

The longer an endotracheal tube or tracheostomy tube is in place, the greater the danger of infection. Frequent oral hygiene and tube care will provide patient comfort and help reduce the risk of infection.

MECHANICAL VENTILATION

Mechanical ventilation is indicated for one of three reasons: to improve or support alveolar ventilation; to reduce the work of breathing; or to aid in supporting oxygenation. Improvement of alveolar ventilation (VA) is most obviously needed when $PaCO_2$ levels are decreasing along with a rising Ph. Reducing the work of breathing may be necessary when respiratory rates are in excess of 30 breaths/min (Table 16–4). All modes of mechanical ventilation are designed to support one of these three functions.

Mechanical ventilation is delivered by either negative or positive pressure. Negative pressure ventilators include the iron lung or thoracic cuirass, usually not used in acute respiratory failure. Positive pressure ventilators force air into the lungs, reversing normal breathing pressures and successfully supplying alveolar ventilation support.

The reversal of the normal negative inspiratory pressure to a positive pressure has a direct effect on the cardiovascular system. The increased intrathoracic pressure impedes venous return to the right heart, reducing stroke volume and cardiac output. The initial response may be a reflex increase in the heart rate to maintain output.

A complication of positive pressure ventilation is pulmonary barotrauma. The peak airway pressure

TABLE 16–4. SIGNS OF FAILURE OF SPONTANEOUS BREATHING

Respiratory rate	> 35 breaths/min
Tidal volume (VT)	<2 ml/kg
Minute ventilation (VE)	<5 or >12 L/min
PaCO$_2$	Increasing by more than 10 mm Hg from baseline
pH	<7.30 with a rising Paco$_2$
Blood pressure	Increase in systolic of 20 mm Hg
Heart rate	Increase of >20 beats/min over resting heart rate

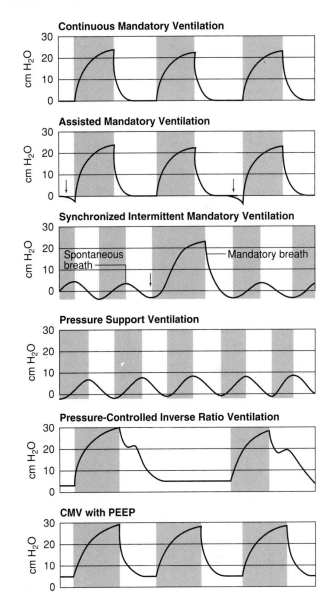

Figure 16–1. Pressure waveforms of differing modes of mechanical ventilation.

manometer on the ventilator should be monitored to assess excessive airway pressures. High peak airway pressures can be monitored through dynamic compliance by dividing peak airway pressure into the tidal volume. Normal dynamic compliance is 40–55 cm/ml. Values lower than 30 cm/ml place the patient at increased risk for barotrauma.

Modes of Mechanical Ventilation

Ventilator breaths can be delivered by several modes. The most common modes are continuous mandatory ventilation (CMV), assisted mandatory ventilation (AMV or assist/control), synchronized intermittent mandatory ventilation (SIMV), and pressure support ventilation (PSV) (Fig. 16–1).

Tidal volume (VT) on all modes is initially set at 10–15 ml/kg with a respiratory rate between 10 and 20 breaths/min. Respiratory rate and tidal volume are manipulated to achieve specific end points such as levels of oxygenation or ventilation.

Continuous Mandatory Ventilation

Continuous mandatory ventilation (CMV) is used to support patients with little or no ventilatory drive or gain control over excessive ventilatory drive. The ventilator delivers the preset tidal volume at the preset rate without sensitivity to patient inspiratory effort. The patient is unable to initiate breaths or change the breathing pattern in any way. CMV is used in patients under anesthesia or in those who are totally paralyzed.

Assisted Mandatory Ventilation

Assisted mandatory ventilation (AMV; assist/control) delivers constant preset tidal volumes and a minimum number of breaths determined by the preset respiratory rate. The patient can initiate more breaths; however, they will be delivered at the preset

tidal volume. The patient can alter the respiratory rate and pattern, not the tidal volume. The advantage of AMV is a reduction in the work of breathing. AMV can be used in weaning from mechanical ventilation by incorporating spontaneous breathing with T-piece trials.

Synchronized Intermittent Mandatory Ventilation

Synchronized intermittent mandatory ventilation (SIMV) delivers a preset respiratory rate and tidal volume but allows the patient to breathe spontaneously between the preset tidal volume and rate.

The ventilator is synchronized with the patient's ventilatory effort in an attempt to reduce competition between the ventilator and the patient. SIMV may prevent respiratory muscle atrophy and aid in the weaning from mechanical ventilation.

There are many controversies about SIMV. It has been shown to actually increase the work of breathing at a low respiratory rate of 6 breaths/min or less because the patient performs most of the work of breathing through the high-resistance ventilator circuit. SIMV rates at 24 breaths/min or higher approximate AMV, as there is no time for the patient to initiate a spontaneous breath at his or her own tidal volume.

Pressure Support Ventilation

In pressure support ventilation (PSV), the ventilator delivers a preset positive pressure as the patient determines the inspiratory time, rate, and inspiratory flow rate. The patient is assisted during the inspiratory phase. When inspiration ceases, the pressure support drops to ambient or PEEP. The level of pressure support is set to achieve a tidal volume of 10–15 ml/kg. When PSV levels greater than 30 cm H_2O are needed, SIMV or AMV may be added to provide a backup of consistent tidal volumes. PSV is valuable as an adjunct to overcoming endotracheal tube resistance and weaning from mechanical ventilation.

Inverse Ratio Ventilation

In severe, refractory hypoxemia a more aggressive form of oxygenation support may be required. One of the most aggressive forms of support is inverse ratio ventilation. The patient must be intubated for this therapy. In inverse ratio ventilation, the inspiratory time from the ventilator is prolonged until it equals or exceeds expiratory time (the opposite of normal). The primary advantage of inverse ratio ventilation is an elevation of mean airway pressure. The elevation of mean airway pressure causes an opening of airways and a subsequent elevation of the PaO_2 and SaO_2. Inverse ratio ventilation is usually given via a pressure controlled mode of ventilation in an attempt to reduce high airway pressures. The term used to describe pressure controlled inverse ratio ventilation is PC-IRV.

When using inverse ratio ventilation, several nursing considerations are essential. First, the patient is usually sedated and paralyzed in order to decrease resistance to the ventilation and to reduce oxygen consumption. Care must be taken to explain to the patient and family the nature of sedation and paralyzation therapy. Second, the risk of barotrauma is increased with inverse ratio ventilation. Both a reduction in cardiac output and increased risk of lung injury (including pneumothorax) are present and should be monitored.

Complications of Ventilator Support

Hypotension may occur secondary to decreased cardiac output when a patient is put on a ventilator or when ventilator adjustments are increased. All positive pressure ventilators exert a continuous positive pressure which decreases venous return to the heart, decreasing cardiac output. The decreased cardiac output may result in a decreased urine output and cardiac dysrhythmias. Cardiac monitoring is essential. Hypotension may be caused by hypovolemia, and intravenous fluids may correct the problem. Vasopressors are indicated if the PCWP is increased and the cardiac output is decreased.

Infection is a most common complication of mechanical ventilation. Strict adherence to sterile technique, ventilator tubing changes every 48 hr, and sputum culture will help to prevent and detect infection. As soon as a culture identifies an infecting organism, specific antibiotic therapy is started. Aggressive pulmonary hygiene procedures are vital nursing interventions in preventing infection.

Atelectasis often occurs with mechanical ventilation. Bronchial hygiene is extremely important to prevent further complications once atelectasis has developed. Accidental disconnection from the ventilator may occur. Immediately reconnect or use a manual resuscitator.

Pneumothorax is not unusual when PEEP is used with mechanical ventilation. Treatment is insertion of a chest tube. Without adequate treatment, pneumothorax can be rapidly fatal.

Overventilation may occur, decreasing $PaCO_2$, more than desired. Reducing rate or VT may be necessary to correct this problem.

Airway Pressure Release Ventilation

Airway pressure release ventilation (APRV) is a noninvasive method used to improve oxygenation by a tightly fitting face mask. Positive pressure is applied throughout the respiratory cycle with short periods of airway pressure release. The release of pressure is designed to improve the elimination of carbon dioxide.

Pressure Controlled Inverse Ratio Ventilation

Pressure controlled inverse ratio ventilation (PC-IRV) reverses the conventional inspiratory to expiratory (I:E) ratio while delivering a pressure controlled breath. PC-IRV is indicated in patients with refractory hypoxemia and high peak airway pressures. Advantages include reduced FIO_2, PEEP, and peak airway pressure, increased lung compliance, reduced minute ventilation and improved oxygenation. Complications associated with PC-IRV include inadequate tidal volume, development of auto-PEEP, increased mean airway pressure, decreased right heart filling, decreased cardiac output, and an increased respiratory rate. Monitoring includes PCWP, cardiac output, blood pressure, exhaled tidal volume, minute ventilation, compliance, PaO_2, $PaCO_2$, and continuous SaO_2.

WEANING FROM MECHANICAL VENTILATION

Weaning is the progressive removal of mechanical ventilatory support to spontaneous breathing. The first step in the weaning process is to determine if the patient is ready for weaning. Assessment includes progress toward correction of the underlying reason for mechanical ventilation and respiratory mechanics; respiratory muscle endurance; and efficiency and work of breathing.

Lung function tests used to assess readiness for weaning include tidal volume, vital capacity, minute ventilation, respiratory rate, and negative inspiratory force (NIF) or peak inspiratory effort (PIP). Minute ventilation is the amount of air exchanged in 1 min. Normal minute ventilation is 5–10 L/min. Negative inspiratory force or peak inspiratory effort is the maximal inspiratory effort the patient can generate, measured by an inspiratory manometer. Normal PIP or NIF is –70 to –90 cm H_2O (Table 16–5). It is important to correct as many of the patient's medical problems as possible before beginning the weaning process (Table 16–6).

There are a number of weaning techniques, including reduction of SIMV rates, alternating AMV with T-piece trials, and PSV. It is not so much the technique that is used, rather the care with which it is applied. Monitoring throughout the weaning process includes assessment of vital signs, respiratory muscle fatigue, oxygenation, $PaCO_2$ and electrocardiographic changes (Table 16–7).

Assisted mandatory ventilation can be used in weaning from mechanical ventilation by incorporating spontaneous breathing (T-piece) trials. In T-piece trials, the patient is removed from the ventilator for progressively increasing periods of time. The patient may start at intervals of 5–10 min four to six times per day and increase to 1–1½ hr two to three times a day. Once the patient can breathe spontaneously through the endotracheal or tracheostomy tube for 1–1½ hr, extubation is likely to be successful. Prolonged breathing through the high-resistance endotracheal or tracheostomy tube is not recommended. CPAP may be added to the T-piece

TABLE 16–5. WEANING PARAMETERS

Muscle Efficiency	
Tidal volume (VT)	2–5 ml/kg
Minute ventilation (VE)	5–10 L/min
Vital capacity	> 10 ml/kg
Respiratory rate	< 30 breaths/min
NIF/PIP	> –20 cm H_2O
Oxygenation	
$PaCO_2$	> 60 mm Hg on FIO_2 < 0.40
Hemoglobin	> 10 g/dl
Cardiac index	> 2.5 L/min
Arterial/alveolar ratio (a/A)	> 30%
Carbon Dioxide Elimination	
$PACO_2$	35–45 mm Hg or at the patient's baseline level to maintain Ph between 7.35 and 7.45
Deadspace/tidal volume (VD/VT)	< 60%

TABLE 16–6. CONSIDERATIONS PRIOR TO INITIATING WEANING

Acid-base abnormalities
Airway secretion management
Cardiac abnormalities
   Arrhythmias
   Decreased cardiac output
   Anemia
Hyperglycemia
Infection
   Fever
Level of consciousness
Pain
Renal failure
   Electrolyte abnormalities
   Fluid imbalance
   Protein loss
Shock
Sleep deprivation

TABLE 16–7. CRITERIA FOR TERMINATION OF WEANING

Change in level of consciousness

Change in vital signs
    Diastolic blood pressure >100 mm Hg
    Fall in systolic blood pressure
    Heart rate >110 beats/min or >20-beats/min increase over baseline
    Respiratory rate >30 breaths/min or >10 breaths/min increase over
      baseline

Falling pulse oximetry saturation

Tidal volume <250 ml

$Paco_2$ increase ≥8 mm Hg

pH <7.35

Electrocardiographic changes
    Premature ventricular contractions (PVCs) >6/min
    Salvos of PVCs
    ST-segment elevation
    Ventricular conduction changes

trial to help maintain oxygenation, improve FRC, and prevent development of microatelectasis.

Synchronized intermittent mandatory ventilation can be used as a weaning tool. The SIMV rate is reduced slowly, about 1–2 breaths every 8–24 hr as tolerated by the patient. The usefulness of SIMV weaning is controversial. Weaning through the SIMV circuit has been shown to actually increase the work of breathing, promote respiratory muscle fatigue, and increase oxygen consumption. SIMV rates of breaths/min or less have been associated with increased airway resistance and chronic respiratory muscle fatigue.

Pressure support ventilation weaning may play a role in promoting endurance training for the respiratory muscles. PSV is initiated at a level to achieve a tidal volume of 10–15 ml/kg of body weight. The PSV is gradually decreased while tidal volume and minute ventilation are monitored. PSV can be used in combination with SIMV to help overcome the in-spiratory work of breathing caused by breathing through the high-resistance ventilator circuit and endotracheal tube. The SIMV rate is gradually reduced to zero, then the PSV is gradually reduced. If the patient can maintain an adequate minute ventilation on 5 cm H_2O or less, the patient can be placed on a T-piece trial. If the patient does well, PSV can usually be discontinued and the patient extubated.

Extubation

Once the patient has been successfully weaned from the mechanical ventilation, the decision to extubate must be addressed. A contraindication to extubation is lack of a gag reflex. Extubation is usually done early in the day to allow for adequate caregiver support and monitoring. Baseline vital signs and ABGs or pulse oximetry are obtained. The head of the bed is elevated to 45–90°. The airway is carefully suctioned to remove any secretions that may have accumulated on top of the cuff. After the cuff is deflated, the patient takes a big breath and coughs forcefully while the tube is removed.

The caregiver must be prepared for reintubation if upper airway obstruction, such as glottic edema, occurs. Inspiratory stridor is treated with inhaled racemic epinephrine 0.5 ml in 1–3 ml normal saline to reduce edema. The dose is repeated at 20–30-min intervals one or two times. If this does not relieve the stridor, immediate intubation is recommended.

The respiratory pattern will change following extubation for approximately 60 min. Minute ventilation increases by as much as 2 L/min, there is a slight increase in the tidal volume, an increase in the respiratory drive and rate, and a decrease in paradoxical abdominal movement. After about an hour, the respiratory pattern will return to pre-extubation patterns.

Acute Respiratory Dysfunction

EDITOR'S NOTE

Several questions on the CCRN exam can be expected to address the concepts of acute respiratory failure and adult respiratory distress syndrome. It is important to understand key physiological events that produce clinical symptoms of these conditions as well as the likely therapeutic events that might improve pulmonary function. This chapter provides a concise review of the major areas that the CCRN exam is likely to cover with respect to these topics.

ACUTE RESPIRATORY FAILURE

Acute respiratory failure (ARF) is the result of abnormalities in ventilation, perfusion, or compliance, leading to hypercapnia and/or hypoxemia. The lungs are unable to maintain adequate oxygenation and carbon dioxide elimination to support metabolism, leading to respiratory acidosis. Identification of the underlying condition is necessary to initiate treatment.

Pathophysiology

Acute respiratory failure presents as an oxygenation or ventilation disturbance that may be life-threatening. An alteration in oxygenation is the most common form of respiratory failure. Perfusion (Q) exceeds ventilation (V) (a low V/Q ratio), causing decreased oxygenation of venous blood and a mixing of less oxygenated blood with arterial blood. The effect is a reduced arterial oxygen pressure (Pao2) value.

In acute respiratory failure due to high V/Q ratios or increased dead space (VD) there is a marked increase in the work of breathing. The patient increases minute ventilation (VE) to compensate for an increased dead space in an effort to maintain adequate alveolar ventilation. Inadequate alveolar ventilation and failure to eliminate carbon dioxide cause acute increases in arterial carbon dioxide ($PaCO_2$) levels, resulting in respiratory acidosis.

Etiology and Risk Factors

Patients at risk for developing ARF include those with chronic obstructive pulmonary disease (COPD), restrictive lung disease, respiratory center depression, pulmonary edema, and pulmonary emboli, among many other conditions (Table 17–1).

Chronic lung disease (COPD) complicated by a pneumonia, left ventricular (LV) failure and pulmonary edema, head injuries producing noncardiogenic pulmonary edema, inhalation injuries, and sepsis are examples of ARF with alterations in oxygenation. ARF caused by a depressed central nervous system (CNS) or a high V/Q ratio causes an increase in $PaCO_2$.

Signs and Symptoms

Ventilation failure due to CNS depression presents with a slowed rate of breathing. Few other obvious physical symptoms may exist. If the ventilation failure is due to increased deadspace, the respiratory rate and depth increase; the respiratory rate may exceed 30 breaths/min. The patient may also complain of shortness of breath and appear anxious.

Assessment findings include tachycardia, atrial cardiac dysrhythmias, pedal edema, tachypnea, dyspnea on exertion or at rest, labored breathing pattern, use of accessory muscles of respiration, crackles, wheezes, and a hyperresonant chest on percussion in patients with advanced COPD (Table 17–2).

TABLE 17–1. CAUSES OF ACUTE RESPIRATORY FAILURE

Oxygenation Disturbances
Respiratory distress syndrome
Pulmonary edema
Pneumonitis
Pneumonia

Alveolar Ventilation Disturbances
Central nervous system depression
Medication or anesthetic effect
Head or cervical cord trauma
Cerebrovascular accident
COPD
Interstitial pulmonary fibrosis
Pneumothorax

Ventilation/Perfusion Disturbances
Pulmonary emboli
Bronchiolitis
COPD
Lung trauma

Left-to-right Shunt
Atelectasis
Oxygen toxicity
Pulmonary edema or emboli
Pneumonia

Invasive and Noninvasive Diagnostic Studies

Arterial blood gas (ABG) values can deteriorate suddenly, indicating acute pulmonary insufficiency. Findings include a PaO_2 less than 60 mm Hg requiring a forced inspiratory oxygen pressure (FIO_2) greater than 0.50 and a $PaCO_2$ greater than 45 mm Hg. Other measures of oxygenation include a decreased a/A ratio (less than 0.25), a widened A–a gradient, and a decreased PaO_2/FIO_2 ratio (below 200). The patient

TABLE 17–2. SYMPTOMS OF OXYGENATION-INDUCED RESPIRATORY FAILURE

Shortness of breath
Orthopnea
PaO_2 <60 mm Hg
SaO_2 <0.90
Anxiety
Increased respiratory rate (>30 breaths/min)
Possible labored breathing
Increased intrapulmonary shunt
Qs/Qt > 20%
a/A ratio < 25%
PaO_2/FIO_2 ratio < 200
A–a gradient > 350 on 100% oxygen

may present with an elevated hematocrit (above 52%) and an elevated hemoglobin (above 18 g/dL) if there is an underlying component of COPD. As the heart rate increases, cardiac output may fall. The pulmonary artery diastolic pressure may be greater than 15 mm Hg if there is underlying lung disease.

Nursing and Collaborative Diagnosis

Potential diagnoses include, but are not limited to:

- impaired gas exchange,
- ineffective breathing patterns,
- activity intolerance,
- inability to sustain spontaneous ventilation,
- potential for ineffective airway clearance,
- anxiety,
- potential for infection.

Goals and Desired Patient Outcomes

Goals and desired patient outcomes include, but are not limited to:

- adequate oxygenation: PaO_2 60–100 mm Hg, SaO_2 greater than 92%.
- adequate ventilation: Ph 7.35–7.45, $PaCO_2$ at baseline or 35–45 mm Hg.
- ability to sustain spontaneous ventilation.

Patient Care Management

Patient care management priorities include correction of hypoxia and acidosis, respiratory muscle rest, control of shock, decreasing risk of developing infection, and nutritional repletion.

Establishment or assurance of an adequate airway is needed to provide supportive treatment. Correction of hypoxia may require the use of oxygen therapy or endotracheal intubation and mechanical ventilation.

When medication is the cause of respiratory failure, discontinuation of the medication may reverse the respiratory depression and is the treatment of choice. When respiratory failure is due to trauma or increased intracranial pressure (ICP), treatment is focused on relieving the increased ICP.

When the problem is a high V/Q ratio, re-establishing perfusion is the key. If a pulmonary embolism exists, thrombolytic therapy, such as with streptokinase or tissue plasminogen activator, may be indicated. If low perfusion is due to a low cardiac output, improving the cardiac output is necessary.

Supportive treatment includes oxygen therapy, positive and expiratory pressure (PEEP), and mechanical ventilation. Treatment of LV failure producing pulmonary edema focuses on resolving the cardiac dysfunction. If a pulmonary infection is the underlying cause, antibiotic therapy is indicated.

Complications

Complications associated with ARF include severe respiratory and metabolic acidosis, infection, failure to wean from mechanical ventilation, and lack of adequate nutritional support.

RESPIRATORY DISTRESS SYNDROME

Respiratory distress syndrome (RDS), also known as acute respiratory distress syndrome (ARDS), is an extreme form of respiratory failure. It is a life-threatening condition manifested by severe hypoxemia and decreased lung compliance. RDS is frequently referred to as noncardiogenic pulmonary edema.

Pathophysiology

There have been many mechanisms and mediators identified for the pathogenesis of RDS. They include neutrophil activation, platelet activation, alveolar macrophage stimulation, complement activation, and release of humoral vasoactive substances (Fig. 17–1).

Respiratory distress syndrome is a response to a direct or indirect injury to the lung that causes increased pulmonary capillary permeability. Normally, the pulmonary capillaries allow only small amounts of fluid to leak into the interstitial compartment that is readily drained by the pulmonary lymphatic system. In RDS, capillary leakage results in a tremendous loss of fluid from the vascular space, primarily due to the loss of vascular proteins. As proteins leave the capillaries, they pull large amounts of fluid into the pulmonary interstitial space, overwhelming the pulmonary lymphatic drainage capability and causing alveolar flooding and impaired oxygen transfer. The result is severe hypoxemia.

Etiology and Risk Factors

The origin of RDS is unclear, although potential causes have been narrowed since the syndrome was first identified. RDS results from direct or indirect injury to the lung. Those at risk for the development of RDS include persons suffering from trauma, oxygen toxicity, drug overdose, disseminated intravascular coagulation (DIC), complications of coronary artery bypass grafting (CABG), inhalation of noxious gases, and sepsis, those having multiple blood transfusions; there are many other causes as well (Table 17–3).

Signs and Symptoms

Respiratory distress syndrome presents with symptoms similar to oxygenation-induced respiratory failure. Rapid deterioration of pulmonary function is a hallmark of RDS. The chest roentgenogram can change within a hour from relatively normal to a white-out picture, reflecting a large accumulation of lung water in a short period of time. Hemodynamic parameters are used to differentiate RDS from pulmonary edema due to LV failure. The pulmonary capillary wedge pressure (PCWP) is generally less than 18 mm Hg in RDS, while LV failure presents with a high PCWP.

Invasive and Noninvasive Diagnostic Studies

Early chest roentgenograms may appear normal. As the lung injury progresses, the chest film will initially show fine infiltrates that progress to diffuse alveolar and interstitial infiltrates, known as a ground-glass appearance.

Arterial blood gases will show a progressive deterioration with a falling PaO_2. As oxygenation worsens, the $PaCO_2$ will begin to rise as compensatory mechanisms, such as an increased respiratory rate, fail. Other measures of oxygenation will reveal an increased V/Q mismatch, increased shunting, decreased oxygen delivery, and decreased oxygen consumption (VO_2).

Placement of a pulmonary artery catheter will reveal a normal, increased, or decreased cardiac output and cardiac index; normal central venous pressure (CVP); increased pulmonary vascular resistance (PVR); and normal, increased, or decreased systemic vascular resistance (SVR). The PCWP will be normal or low with a normal or increased pulmonary artery systolic (PAS) and diastolic (PAD) pressure.

Nursing and Collaborative Diagnoses

Diagnoses include, but are not limited to:

- impaired gas exchange related to oxygenation and ventilation failure.
- ineffective airway clearance related to retained secretions.
- ineffective breathing pattern related to increased dead space ventilation.
- dyspnea relative to increased dead space ventilation.
- anxiety relative to inexperience with procedures and the critical care setting.

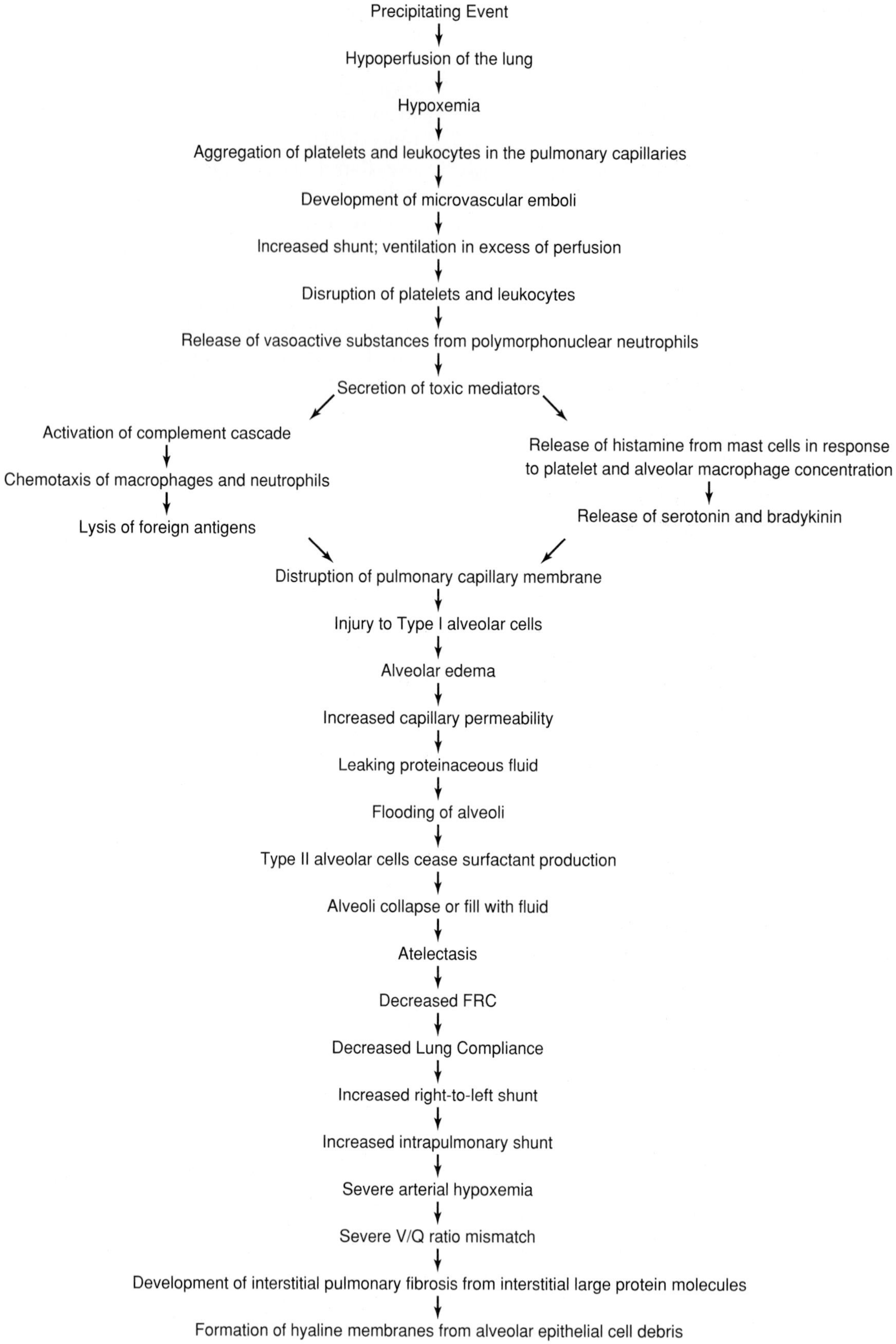

Precipitating Event
↓
Hypoperfusion of the lung
↓
Hypoxemia
↓
Aggregation of platelets and leukocytes in the pulmonary capillaries
↓
Development of microvascular emboli
↓
Increased shunt; ventilation in excess of perfusion
↓
Disruption of platelets and leukocytes
↓
Release of vasoactive substances from polymorphonuclear neutrophils
↓
Secretion of toxic mediators

Activation of complement cascade
↓
Chemotaxis of macrophages and neutrophils
↓
Lysis of foreign antigens

Release of histamine from mast cells in response to platelet and alveolar macrophage concentration
↓
Release of serotonin and bradykinin

Distruption of pulmonary capillary membrane
↓
Injury to Type I alveolar cells
↓
Alveolar edema
↓
Increased capillary permeability
↓
Leaking proteinaceous fluid
↓
Flooding of alveoli
↓
Type II alveolar cells cease surfactant production
↓
Alveoli collapse or fill with fluid
↓
Atelectasis
↓
Decreased FRC
↓
Decreased Lung Compliance
↓
Increased right-to-left shunt
↓
Increased intrapulmonary shunt
↓
Severe arterial hypoxemia
↓
Severe V/Q ratio mismatch
↓
Development of interstitial pulmonary fibrosis from interstitial large protein molecules
↓
Formation of hyaline membranes from alveolar epithelial cell debris

Figure 17–1. Pathogenesis of respiratory distress syndrome.

TABLE 17-3. CONDITIONS ASSOCIATED WITH THE DEVELOPMENT OF RDS

Anaphylaxis
Excessive fluid administration
Sepsis
Inhalation of noxious gases/fumes
Pulmonary infection
Aspiration of gastric contents
Drug overdose
Hemorrhage
DIC
Eclampsia
Near-drowning
Oxygen toxicity
Trauma
    Long bone fractures
    Fat emboli
    Shock
    Pulmonary contusions
    Multiple transfusions
    Sepsis
Multiple organ dysfunction syndrome

- alteration in tissue perfusion related to decreased oxygenation
- alteration in cardiac output related to decreased fluid volume or an adverse effect of PEEP.
- activity intolerance related to hypoxia.
- potential for infection related to artificial airway, immobility, impaired pulmonary defense mechanisms, and retained secretions.
- inability to sustain spontaneous ventilation related to increased intrapulmonary shunt and decreased V/Q ratio.
- impaired communication related to intubation and mechanical ventilation.
- potential for dysfunctional weaning related to prolonged mechanical ventilation.

Goals and Desired Patient Outcomes

Goals and desired patient outcomes include, but are not limited to:

- adequate oxygenation.
- improved ventilation.
- improved intrapulmonary shunt.
- no evidence of infection.
- ability to sustain spontaneous ventilation.
- decreased anxiety.
- ability to maintain adequate cardiac output.
- ability to maintain adequate tissue perfusion.

Patient Care Management

Treatment of RDS is supportive, primarily centering on supporting oxygenation through use of high oxygen concentrations, PEEP, continuous positive airway pressure (CPAP), or inverse ratio ventilation (IRV).

Management of oxygenation is directed at preserving oxygen consumption. Interventions include reduction of fever, and preventing hypothermia and alkalosis. Use of neuromuscular blockade may be instituted to reduce muscle activity and further prevent excessive oxygen consumption. Supplemental oxygen support at an FIO_2 of 0.50 or less with a PaO_2 of 60–70 mm Hg is preferred to limit the risk of development of oxygen toxicity while maintaining adequate oxygenation.

Fluid administration is kept to a minimum, allowing for a PCWP as low as possible to avoid further increases in lung water while maintaining an adequate cardiac output. Both crystalloids and colloids are used in fluid management. Crystalloids are used to decrease alveolar edema caused by albumin crossing the capillary membrane and drawing fluid into the alveoli. Colloids are used to increase circulating albumin to create a gradient to draw fluid from the interstitium to the capillaries. Diuretics and beta adrenergic agonists may be used to remove excessive fluid if the PCWP becomes elevated.

There are many therapies under investigation to treat RDS. Therapies used to treat alveolar damage include antioxidants, arachidonic acid metabolite inhibitors, antiendotoxins, monoclonal antibodies, anticytokines, and cyclooxygenase inhibitors. Other drugs include nonsteroidal anti-inflammatory drugs, antifungal agents (e.g., ketoconazole), exogenous surfactant, prostaglandins, nitric oxide therapy, and corticosteroids in the later stages of RDS. Some centers have advocated the use of extracoporeal membrane oxygenation (ECMO) as a therapy for RDS; however, it is not yet widely employed in the treatment of RDS. Extracorporeal carbon dioxide removal ($ECCO_2R$) is a new therapy under investigation to support tissue oxygenation.

Complications

Complications associated with RDS include metabolic and respiratory acidosis, cardiac arrest, barotrauma, and oxygen toxicity. Long-term complications include permanent reduction in pulmonary functions (e.g., decreased vital capacity and obstruction to airflow). Some patients may develop bronchopulmonary dysplasia—an obliteration of the bronchioles and formation of large cystic air spaces and thick fibrotic walls. Death is usually the result of the precipitating event of RDS, not RDS alone.

ACUTE RESPIRATORY INFECTIONS

Acute respiratory infections include pneumonia and influenza. Pneumonia is an acute inflammatory response of the lungs caused by a bacterial or viral organism. Influenza is a viral upper respiratory tract infection. The organisms can enter the lung directly, by inhalation, or infect the lung via the blood.

The majority of acute respiratory illness are viral in origin and involve the upper respiratory tract (Table 17–4). Viral pneumonias are usually community acquired, transmitted by airborne droplets, although they can be nosocomial. Patients with a viral upper respiratory tract illness (URI) are at risk for development of a secondary bacterial infection.

Pathophysiology

When an organism enters the lung, macrophages and the lymph system work to remove them and prevent infection. When the lung's normal defense mechanisms fail, the organisms multiply, filling the alveoli with exudate. This results in areas of low ventilation and normal perfusion, but increased shunt. Hypoxic vasoconstriction reduces blood flow to the affected area. The organisms cause edema of the airway and stimulate goblet cells to increase mucus production. The increase in secretions and airway edema increase airway resistance, leading to an increased work of breathing.

Etiology and Risk Factors

Patients at risk for development of pneumonia include older adults; persons with dehydration, immobility, malnutrition, or COPD; the immunosuppressed, and those taking drugs that impair airway clearance.

Signs and Symptoms

Signs and symptoms of bacterial pneumonia include fever, shaking chills, pleuritic chest pain that is worse on inspiration, and cough. Sputum ranges from reddish to green.

Viral pneumonia presents with sudden onset of fever; dry cough; headache; myalgia; retrosternal chest pain unaffected by respiration; dyspnea; and cough.

Invasive and Noninvasive Diagnostic Studies

The chest film will reveal lobar infiltrates and may show pleural effusion. The location and type of infiltrates is often a clue to the type of organism present (Table 17–5).

Arterial blood gases may show a decreased PaO_2. Elevated leukocyte counts with a left shift and elevated bands may be seen. Sputum cultures may be done to identify the organism; however, routine sputum cultures are not recommended for community-acquired pneumonia unless the patient does not respond to therapy or is immunocompromised.

TABLE 17–4. ACUTE RESPIRATORY INFECTIONS: CAUSATIVE ORGANISMS

Bacterial
Community-acquired
Pneumococcus
Streptococcus
Klebsiella
Haemophilus influenzae
Nosocomial
Staphylococcus
Pseudomonas

Viral
Community-acquired
Mycoplasma
Cytomegalovirus (CMV)
Respiratory syncytial virus (RSV)
Pneumocystis carinii
Influenza
Adenovirus
Legionella pneumophila (Legionnaires' disease)

TABLE 17–5. CHEST ROENTGENOGRAPHIC FINDING BY ORGANISM

Organism	Chest Film Findings
Pneumococcus	Lobar infiltrates, ipsilateral pleural effusion
Staphyloccus	Bilateral segmental consolidation, bilateral multisegmental or multilobar infiltrates with consolidation
Streptococcus	Infiltrates, pleural effusion
Klebsiella	Lobar consolidation, multiple upper lobes, bulging fissures, volume loss, abscess formation, necrosis with fibrosis, cavity formation, and bronchiectasis
Pseudomonas	Lower lobe infiltrates and consolidation, focal or diffuse infiltrates, abscesses, pleural effusions
Mycoplasma	Nodular, patchy or perihilar infiltrates; two or more lobes are commonly affected
Influenza	Normal
Adenovirus	Patchy infiltrates
Cytomegalovirus	Patchy infiltrates
Pneumocystis carinii	Atypical patchy infiltrates, nodular or perihilar infiltrates involving two or more lobes

Nursing and Collaborative Diagnoses

Diagnoses include, but are not limited to:

- impaired gas exchanged related to increased shunt.
- ineffective airway clearance related to retained secretions.
- activity intolerance related to breathlessness.
- dyspnea related to alveolar hypoventilation.

Goals and Desired Patient Outcomes

Goals and desired patient outcomes include, but are not limited to:

- improved oxygenation; $PaO_2 \geq 60$ mm hg, $SaO_2 \geq 92\%$.
- increased activity tolerance.
- reversal of dyspnea.
- decreased breathlessness on exertion.
- clearance of airway secretions.

Patient Management

Management includes administration of the appropriate antibiotic by intravenous, oral, or intramuscular (Table 17–6) routes. Hydration is important to keep secretions thin and prevent them from becoming thick and tenacious. Aggressive pulmonary hygiene, such as deep breathing, coughing, and aerosol treatments, are used to help remove secretions. Bronchodilators are used to increase airway size and relax airway muscles. Analgesics are recommended to treat muscle aches and fever.

Complications

Complications of pneumonia include hypotension, sepsis, and death.

STATUS ASTHMATICUS

Status asthmaticus is a severe continuing attack of asthma that fails to respond to conventional drug therapy. It can last for days to weeks; even with optimal therapy, it may be fatal.

Pathophysiology

Status asthmaticus is a disease characterized by airway hyperreactivity or hyperresponsiveness, airway obstruction, and airway inflammation. The increased airway responsiveness is manifested by narrowing of airways secondary to bronchial constriction and excessive mucous obstruction, increas-

TABLE 17–6. RECOMMENDED ANTIMICROBIAL AGENTS

Organism	Antimicrobial Agent
Klebsiella pneumoniae	Parenteral cephalosporin, ciprofloxacin
Legionella	Erythromycin, rifampin
Mycoplasma pneumoniae	Erythromycin, azrithromycin, clarithromycin
Pseudomonas pneumoniae	Vancomycin, parenteral cephalosporin, imipenem + cilastatin, tobramycin, ciprofloxacin
Staphylococcus pneumoniae	Vancomycin, parenteral cephalosporin
Streptococcus pneumoniae	Penicillin G, ciprofloxacin, anti-pseudomonal aminoglycosides

ing the work of breathing, interfering with gas exchange, and producing hypoxemia (Figure 17–2). Air trapping with resulting hyperinflation of the lungs is a common clinical feature.

When an inhaled substance elicits a hypersensitive response, Immunoglobulin E (IgE) antibodies stimulate mast cells in the lung to release histamine. Histamine causes inflammation, irritation, and edema in the smooth muscles by attaching to receptor sites in

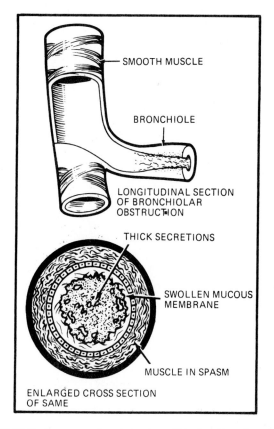

Figure 17–2. Appearance of respiratory bronchioles in asthma (bronchiole obstruction on expiration by muscle spasm, swelling of mucosa, and thick secretions).

the bronchi. There is a release of inflammatory mediators from the epithelial cells, the epithelial mast cells and macrophages. Eosinophils and neutrophils alter the integrity of the epithelium, and changes occur in the autonomic neural control of the airway, the mucociliary function and airway responsiveness. Prostaglandin production is stimulated and further enhances the effects of histamine, stimulating goblet cells to secrete excessive tenacious mucous, leading to airway narrowing (Fig. 17–3).

As the attack continues unabated, the bronchial walls hypertrophy and secretion clearance is diminished, causing bronchiolar obstruction and reducing alveolar ventilation, and causing hyperinflation of the lung.

Early airway closure causes increased intrathoracic pressure on exhalation, inhibiting alveolar ventilation. As alveoli fill with the excessive mucus, intrapulmonary shunt increases as blood is shunted by nonfunctioning alveoli. Diminished ventilation results in a respiratory acidosis.

Etiology and Risk Factors

Status asthmaticus is a complication of asthma. The three most common causes of status asthmaticus are (1) exposure to allergens; (2) noncompliance with the medication regimen; and (3) respiratory infections. It can result from a reaction to an allergen or nonallergen such as exercise and can be precipitated by irritants such as cold air, odors, chemicals, or changes in the weather. Environments which become unusually hot, cold, or dusty often trigger status asthmaticus because of the effect of inspired air on the lungs. Other triggers include psychological and emotional stimuli, aspirin, nonsteroidal anti-inflammatory drugs, beta adrenergic agents, overuse of bronchodilators, and autonomic nervous system imbalance.

Signs and Symptoms

Patients in status asthmaticus are extremely dyspneic, with a hyperpneic respiratory pattern, and a sensation of chest tightness. Inspiratory and expiratory wheezing is usually audible, with a prolonged expiratory phase as the patient tries to exhale the trapped air through narrow airways. Physical examination reveals tachypnea, tachycardia, rapid, thready pulse, use of accessory respiratory muscles, distant heart sounds, hyperresonance on percussion, flaring nares, pallor, cyanosis, increased work of breathing, and fatigue. The disappearance of wheezing may be an ominous sign as the airway may have become completely obstructed. The patient may have pulsus paradoxus, a drop in the systolic blood pressure of 12 mm Hg or more during inspiration.

Invasive and Noninvasive Diagnostic Studies

Arterial blood gases may reveal a normal or increased $PaCO_2$ and a falling PaO_2. Chest roentgenography will probably not be helpful, showing a hyperinflated lung that is normal or translucent. Pulmonary function test are not useful during the acute phase, as the patient is unable to move enough air to complete the test.

Nursing and Collaborative Diagnoses

Diagnoses include but are not limited to:

- impaired gas exchange related to alveolar hypoventilation.
- ineffective airway clearance related to excessive mucus production.
- ineffective breathing pattern related to increased work of breathing.
- at risk of inability to sustain spontaneous ventilation related to respiratory muscle fatigue.

Goals and Desired Patient Outcomes

Goals and patient outcomes include, but are not limited to:

- maintenance of a patent airway.
- reversal of respiratory acidosis; pH greater than 7.35.

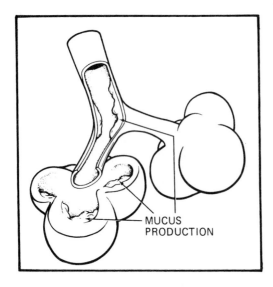

Figure 17–3. Airway lumen in bronchitis.

- control of airway secretions.
- spontaneous ventilation.
- reversal of bronchospasm.
- adequate oxygenation; PaO_2 greater than 60 mm Hg

Patient Care Management

Management includes support of ventilation and respirations. Because of the extreme life-threatening aspects of status asthmaticus, continuous administration of intravenous theophylines, usually aminophylline (e.g., methylxanthines), is instituted. Other treatments include sympathomimetic aerosol therapy, subcutaneous epinephrine, corticosteroids, and beta agonist bronchodilators. Mechanical ventilation may be necessary to support respiration while the above therapies take effect. Additional therapies include hydration, monitoring of oxygenation with ABGs or pulse oximetry, systemic corticosteroids, and antibiotics if signs of infection are present.

Be aware of a decreasing level of consciousness, diminished wheezing, or a rising $PaCO_2$. These may signal a worsening of the asthma episode.

Complications

Complications include pneumothorax, hypoxemia, respiratory acidosis, and hypoxia. Status asthmaticus can cause respiratory failure and death.

Acute Pulmonary Embolism and Aspiration

EDITOR'S NOTE

Pulmonary embolism is a likely content area for questions in the CCRN exam. Pulmonary emboli are best understood when applied to concepts in pulmonary physiology relative to disturbances of ventilation and perfusion (Chapter 14). However, the physical presentation and treatment discussed in this chapter are necessary to remember for purposes of the test.

ACUTE PULMONARY EMBOLISM

An acute pulmonary embolus is a thrombus that occurs in the body, travels through the venous circulation to the pulmonary circulation, and partially or completely occludes a pulmonary artery. A massive pulmonary embolism is one in which more than 50% of the pulmonary artery bed is occluded.

Pathophysiology

The lung is capable of filtering small clots and other substances through fibrolytic mechanisms in the lung. The lung cannot dissolve large clots or multiple small clots. Most pulmonary emboli occur when a lower-extremity, deep-vein thrombus breaks loose from its attachment and flows through the venous circulation, entering the right ventricle and then lodging in small pulmonary arteries (Fig. 18–1). The embolus will most often lodge in the right lower lobe because of increased regional blood flow. Once in the lung, the embolus may be dissolved, grow in size, or fragment

into many smaller pieces. An embolus can be composed of platelets, thrombin, erythrocytes, leukocytes, air, fat, fluid, tumors, or amniotic fluid (Table 18–1). Nonthrombotic emboli have a greater potential for entering the left heart because they can change shape easily and pass through the pulmonary capillary bed into the systemic circulation. Compromise will occur more readily if there is underlying chronic obstructive pulmonary disease (COPD), congestive heart failure (CHF), or other chronic conditions.

Obstruction of the pulmonary vasculature stimulates neurohumoral stimuli, increasing pulmonary artery pressure and the pulmonary vascular resistance. Because there is a disruption in the blood flow to alveoli, they become nonfunctioning units, not participating in the exchange of carbon dioxide and oxygen; increased deadspace. In an effort to maintain adequate gas exchange, ventilation is preferentially shifted to the noninvolved areas of the lung. This results in constriction of the distal airways, leading to alveolar collapse and atelectasis.

Etiology and Risk Factors

Patients at risk for development of thrombus formation include persons with three factors referred to as Virchow's triad: (1) damaged vascular endothelium; (2) venous stasis; and (3) hypercoagulability of the blood. Natural processes of clot dissolution may cause release of fragments, or external mechanisms such as direct trauma, muscle contraction, or changes in perfusion may contribute to the release of the thrombus.

Pulmonary emboli may develop in patients with no predisposing factors. Some predisposing factors include stasis of venous blood resulting from immobilization, varicose veins, obesity, pregnancy, and

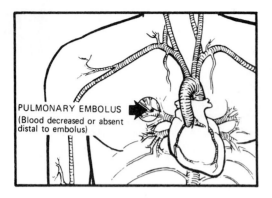

Figure 18–1. Pulmonary embolism.

CHF. Aging, vasculitis, trauma to the vessel wall during venipuncture or prolonged intravenous therapy, venous wall damage due to soft tissue trauma, fractures, or infiltration by malignant cells may also cause thrombi. Hypercoagulability is related to thrombocytosis, increased platelet activity following surgery, trauma, parturition, polycythemia, and hemoconcentration. Rare occasions of thrombus formation include thrombus formation in the heart secondary to acute myocardial infarction, atrial fibrillation, subacute bacterial endocarditis, and cardioversion.

Signs and Symptoms

Increased respiratory rate and tachycardia are the most common signs of pulmonary embolism. The signs and symptoms of pulmonary emboli must be divided into the clinical pictures of a massive embolism and a submassive embolism. Massive embolism occurs suddenly. The patient may have crushing, substernal chest pain and appear to be in shock, with hypotension, dyspnea, cyanosis, apprehension, or coma. Respirations are rapid, shallow, and gasping. Arterial pulse is rapid and the volume is diminished. If awake, the patient may express feelings of impending doom.

Submassive embolism may present only fleeting minimal symptoms. If the submassive embolism has occluded a medium-size artery, tachypnea, dyspnea, tachycardia, generalized chest discomfort, and pleu-ritic-type chest pain may develop within a few hours. Fever, cough, and hemoptysis may occur over several hours or days. A pleural friction rub and a pleural effusion may develop.

Invasive and Noninvasive Diagnostic Studies

Routine chest films may be normal but about 20% of such cases may show some consolidation. The chest film may be inconclusive within the first few hours after embolism. Things to look for on the chest film include pulmonary disease, atelectasis, pleural effusion, elevated diaphragm, and a prominent pulmonary artery.

The electrocardiogram (ECG) may be normal but most often shows sinus tachycardia or right ventricular (RV) strain. In an extensive pulmonary emboli the ECG will show right axis deviation, transient right bundle branch block, ST-segment depression, T-wave inversion in leads V1 and V4, and tall peaked P waves in leads II, III, and AVF. If the emboli is massive, the ECG may show electromechanical dissociation (EMD).

Arterial blood gases (ABGs) are unreliable indicators of pulmonary embolism. If the arterial oxygen pressure (PaO_2) is above 80 mm Hg on room air, a pulmonary embolism is less likely, although one may exist and not occlude major arteries. The ABGs may show a decrease PaO_2 and $PaCO_2$.

The most useful tests are nuclear studies and pulmonary angiography. A ventilation/perfusion (V/Q) lung scan that is normal usually rules out a pulmonary embolism. If a lung scan shows perfusion defects on segments that appear normal on chest roentgenography, then pulmonary embolism is likely. A lung scan may be abnormal due simply to COPD.

Pulmonary angiography is the most accurate way to diagnose pulmonary embolism. A positive angiogram will reveal filling deficits or sharp cut-offs in blood flow. A magnetic resonance imaging scan can also be used to detect changes in pulmonary blood flow or pin point an embolus.

Nursing and Collaborative Diagnoses

Diagnoses include, but are not limited to:

- impaired gas exchange related to increased deadspace ventilation.
- ineffective breathing pattern related to alveolar hypoventilation.
- anxiety related to difficulty breathing.
- decreased cardiac output related to RV failure.

TABLE 18–1. ETIOLOGY OF PULMONARY EMBOLI

Deep-vein thrombosis
Air embolus
Septic embolus
Fat embolus
Tumor embolus
Amniotic fluid embolus

- altered peripheral tissue perfusion related to thrombus formation.
- at risk for inability to sustain spontaneous ventilation related to increased deadspace and decreased alveolar ventilation.

Goals and Desired Patient Outcomes

Goals and desired patient outcomes include, but are not limited to:

- adequate oxygenation.
- reversal of the clot.
- reduction in risk for additional clot formation.
- prevention of pulmonary infarction.
- improved V/Q ratio.

Patient Care Management

Heparin is the immediate drug of choice. Heparin impedes clotting by preventing fibrin formation. Within 30 min of a bolus administration, anticoagulation should be documented. A partial thromboplastin time (PTT) of 55–85 sec is adequate anticoagulation. Anticoagulation is continued by a heparin bolus every 4–6 hr or a continuous intravenous heparin drip. Continuous intravenous heparin is preferred for patients at high risk or with a massive embolus. A continuous infusion maintains a steady therapeutic blood level in contrast to the heparin bolus every 4–6 hr. The bolus causes peak levels for short times and subtherapeutic levels for the remaining time before another bolus is due. Heparin is usually continued for several days or when oral anticoagulation can become effective.

Oral anticoagulants are often started 3–4 days before stopping the heparin to avoid a period of no anticoagulant therapy. Oral anticoagulants are usually given for 6–8 weeks if the patient is asymptomatic. They may be given indefinitely or for the remainder of the patient's life for multiple reasons.

Streptokinase, urokinase, and tissue plasminogen activator (TPA) are thrombolytic enzymes being used to dissolve or lyse the emboli. These three thrombolytic agents are administered only by intravenous infusion. Therapeutic action begins immediately and ceases with the interruption of the intravenous administration. However, residual effects may last for as long as 12–24 hr.

Surgery is reserved for those patients who do not respond to anticoagulants, who have rebound effects to heparin, or who have recurrent emboli. Procedures may include ligation or clipping of the inferior vena cava, filter placement in the vena cava,

and embolectomy. Embolectomy is a serious operation and is usually reserved for the massive emboli or for the decompensating patient that cannot be stabilized. The vena caval umbrella inserted in the inferior vena cava may filter emboli and eliminate the necessity of major surgery in select patients.

Prevention of thrombus formation is critical. Ambulate patients as much as their clinical condition allows. Elevating legs, use of pneumatic devices, the use of antiembolic hose, and active and passive exercises, including range-of-motion, will help prevent stasis of venous blood in nonambulating patients. Patient and family education about risk factors of embolism development and prevention measurements are important.

Complications

A complication of pulmonary embolism is pulmonary hypertension from pulmonary arterial obstruction. If the obstruction is partial or develops slowly, the patient may survive to be treated. However, if the obstruction is rapid and total, the patient may suffer sudden death. Chronic pulmonary hypertension does not usually occur with a single embolus. It usually results from multiple emboli of middle-sized vessels.

Complications of pulmonary embolism may include pulmonary infarction due to extension of emboli. Any embolus that is large enough to alter hemodynamics can result in complications. These include stroke, myocardial infarction, cardiac dysrhythmias that are not amenable to therapy, liver failure and necrosis secondary to congestion, pneumonia, pulmonary abscesses, adult respiratory distress syndrome, shock, and death.

PULMONARY ASPIRATION

Pulmonary aspiration is the inhalation of foreign fluid or particulate matter into the lower airways.

Pathophysiology

Aspiration of foreign substances into the lung results in a chemical pneumonitis. This provides a medium for bacterial growth. If not treated, it can progress to a necrotizing process, resulting in lung abscess and empyema.

Etiology and Risk Factors

Pulmonary aspiration can be the result of inhalation of gastric contents, fluids (as in a near drowning), or saliva. Patients at risk for aspiration include the elderly and patients with neurological compromise (e.g., a cerebral vascular accident, seizures, or dementia). Head trauma, drug and alcohol overdose, vomiting, intestional obstruction, and gastro-esophageal reflux are all risk factors for aspiration.

Signs and Symptoms
Signs and symptoms include fever, breathlessness, tachycardia, tachypnea, wheezing, cough, and pleuritic pain.

Invasive and Noninvasive Diagnostic Studies
Chest roentgenography may reveal patchy infiltrates or large areas of fluid in the lung. ABGs may be normal or show a falling PaO_2, depending on the amount of the lung involved. Gram's stain and sputum cultures may be used to identify the organism.

Nursing and Collaborative Diagnoses
Diagnoses include, but are not limited to:

- impaired gas exchange related to increased shunt.
- high risk for infection related to aspiration of foreign material.
- ineffective breathing pattern related to breathlessness.
- ineffective airway clearance related to retained secretions.

Goals and Desired Patient Outcomes
Goals and desired patient outcomes include, but are not limited to:

- improved oxygenation.
- elimination of infection.
- reversal of breathlessness.
- removal of secretions.

Patient Care Managment
Management includes bronchodilators, intravenous fluids, and aggressive pulmonary hygiene. Routine use of antibiotics is not recommended. Steroids are not recommended because they have not been shown to be effective.

Complications
Complications include development of pneumonia, necrotizing pneumonitis, lung abscess, and empyema.

Thoracic Trauma and Air Leak Syndromes

EDITOR'S NOTE

Chest trauma is reviewed in this chapter to provide adequate information about the assessment and treatment of chest injuries. Chest trauma, particularly from an assessment point of view, is also better understood if considered along with concepts in pulmonary physiology. The goal of this chapter is to provide enough information to help you understand how to assess and treat key pulmonary but not overwhelm you with unnecessary information.

THORACIC TRAUMA

Thoracic injuries are common in multiple trauma. The more systems involved in the trauma, the more critical each injury becomes. Thoracic injuries are especially serious in the elderly, the obese, and patients with cardiac or pulmonary disease. The older the patient, the more likely underlying health problems and diminished physiological reserve. Statistically, if there is a thoracic injury alone, there is a 5–10% mortality rate. If there is a thoracic injury and another injury, the mortality rate is 30%. Thoracic trauma occurs in 6 out of 10 motor vehicle accidents.

Pulmonary Contusion

The most common visceral injury is pulmonary contusion. The next most common visceral injury is pulmonary laceration.

Pathophysiology

Pulmonary contusion is damage to the lung parenchyma, resulting in localized edema and hemorrhage. The thorax hits an object such as the steering wheel, compressing the thoracic cage, diminishing its size, and compressing the lungs as a result of the increased intrathoracic pressure. As the thorax rebounds from the steering wheel, the thoracic cage increases in size, decreasing the intrathoracic pressure and the pressure on the lung parenchyma. The lung parenchyma, under pressure, expands, rupturing capillaries and resulting in hemorrhage (Fig. 19–1).

If the force of the injury is sufficient to lacerate the lungs, bleeding is common and potentially dangerous. Laceration may occur from tearing due to rib fractures or direct puncture.

Etiology and Risk Factors

Contusions may occur as the result of blunt thoracic trauma or penetrating lung trauma. Motor vehicle accidents are the most common cause of lung contusion.

Signs and Symptoms

Depending on the severity of the trauma, symptoms may include tachypnea, tachycardia, and blood-tinged secretions. Crackles may be heard throughout all lung fields as a result of retained secretions.

Invasive and Noninvasive Diagnostic Studies

The diagnosis of pulmonary contusion due to blunt trauma is difficult since symptoms may not occur for from 4–72 hr post trauma. Chest roentgenograms may be normal or may reveal localized opacification in the injured area. The affected area may be larger

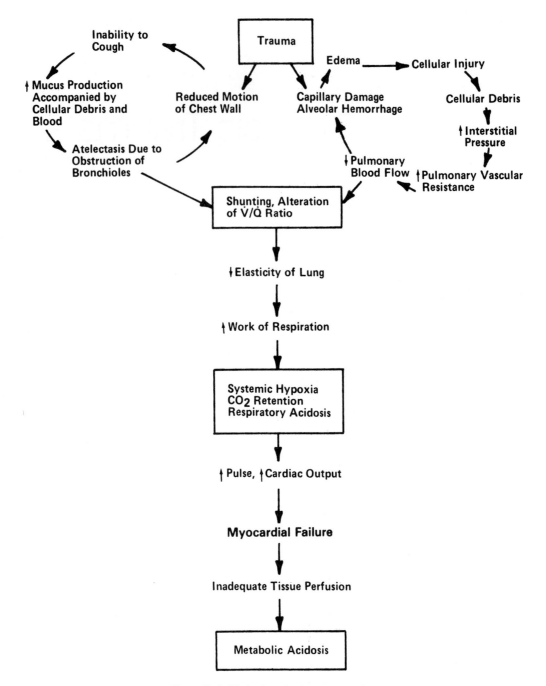

Figure 19–1. Mechanism of pulmonary contusion.

than revealed by the chest film. Arterial blood gases (ABGs) will show a decreased carbon dioxide ($PaCO_2$) and oxygen pressures (PaO_2) and a worsening of the PaO_2/FIO_2 ratio (or a/A) ratio, indicating increasing Qs/Qt.

Nursing and Collaborative Diagnoses
Diagnoses include, but are not limited to:

- Impaired gas exchange related to in-creased ventilation/perfusion (V/Q) mismatch.
- Ineffective breathing pattern related to chest

pain.
- Pain related to thoracic injury.
- Risk for fluid volume imbalance related to lung parenchymal injury.
- Ineffective airway clearance related to retained secretions.

Goals and Desired Patient Outcomes

- Patent airway.
- Improved oxygenation: PaO_2 above 60 mm Hg, oxygen saturation (SaO_2) at least 92%.
- Adequate pain control without respiratory

depression.
- Improved shunt fraction.
- Restoration of normal lung function.
- Effective airway clearance.
- Fluid balance; central venous pressure (CVP) and pulmonary capillary wedge pressure (PCWP) within normal levels.

Patient Care Management

If the contusion is mild, monitoring and supplemental oxygen by mask may be sufficient. Severe pulmonary contusions are treated like respiratory distress syndrome (RDS) because of the large amount of lung tissue damage, refractory hypoxemia, and decreased lung compliance. Agitation and anxiety may indicate the presence of hypoxia and may be a first sign of impending deterioration.

Since moderate to severe pulmonary contusions are often accompanied by multisystem injuries, the fluid administration must be balanced against hemodynamic and pulmonary function. Fluid overload is associated with poor outcomes. Intake and output, CVP, and pulmonary artery pressure (PAP) should be monitored. Steroids have been used to reduce lung edema; however, they are no longer recommended because of their lack of effectiveness.

Nasotracheal suctioning and humidification may help with removal of secretions.

Complications

Complications include pulmonary laceration, hemothorax and development of RDS. A pulmonary laceration occurs when the force of the injury is sufficient to lacerate the lung from a rib fracture or direct puncture, causing bleeding and hemothorax. Tracheal lacerations can occur which are life threatening and require immediate surgery.

Fractured Ribs

One of the most common closed thoracic injuries is rib fractures.

Pathophysiology

It is not common to have a fracture of the first rib. Fracture of the first rib is life-threatening and indicates severe underlying thoracic and/or abdominal injuries. When a very strong force is applied to the upper thoracic cage, the result is a "star burst" fracture, that is, pieces of bone going in all directions. Sternal fracture is suspected when there is paradoxical movement of the anterior chest wall.

Fracture of the second rib is commonly termed the hangman's fracture. Ribs 3–8 are the most commonly fractured. If a single rib is fractured pain

relief is usually the only treatment necessary. The intact rib on each side of the fractured rib stabilizes the fracture and keeps it in alignment for healing. Fractures of ribs 9–12 arouse suspicion of the possibility of laceration and/or rupture of the spleen and liver.

Etiology and Risk Factors
Rib fractures occur as the result of a blunt force which does not penetrate the chest wall. Motor vehicle accidents, falls, and violent assault are the common causes of closed thoracic injury.

Signs and Symptoms
Symptoms include pain, dyspnea, ecchymosis, and splinting on movement. The patient should be examined for neck injuries, brachial plexus injury, pneumothorax, aortic rupture or tear, and thoracic outlet syndrome.

Invasive and Noninvasive Diagnostic Studies
Rib fractures can be diagnosed by chest roentgenography. It may be difficult to see hairline fractures initially. Simple rib fractures are more easily seen as they begin to repair and lay down additional calcium at the injury site. Compound rib fractures and fractures with overlying bone are more easily detected by chest roentgenography.

Nursing and Collaborative Diagnoses
Diagnoses include, but are not limited to:

- Pain related to thoracic cage injury.
- Ineffective breathing pattern related to splinting of injured area.
- Impaired gas exchange related to alveolar hypoventilation.

Goals and Desired Patient Outcomes
Goals and desired patient outcomes include, but are not limited to:

- Pain control without ventilatory compromise.
- Adequate oxygenation: PaO_2 above 60 mm Hg, SaO_2 at least 92%.
- Stabilization of the rib fractures.
- Prevention of atelectasis and pneumonia.

Patient Management
Management includes relief of pain and pulmonary hygiene. Intercostal nerve block is most efficient in relieving pain, yet does not interfere with coughing, sighing, and deep breathing. Bronchial hygiene and physical therapy are used to prevent development of

atelectasis. Binders are not recommended because they decrease excursion over a wide area of the thorax, predisposing the patient to hypoxemia and atelectasis. Sternal fractures may be stabilized with traction or with endotracheal intubation, mechanical ventilation, and positive end expiratory pressure (PEEP).

Complications

Complications include atelectasis, fever, pneumonia, and retained pulmonary secretions.

Flail Chest

Flail chest refers to two or more adjacent ribs with two or more fractures, anteriorly or laterally. The flail thorax may be especially severe if it is associated with a transverse fracture of the sternum. Sternal fracture is suspected when there is paradoxical movement of the anterior thoracic wall.

Pathophysiology

A section of the chest wall becomes detached from the thoracic cage. The involved portion of the thoracic wall may be so unstable that it will move paradoxically or opposite to the rest of the thoracic wall when the patient breathes (Fig. 19–2). During inspiration, negative intrathoracic pressure increases and the chest wall moves outward. With a flail chest, the injured segment moves inward. On expiration, intrathoracic pressure decreases, the chest wall moves inward, and the flail section moves outward. This results in atelectasis and alveolar collapse as the alveoli cannot fill with air.

Etiology and Risk Factors

Causes include fights, motor vehicle accidents, blast injuries, and athletic injuries.

Signs and Symptoms

Symptoms of flail thoracic include rapid, shallow respirations, cyanosis, severe thoracic wall pain, shock, bony crepitation at the site of fracture, and paradoxical thoracic movement. There may be signs of pulmonary contusion, bruised thorax, and tender chest on palpation. Hypotension, tachycardia, and hemoptysis may also be present.

Invasive and Noninvasive Diagnostic Studies

Chest roentgenography confirms the diagnosis of flail chest. ABGs may show a falling PaO_2, increasing $PaCO_2$ and a pH below 7.35—respiratory acidosis.

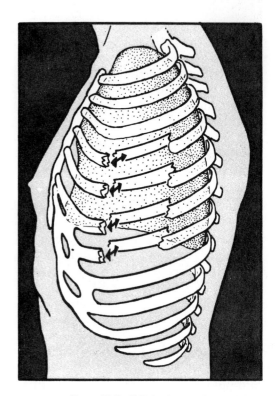

Figure 19–2. Flail chest segment.

Nursing and Collaborative Diagnoses

Diagnoses include, but are not limited to:

- Impaired gas exchange related to alveolar hypoventilation.
- Ineffective breathing pattern related to flailing chest wall segment.
- Pain related to chest wall injury.

Goals and Desired Patient Outcomes

Goals and desired patient outcomes include, but are not limited to:

- Adequate oxygenation: PaO_2 at least 60 mm Hg, SaO_2 at least 92%.
- Stabilization of flail segment.
- Prevention of atelectasis and pneumonia.
- Maintain fluid balance.
- Lack of retained secretions.

Patient Management

Specific treatment is stabilization of the flail segment and restoration of normal breathing. In an emergency, anything can be used to stabilize the thoracic wall and help immobilize the segment, (e.g., sandbags or hands). In the critical care unit, intubation, positive pressure ventilation, and PEEP may be used to stabilize the flailing segment. Neuromuscular blockade may be used to paralyze the patient and allow the ventilator to help stabilize the chest wall. Adequate sedation must be provided when using a neuromuscular blockade.

Pain control is a top priority. Patients are medicated to achieve adequate pain control and reduce the work of breathing.

Complications

Complications include pulmonary contusion, pneumothorax, hypoxia, pulmonary laceration, and cardiac contusion.

Hemothorax

Hemothorax is an accumulation of blood in the thorax. It is often accompanied by a pneumothorax.

Pathophysiology

The two major effects of a hemothorax are the accumulation of blood in the lungs, collapsing alveoli, and systemic hypovolemia. Shock can occur quickly with the development of a hemothorax. Trauma to the thorax may cause bleeding from the intercostal, pleural, lung parenchymal, or mediastinal vessels or from the internal mammary artery. As blood fills the pleural space, the underlying lung tissue is compressed, causing alveolar collapse. A hemothorax may be self-limiting. As the blood accumulates in the chest, the increasing pressure may reduce or stop the source of bleeding.

Etiology

Hemothorax is caused by blunt or penetrating thoracic trauma, iatrogenic causes, lacerated liver, or perforated diaphragm. It may also result from thoracic surgery, anticoagulant therapy, or a dissecting thoracic aneurysm.

Signs and Symptoms

The symptoms of a hemothorax depend on the size of the blood accumulation. Small amounts of blood (i.e., 400 mL or less) will cause minimal symptoms. Larger amounts of blood (i.e., 400 mL or more) usually present with signs of shock: tachycardia, tachypnea, hypotension, and anxiety. Breath sounds may be diminished or absent, and the chest is dull on percussion.

Invasive and Noninvasive Diagnostic Studies

The chest film may show pleural fluid or a mediastinal shift. ABGs will show a normal or decreased PaO_2, an increased $PaCO_2$, and a falling pH. If there has been a large amount of bleeding, the hematocrit and hemoglobin levels may be decreased. CVP or PAP may be low if fluid volume depletion is evident.

Thoracentesis is used for both diagnosis and treatment. A large-bore needle is inserted into the chest and aspirated for blood or serosanguineous fluid.

Nursing and Collaborative Diagnoses

Diagnoses include, but are not limited to:

- Impaired gas exchange related to alveolar hypoventilation.
- Ineffective breathing pattern related to decreased lung volume.
- Fluid volume deficit related to hemorrhage.
- Pain related to thoracic injury.
- High risk for infection related to traumatic injury.
- Anxiety related to pain and traumatic injury.

Goals and Desired Patient Outcomes

Goals and desired patient outcomes include, but are not limited to:

- Stabilizing the patient's hemodynamic status.
- Adequate oxygenation: PaO_2 at least 60 mm Hg, SaO_2 at least 92%.
- Restoring and maintaining fluid balance.
- Re-expansion of the affected lung.
- Control of pain.
- Reduction of anxiety.

Patient Management

Small hemothoraces may resolve spontaneously because of low pulmonary system pressure and the presence of thromboplastin in the lungs. Large hemothoraces are treated with the insertion of one or more thoracic tubes in the fifth or sixth intercostal space in the midaxillary line (Fig. 19–3). The thoracic tube is sutured in place and covered with a sterile dressing after connection to an underwater seal with suction. Autotranfusion may be used for patients with a blood loss of 1 L or more. Severe or uncontrollable hemothorax may require thoracotomy to remove the blood and fluid from the lung and correct the source of bleeding.

Monitoring the patient's ability to expel secretions and suctioning when necessary are important in preventing hypoxia and atelectasis. Analgesics are recommended for relief of pain.

Complications

Complications of a hemothorax include atelectasis, lung collapse, hypoxemia, and mediastinal shift.

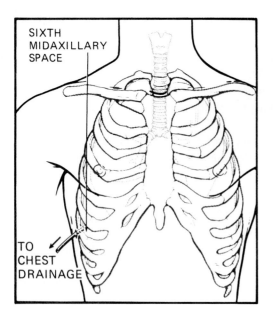

SIXTH MIDAXILLARY SPACE

TO CHEST DRAINAGE

Figure 19–3. Chest tube insertion for hemothorax.

Diaphragmatic Rupture

Pathophysiology
The immediate result of a significant tear in the diaphragm is the herniation of the abdominal contents into the thoracic cavity. The rupture allows air to enter the thorax, causing increasing intrathoracic pressure. In the majority of cases, the left hemidiaphragm is injured, perhaps because of the protection by the liver on the right side.

Etiology and Risk Factors
Rupture of the diaphragm is associated with both blunt and penetrating trauma, especially gunshot wounds of the lower abdomen and chest. The incidence of diaphragmatic rupture is doubled in patients with a fractured pelvis. It is almost always accompanied by intraperitoneal and multisystem injuries.

Signs and Symptoms
Primary symptoms of a ruptured or herniated diaphragm include auscultation of bowel sounds in the chest, increasing shortness of breath, unequal diaphragmatic movement on palpation, elevated diaphragm and hyperresonance to percussion, marked or increasing respiratory distress, severe shoulder pain on the same side as the tear, and shock.

Invasive and Noninvasive Diagnostic Studies
The chest film may reveal an elevated, arched shadow of a high left hemidiaphragm, a mediastinal shift to the right, shadows above the diaphragm, and abnormal air/fluid levels. The chest film may also reveal a nasogastric tube in the left thorax, or air bubbles in the left chest, indicating visceral herniation. Diagnosis is aided by peritoneal lavage and fiberoptic endoscopy. Inability to insert a nasogastric tube may also help diagnosis a rupture, as the tube cannot pass the kinked esophagus.

Nursing and Collaborative Diagnoses
Diagnoses include, but are not limited to:

- Impaired gas exchange related to alveolar hypoventilation.
- Ineffective breathing pattern related to increased intrathoracic pressure.
- Fluid volume deficit related to hemorrhage.
- Pain related to thoracic injury.
- High risk for infection related to traumatic injury.
- Anxiety related to pain and traumatic injury.

Goals and Desired Patient Outcomes
Goals and desired patient outcomes include, but are not limited to:

- Stabilizing the patient's hemodynamic status.
- Adequate oxygenation: PaO_2 at least 60 mm Hg, SaO_2 at least 92%.
- Control of pain.
- Reduction of anxiety.
- Surgical repair of the rupture.

Patient Care Management
Immediate treatment is to establish adequate respiratory function. This is most frequently accomplished by endotracheal intubation and mechanical respiration. Stabilizing a patient in shock prior to surgery may or may not be possible, depending on the severity of the rupture. Definitive therapy consists of surgical repair of the torn diaphragm and replacement of the abdominal organs in the abdominal cavity.

The patient's respiratory status should be monitored to ensure adequate oxygenation. Increased intrathoracic pressure and abdominal contents in the thoracic cavity will usually cause marked hemodynamic compromise.

Complications
Complications include strangulation of the bowel or bowel obstruction, cardiovascular collapse, and death.

AIR-LEAK SYNDROMES

A pneumothorax is accumulation of air in the pleural space. It may be the result of blunt or penetrating trauma, or rupture of a bleb or emphysematous bulla, or have an iatrogenic cause, such as mechanical ventilation or high levels of PEEP (Table 19–1). There are three types of pneumothorax; closed, open, and tension pneumothorax.

The closed pneumothorax occurs when air enters the pleural space through the airways. If the air cannot escape the chest, intrapleural pressure increases, pressure on the other lung and heart will continue, and a tension pneumothorax is possible.

An open pneumothorax is caused by a penetrating injury which allows air to enter and exit the pleural space (Fig. 19–4). The open pneumothorax is less dangerous than closed pneumothorax because of the reduced likelihood of developing a tension pneumothorax.

Tension pneumothorax is potentially life-threatening. Air accumulates in the pleural space, but cannot escape. During inhalation air is sucked into the pleura through a tear; on exhalation, the torn pleura closes against the parenchyma, creating a one-way valve system that prevents the air from being exhaled (Fig. 19–5).

Pathophysiology

The lungs are contained in the visceral pleural. The parietal pleura line the thorax. The potential area between these two pleura, the pleural space, is filled with a thin layer of lubrication. If air or fluid enter the space, the surfaces are separated. The pressure of the intrapleural space is –5 cm H_2O. When air or fluid enter the pleural space, the pressure becomes positive. This positive pressure leads to lung collapse, decreased lung compliance, decreased total lung capacity, and decreased vital capacity. Hypoxia is the result of the increasing V/Q mismatch. If the pressure cannot escape, as in tension pneumothorax, the intrathoracic pressure continues to build, leading to hemodynamic compromise and possible cardiovascular collapse.

The tension pneumothorax quickly produces hemodynamic and cardiopulmonary compromise. On inspiration, more air is drawn in through the tear, however, it has nowhere to escape. The accumulation of air in the thorax causes increasing intrathoracic pressure that results in severe hemodynamic imbalances.

Signs and Symptoms

A simple pneumothorax may present with only mild respiratory distress, asymmetrical chest wall expansion, vague complaints of difficulty catching one's breath, and chest pain (see Table 19–1).

Tension pneumothorax produces symptoms that include dyspnea and restlessness, progressive cyanosis, diminished or absent breath sounds on the affected side, decreased chest wall movement, signs of increasing respiratory distress, chest pain and tracheal shift toward the *unaffected* side, asymmetrical chest wall movement, and rigidity on the affected side. The mediastinum, the trachea, and the point of maximum intensity (PMI) all shift away from the affected side. A tension pneumothorax is a medical emergency that requires immediate treatment.

Invasive and Noninvasive Diagnostic Studies

The chest film will show accumulation of air in the pleural space. A mediastinal shift may be evident. ABGs will show a decreased PaO_2, an increased $PaCO_2$, and an increased pH (respiratory alkalosis).

Nursing and Collaborative Diagnoses

Diagnoses include, but are not limited to:

- Impaired gas exchange related to decreased lung tissue for ventilation.
- Ineffective breathing pattern related to collapsed lung.
- Anxiety related to increasing difficulty breathing.
- Dyspnea related to decreased alveolar ventilation.
- At risk for decreased cardiac output related to increased intrapulmonary pressures.

TABLE 19–1. SIGNS AND SYMPTOMS OF PNEUMOTHORAX

Inspection
Asymmetrical chest wall movement
Hyperexpansion
Chest wall rigidity on the affected side

Palpation
Subcutaneous emphysema
Decreased vocal fremitus
Mediastinal shift
Tracheal deviation
Tympany on the affected side

Percussion
Hyperresonance on the affected side

Auscultation
Decreased or absent breath sounds on the affected side

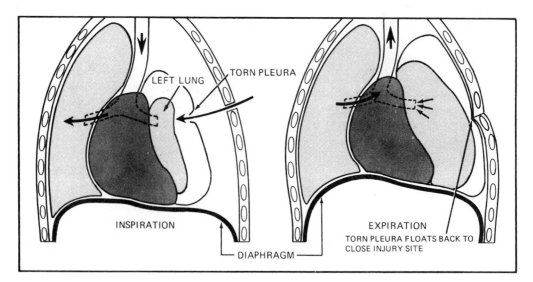

Figure 19–4. Open pneumothorax.

Goals and Desired Patient Outcomes

Goals and desired patient outcomes include, but are not limited to:

- Re-expansion of the collapsed lung.
- Adequate oxygenation.
- Maintain cardiac output.
- Reduction and control of pain.
- Maintenance of chest drainage system.

Patient Management

Drainage of air and fluid from the pleural space requires an evacuation system that allows air and fluids to exit but not re-enter. If the pneumothorax is small enough, needle aspiration or thoracentesis may be sufficient treatment to re-expand the lung. Smaller catheters are being used to evacuate air from the thorax, resulting in a less traumatic puncture and increased patient comfort. A catheter with a flutter valve may be used to allow the air to escape without reaccumulating. Because of the small diameter of the tubes, they are not recommended for draining fluid or blood.

If a chest tube is used it is inserted in the second or third intercostal space at the midclavicular line to remove the air (Fig. 19–6). Chest tubes are sutured in place and connected to a water seal or suction drainage system. The insertion site of the tube is cov-

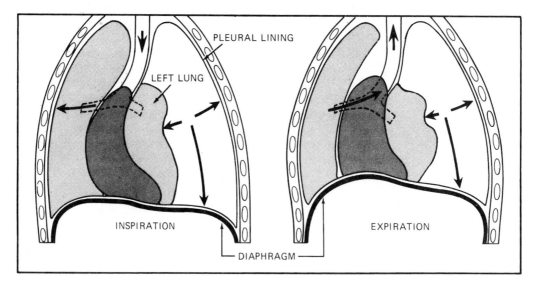

Figure 19–5. Tension pneumothorax.

ered with a sterile dressing and connected to a water-sealed drainage system.

The most common pleural units are single plastic units that can serve as one-, two-, or three-chamber units, depending on the patient's needs. Some pleural units place a collection chamber before the water seal chamber to avoid the effect of increasing resistance to air evacuation. As fluid accumulates in the water seal, the hydrostatic resistance to air leaving the pleural space increases. The collection chamber before the water seal chamber reduces this problem. The water seal is situated at the end of the pleural tube to provide minimal resistance to pressure changes in the pleural space. Suction chambers have been developed to accelerate re-expansion of the pleural space. While the value of suction is controversial, many physicians routinely order low suction levels between 10 and 40 cm H_2O. Low levels are employed to avoid injury to pulmonary parenchymal tissue.

Air leaving the pleural space is readily seen by the bubbling in the water seal chamber. When air has ceased leaking from the pleural space, bubbling in the water seal chamber ceases. Evacuation of fluid is noted by measuring the amount of fluid in the collection chamber.

For evacuation of air, chest tubes are placed superiorly and anteriorly in a patient lying flat, near the second intercostal space in the midclavicular line. Chest tubes are placed in gravity dependent positions to facilitate fluid evacuation; near the fifth intercostal space in the midaxillary line. Placement

lower than the fifth intercostal space increases the risk of puncturing abdominal viscera.

Chest tubes should not be clamped if bubbling is present in the water seal chamber. The potential for a tension pneumothorax exists in a situation where a tube is clamped while air is still exiting the pleural space. If no air is leaking from the pleural space, the clamping of a chest test is generally not a problem, provided no major blood accumulation is also present.

Milking and stripping of chest tubes is not recommended, as it has been shown to create suction pressures of up to −400 cm H_2O. This can cause damage to lung tissue and disruption of suture lines.

Chest films are used to verify position of the chest tubes and monitor the re-expansion of the lung.

Complications

Complications of pneumothorax are dependent on the size, rate of development, and underlying cardiopulmonary status of the patient. Cardiac and pulmonary failure can result from the sudden development of a large pneumothorax or a tension pneumothorax.

PULMONARY BIBLIOGRAPHY

Ahrens, T.S. (1993). Changing perspectives in the assessment of oxygenation. *Crit Care Nurse, 13,* 4, 78–83.

Aloi, A., & Burns, S.M. (1995). Continuous airway pressure monitoring in the critical care setting. *Crit Care Nurse, 15,* 2, 66–74.

American Thoracic Society (1993). Guidelines for the initial management of adults with community-acquired pneumonia: diagnosis, assessment of severity, and initial antimicrobial therapy. *Am Rev Resp Dis, 148,* 1418–1426.

Dickson, S.L. (1995). Understanding the oxyhemoglobin dissociation curve. *Crit Care Nurse, 15,* 5, 54–58.

Dirkes, S., Dickinson, S., & Valentine, J. (1992). Acute respiratory failure and ECMO. *Crit Care Nurse, 12,* 7, 39–47.

Freichels, T. (1993). Orchestrating the care of mechanically ventilated patients. *Am J Nurs, 93,* 10, 26–35.

Goodnough Hammeman, S.K., Ingersoll, G.L., et al. (1994). Weaning from short-term mechanical ventilation: a review. *Am J Crit Care, 3,* 6, 421–441.

Hagler, D.A., & Traver, G.A. (1994). Endotracheal saline and suction catheters: sources of lower airway contamination. *Am J Crit Care, 3,* 6, 444–447.

Hammer, J. (1995). Challenging diagnosis: adult respiratory distress syndrome. *Crit Care Nurse, 15,* 5, 46–51.

Juarez, P. (1992). Mechanical ventilation for the patient with severe ARDS: PC-IRV. *Crit Care Nurse, 12,* 4, 34–39.

Kandra, T.G., & Rosenthal, M. (1993). The pathophysiology of respiratory failure. *Int Anesth Clin, 31,* 2, 119–147.

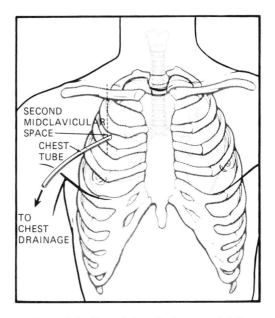

SECOND MIDCLAVICULAR SPACE

CHEST TUBE

TO CHEST DRAINAGE

Figure 19–6. Chest tube insertion for removal of air.

Kim, M.J., McFarland, G.K., & McLane, A.M. (1995). *Pocket Guide to Nursing Diagnosis*, ed 6. St. Louis; C.V. Mosby.

Kinney, M.R., Packa, D.R., & Dunbar S.B. (1993). *AACN's Clinical Reference for Critical-Care Nursing*. St. Louis: C.V. Mosby.

Knebel, A.R., Shekleton, M.E., Burns, S., et al. (1994). Weaning from mechanical ventilation: concept development. *Am J Crit Care, 3*, 6, 416–420.

Laskowski-Jones, L. (1995). Meeting the challenge of chest trauma. *Am J Nurs, 95*, 9, 23–30.

Mancinelli-Van Atta, J., & Beck, S.L. (1992). Preventing hypoxemia and hemodynamic compromise related to endotracheal suctioning. *Am J Crit Care, 1*, 3, 62–79.

Milic-Emili, J. (1992). How to monitor intrinsic PEEP—and why. *J Crit Illness, 7*, 1, 25–32.

Redick, E.L. (1993). Closed-system, in-line endotracheal suctioning. *Crit Care Nurse, 13*, 4, 47–51.

Ruggles, L. (1995). Auto-Peep: measurement issues and nursing interventions. *Crit Care Nurse, 15*, 2, 30–38.

Shlafer, M. (1993). *The Nurse, Pharmacology and Drug Therapy*. Redwood City, California: Addison-Wesley.

Sinski, A., & Corbo, J. (1994). Surfactant replacement in adults and children with ARDS—an effective therapy. *Crit Care Nurse, 14*, 6, 54–59.

Stiesmeyer, J.K. (1993). A four-step approach to pulmonary assessment. *Am J Nurs, 93*, 8, 22–31.

Swearingen, P.L., & Keen, J.H. (1995). *Manual of Critical Care, Applying Nursing Diagnoses to Adult Critical Care*. St. Louis: C.V. Mosby.

Urban, N.A., Greenlee, K.K., Krumberger, J.M., & Winkelman, C. (1995). *Guidelines for Critical Care Nursing*, St. Louis: C.V. Mosby.

West, J.B. (1992). *Pulmonary Pathophysiology—the Essentials*. Baltimore: Williams & Wilkins.

Weilitz, P.B. (1993). Weaning a patient from mechanical ventilation. *Crit Care Nurse, 13*, 4, 33–43.

Pulmonary Practice Exam

Questions 1 and 2 refer to the following scenario:

A 56-year-old female is admitted to the unit with acute shortness of breath. She has a history of chronic obstructive pulmonary disease (COPD), congestive heart failure (CHF), and sleep apnea. Her current weight is 125 kg and she is 157 cm (5'2") tall. On arrival to the emergency room, she is very short of breath and requires intubation. Her arterial blood gases (ABGs) and vital signs reveal:

pH	7.29
PaO_2	59
$PaCO_2$	74
HCO_3^-	35
blood pressure	134/86
pulse	122
respiratory rate	33

She is placed on mechanical ventilation at the following settings:

Mode	assisted mandatory ventilation (AMV)
V_T	850
Respiratory rate	12
FIO_2	0.40
PAP	42 cm H_2O
PEEP	+3 cmH_2O

She is given the following medications:

albuterol	4 mg q2h
dobutamine	3 μg/kg/min
IV fluids	50 ml/hr
lorazepam	3 mg/hr

She is drowsy but responds to hearing her name called. After therapy, her vital signs are:

blood pressure	98/56
pulse	112 (atrial fibrillation)
respiratory rate	12 (not breathing above the ventilator)

temperature	37.8
pulse oximetry (SpO_2)	0.95

Her ABGs reveal:

pH	7.55
PaO_2	78
$PaCO_2$	38
HCO_3^-	36

Her electrolytes are:

Sodium	136
Potassium	3.7
Chlorine	85

1. Based on the above information, what is your interpretation of her current ABGs compared to her initial ABG?
   (A) respiratory alkalosis with a compensating metabolic acidosis and the presence of an increased anion gap
   (B) primary uncompensated metabolic alkalosis
   (C) respiratory acidosis, corrected with mechanical ventilation—the compensating metabolic alkalosis remains
   (D) uncompensated respiratory acidosis

2. What would be your response to the above ABGs?
   (A) reduce the ventilator rate
   (B) increase the PEEP
   (C) change the albuterol from 4 to 5 mg
   (D) add pressure support ventilation (PSV)

Questions 3 and 4 refer to the following scenario:

A 51-year-old male is in the intensive care unit with the diagnosis of acute respiratory failure (ARF), possibly secondary to sepsis. His last vital signs and laboratory data were as follows:

blood pressure	108/60
pulse	70 (normal sinus rhythm)
respiratory rate	12

temperature	38.8
pulse oximetry (SpO$_2$)	0.99
pH	7.52
PaO$_2$	109
PaCO$_2$	29
HCO$_3^-$	29

He is currently on mechanical ventilation with the following settings:

mode	assisted mandatory ventilation
VT	800
respiratory rate	10
PAP	38 cm H$_2$O
PEEP	+5 cm H$_2$O
FIO$_2$	100%

He also has an end tidal carbon dioxide (PetCO$_2$) analyzer in place. It is reading 27 mm Hg.

Based on the above information, the physician changes the VT from 800 to 750. He requests ABGs in 30 min. Thirty minutes after the ventilator change, the PetCO$_2$ is 35.

3. Are ABGs still necessary?
   (A) yes, based on the inaccuracy of the PetCO$_2$ technology
   (B) no, the PetCO$_2$ will probably accurately trend the PaCO$_2$
   (C) yes, since PetCO$_2$ does not reveal changes in blood gases
   (D) no, since the PetCO$_2$ will accurately reflect changes in the PaO$_2$ and SpO$_2$ values

4. Based on the above ABGs, what is your interpretation of this patient's condition?
   (A) uncompensated respiratory alkalosis
   (B) respiratory acidosis with a compensating metabolic alkalosis
   (C) compensated metabolic alkalosis
   (D) uncompensated respiratory acidosis

5. The upper airway serves three of the key functions listed below. Select the one function that is NOT served by the upper airway.
   (A) humidification of air
   (B) removal of particles
   (C) warming of inspired air
   (D) participation in gas exchange

6. Which part of the trachea is relatively avascular, allowing for emergency placement of artificial airways in this area?
   (A) thyroid cartilage
   (B) cricothyroid cartilage
   (C) laryngopharynx
   (D) glottis

7. The left and right mainstem bronchi divide from the trachea at which of the following locations?
   (A) carina
   (B) sternoclavicular junction
   (C) lingula
   (D) larynx

8. Right mainstem bronchus intubations are more likely to be performed than left bronchus intubations for which of the following reasons?
   (A) The right mainstem bronchus has more ciliary clearance of mucus, facilitating passage of the endotracheal tube.
   (B) The left mainstem bronchus is located several inches lower than the right.
   (C) The left mainstem bronchus, although wider than the right, sits posterior to the right mainstem bronchus.
   (D) The right mainstem bronchus is wider and has less angulation than the left.

Questions 9 through 11 refer to the following scenario:

A 69-year-old female is admitted at 0700 with persistent right-sided chest pain that is not affected by respiration or position. She had a V/Q scan at 0900 that showed intermediate probability for a pulmonary embolism. The pain fluctuates and is now not very severe. She has crackles in her right middle lobe. Her ECG shows no signs of ischemia. She is not intubated, but is on a 35% high-humidity face mask. She has the following vital signs and ABGs:

blood pressure	94/56
pulse	108 (sinus tachycardia)
respiratory rate	26
temperature	36.7
SpO$_2$	.98
pH	7.26
PaO$_2$	98
PaCO$_2$	30
HCO$_3^-$	18
lactate	4.8

Her physician has told you he will call about 1600 (4 PM). The current time is 1100. You are to call him only if something is *SIGNIFICANTLY* abnormal with her physical or laboratory values.

9. Based on the above information, interpret the ABGs.

(A) respiratory alkalosis with a compensating metabolic acidosis

(B) metabolic acidosis with a compensating respiratory alkalosis

(C) uncompensated respiratory alkalosis

(D) uncompensated metabolic acidosis

10. Based on the above information, what is your interpretation of her oxygenation status?
(A) She shows signs of poor tissue oxygenation based on the elevated lacate, low HCO_3^- and pH.
(B) Her oxygenation is presently adequate based on the normal SpO_2 and PaO_2.
(C) Her oxygenation is inadequate based on the FIO_2 of 0.35 only generating a PaO_2 of 98.
(D) Presently her oxygenation is adequate based on the FIO_2 of 0.35 only generating a PaO_2 of 98 and an SpO_2 of 0.98.

11. What intervention should you take at this time?
(A) Do not notify the physician but increase the FIO_2 per standing orders.
(B) Notify the physician because of significantly abnormal values.
(C) Wait until the physician calls at 1600 to report because while some values are abnormal, they are not significantly abnormal.

12. What is the name of the lipoprotein secreted by alveolar type II cells that promotes alveolar expansion by increasing the surface tension of the alveoli?
(A) surfactant
(B) phagocytes
(C) alveolar epithelium
(D) pulmonary parenchyma

13. From which structure does the hypoxemic drive to breathe originate?
(A) aortic and carotid arteries
(B) pons
(C) medulla
(D) basal ganglia

14. Cheyne-Stokes breathing is characterized by which of the following respiratory patterns?
(A) rapid, shallow breathing
(B) short periods of apnea followed by respirations of increasing depth that then slow again to apnea
(C) regular, deep breathing patterns that alternate with shallow breathing patterns over a period of several minutes
(D) slow, deep breaths

Questions 15 and 16 refer to the following scenario:

After consultation with the physician, you have decided to begin weaning a 71-year-old female from mechanical ventilation. She is placed on pressure support ventilation (PSV) of 5 cm H_2O with a PEEP of +3 cm H_2O. After the weaning trial has been in progress for an hour, you obtain ABGs. The ABGs and vital signs are as listed below:

blood pressure	140/78
pulse	94 (sinus tachycardia)
respiratory rate	22
temperature	37.3
SpO2	.98
pH	7.23
PaO_2	91
$PaCO_2$	59
HCO_3^-	24

15. Based on the above information, what is your interpretation of the ABGs?
(A) respiratory acidosis with a compensating metabolic alkalosis
(B) metabolic acidosis with a compensating respiratory alkalosis
(C) uncompensated respiratory acidosis
(D) uncompensated metabolic alkalosis

16. Based on the above information, what action should you take?
(A) extubate at this time because she is doing well enough
(B) return to the ventilator since the ABGs indicate that she is failing the spontaneous breathing attempt
(C) continue the trial for another hour and then repeat the ABGs

17. In order to avoid ischemia of the trachea during endotracheal intubation, endotracheal cuff pressures should remain below venous drainage pressures. Normal pressures in the cuff should be kept in which range?
(A) 0 to 5 mm Hg
(B) 5 to 10 mm Hg
(C) 10 to 15 mm Hg
(D) 15 to 20 mm Hg

18. Normal arterial PO_2 levels (at sea level) fall within which of the following ranges?
(A) 20 to 35 mm Hg
(B) 35 to 45 mm Hg
(C) 60 to 80 mm Hg
(D) 80 to 100 mm Hg

19. Normal venous P_{O_2} levels (at sea level) fall within which of the following ranges?
    (A) 20 to 35 mm Hg
    (B) 35 to 40 mm Hg
    (C) 60 to 80 mm Hg
    (D) 80 to 100 mm Hg

20. Normal arterial hemoglobin saturation (Sa_{O_2}) fall within which of the following ranges?
    (A) 0.40 to 0.60
    (B) 0.60 to 0.80
    (C) 0.80 to 0.90
    (D) >0.95

21. Normal mixed venous hemoglobin saturation (Sv_{O_2}) fall within which of the following ranges?
    (A) 0.40 to 0.60
    (B) 0.60 to 0.75
    (C) 0.80 to 0.90
    (D) >0.95

22. When comparing finger oximetry values (Sp_{O_2}) to Sa_{O_2} levels, which of the following statements is most accurate?
    (A) Sp_{O_2} values underestimate Sa_{O_2} values.
    (B) Sp_{O_2} values overestimate Sa_{O_2} values.
    (C) Sp_{O_2} values should equal Sa_{O_2} values.
    (D) Sp_{O_2} values do not correlate with Sa_{O_2} values.

Questions 23 and 24 refer to the following scenario:

A 75-year-old male is admitted to the unit with the diagnosis of pneumonia. He is short of breath and has circumoral cyanosis. He has crackles throughout both lungs. His initial ABGs and vital signs are:

blood pressure	122/62	pH	7.25
pulse	114	Pa_{O_2}	34
respiratory rate	30	Pa_{CO_2}	53
temperature	37.4	HCO_3^-	25
Sp_{O_2}	.77		

The physician requests the following:

I. Place him on 40% oxygen via a face mask
II. start gentamicin 80 mg IV tid
III. do not give sedatives

She asks that you should inform her of any changes which indicate that his condition is worsening. After you start the oxygen, the circumoral cyanosis goes away. He states he feels about the same. His repeat ABGs and vital signs reveal:

blood pressure	116/58	pH	7.21
pulse	115	Pa_{O_2}	61

respiratory rate	30	Pa_{CO_2}	59
temperature	37.5	HCO_3^-	25
Sp_{O_2}	.91		

23. Based on the above information, what do you think of the above patient's condition?
    (A) He is getting better based on his improved Sp_{O_2} and Pa_{O_2}.
    (B) He is about the same based on his blood pressure, pulse, respiratory rate, and HCO_3^-
    (C) He is getting worse based on his pH and Pa_{CO_2}

24. What action is necessary, if any, for the above situation?
    (A) No action is necessary, since he is improved.
    (B) Call the physician based on the abnormal data.
    (C) Repeat ABGs in 1 hr but do not call the physician since his physical condition has not markedly changed.

25. Which of the following does NOT worsen dynamic compliance?
    (A) obesity
    (B) airway secretions
    (C) third-trimester pregnancy
    (D) loss of airway rigidity

26. Which of the following best describes vital capacity?
    (A) maximal inspiration followed by maximal expiration
    (B) normal inspiratory volumes
    (C) the amount of air vital to the person in 1 min
    (D) the amount of air in the lungs at rest

27. The amount of air that does NOT participate in gas exchange is referred to by which of the following terms?
    (A) minute ventilation
    (B) alveolar ventilation
    (C) dead space ventilation
    (D) bronchial ventilation

28. Alveolar ventilation is described by which of the following formulas?
    (A) dead space ventilation + tidal volume
    (B) minute volume – dead space ventilation
    (C) tidal volume + minute ventilation
    (D) respiratory rate × tidal volume

29. Which level of dead space is considered normal?
    (A) 25 to 35%
    (B) 40 to 50%

(C) 55 to 65%
(D) 70 to 80%

Questions 30 and 31 refer to the following scenario:

A 28-year-old female is admitted with acute shortness of breath. Her respiratory rate is 29, V_T 500, pulse 126, blood pressure 140/88. She has a history of asthma and is compliant with her medication regimen. Her ABGs reveal the following information:

PaO_2	71
$PaCO_2$	27
pH	7.50
HCO_3^-	24

30. Based on the preceding information, what would you estimate her dead space to be?
(A) normal
(B) probably low
(C) probably elevated
(D) cannot be estimated based on ABGS and minute ventilation.

31. What is her minute ventilation?
(A) elevated
(B) low
(C) normal
(D) cannot be estimated

32. Which of the following is the most common cause of hypoxemia?
(A) diffusion barriers
(B) hypoventilation
(C) changes in barometric pressure
(D) intrapulmonary shunts

33. Which of the following is an estimate of intra-pulmonary shunting?
(A) arterial/alveolar ratio
(B) diffusion capacity
(C) mixed venous oxygen tensions
(D) FEV_1 (forced expiratory volume in 1 sec)

34. Which of the following is the best description of FIO_2 (fraction of inspired oxygen)?
(A) the molecular weight of oxygen
(B) the percent of oxygen during inspiration
(C) the amount of oxygen (in cc) during inspiration
(D) the fraction of oxygen versus carbon dioxide during inspiration

35. Which of the following would be a normal oxygen tension (PaO_2) on exposure to 100% oxygen?

(A) 60 to 100 mm Hg
(B) 100 to 250 mm Hg
(C) 250 to 400 mm Hg
(D) 400 to 600 mm Hg

Question 36 and 37 refer to the following scenario:

A 48-year-old male is admitted with the diagnosis of noncardiogenic pulmonary edema. Analysis of his ABGs reveals the following:

PaO_2	86
$PaCO_2$	36
pH	7.37
FIO_2	50%

36. Estimate the intrapulmonary shunt from the preceding data.
(A) normal
(B) low
(C) elevated
(D) cannot be estimated if the patient is on oxygen

37. Assume that the patient is on a regular diet. Based on the preceding data, would it be safe to remove his oxygen in order to allow him to eat?
(A) no
(B) yes
(C) only if his nutritional status were depleted
(D) yes, providing he rests during the meal

38. Normal intrapulmonary shunts fall within which of the following ranges?
(A) 0 to 5%
(B) 6 to 15%
(C) 16 to 21%
(D) >21%

39. Which of the following is the most important determinant of oxygen transport?
(A) PaO_2
(B) SaO_2
(C) hemoglobin level
(D) cardiac output

40. Which of the following is an indicator of the balance between oxygen transport and consumption?
(A) PaO_2
(B) SaO_2
(C) SvO_2
(D) oxygen delivery

Questions 41 and 42 refer to the following scenario:

A 62-year-old female is admitted to the unit with respiratory failure following hip replacement surgery. She complains of shortness of breath and orthopnea. She has the following laboratory data available:

PaO_2	61
SaO_2	0.90
SvO_2	0.65
$PaCO_2$	39
pH	7.35
FIO_2	60%

41. Based on the preceding information, which condition is likely to be developing?
    (A) severe intrapulmonary shunt
    (B) severe imbalance between oxygen transport and cellular oxygen demand
    (C) increased oxygen extraction rates
    (D) hypercarbic respiratory failure

42. Does the FIo2 need to be increased, based on her oxygenation status?
    (A) no, the SvO_2 indicates adequate oxygenation
    (B) yes, the PaO_2 is low and warrants further oxygen therapy
    (C) yes, the SvO_2 is low and warrants further oxygen therapy
    (D) no, since her intrapulmonary shunt is near normal

43. If the Svo2 level decreases, all of the following parameters but one should be investigated by the nurse. Which parameter does NOT warrant investigation?
    (A) oxygen content (CaO_2)
    (B) SMA-6 (electrolytes)
    (C) cardiac output
    (D) oxygen consumption

44. Which of the following corresponds most closely to the normal oxygen transport level?
    (A) 250 to 550 cc/min
    (B) 600 to 1000 cc/min
    (C) 1200 to 1600 cc/min
    (D) 1600 to 2000 cc/min

45. Which of the following exerts the primary chemical control over breathing?
    (A) oxygen tension
    (B) carbonic acid level
    (C) carbon dioxide level
    (D) bicarbonate level

46. Which of the following corresponds most closely to the normal minute ventilation (V_E)?
    (A) 1 to 4 L/min
    (B) 5 to 10 L/min
    (C) 11 to 15 L/min
    (D) >15 L/min

47. The oxyhemoglobin dissociation curve is best described as illustrating which of the following?
    (A) the ability of oxygen to dissociate into different ions
    (B) the amount of oxygen carried in the blood per minute
    (C) the amount of oxygen carried in the dissolved state
    (D) the ability of hemoglobin to bind with oxygen

48. An acid is best described as which of the following?
    (A) a substance that gives up a hydrogen ion
    (B) a substance that accepts a hydrogen ion
    (C) an entity preventing oxygen from taking the electron split from hydrogen
    (D) a substance that depletes free floating hydrogen from the blood

49. The pulmonary response to a change in hydrogen ion concentration occurs in which time frame?
    (A) within 24 hr
    (B) within 48 hr
    (C) within 1 week
    (D) within 5 min

50. The renal response to a change in hydrogen ion concentration occurs in which time frame?
    (A) within 24 hr
    (B) within 48 hr
    (C) within 1 week
    (D) within 5 min

51. Which of the following is the basis for the primary renal buffering mechanism for a change in hydrogen ion level?
    (A) bicarbonate
    (B) phosphate
    (C) protein
    (D) sulfate

Questions 52 through 57 require you to interpret a set of blood gas values:

52. What would be the correct interpretation of the following blood gas values?

pH	7.35
$PaCO_2$	72
HCO_3^-	41

(A) respiratory acidosis alone
(B) respiratory acidosis with compensating metabolic alkalosis
(C) metabolic alkalosis alone
(D) metabolic acidosis with compensating respiratory alkalosis

53. What would be the correct interpretation of the following blood gas values?

pH	7.22
$PaCO_2$	64
HCO_3^-	24

(A) respiratory acidosis alone
(B) respiratory acidosis with compensating metabolic alkalosis
(C) metabolic alkalosis alone
(D) metabolic acidosis with compensating respiratory alkalosis

54. What would be the correct interpretation of the following blood gas values?

pH	7.53
$PaCO_2$	36
HCO_3^-	35

(A) respiratory acidosis alone
(B) respiratory acidosis with compensating metabolic alkalosis
(C) metabolic alkalosis alone
(D) metabolic acidosis with compensating respiratory alkalosis

55. What would be the correct interpretation of the following blood gas values?

pH	7.55
$PaOCO_2$	21
HCO_3^-	26

(A) respiratory alkalosis alone
(B) respiratory alkalosis with compensating metabolic acidosis
(C) metabolic alkalosis alone
(D) metabolic acidosis with compensating respiratory alkalosis

56. What would be the correct interpretation of the following blood gas values?

pH	7.36
$PaCO_2$	24
HCO_3^-	14

(A) respiratory alkalosis alone
(B) respiratory alkalosis with compensating metabolic alkalosis

(C) metabolic alkalosis alone
(D) metabolic acidosis with compensating respiratory alkalosis

57. What would be the correct interpretation of the following blood gas values?

pH	7.15
$PaCO_2$	37
HCO_3^-	11

(A) respiratory acidosis alone
(B) respiratory acidosis with compensating metabolic alkalosis
(C) metabolic acidosis alone
(D) metabolic acidosis with compensating respiratory alkalosis

Questions 58 and 59 refer to the following scenario:

A 58-year-old male admitted with the diagnosis of COPD (chronic obstructive pulmonary disease) presents with shortness of breath, circumoral cyanosis, and orthopnea. He is alert and oriented, stating that these symptoms started a few days earlier. He presents with the following blood gas values:

pH	7.36
$PaCO_2$	66
PaO_2	50
HCO_3^-	37
FIO_2	room air

58. Based on the preceding information, which condition is likely to be developing?
(A) acute oxygenation failure
(B) acute ventilation failure
(C) metabolic acidosis
(D) pure respiratory acidosis

59. Which treatment would be indicated for this patient?
(A) intubation and mechanical ventilation
(B) PEEP (positive end expiratory pressure) therapy
(C) inverse ratio ventilation
(D) high-flow, low-FIO_2 oxygen therapy

60. A patient with the diagnosis of asthma is admitted to your unit. He has received initial bronchodilator therapy in the emergency room. His blood gas values at that time were as follows:

pH	7.39
$PaCO_2$	25
PaO_2	62
HCO_3^-	25
FIO_2	0.30

Which of the following sets of blood gas values would indicate a worsening of the asthmatic episode due to diminished alveolar air flow?

(A) pH 7.30, $PaCO_2$ 48, PaO_2 70, FIO_2 0.40
(B) pH 7.35, $PaCO_2$ 29, PaO_2 69, FIO_2 0.40
(C) pH 7.48, $PaCO_2$ 18, PaO_2 60, FIO_2 0.40
(D) pH 7.39, $PaCO_2$ 24, PaO_2 58, FIO_2 0.40

61. Which of the following parameters is used as an estimate of alveolar ventilation (VA)?

(A) PaO_2
(B) $PaCO_2$
(C) pH
(D) alveolar–arterial oxygen gradient

62. At which pH is an acidosis generally treated?

(A) <7.25
(B) 7.25 to 7.35
(C) 7.35 to 7.45
(D) any pH >7.45

63. Which of the following is NOT a cause of acute respiratory failure?

(A) CNS (central nervous system) injury
(B) right-ventricular failure
(C) excessive use of narcotics
(D) left-ventricular failure

64. You are assisting another nurse with moving a patient up in bed when the low-pressure alarm on the ventilator goes off. It also indicates a low tidal volume is present. The patient is becoming short of breath and his SpO_2 has dropped from 0.95 to 0.84. The endotracheal tube appears to be in place and no obvious disconnection from the ventilator is present. The other nurse goes to call respiratory therapy. What should you do?

(A) increase the tidal volume on the ventilator while instructing the patient to remain calm
(B) increase the FIO_2 on the ventilator while instructing the patient to remain calm
(C) remove the ventilator and begin manual respiration (Ambu bag)
(D) increase the ventilator respiratory rate and peak flow

65. A 34-year-old female is in the unit with acute respiratory distress secondary to sepsis following a motor vehicle accident. She currently has a chest tube in place, set at 20 cm H_2O suction. There is no bubbling in the water seal although there is bubbling in the suction control chamber. While you were at lunch, one of the unit technicians tells you they clamped the chest tube to determine if the suction level was still at 20 cm H_2O. It is still clamped when you go into the room. The patient does not complain of any symptom change. About the same time, the patient's physician comes into the room and notices the clamped tube. He becomes very upset and says to get an immediate chest roentgenogram to see if a tension pneumothorax has occurred. What should you do?

(A) unclamp the tube and get the chest film as soon as possible
(B) excuse yourself while you find the technician
(C) explain that there is no need for the chest film since the water seal chamber was not bubbling
(D) explain that there is no need for the chest film since the patient has no symptom change

66. How is the PCWP (pulmonary capillary wedge pressure) used in the differentation of ARDS (adult respiratory distress syndrome) from cardiogenic-induced pulmonary edema?

(A) A low PCWP with large intrapulmonary shunts suggests ARDS.
(B) The PCWP rises in both ARDS and pulmonary edema but the PCWP in ARDS is usually over 30 mm Hg.
(C) The PCWP is low in ARDS but the CVP (central venous pressure) is elevated.
(D) The PCWP equals the CVP in ARDS but not pulmonary edema.

Questions 67 and 68 refer to the following scenario:

A 64-year-old female is admitted to your unit two days after CABG (coronary artery bypass graft) surgery. Symptoms include severe shortness of breath, which has developed over the past 2 hr; its cause is unknown. A chest roentgenogram shows marked amounts of fluid in both lungs. Blood gas and pulmonary artery catheter information is as follows:

PULMONARY ARTERY CATHETER

blood pressure	98/64
pulse	114
pulmonary arterial pressure	44/23
PCWP	12
CVP	3
cardiac output	5.4
cardiac index	2.9

BLOOD GASES

pH	7.35
$PaCO_2$	35
PaO_2	73
FIO_2	70%

67. Based on the preceding data, which condition is likely to be developing?
    (A) congestive heart failure (CHF)-induced pulmonary edema
    (B) sepsis from pulmonary infection
    (C) hypovolemia-induced left heart failure
    (D) adult respiratory distress syndrome (ARDS)

68. Which treatment is most likely indicated to support the preceding condition?
    (A) oxygen and PEEP (positive end expiratory pressure) therapy and fluid administration
    (B) oxygen and PEEP therapy and fluid restriction
    (C) mechanical ventilation and dobutamine
    (D) intubation, bicarbonate administration, and dopamine

69. Mortality with adult respiratory distress syndrome (ARDS) can be high, as much as 50%. What is the usual cause of death?
    (A) hypoxemia from the ARDS-induced intrapulmonary shunt
    (B) left ventricular failure induced by the ARDS
    (C) hypotension induced by the pulmonary capillary leak syndrome
    (D) the precipitating event that initiated the ARDS

Questions 70 and 71 refer to the following scenario:

A 74-year-old, 70-kg male is admitted to your unit with a diagnosis of respiratory failure secondary to pneumonia. He is currently intubated and on assisted mandatory ventilation (AMV), with a V_T of 750 cc, ventilator respiratory rate of 10, total rate of 29. His blood gas values are as follows:

pH	7.48
$PaCO_2$	30
PaO_2	64
FIO_2	80%

70. Based on the preceding information, which type of respiratory failure exists?
    (A) oxygenation failure
    (B) ventilation failure
    (C) combined oxygenation and ventilation failure
    (D) neither oxygenation nor ventilation failure

71. Which treatment would be indicated based on the blood gas values given?

    (A) increase the ventilator V_T
    (B) decrease the ventilator rate
    (C) add PEEP (positive end expiratory pressure) therapy to reduce the FIO_2
    (D) reduce the FIO_2 while increasing the ventilator peak flow rate

72. Which system gives more stable FIO_2 therapy?
    (A) simple face mask
    (B) nasal cannula
    (C) rebreathing mask
    (D) Venturi mask

73. At which level of FIO_2 support is oxygen toxicity thought to develop?
    (A) 30 to 40% for longer than 48 hr
    (B) 40 to 50% for longer than 2 hr
    (C) >50% for longer than 24 hr
    (D) FIO_2 does not cause oxygen toxicity; high PaO_2 values are the cause of toxicity.

74. Which of the following is an indication for PEEP (positive end expiratory pressure) therapy?
    (A) to improve carbon dioxide elimination
    (B) to treat a metabolic acidosis
    (C) to reduce postoperative bleeding
    (D) to allow reduction in FIO_2 levels

75. When PEEP (positive end expiratory pressure) or CPAP (continuous positive airway pressure) is used, which of the following values is monitored by the nurse to assess the effectiveness of therapy?
    (A) mean arterial pressure
    (B) right atrial pressure
    (C) $PaCO_2$ levels
    (D) SaO_2 values

76. During a code, the physician is attempting to intubate the patient but is uncertain if the endotracheal tube is in the lungs. Breath sounds are present but difficult to hear. What should you do to help the physician?
    (A) Call for a stat chest film and keep bagging the patient.
    (B) Attach a carbon dioxide monitor to confirm tube placement.
    (C) Call for someone for anesthesia to come intubate.
    (D) Suggest he pull the tube and start over.

Questions 77 and 78 refer to the following scenario:

A 38-year-old female is admitted with respiratory failure secondary to viral pneumonitis. She is currently on assisted mandatory ventilation (AMV) with a ventilator rate of 12, total rate of 26, V_T of 800, FIO_2 of 80%, and peak airway pressures of 38. Finger oximetry (SpO_2) values are about 0.93. She suddenly becomes restless and indicates that she is short of breath. Her SpO_2 decreases to 0.83. Breath sounds are diminished on the right with peak airway pressures of 52 cm H_2O.

77. Based on the preceding information, which condition is likely to be developing?
   (A) adult respiratory distress syndrome (ARDS)
   (B) pneumonia
   (C) pneumothorax
   (D) pericardial tamponade

78. Treatment would most likely include which of the following measures?
   (A) administration of morphine and furosemide (Lasix)
   (B) addition of 5 cm of PEEP (positive end expiratory pressure)
   (C) administration of dobutamine
   (D) insertion of a chest tube

79. Pressure support ventilation (PSV) differs from intermittent mandatory ventilation (IMV) and assisted mandatory ventilation (AMV) in which of the following ways?
   (A) PSV includes a level of PEEP (positive end expiratory pressure) with each breath.
   (B) PSV is negative pressure regulated.
   (C) IMV and AMV are volume limited, PSV pressure limited.
   (D) IMV and AMV do not reduce the work of breathing, whereas PSV reduces the work of breathing and is therefore a better weaning tool.

80. Which of the following is an indication of potential ability to breathe spontaneously when removed from the ventilator?
   (A) vital capacity of 5 cc/kg
   (B) tidal volume of 1 to 2 cc/kg
   (C) peak inspiratory pressures less than 20 cm H_2O
   (D) minute ventilation of 5 to 10 L/min

Questions 81 and 82 refer to the following scenario:

A 58-year-old, 80-kg male is recovering from acute respiratory failure. He has been on mechanical ventilation for 5 days and was previously in good health. He currently has no shortness of breath and is on an intermittent mandatory ventilation (IMV) of 12 with a total respiratory rate of 18. His FIO_2 is 0.40

with a PaO_2 of 98, a $PaCO_2$ of 36, pH of 7.42. He has the following weaning parameters:

V_T	410 cc
V_C	950 cc
PIP	−29 cm H_2O
V_E	9 L/min
respiratory rate	22

81. Based on the preceding information, which form of weaning is most likely to be implemented?
   (A) intermittent mandatory ventilation (IMV)
   (B) inverse ratio ventilation (IRV)
   (C) T-piece trial
   (D) pressure support ventilation (PSV)

Before answering question 82, read the following additional information:

After 1 hr on a T-piece trial, the following additional information is available:

V_T	450 cc
V_C	950 cc
PIP	−38 cm H_2O
V_E	8.3 L/min
respiratory rate	18
SaO_2	96%
PaO_2	85
$PaCO_2$	39
pH	7.39

82. Based on the additional information, what should be the next step in weaning this patient?
   (A) Place him back on the ventilator and repeat the attempt later.
   (B) Change to pressure support ventilation (PSV) weaning.
   (C) Extubation is indicated.
   (D) Rest one more day, then extubate.

Questions 83 through 85 refer to the following scenario:

A 63-year-old male is admitted with acute respiratory distress. Symptoms include marked shortness of breath and circumoral cyanosis. He is awake but is beginning to be less responsive. He has a history of chronic obstructive pulmonary disease (COPD). Blood gases reveal the following information:

pH	7.22
$PaCO_2$	62
PaO_2	54
SaO_2	0.81
HCO_3^-	25
FIO_2	30%

83. Based on the preceding information, which condition is likely to be developing?
    (A) congestive heart failure (CHF)
    (B) adult respiratory distress syndrome (ARDS)
    (C) acute respiratory failure (ARF)
    (D) pulmonary emboli

84. What would be the first treatment indicated at this time?
    (A) increase the FIO_2
    (B) intubate and place on mechanical ventilation
    (C) postural drainage treatment
    (D) aminophylline aerosol treatment

85. A 42-year-old male is in the unit with hepatic failure secondary to ETOH (alcohol) abuse. He is currently intubated for airway protection and requires sedation to keep him from fighting the ventilator. He has the following ventilator settings and vital signs:

mode	IMV
blood pressure	124/76
rate	12
pulse	92
V_T	750
respiratory rate	18
FIO_2	0.30
SpO_2	.97

    He is combative (or restless) at times and requires restraints. When you go into the room to check on him, he is just in the process of extubating himself. He yells "Thank God that is out." His vital signs are:

blood pressure	148/88
pulse	112
respiratory rate	22
SpO_2	.98

    You tell the secretary to call the physician. It will take 10 min for the physician to get there. What should you do in the meantime?
    (A) Attempt to reintubate with a new endotracheal tube.
    (B) Manually bag him with 100% oxygen.
    (C) Place a 40% face mask on him and observe his response.
    (D) Give a midazolam (Versed) bolus to sedate him in preparation for reintubation.

86. Which of the following is a complication of mechanical ventilation and PEEP (positive end expiratory pressure) therapy?

    (A) atelectasis
    (B) oxygen toxicity
    (C) reduced cardiac output
    (D) adult respiratory distress syndrome (ARDS)

87. What is the highest FIO_2 that can generally be achieved with a nasal cannula?
    (A) 30%
    (B) 40%
    (C) 60%
    (D) 100%

Questions 88 and 89 refer to the following scenario:

A 70-year-old male is in your unit with a diagnosis of exacerbation of chronic obstructive pulmonary disease (COPD), probably a pneumonia-induced event. He has very thick secretions, which have been difficult to remove during endotracheal suctioning.

88. Which of the following is the best method to aid in removal of thick secretions?
    (A) instillation of saline
    (B) increasing the suction pressure
    (C) stimulation of his cough reflex
    (D) increasing the humidity of his oxygen

89. Failure to remove the secretions will produce which effect on blood gases?
    (A) decrease in $PaCO_2$
    (B) decrease in PaO_2
    (C) increase in pH
    (D) increase in HCO_3^- levels

90. What is the optimal level of PEEP (positive end expiratory pressure) therapy?
    (A) the highest level of PEEP that increases cardiac output
    (B) the highest level of PEEP that stabilizes $PaCO_2$ and PaO_2
    (C) the lowest level of PEEP that improves cardiac output and SaO_2
    (D) the lowest level of PEEP that increases the PaO_2 without depressing the cardiac output

91. Which of the following conditions produces both ventilation and perfusion disturbances?
    (A) emphysema
    (B) asthma
    (C) superior vena caval syndrome
    (D) chronic bronchitis or COPD

92. Which of the following is an example of the bronchodilator category of methylxanthines?

(Answers cont'd.)

(A) terbutaline
(B) albuterol
(C) metaproterenol
(D) theophylline

93. Low PaO$_2$ levels produce at least three physiological reactions. Which of the following is NOT a consequence of low PaO$_2$ levels?
(A) pulmonary hypertension
(B) increased drive to breathe
(C) low SaO$_2$ levels
(D) left shift of the oxyhemoglobin dissociation curve

94. If the finger oximeter is reading 0.97 and the PaO$_2$ is 63, what may we infer about the oxyhemoglobin dissociation curve?
(A) A left shift in the oxyhemoglobin dissociation curve exists.
(B) A right shift in the oxyhemoglobin dissociation curve exists.
(C) The oxyhemoglobin dissociation curve is in a normal position.
(D) The oxyhemoglobin dissociation curve cannot be correlated with SaO$_2$ and PaO$_2$ values.

95. If the oxyhemoglobin dissociation curve shifts to the right, what is the clinical implication?
(A) Oxygen is more readily dissociated from hemoglobin.
(B) Hemoglobin binds oxygen more tightly.
(C) Erythropoietin stimulation will increase hemoglobin levels.
(D) Phosphate levels will be depleted.

Questions 96 and 97 refer to the following scenario:

A 70-year-old female is admitted to your unit with the diagnosis of exacerbation of COPD (chronic obstructive pulmonary disease). She is currently short of breath, is using accessory muscles to breathe, and complains of difficulty eating over the past several weeks because of her shortness of breath. Her blood pressure is 142/88, pulse rate 108. She has the following laboratory information:

pH	7.39
PaCO$_2$	32
PaO$_2$	59
FIO$_2$	room air
hemoglobin	10

96. Based on the preceding information, which condition is likely to be present?

(A) oat cell carcinoma
(B) emphysema
(C) asthma
(D) pulmonary emboli

97. Which of the following treatments would most improve her oxygen transport status?
(A) oxygen therapy
(B) blood transfusion
(C) continuous positive airway pressure (CPAP) therapy
(D) intermittent positive pressure breathing (IPPB) treatment

98. Which combination of treatments would be most effective in treating status asthmaticus?
(A) corticosteriods and bronchodilators
(B) methylxanthines and antibiotics
(C) postural drainage and bronchodilators
(D) oxygen and bronchodilators

Questions 99 through 101 refer to the following scenario:

A 24-year-old female is admitted to your unit in acute respiratory distress with the diagnosis of asthma. Lung auscultation reveals generalized wheezing. She is compliant with medications at home. She has received epinephrine and aminophylline in the emergency room with no improvement of her symptoms. Her blood gases reveal the following:

pH	7.48
PaCO$_2$	27
PaO$_2$	59
FIO$_2$	4 L/min via nasal cannula
HCO$_3^-$	23

99. Based on the preceding information, which condition is likely to be developing?
(A) pneumonia
(B) status asthmaticus
(C) pulmonary emboli
(D) adult respiratory distress syndrome (ARDS)

100. Assume the FIO$_2$ is increased to 6 L/min. Which of the following blood gas values would be an indication of a worsening status?

	(A)	(B)	(C)	(D)
pH	7.36	7.52	7.44	7.44
PaCO$_2$	40	24	27	29
PaO$_2$	70	64	72	59

101. Physical assessment by the nurse is one of the keys to evaluation of therapy. During auscultation of the patient's lungs, what should the nurse be aware of if a reduction in the degree of wheezing were to occur?
    (A) Her condition may be worsening or improving.
    (B) Reduction in wheezing always indicates improvement.
    (C) Right-ventricular failure is developing.
    (D) Pulmonary hypertension is being alleviated.

102. What is the definition of status asthmaticus?
    (A) the first episode of a newly diagnosed asthmatic
    (B) the preterminal asthmatic episode
    (C) an asthma episode that has failed to improve with conventional treatment
    (D) an asthma episode that is complicated by congestive heart failure (CHF)

103. Pulmonary emboli produce all of the following physiologic changes but one. Which of the following is NOT likely to occur with pulmonary emboli?
    (A) pulmonary hypertension
    (B) arterial hypoxemia
    (C) hypocarbia (low $PaCO_2$)
    (D) congestive heart failure

104. Which of the following tests is most diagnostic for pulmonary emboli?
    (A) blood gas analysis
    (B) ventilation/perfusion scans
    (C) pulmonary angiography
    (D) pulmonary function tests

105. Effects from recurrent emboli due to deep venous thrombosis can be avoided by which one of the following therapies?
    (A) use of a Greenfield (inferior vena caval) filter
    (B) heparin
    (C) coumadin
    (D) use of lower-extremity alternating compression devices

Questions 106 and 107 refer to the following scenario:

A 34-year-old female is admitted to your unit 3 weeks following caesarean delivery with acute shortness of breath and right chest pain. She has no prior cardiopulmonary medical history. She has the following blood gas values:

pH	7.46
$PaCO_2$	30
PaO_2	62
FIO_2	3 L/min

106. Based on the preceding information, which condition is likely to be developing?
    (A) adult respiratory distress syndrome (ARDS)
    (B) dissecting thoracic aneurysm
    (C) pleuritis
    (D) pulmonary emboli

107. Which treatment would most likely improve her immediate symptoms?
    (A) heparin
    (B) oxygen therapy
    (C) tissue plasminogen activator (tPA) or streptokinase
    (D) aminophylline

108. Which of the following features of pleural drainage systems indicates an active pleural leak?
    (A) bubbling in the water seal chamber
    (B) bubbling in the suction control chamber
    (C) fluctuation of water level in the water seal chamber with respiration
    (D) no fluctuation of water level in the water seal chamber with respiration

109. Which type of condition can lead to a tension pneumothorax?
    (A) closed pneumothorax
    (B) open pneumothorax
    (C) subcutaneous emphysema
    (D) pneumomediastinum

110. Which type of rib fracture has the highest complication rate?
    (A) first rib
    (B) third rib
    (C) fifth rib
    (D) seventh rib

Questions 111 and 112 refer to the following scenario:

A 42-year-old female is admitted to your unit following a motor vehicle accident. She has injuries to the sternum and neck. Roentgenograms in the emergency room reveal no obvious injuries. After 1 hr in the unit, she complains of sudden, severe shortness of breath. She is extremely anxious. On examination, you notice that she has developed subcutaneous emphysema across her chest. Her breath sounds are equal but markedly diminished. The trachea is midline.

111. Based on the preceding information, which condition is likely to be developing?
    (A) tension pneumothorax
    (B) tracheal laceration
    (C) closed pneumothorax
    (D) pneumomediastinum

112. Which treatment is indicated for this condition?
    (A) immediate surgery
    (B) chest tube insertion
    (C) pericardiocentesis
    (D) thoracocentesis

113. Which of the following findings would be an indication of a ruptured diaphram?
    (A) diminished bowel sounds
    (B) tracheal shift toward the affected diaphragm
    (C) irregular breathing
    (D) bowel sounds in the chest

Questions 114 and 115 refer to the following scenario:

A 26-year-old male is admitted to your unit from the emergency room with chest injuries following a motor vehicle accident. He complains of chest pain and shortness of breath. The right side of his chest (between the fourth and seventh intercostal spaces) moves in on inspiration and out on expiration. A chest film shows fractured ribs of the third through eighth intercostal spaces.

114. Based on the preceding information, which condition is likely to be developing?
    (A) tension pneumothorax
    (B) hemopneumothorax
    (C) pericardial tamponade
    (D) flail chest

115. Which treatment would be best advised for this patient?
    (A) open thoracotomy
    (B) positive pressure ventilation
    (C) external rib fixation with sandbags
    (D) supportive therapy, such as oxygen therapy and pain relief

Questions 116 to 118 refer to the following scenario:

A 41-year-old female is admitted to your unit following a fall from the roof of her single-story house, having landed on her left chest. She complains of left chest pain which increases in intensity with deep inspirations. An admission chest roentgenogram is unremarkable. She is coughing small amounts of blood-tinged sputum. Her trachea is mid-line. Her ECG and heart tones are normal. Blood pressure is 140/80, pulse 120, respiratory rate 28. SaO_2 is 92% on room air.

116. Based on the preceding information, which condition would need to be ruled out?
    (A) cardiac rupture
    (B) cardiac tamponade
    (C) pulmonary contusion
    (D) Pneumomediastinum

Four hours after admission the patient appears agitated and complains of increasing shortness of breath. Her pulse rate is now 140 and her respiratory rate is 38. The pulse oximeter displays a reading of 85% on room air.

117. What further treatment would be indicated based on this scenario?
    (A) repeat chest film and supplemental oxygen
    (B) insertion of a left chest tube
    (C) pericardiocentesis
    (D) emergent intubation

118. Which of the following would best support the diagnosis of pulmonary contusion?
    (A) a deteriorating PaO_2 value
    (B) 12-lead ECG
    (C) distant heart tones and hyperventilation

Questions 119 and 120 refer to the following scenario:

A 23-year-old female is admitted to your unit from the emergency room following a motor vehicle accident. She has no apparent injuries, although a chest film indicated a fourth-rib fracture on the left and a fifth-rib fracture on the right. Shortly after arrival in the unit, she develops marked shortness of breath and manifests a rightward deviation of the trachea and diminished breath sounds on the left. Her blood pressure is 94/62, pulse 120, respiratory rate 32.

119. Based on the preceding information, what condition is likely to be developing?
    (A) open pneumothorax
    (B) tension pneumothorax
    (C) cardiac tamponade
    (D) flail chest

120. What would be the best treatment for this condition?
  (A) insertion of pleural chest tubes
  (B) insertion of mediastinal chest tubes
  (C) open thoracotomy
  (D) pericardiocentesis

121. A 38-year-old male is admitted to your unit following a fall from a bicycle. He has sustained possible fractures of the sixth through ninth ribs on the right. Which of the following could be physical signs of fractured ribs without a pneumothorax?
  I. decreased breath sounds over the area
  II. shallow breathing
  III. splinting of the affected side
  (A) I and II
  (B) I and III
  (C) II and III
  (D) I, II, and III

Pulmonary Practice Exam

1. _____
2. _____
3. _____
4. _____
5. _____
6. _____
7. _____
8. _____
9. _____
10. _____
11. _____
12. _____
13. _____
14. _____
15. _____
16. _____
17. _____
18. _____
19. _____
20. _____
21. _____
22. _____
23. _____
24. _____
25. _____
26. _____
27. _____

28. _____
29. _____
30. _____
31. _____
32. _____
33. _____
34. _____
35. _____
36. _____
37. _____
38. _____
39. _____
40. _____
41. _____
42. _____
43. _____
44. _____
45. _____
46. _____
47. _____
48. _____
49. _____
50. _____
51. _____
52. _____
53. _____
54. _____

55. _____
56. _____
57. _____
58. _____
59. _____
60. _____
61. _____
62. _____
63. _____
64. _____
65. _____
66. _____
67. _____
68. _____
69. _____
70. _____
71. _____
72. _____
73. _____
74. _____
75. _____
76. _____
77. _____
78. _____
79. _____
80. _____
81. _____

82. _____
83. _____
84. _____
85. _____
86. _____
87. _____
88. _____
89. _____
90. _____
91. _____
92. _____
93. _____
94. _____
95. _____
96. _____
97. _____
98. _____
99. _____
100. _____
101. _____
102. _____
103. _____
104. _____
105. _____
106. _____
107. _____
108. _____

109. _____

110. _____

111. _____

112. _____

113. _____

114. _____

115. _____

116. _____

117. _____

118. _____

119. _____

120. _____

121. _____

1. __C__ _p 178, 184_
2. __A__ _p 194_
3. __B__ _p 188_
4. __A__ _p 184_
5. __D__ _p 162–163_
6. __B__ _p 164_
7. __A__ _p 166_
8. __D__ _p 166_
9. __B__ _p 184_
10. __A__ _p 179_
11. __B__ _p 179_
12. __A__ _p 167_
13. __A__ _p 169_
14. __B__ _p 181_
15. __C__ _p 184_
16. __B__ _p 193_
17. __D__ _p 192_
18. __D__ _p 184_
19. __B__ _p 184_
20. __D__ _p 184_
21. __B__ _p 187_
22. __B__ _p 187_
23. __C__ _p 178_
24. __B__ _p 178_
25. __D__ _p 169, 170_
26. __A__ _p 171_
27. __C__ _p 171_

28. __B__ _p 171_
29. __A__ _p 171_
30. __A__ _p 171_
31. __A__ _p 171_
32. __D__ _p 174_
33. __A__ _p 175_
34. __B__ _p 189_
35. __D__ _p 190_
36. __C__ _p 175_
37. __A__ _p 189_
38. __A__ _p 174_
39. __D__ _p 172_
40. __C__ _p 187_
41. __A__ _p 175_
42. __A__ _p 187, 189_
43. __B__ _p 187, 188_
44. __B__ _p 173_
45. __C__ _p 168_
46. __B__ _p 171_
47. __D__ _p 173–174_
48. __A__ _p 176_
49. __D__ _p 176_
50. __B__ _p 177_
51. __A__ _p 177_
52. __B__ _p 184_
53. __A__ _p 184_
54. __C__ _p 184_

55. __A__ _p 184_
56. __D__ _p 184_
57. __C__ _p 184_
58. __A__ _p 189_
59. __D__ _p 189_
60. __A__ _p 204, 205_
61. __B__ _p 171_
62. __A__ _p 178_
63. __B__ _p 197_
64. __C__ _p 194_
65. __C__ _p 219_
66. __A__ _p 199_
67. __D__ _p 199_
68. __B__ _p 201_
69. __D__ _p 201_
70. __A__ _p 198_
71. __C__ _p 190_
72. __D__ _p 189_
73. __C__ _p 189_
74. __D__ _p 190_
75. __D__ _p 190_
76. __B__ _p 188_
77. __C__ _p 217_
78. __D__ _p 218_
79. __C__ _p 193, 199_
80. __D__ _p 195_
81. __C__ _p 195_

82. __C__ _p 195_
83. __C__ _p 198_
84. __B__ _p 198_
85. __C__ _p 195_
86. __C__ _p 191_
87. __B__ _p 190_
88. __C__ _p 191_
89. __B__ _p 174_
90. __D__ _p 190_
91. __D__ _p 198_
92. __D__ _p 205_
93. __D__ _p 174_
94. __A__ _p 174_
95. __A__ _p 174_
96. __B__ _p 198_
97. __A__ _p 189_
98. __A__ _p 205_
99. __B__ _p 203–204_
100. __A__ _p 205_
101. __A__ _p 205_
102. __C__ _p 203_
103. __D__ _p 208–209_
104. __C__ _p 208_
105. __A__ _p 209_
106. __D__ _p 208_
107. __C__ _p 209_
108. __A__ _p 219_

109. ___A___ p 217

110. ___A___ p 213

111. ___B___ p 213

112. ___A___ p 213

113. ___D___ p 216

114. ___D___ p 214

115. ___D___ p 214

116. ___C___ p 211

117. ___A___ p 212–213

118. ___A___ p 212

119. ___B___ p 217

120. ___A___ p 218

121. ___D___ p 213

III

ENDOCRINE

Karen Sudhoff Allard

20

Introduction to the Endocrine System

EDITORS' NOTE

Endocrine concepts make up about 4% (eight questions) of the CCRN test. According to the CCRN guideline from the AACN Certification Corporation, the key areas of endocrine dysfunction covered in the exam include the following: (1) diabetes insipidus; (2) inappropriate secretion of antidiuretic hormone (SIADH); (3) hyperglycemic hyperosmolar nonketotic coma (HHNK); (4) diabetic ketoacidosis; and (5) acute hypoglycemia. Considering these five areas will be covered in only eight questions on the CCRN exam, it is unlikely that detailed attention will be given to each content area.

While recent CCRN exams have not specifically addressed items which have in the past been on the exam, such as thyrotoxic crisis, myxedema coma, and acute adrenal insufficiency/pheochromocytoma, we have left in the chapters on these topics for two reasons. First, a review of these chapters may help give you insight into endocrine disturbances in general. Second, while questions on the exam may not specifically address these disorders, an understanding of the content may help answer questions which are indirectly related to these concepts.

As you review the following chapters on the endocrine system, focus on key concepts rather than minor details. Endocrine dysfunction is a difficult area for many nurses taking the CCRN exam. Do your best to acquaint yourself with the information

in these chapters while also noting patients in your units with endocrine disturbances. Relating material in this text to patients in your unit will strengthen your ability to recall key concepts in endocrinology and increase the likelihood of correctly answering most of the questions on endocrinology.

HORMONAL PURPOSE & FUNCTION OF THE ENDOCRINE SYSTEM

The primary function of the endocrine system is to regulate metabolic functioning of the body. Metabolic functioning includes chemical reactions and the rates of these reactions, growth, transportation of chemicals, secretions, and cellular metabolism.

A close interrelationship exists between the nervous system (responsible for integration of body processes) and the endocrine system (responsible for appropriate metabolic activity). Neuronal stimulation is required for some specific hormones to be secreted and/or to be secreted in adequate amounts.

The endocrine system is composed of specific glands (Fig. 20–1) which secrete their chemical substances directly into the bloodstream. The major single endocrine glands are the pituitary (also called the hypophysis) (Fig. 20–2) and the thyroid. The parathyroids are usually four glands, not two sets of paired glands. The adrenals form one pair of endocrine glands. Other glands that contain endocrine components and function in both the endocrine system and another system are the ovaries and testes (collectively termed the gonads) and the pancreas. The thymus gland has a major role in

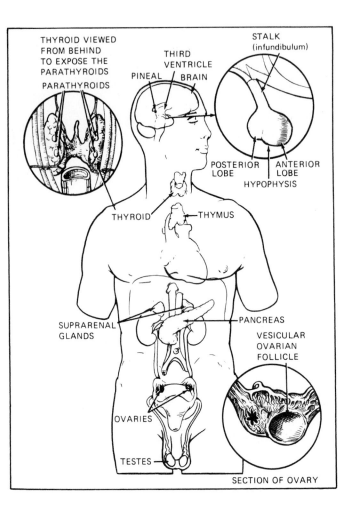

Figure 20–1. Overview of the endocrine system.

immunology but is sometimes included in discussions of the endocrine system.

All endocrine glands are very vascular. The endocrine glands function by extracting substances from the blood to synthesize into complex hormones. Hormones are released from the specific endocrine glands into the veins that drain the glands themselves. The circulatory system is used to transport endocrine substances to target glands and tissues throughout the body.

CLASSIFICATION OF HORMONES

The substances secreted by endocrine glands are chemicals called hormones. Hormones exert a physiological control on body cells. Local hormones are those released in specific areas (or tissues) and they exert a limited, local effect. Acetylcholine is an example of a local hormone having physiological control at some synapses in the nervous system. General hormones are secreted by a specific endocrine gland and transported by the vascular system to a specific, predetermined site.

Important General Hormones

All of the general hormones are important for regulatory action on functions in the body. However, dysfunctional secretion of certain hormones would rarely, if ever, be a reason for admission to a critical care unit. General hormones include oxytocin, follicle-stimulating hormone (FSH), luteinizing hormone (LH), prolactin, melanocyte-stimulating hormone (MSH), corticosterone, deoxycorticosterone, and androgens (including estrogens, progesterone, and testosterone). These hormones will not be detailed in this text.

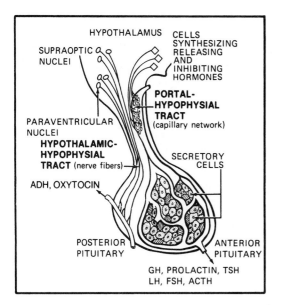

Figure 20–2. Paraventricular nucleus and supraoptic nucleus of the hypothalamus.

The general hormones which the dysfunctional secretion of may precipitate admission to a critical care area are listed in Table 20–1 and will be covered in the following three chapters.

TYPES OF HORMONES

Hormones may be amines, peptides, proteins (or protein derivatives), or steroids. Prostaglandins are often considered tissue hormones. The first three types of hormones are water soluble and do not require a carrier molecule for transportation throughout the body. Steroids and thyroxine are not water soluble and must rely on a carrier substance to transport them to their site of action, known as the target cell.

TABLE 20–1. ENDOCRINE GLANDS AND HORMONES OF SIGNIFICANT IMPORTANCE

Glands	Hormones
Adenohypophysis (anterior pituitary)	Adrenocorticotropin, somatotropin or growth hormone, thyroid-stimulating hormone
Neurohypophysis (posterior pituitary)	Antidiuretic hormone, oxytocin
Thyroid	Thyroxine, triiodothyronine, calcitonin
Parathyroid	Parathyroid hormone (parathormone)
Adrenal medulla	Epinephrine, norepinephrine
Adrenal cortex	Glucocorticoids (cortisol), mineralo-corticoids (aldosterone)
Pancreas	Insulin, glucagon

Prostaglandins are unsaturated fatty acids, of which three types have been identified on the basis of their chemical structure. They are synthesized in the seminal vesicles, brain, liver, iris, kidneys, lungs, and other areas. Prostaglandins have a potent effect but are considered local hormones, not general hormones.

EDITORS' NOTE

While the actions of hormones are important, remember that you should concentrate on general concepts rather than specific information. Terms such as amine hormone are for purposes of explanation. Do not expect to see this type of information on the CCRN exam.

ACTION OF HORMONES

Amine, Protein, and Peptide Hormones

Amine, protein, and peptide hormones include growth hormone (GH), adrenocorticotropin (ACTH), thyroid-stimulating hormone (TSH), parathyroid hormone (PTH), calcitonin, insulin, the catecholamines, glucagon, antidiuretic hormone (ADH), FSH, LH, and prolactin. Since these hormones are water soluble and do not require a carrier substance, their concentrations may fluctuate rapidly and widely. These hormones are thought to react with specific surface receptors on the target cell membrane. This alters the membrane enzymes and leads to a change in the intracellular concentration of an enzyme. The hormone is called the first messenger and the intracellular enzyme is called the second messenger. The second messengers are cyclic 3', 5' adenosine monophosphate (cAMP), cyclic guanosine monophosphate (cGMP), calcium–calmodulin complex, and prostaglandins. Cyclic AMP (within the cell) activates enzymes, causes protein synthesis, alters cell permeability, causes muscle relaxation/contraction, and causes secretion. It is by the action of cAMP that many hormones exert control over the cells.

Steroids and Thyroxine

Steroids (sex hormones, aldosterone, and cortisol) and thyroxine are non-water-soluble hormones.

These hormones are able to cross the cell membrane easily and then bind with an intracellular receptor. The hormone–receptor complex reacts with chromatin in the cell nucleus to synthesize specific proteins. Because these hormones are lipid chemicals, the reactions take longer to occur, but are no less potent than the amine, protein, and peptide hormone reactions.

THE NEGATIVE-FEEDBACK SYSTEM

Some hormones are needed in very minute amounts in the body for variable amounts of time; some have prolonged action periods; and some affect and interact with other hormones, producing a very complex, intricate system. A control system must exist to maintain this complex system.

Most control systems, including the endocrine system, act by a negative-feedback mechanism. When there is an increased hormone concentration, physiological control is increased. The stimulus for hormone production received in the hypothalamus is decreased. This results in an inhibition of hormone-releasing factors which is negative in relation to the stimulus. In the same manner, when there is deficient or absent hormone concentrations, a stimulus is received in the hypothalamus which results in an increased release of hormone-stimulating factors. This again is a negative (or opposite) response to the stimulus sent to the hypothalamus. The greater the need for the hormone, the greater the intensity of the stimulus, and similarly, the greater the concentration of the hormone, the lower the intensity of the stimulus.

When a hormone concentration is deficient, as more hormone is produced and/or secreted, the physiological control of the body cells increase. With an increase in physiological control, the feedback stimulus relayed to the endocrine gland decreases in intensity and release of the hormone decreases as homeostasis is achieved. The reverse process applies when the hormone concentration is excessive.

It is known that the hypothalamus produces releasing and inhibiting hormones (or factors) whose single target is the adenohypophysis, the so-called master gland. It is believed that all hormones have releasing and inhibiting factors produced by the hypothalamus, but only eight are known at this time (Table 20–2).

The principles of achieving regulatory control are similar with all the hormones listed in Table 20–1, with the exception of the hormones of the adrenal medulla.

The hormones of the adrenal medulla—epinephrine and norepinephrine—are under control of the autonomic nervous system. The hormones of the neurohypophysis (the posterior pituitary) are controlled by the concentration of the substance released from the target cell "feeding back" on the hypothalamus. The release of the hormone leads to a change in a plasma constituent that regulates hypothalamic activity rather than the gland itself. Tropic hormones, secreted only by the adenohypophysis (the anterior pituitary), cause an increase in size and secretion rates of other endocrine glands and are

TABLE 20–2. RELEASING AND INHIBITING FACTORS PRODUCED BY THE HYPOTHALAMUS

Releasing Hormones	Inhibiting Hormones	Peripheral Hormones
Growth hormone-releasing hormone	Growth hormone-inhibiting hormone	Growth hormone
Prolactin-releasing hormone	Prolactin-inhibiting hormone	Prolactin
Corticotropin-releasing hormone	—	Adrenal steroids
Follicle-stimulating hormone-releasing hormone	—	Gonadal steroids
Luteinizing hormone-releasing hormone	—	Gonadal hormones
Thyrotropin-releasing hormone	—	Thyroid hormones

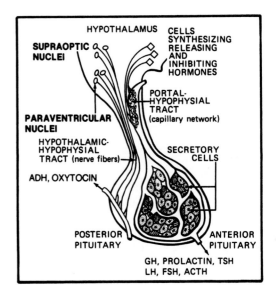

Figure 20–3. Portal-hypophysial tract and hypothalamic-hypophysial tract of the hypothalamus.

controlled by the negative-feedback system as well as other factors.

All adenohypophysial hormone-releasing and -inhibitory factors (except the adrenal medulla) are carried by the hypothalamo-hypophysial tract from the hypothalamus into the median eminence (Fig. 20–3) and then into the hypophysial stalk.

EDITORS' NOTE

Remember, basic anatomy concepts such as the pituitary stalk are usually not addressed on the CCRN exam. It may be helpful to understand basic anatomy concepts for general understanding, but do not spend too much time attempting to memorize this type of detail.

In the stalk, the hypophysial portal system carries the releasing and inhibitory factors into the adenohypophysis for storage until needed.

The two neurohypophysial hormone-releasing and -inhibiting factors are formed in the paraventricular nucleus and supraoptic nucleus in the hypothalamus (see Fig. 20–3). They are then carried by nerve fibers into the neurohypophysis for storage.

Anatomy, Physiology, and Dysfunction of the Pituitary Gland

EDITORS' NOTE

As you review the functions of the pituitary gland, do not attempt to memorize basic anatomical features. Rarely would anatomy questions, such as the type of tissue from which the pituitary arises, be on the CCRN exam. Skim these areas with the goal being to acquaint yourself with terms and concepts. Focus your attention on the key functions of the gland and how they may cause clinical disturbances.

The pituitary gland, or hypophysis, is a small gland about 1 cm in diameter and weighing about 0.5 g. It is located in the sella turcica, a depression in the sphenoid bone of the skull (Fig. 21–1), and is attached to the hypothalamus by the hypophysical stalk.

ANATOMY OF THE HYPOPHYSIS

The hypophysis has two lobes, each of which derives from a different type of tissue. The anterior lobe, or adenohypophysis, is an outgrowth of pharyngeal tissue, which grows upward toward the brain in the embryo. The posterior lobe, or neurohypophysis, is an outgrowth of the hypothalamus, which grows downward in the embryo. A mnemonic may help you to keep these terms straight: the anterior pituitary starts with the letter "a" as does adenohypophysis (adeno- = anterior). The two lobes are separated by the pars intermedia, a small, almost avascular band of fibers whose function, other than keeping the two lobes separate, is unknown (Fig. 21–2).

The hypophysis is often referred to as the body's master gland because the hormones it secretes regulate many other endocrine glands.

Structure of the Adenohypophysis

The adenohypophysis is composed of epithelial-type cells (embryologic extension of pharyngeal tissue). Many different types of epithelial cells have been identified for each hormone formed.

In the adenohypophysis are microscopic blood vessels composing the hypothalamic-hypophysial portal vessels (Fig. 21–3). These vessels connect the hypothalamus and the adenohypophysis (by passage through the pituitary stalk) and terminate in the anterior pituitary sinuses.

Substances carried in the hypothalamic-hypophysial vessels are actually hormone factors and not hormones per se. These factors are releasing and inhibiting factors (see Table 20–2). For each adenohypophysial hormone, there is an associated releasing factor. For some adenohypophysial hormones, there are inhibitory factors.

Structure of the Neurohypophysis

Many cells of the neurohypophysis are called pituicytes. Pituicytes are like the glial cells of the nervous system. The pituicytes provide supporting tissue for nerve tracts that arise from the supraoptic nuclei and paraventricular nuclei of the hypothalamus. The supraoptic nuclei and the paraventricular nuclei form the neurohypophysial hormones. These hormones are carried by the nerve tracts through the

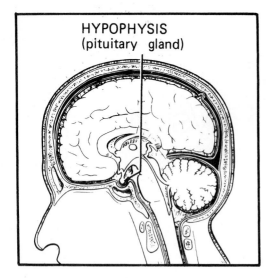

Figure 21–1. Location of the hypophysis (pituitary gland).

hypophysial stalk and terminate in bulbous knobs in the neurohypophysis. The knobs lie on the surface of capillaries. As a hormone that is formed in the hypothalamus and stored in the bulbous knobs is needed, exocytosis occurs. Exocytosis is the discharge of substances from a cell that are too large to diffuse through the cell membrane. The hormone is thus secreted from the bulbous knobs onto the capillaries and is absorbed into the vascular system. The adenohypophysis has a vascular relationship to the hypothalamus, whereas the neurohypophysis has a neural relationship.

PHYSIOLOGY

The action of the various hormones is to control the activity of the target glands and target tissues. Hormones exert an effect on target tissues by altering the rates at which cellular processes occur. There are two basic mechanisms of hormone action: cyclic 3′, 5′ adenosine monophosphate (cAMP) and genetic activation. Cyclic AMP initiates actions characteristic of the target cell. For example, parathyroid hormone cells activated by cAMP form and secrete parathyroid hormone (parathormone); specific cells in the pancreas activated by cAMP form and secrete glucagon. Known hormones affected by cAMP include secretin, glucagon, parathormone, vasopressin, catecholamines, adrenocorticotropin, follicle-stimulating hormone, thyroid-stimulating hormone, and hypothalamic releasing factors.

Hormones of the Adenohypophysis

Hormone factors, all formed in the hypothalamus, are secreted by the adenohypophysis.

1. The thyrotropin-releasing hormone (TRH): causes the release of thyroid-stimulating hormone (TSH).
2. The growth hormone-releasing hormone (GRH): causes release of the growth hormone (GH), or somatotropin (STH). The

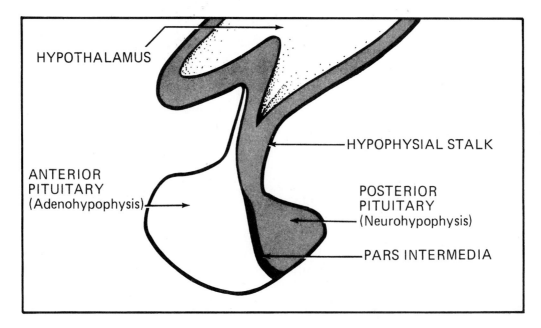

Figure 21–2. Lobes of the hypophysis.

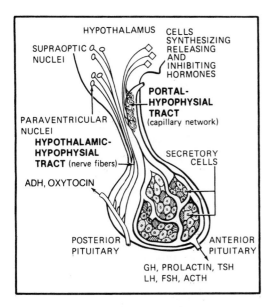

Figure 21–3. The hypothalamic-hypophysial portal vessel.

growth hormone-inhibiting hormone (GIF), or somatostatin, inhibits the release of growth hormone.

3. Corticotropin-releasing hormone (CRH): causes release of adrenocorticotropin (ACTH).
4. Gonadotropin-releasing hormone (GnRH): causes release of luteinizing hormone (LH) and follicle-stimulating hormone (FSH).
5. Prolactin-inhibiting hormone (PIH): causes inhibition of prolactin secretion.
6. Human chorionic gonadotropin (HCG).
7. Human placental lactogen (HPL).

All of the major adenohypophysial hormones have an effect upon a target gland except growth hormone.

Growth Hormone and Metabolism
Growth hormone is also called somatotropin. Somatotropin has a general effect upon bones, organs, and soft tissues; it is, therefore, considered a peripheral hormone. It influences the growth of body tissues.

Growth hormone has an important role in all aspects of metabolism. Growth hormone increases the rate of intracellular protein synthesis throughout the body. It is a factor in the mobilization of fatty acids from adipose tissue and in the conversion of these fats into energy. Growth hormone conserves carbohydrates by decreasing glucose utilization in the body.

Growth Hormone Factors
There are specific factors which stimulate or inhibit the release of growth hormone.

The most common factors inhibiting the release of GH include hyperglycemia, sustained corticosteroid therapy at high levels, and the release of growth hormone-inhibiting factor (GIF) from the hypothalamus.

Common factors promoting release of the growth hormone include pituitary tumors, hypoglycemia, exercise, decreased amino acid levels, and the release of growth hormone-releasing hormone (GRH) from the hypothalamus.

Growth hormone secretion follows a diurnal pattern, with most release occurring in the first 2 hr of deep sleep. This follows the non-REM (rapid eye movement) stage of sleep pattern.

Hormones of the Neurohypophysis

There are two hormones released by the neurohypophysis. Antidiuretic hormone (ADH), also called vasopressin, and oxytocin. Oxytocin will not be discussed in this text.

EDITORS' NOTE

One or two questions may be expected on the influence of ADH on clinical conditions.

Antidiuretic hormone (ADH) is formed mainly in the supraoptic nuclei of the hypothalamus. (The paraventricular nuclei mainly form oxytocin. The ratio of ADH to oxytocin formed in the supraoptic nuclei is 6:1, whereas the ratio is 1:6 in the paraventricular nuclei.) ADH is transported from the supraoptic nuclei by neurophysins. Neurophysins are protein carriers that bind very loosely with ADH and oxytocin to transport these hormones to the neurohypophysis for storage until needed.

Action of Antidiuretic Hormone
Antidiuretic hormone works on the distal convoluted tubules and the collecting ducts of the kidney. ADH alters the permeability of these tubules and ducts. Without ADH, the tubules and ducts are impermeable to water. In the presence of ADH, these tubules and ducts become permeable to

water, thus allowing large quantities of water to leave the tubules and collecting ducts and to re-enter the hypertonic medullary interstitial fluid. This helps to conserve and balance the fluid content of the body.

Control of Antidiuretic Hormone

Serum sodium levels and extracellular fluid osmolality exert a major influence on ADH. Osmoreceptors shrink when hypertonicity of the extracellular fluid exists. The osmoreceptors emit impulses to the hypothalamus and ADH is released from the neurohypophysis to reabsorb water from the kidneys and to re-establish homeostasis. When body fluids become diluted, stimulated osmoreceptors result in the inhibition of ADH, and water is *not* reabsorbed from the kidneys. Many factors control ADH in addition to the serum sodium and extracellular osmolality. Inadequate blood volume stimulates volume receptors in the periphery, the carotid sinus, the left atrium of the heart, and the aortic arch, stimulating release of ADH. ADH response is much greater in hemorrhagic states than in altered-osmolality states. Trauma, stress, anxiety, exercise, pain, exposure to heat, nausea, hypoxia, nicotine and dilantin enhance ADH release. ADH release is inhibited by a decreased plasma osmolality, increased intravascular volume, alcohol ingestion, and pituitary surgery.

NEUROHYPOPHYSIAL DYSFUNCTION

There are two main neurohypophysial disorders: diabetes insipidus and the syndrome of inappropriate ADH (SIADH).

Diabetes Insipidus

When there are decreased levels of ADH, diuresis and dehydration occur. Decreased levels of ADH are found when there is damage or destruction of the ADH neurons in the supraoptic and paraventricular neurons of the hypothalamus. Diabetes insipidus results.

Symptoms

Diabetes insipidus symptoms include dilute urine (until severe dehydration occurs), with a specific gravity between 1.001 and 1.005. Urinary output varies from 2 to 15 L/day regardless of fluid intake. Polyuria is often of sudden onset. Polyuria may not occur until 1–3 days postinjury due to the utilization of stored ADH in the neurohypophysis. Polydipsia will occur unless the thirst center has been damaged. There is an increased serum osmolality and a decreased urine osmolality (100–200 mOsm/kg). A relative diabetes insipidus may occur in cases of high dose, lengthy steroid therapy with a specific gravity of the urine ranging from 1.000 to 1.009, urine osmolality less than 500 mOsm, and urinary volume about 6–9 L/day. Urine output greater than 200 mL/hr for 2 hr should be reported to a physician.

Etiology

The two leading causes of diabetes insipidus are hypothalamic or pituitary tumor and closed-head injuries with damage to the supraoptic nuclei and/or hypothalamus. Postoperative diabetes insipidus is usually transient. Other causes include inflammatory and degenerative systemic conditions, but these are not common.

Treatment

The objective of therapy is first to prevent dehydration and electrolyte imbalances while determining and treating the underlying cause. A variety of replacement therapy modalities are available. Fluid support with hypotonic Dextrose in water is essential. The goal is to return the urine volume milliliter for milliliter plus any insensible loss. The patient who is unable to manage his thirst may have a decreased level of consciousness or defective hypothalamic thirst center. Obtaining the patient's weight daily to assess fluid loss is essential. Aqueous pitressin may be given as an intravenous bolus, or continuous infusion, or subcutaneously. It is a short-acting ADH therapy with vasopressor activity. Desmopressin acetate (DDAVP, 1, desamino-8-D-arginine vasopressin) is a synthetic ADH that can be used as an intravenous (central line only), subcutaneous, or nasal spray therapy. The advantage of DDAVP is a longer duration of action and negligible vasoactive properties. Following head trauma or neurosurgery, an aqueous vasopressin infusion or 5–10 units subcutaneously may be used to decrease the risk of dehydration and hypotension. If related to pituitary manipulation in surgery, diabetes insipidus may resolve in only a few days. In 50% of post-traumatic cases of diabetes insipidus, a three-phase cycle may occur. An initial diuretic phase is followed in 2–14 days by a period of antidiuresis. The oliguria is believed to be related to the release of stored vasopressin from the posterior pituitary with the resolution of the cerebral edema. The patient then demonstrates a permanent diabetes insipidus.

Nursing Interventions

Of prime importance is the accurate recording of the patient's intake and output. Monitoring body weight, electrolytes (especially potassium and sodium), urine specific gravity, osmolality, blood urea nitrogen, and for signs of dehydration and hypovolemic shock will allow for early intervention in cases prone to deterioration.

The Syndrome of Inappropriate Secretion of Antidiuretic Hormone

The syndrome of inappropriate secretion of ADH (SIADH) is the second dysfunction of ADH. In SIADH there is either increased secretion or increased production of ADH. This increase is unrelated to osmolality and causes a slight increase in total body water. Sodium (hyponatremia) and osmolar (hypoosmolality) concentration in extracellular fluid and serum is severely decreased.

Etiology

The syndrome of inappropriate secretion of ADH is occasionally caused by pituitary tumor, but is much more commonly caused by a bronchogenic (oat cell) or pancreatic carcinoma. Head injuries, other endocrine disorders (such as Addison's disease and hypopituitarism), pulmonary disease (such as pneumonia, lung abscesses, tuberculosis), central nervous system infections (and tumors), and drugs such as tricyclics, oral hypoglycemic agents, diuretics, and cytotoxic agents are all possible causes.

Symptoms and Complications

Symptoms produced by SIADH reflect the interaction between the underlying condition and excessive water retention. Symptoms are mainly neurologic, and nonspecific. The most common symptoms of SIADH are personality changes, headache, decreased mentation, lethargy, nausea, vomiting, diarrhea, anorexia, decreased tendon reflexes, seizures, and coma. Complications of SIADH include seizures, coma, and death.

Laboratory Recognition

The cardinal laboratory abnormality in SIADH consists of plasma hyponatremia (less than 130 mmol/L) and hypo-osmolality (275 mOsm/kg) occurring simultaneously with inappropriate hyperosmolality of the low-volume urine. Urine will have an osmolality of more than 900 mOsm/kg with an increase in urine sodium. Another feature that separates SIADH from other conditions that produce hyponatremia is the high urinary sodium excretion. Other laboratory findings are nonspecific. Central nervous system symptoms are more evident as the serum sodium drops below 125 mmol/L. Seizures and coma are more likely to be present in the patient with a serum sodium less than 115 mmol/L.

Treatment

The first step in treating SIADH is to restrict fluid intake to prevent water intoxication. The objective of therapy is to correct electrolyte imbalances. Daily weights are important measures of fluid gain. In severe cases, 3% hypertonic saline and intravenous furosemide (Lasix) are used. Supplemental potassium is usually necessary with follow-up frequent monitoring of serum potassium and sodium level. Demeclocycline (less than 2400 mg/day) and lithium carbonate (up to 900 mg/day) have proven useful by interfering with the normal ADH effect of increasing cAMP in the distal tubules and collecting ducts.

Nursing Interventions

With SIADH it is necessary to maintain strict fluid restrictions and to monitor the patient for electrolyte imbalances as indicated by confusion, weakness, lethargy, vomiting, and/or seizures. Fluid limitation may be set at 800–1000ml/day. The oral intake should be equal to the urine output until normalization of the serum sodium. Fluids high in sodium should be selected. If hypertonic saline is given, it should be given slowly (1–2 ml/kg/hr) and the patient monitored for congestive heart failure. All drips should be in a saline base. The nasogastric tube should be irrigated with normal saline instead of water, and enemas should be avoided. Accurate intake and output, daily weights, and laboratory monitoring of urine specific gravity and electrolyte levels are important.

Neurological status should be assessed for subtle signs of decreasing level of consciousness and seizure precautions should be taken. If the patient is comatose, turning, suctioning as needed, and standard nursing care procedures are required. Frequent oral care, mouth-rinsing without swallowing, and snacking on hard candy and chilled beverages are necessary during fluid restriction. Mouthwashes with an alcohol base and lemon and glycerine swabs should be avoided because of their drying effects. Cardiac monitoring will allow for early identification of impending hyperkalemia and its associated cardiac problems. Nutritional needs of the patient must be met without increasing fluid intake. Providing emotional support to the alert patient by stating that this condition can be treated successfully will help to obtain the patient's cooperation unless he or she has an untreated psychological problem.

Anatomy, Physiology, and Dysfunction of the Thyroid and Parathyroid Glands

EDITORS' NOTE

The most recent CCRN guidelines do not discuss the care of patients with thyroid and parathyroid disturbances as part of the CCRN exam. However, understanding of thyroid and parathyroid function is useful for understanding other clinical conditions, particularly electrolyte and cardiovascular responses. You may be able to concentrate less heavily on this chapter, however, than in the past.

ANATOMY OF THE THYROID GLAND

Location and Shape

The thyroid gland is in the anterior portion of the neck at the lower part of the larynx and the upper part of the trachea (Fig. 22–1). The thyroid has two lobes which, with a little imagination, resemble a butterfly's wings. The lobes lie on either side of the trachea and are connected by a narrow band of tissue called the isthmus, which lies anteriorly across the second and third tracheal rings.

Internal Structure

Each lobe of the thyroid is divided into lobules by dense connective tissue. Each lobule (Fig. 22–2) is composed of sac-like structures called follicles. The follicles are lined with cuboidal epithelium.

The follicular sacs are filled with a thick, viscous material called colloid. Colloid is actually thyroglobulin, which is converted to thyroxine as needed. Storage, synthesis, and release of thyroxine is controlled by the hypothalamic-releasing hormone (factor) and the thyroid-stimulating hormone of the adenohypophysis.

PHYSIOLOGY OF THE THYROID GLAND

The thyroid gland secretes three important hormones: thyroxine, triiodothyronine, and thyrocalcitonin. Approximately 90% of the hormone is thyroxine (T4) and 10% is triiodothyronine (T3). In peripheral tissues, thyroxine is converted to triiodothyronine. The functions of these two hormones are essentially the same. Thyroid hormones stimulate metabolism of all body cells and produce effective function of multiple body systems. The intensity, speed of action, and formation of these hormones differ.

Iodide Trapping (the Iodide Pump)

To form thyroid hormones, iodides must be removed from blood and extracellular fluids and transported into the thyroid gland follicles. The basal membrane of the thyroid gland has the ability to transfer iodide into the thyroid cells. The iodide then diffuses throughout the thyroid cells and follicular sacs. This process in known as iodide

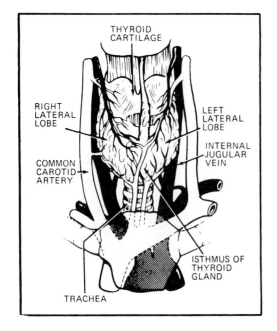

Figure 22–1. Location and shape of the thyroid gland.

trapping. The iodide is stored until thyroglobulin is needed. It then becomes ionized by the enzyme peroxidase and hydrogen peroxide, converting the iodide into iodine at the point where thyroglobulin is released intracellularly. If the peroxidase system is blocked, thyroid hormone production ceases.

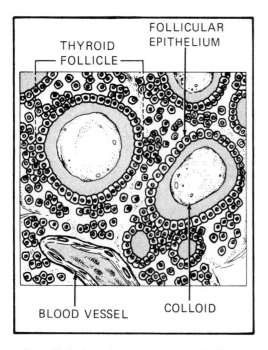

Figure 22–2. Internal structure of the thyroid follicles.

Organification of Thyroglobulin

Thyroglobulin is the major component reacting with iodide to form thyroxine. Thyroid cells synthesize the glycoprotein thyroglobulin, which is the colloid filling the follicular sacs. The binding of iodide with the glycoprotein is termed the organification of thyroglobulin. The iodide is then an oxidized iodine. The oxidized iodine slowly bonds with tyrosine (an amino acid). In the presence of enzymes, this bonding is very rapid. Chemical reactions progress to yield thyroxine and triiodothyronine. The thyroid hormones are stored in an amount that is equal to the normal body requirements for 1–3 months.

Release of Thyroxine and Triiodothyronine

These two thyroid hormones separate from the thyroglobulin molecule. Separation is a multistep process involving several intermediate chemicals. The end result is that thyroxine and triiodothyronine are lysed from the glycoprotein. Once freed, these thyroid hormones enter the venous circulatory system of the thyroid gland itself and are carried into the systemic circulation. The strongest stimulation to release these hormones is cold temperature. Thyrotropin-releasing hormone factors (TRH) will stimulate release of thyroid-stimulating hormone (TSH), and thyroxine and triiodothyronine will be released from the thyroid gland (but not as rapidly as in response to cold).

The release of these hormones is inhibited by heat, insufficient hypothalamic-releasing factors (which result in insufficient thyroid-stimulating hormones), and/or increases in plasma glucocorticoids.

Action of Thyroxine and Triiodothyronine

An interesting "rule of four" exists. Once these two hormones are in the peripheral tissues, triiodothyronine is four times as strong in initiating metabolic activities as thyroxine. Thyroxine's effect upon the tissues will last four times as long as triiodothyronine's effect. So these two hormones balance each other very well.

Thyroxine Function

Approximately 1 mg of iodine per week is needed for normal thyroxine formation. Iodides are absorbed from the gastrointestinal tract. Two-thirds of ingested iodides are excreted in the urine and the remaining one-third is used by the thyroid gland to form the glycoprotein thyroglobulin.

The major effect of the thyroid hormones is to increase all metabolic activities of the body, excluding those of the brain, spleen, lungs, retina, and testes. In children, the thyroid hormones also promote growth.

Production, Release, and Action of Calcitonin

Calcitonin is manufactured in special thyroid cells called parafollicular cells or C cells. These cells are found in the interstitial tissue between the follicles of the thyroid gland.

An increase in plasma concentration of calcium stimulates the release of calcitonin, as will the ingestion or administration of magnesium and/or glucagon.

Calcitonin functions in a relationship with parathyroid hormone more so than with the thyroid hormones. Calcitonin's major effect is on bones. Calcitonin reduces plasma calcium levels by immediate decrease in osteoclastic activity, a transient increase in osteoblastic activity, and a prolonged prevention of new osteoclast formation. Calcitonin also interacts with parathormone in the urinary excretion of calcium, magnesium, phosphates, and other electrolytes.

ANATOMY OF THE PARATHYROID GLANDS

Size and Location

The parathyroid glands are four small, flat, roundish glands located on the posterior surface of the lateral lobes of the thyroid (Fig. 22–3). Usually one parathyroid gland is located at the superior end of each thyroid lobe, and another gland is located at the inferior end of each lateral lobe of the thyroid. This location may vary considerably. It is normal to have four glands; however, there may be fewer or more than four glands.

Internal Structure

Two types of cells have been identified in the adult parathyroid gland. Chief cells (Fig. 22–4) are the

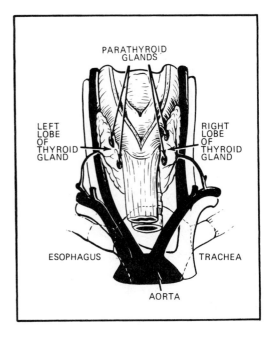

Figure 22–3. Location of the parathyroid glands (posterior view).

main cells in the adult. Oxyphil cells (Fig. 22–4) are present in adults but are frequently absent in children. The function of oxyphil cells is unknown. There is a possibility that oxyphil cells are modified chief cells.

PHYSIOLOGY OF THE PARATHYROID GLANDS

Hormone Secretion

The parathyroid glands secrete a hormone termed parathormone (PTH). If two of the glands are inadvertently removed during a subtotal thyroidectomy, the remaining glands will produce sufficient parathormone for the body's needs. Some parathyroid tissue should be preserved. This tissue will hypertrophy and continue to secrete parathormone. Chief cells in the parathyroid gland are responsible for the secretion of parathormone.

When hypothalamic releasing factors are stimulated by a decreased serum calcium level or an increased serum magnesium/phosphate concentration, a series of reactions occur, resulting in the secretion of parathormone.

Parathormone release is also inhibited by hypothalamic factors when serum calcium is increased or when there is an excessive concentration of vitamin D.

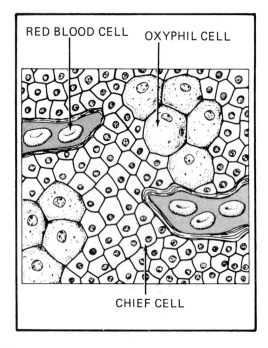

RED BLOOD CELL   OXYPHIL CELL

CHIEF CELL

Figure 22–4. Chief cells and oxyphil cells of a parathyroid gland.

Action of Parathyroid Hormone

The main action of parathormone and calcitonin is conservation of normal blood calcium levels. Parathormone decreases renal tubular reabsorption of phosphates, sodium, potassium, and amino acids. It increases reabsorption of calcium, magnesium, and hydrogen ions.

Activated vitamin D is essential for parathormone to function appropriately. The release of parathyroid hormone is controlled by a negative feedback mechanism between the blood calcium levels, the hypothalamus, and the parathyroid glands.

Target cells of the parathyroid glands include those of all bones (in a reciprocal relationship with calcium), the kidneys, and the gastrointestinal tract, if there is sufficient ingestion of vitamin D.

THYROID DYSFUNCTION

Common thyroid disorders result from too little (hypothyroidism) or too much (hyperthyroidism) secretion of the thyroid hormone. Hypothyroidism, also called myxedema, results from a lack of thyroid hormones. Myxedema coma is the result of severe deficiency or total absence of thyroid hormones. Hyperthyroidism is also called Graves' disease. The fulminant form of hyperthyroidism is called thyroid storm or thyrotoxic crisis. Storm or crisis may occur at any time.

Hypothyroidism (Myxedema)

Hypothyroidism is present when there is insufficient secretion of thyroid hormone. In hypothyroidism, the thyroid gland is usually small and consists of large amounts of fibrous tissue. Some 60% of all cases have autoantibodies present, caused by an autoimmune process.

Hypothyroidism is a chronic disease that is 10 times more common in females than in males and occurs in all age groups, but most commonly after the age of 50. Physiological signs and symptoms of hypothyroidism are the same regardless of the etiologic basis.

Etiology
Hypothyroidism can result from a thyroidectomy. A more common cause is inadequate dosage of thyroid medications in the known hypothyroid patient and post-thyroidectomy patient. Lack of compliance with the prescribed medical regimen, cessation of medication, pituitary tumors, autoimmune processes, and idiopathic factors are other causes of hypothyroidism. Myxedema coma can develop from a decompensation of a pre-existing hypothyroid state due to infection, trauma, exposure to cold, administration of sedatives, physical stress, or anesthesia.

Signs and Symptoms
A common symptom is edema of the face and a puffiness of the eyelids (Fig. 22–5). Bloating of the face produces a broad, round shape. Lips become thickened and develop a cyanotic hue. Weakness, fatigability, exertional dyspnea, sensation of cold, paresthesia of the fingers, and loss of hearing are frequent symptoms. Lethargy, lack of concentration, failing memory, and alteration in mentation occur. Skin and hair changes are often early signs of hypothyroidism. The skin becomes dry and scaly and the hair becomes friable and dry, and falls out. Total body hair may be involved. These signs increase as the condition progresses to myxedema coma.

Complications
The most serious complication of hypothyroidism is its progression to myxedema coma and death if untreated. Hypothyroidism is associated with an increased incidence of early, severe arteriosclerosis. Anemia and increased sensitivity to hypnotic and sedative drugs may become serious problems. Resistance to infection is suppressed and response to

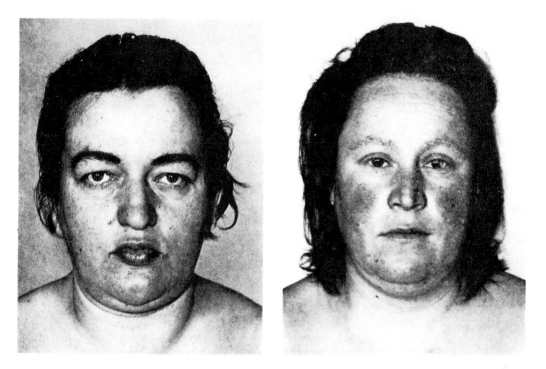

Figure 22–5. Facial appearance of two patients with myxedema.

treatment of infection is poor. Angina and myocardial infarction are especially common after starting replacement thyroid therapy. The therapy improves and increases myocardial action, but the arteriosclerosis prevents increased delivery of oxygen to the myocardium. Commonly, this results in ischemia and infarction.

Treatment

The optimum treatment for hypothyroidism is early intervention. The only possibility for prevention of complications is the early recognition of hypothyroidism and close monitoring of medical therapy for the remainder of the patient's life. This, of course, necessitates the patient's compliance with the medical regimen.

Usual thyroid hormone replacement may be accomplished with any of the following: (1) Desiccated thyroid extract (Thyroid USP) in daily doses of 60 mg PO with an increase every 15–30 days to a daily maximum of 180 mg PO. (2) Levothroxine sodium (L-thyroxine sodium; Synthroid) in doses of 0.025–0.1 mg PO daily with an increase of 0.05–0.1 mg every 1–4 weeks until stable. Maintenance dose is 0.1–0.4 mg daily PO. (3) Liothyronine sodium (T3) (Cytomel) in doses of 25 μg PO daily with an increase of 12.5–25 μg daily every 1–2 weeks until stable. The usual maintenance dose is 25–75 μg daily PO.

EDITORS' NOTE

Do not attempt to remember all these dosages. For the CCRN test, keep in basic concepts such as hypothyroidism (if addressed at all) simply requires thyroid hormone replacement.

Myxedema Coma

Myxedema coma is a life-threatening emergency that is fatal without treatment.

Clinical Presentation

Myxedema coma is characterized by hypothermia, hypoventilation, hyponatremia, hyporeflexia, hypotension, and bradycardia. The crisis is more common in winter than in summer because it occurs in response to exposure to cold. Myxedema crisis also occurs frequently following trauma, infection, and central nervous system depression.

The most frequent complication not already mentioned is seizures, which may be almost continuous as death becomes imminent.

Treatment

A multiple-systems approach must be used in treating this emergency. Mechanical ventilation is used to control hypoventilation, carbon dioxide narcosis, and respiratory arrest. Intravenous hypertonic normal saline and glucose will correct the dilutional hyponatremia and hypoglycemia. Warming blankets should be used to increase temperature gradually. Hydrocortisone (100–300 mg daily) may be used to treat a possible adrenocortical insufficiency (a commonly associated problem). Thyroid therapy is started immediately without waiting for laboratory confirmation of the diagnosis. Levothyroxine sodium (L-thyroxine sodium) is the most commonly used drug in this emergency. Intravenous doses of 0.2–0.5 mg are given during the first 24 hr. Oral doses may then be tolerated. Vasoactive drugs may be used to support blood pressure. Bradycardia may require treatment with drugs or with a temporary pacemaker.

Hyperthyroidism

Toxic goiter and thyrotoxicosis are synonyms for hyperthyroidism. Hyperthyroidism due to Graves' disease is thought to be an autoimmune process, although the terms are used interchangeably.

Etiology

In hyperthyroidism, the thyroid gland enlarges, usually to two or more times the normal size. This releases excess thyroid hormones into the body, increasing the systemic adrenergic activity. Hyperthyroidism is thought to be caused by a failure of the negative-feedback system. Some cases are due to thyroid adenomas, goiters, or familial traits.

Clinical Presentation

Exophthalmos (protruding eyeballs) is a clinical sign of hyperthyroidism or Graves' disease (Fig. 22–6). The common signs and symptoms are marked fatigue accompanied by insomnia, tachycardia, heat intolerance, emotional lability, irritability, nervousness, and weight loss (often extreme).

Diagnosis and Treatment

The diagnosis is confirmed by the finding of increased thyroxine and triiodothyronine levels and an increased Iodine-131 (^{131}I) uptake by the thyroid. Some physicians maintain that the ^{131}I test is the only reliable index, along with the patient's symptoms, to establish a diagnosis of hypo- or hyperthyroidism. Treatment may be medical or surgical. Propylthiouracil or methimazole is given orally for 6 weeks

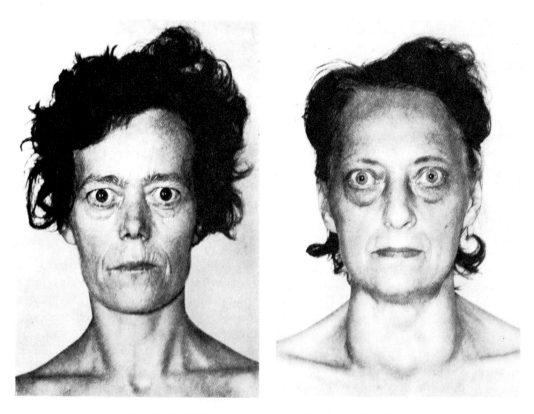

Figure 22–6. Facial appearance of two patients with hyperthyroidism.

to decrease synthesis and secretion of hormones from the thyroid. Once the patient is euthyroid, ^{131}I or a subtotal thyroidectomy may be used as definitive therapy. The patient usually requires daily thyroid medication (for life) after surgery.

Complications

Heart failure, malnutrition, and ventilatory failure (due to exhaustion) are common. A more life-threatening complication is thyroid storm.

Thyrotoxic Crisis (Thyroid Storm)

Thyrotoxic crisis is a metabolic emergency and has a greater than 20% mortality rate.

Pathophysiology

This is the same as for hyperthyroidism.

Etiology

Any factor that increases synthesis and secretion of thyroid hormones may cause a storm. Etiologic factors include subtotal thyroidectomy (due to release of thyroid hormones during the surgery), ketoacidotic states, abruptly stopping antithyroid drugs, or overdosing on thyroid medications (intentional or otherwise). Trauma, stress, and/or infection may precipitate a crisis.

Clinical Presentation

The thyroid storm syndrome characteristically includes hyperthermia (up to 106°F), hypertension with widened pulse pressure, and tachydysrhythmias (atrial fibrillation and paroxysmal atrial tachycardia). An S_3 gallop may appear with pulmonary edema. Diarrhea, dehydration, diaphoresis, and altered neurological status, including agitation, tremors, hyperkinesia, delirium, and stupor/coma, are common. Increase appetite, fatigue, proximal muscle weakness, atrophy, and amenorrhea are common. Nausea and vomiting with weight loss are common.

Treatment

Treatment of thyroid storm is of an emergency nature. Treatment is started without waiting for laboratory confirmation of the diagnosis. The *first* objective is to support vital functions, which necessitates respiratory, cardiac, and renal monitoring and lowering body temperature. Nonaspirin antipyretics are used with a cooling blanket and ice packs to assist in reducing the fever. (The core temperature should be monitored.) Second, a reversal of peripheral effects of excessive thyroid hormone is achieved by intravenous propranolol hydrochloride (Inderal) to decrease the hypermetabolic activity. Propranolol is a beta adrenergic blocker used to control tachycardias, which are often resistant to digitalis therapy. Propranolol is changed to oral doses as soon as possible since effects may last 4–8 hr. If propranolol fails, calcium ion antagonist (i.e., verapamil) may be used. If hypertension does not respond to beta adrenergic blocking drugs, reserpine and guanethidine are alternative drugs which deplete the catecholamine stores. Reserpine in doses of 0.5–1 mg IM, then 1–2.5 mg IM q4–6h helps reverse peripheral effects, provides sedation, decreases anxiety, and may help reduce the tachycardia. Maximum dose is 4 mg. When tolerated, a daily dose of 0.1–0.5 mg PO is given for maintenance.

Third, the reduction of the available and circulating thyroid hormones must be achieved. Iodine solutions may slow the release of thyroid hormones. The two most commonly used are Lugol's solution and sodium iodide. Lugol's solution is 30 drops of iodine mixed in milk or juice and given orally through a straw to prevent staining of the teeth. Slow intravenous administration of sodium iodide 1–2 g may block release of thyroid hormone. Propylthiouracil and methimazole will reduce iodide uptake and decrease synthesis of thyroid hormones.

Fourth, high doses of hydrocortisone will help support body functions in this extreme-stress situation. Doses as high as 300 mg/day may be needed.

Fifth, large amounts of vitamin B complex are required, along with glucose, protein, and carbohydrates, to provide the body with necessary nutrients for its extreme catabolic state.

Nursing Interventions

General symptomatic supportive care is appropriate. A quiet environment with limited visitors helps decrease external stress. Physiological stress is often treated with hydrocortisone daily.

Cooling blankets are useful in hyperpyrexia. Cooling to the extent of shivering and piloerection (hair on arms standing up, i.e., goose bumps) may have a rebound effect of raising the temperature even higher and increasing metabolic activity. Adjustment of room temperature is necessary; a cool room is desirable.

Fluids, electrolytes, and glucose are given to prevent dehydration and imbalances, and to provide energy to meet metabolic needs. Sodium iodine may be given by nasogastric tube or intravenously to prevent release of thyroid hormones.

Complications

If untreated, thyroid storm results in heart failure, exhaustion, coma, and death. With treatment, the sequence is frequently the same. Thyroid storm is most often seen in the summer in undiagnosed or inadequately treated hyperthyroid persons. The presence of stress, infection, nonthyroid surgery, diabetic ketoacidosis, and trauma may result in thyroid storm so intense that it is not amenable to reversal.

PARATHYROID DYSFUNCTION

Hypoparathyroidism

A major parathyroid dysfunction is hypoparathyroidism. This state is a metabolic crisis. Hypoparathyroidism is often seen with hypocalcemia.

Pathophysiology

A deficiency of the parathormone causes a hypocalcemic state, resulting in abnormal neuromuscular activity (calcium level less than 8.5 mg/dl). It is thought that this deficiency occurs secondary to a dysfunction in the calcium and phosphate concentration feedback loops' control systems.

Etiology

Acute hypocalcemia and hyperphosphatemia is usually secondary to ischemia or damage of the parathyroid gland during a thyroidectomy. Hypomagnesemia caused by malnutrition and malabsorption, increased renal secretion, and chemotherapeutic agents may also cause hypoparathyroidism. Very rarely, radiation therapy (^{131}I) of the thyroid may cause hypoparathyroidism, as can acute pancreatitis. It may also be idiopathic.

Clinical Presentation

Nausea, vomiting, and abdominal cramps are common. Dyspnea may be accompanied by a laryngeal stridor and cyanosis. Neurological signs and symptoms are prominent. There may be confusion, emotional lability, paresthesias of fingers and toes, and muscular twitching progressing to tetany and convulsions. (A decrease in the threshold for nerve and muscle excitation leads to muscle spasms, hyperreflexia, clonic-tonic convulsion, and laryngeal spasm.)

Diagnosis

Laboratory blood work will show hypocalcemia. Urine tests will reveal hypophosphaturia and perhaps hypocalcuria. Two signs are a positive Trousseau and a positive Chvostek sign, although these signs are not always present.

Treatment

The objective of treatment is to raise serum calcium levels to normal. If seizures and tetany have not developed, oral calcium supplements are indicated with additional vitamin D to promote calcium absorption. (Calcium may be given with food but not with milk since milk products will decrease calcium absorption.)

Some types of calcium chloride should only be given through a central line, as infiltration in a peripheral line will result in tissue necrosis and sloughing. Calcium cannot be infused in saline because that would cause precipitation formation with sodium bicarbonate, forcing calcium ion excretion in the kidneys.

Cardiac status must be monitored, especially if the patient is on digitalis. Digitalis and calcium have a synergistic action.

Complications

Complications include seizures, tetany, laryngeal spasm, shock, and death. A quiet environment with supportive equipment (ventilator, pacemaker) on standby may be useful in preventing potential complications.

Nursing Interventions

Preventive nursing care in hypoparathyroidism may avoid the complications of seizures and tetany. The environment should be modified to be as quiet as possible including the limiting of visitors until the patient is well stabilized.

A respirator on standby will provide for immediate intervention in the advent of hypoventilation or deteriorating respiratory status as shown by serial arterial blood gas values. Emotional and physical stress often cause hyperventilation. In turn, hyperventilation causes alkalosis, which may precipitate tetany.

Cardiac monitoring is essential since calcium therapy may alter cardiac conduction times, with resultant dysrhythmias. Standard monitoring of intake/output, response to medication therapy, neurological status, and such are applicable to these patients as the medication therapy will cause a change in the patient's electrolytes and fluid balance.

Administration of calcium as ordered, with special attention to possible infiltration and precipitation if being given intravenously, and *avoiding* milk products if being given orally will help ensure maximum benefit with minimal side effects of the drugs.

Trousseau's sign is elicited by occluding circulation to the arm. This is done by inflating a blood pressure cuff to just above the systolic pressure level. If positive, the patient's hand will develop a carpopedal spasm within 3 min. A carpopedal spasm results in a hollow palm position and fingers rigid and flexed at the metacarpophalangeal joints. Chvostek's sign is elicited by lightly tapping the facial nerve in front of the ear. If positive, there is a unilateral contraction of the facial muscles.

Anatomy, Physiology, and Dysfunction of the Pancreas

The pancreas has a dual classification. It is considered an accessory digestive gland because it produces many enzymes essential to digestion. These enzymes are released through exocrine glands (glands that release substances through ducts). The pancreas (Fig. 23–1) is also classified as an endocrine gland because it releases two hormones, insulin and glucagon, directly into the bloodstream.

ANATOMY

There are two major types of tissues found in the pancreas: the acini and the islets of Langerhans. The acini secrete digestive enzymes into the duodenum by exocrine glands. The islets of Langerhans are scattered throughout the pancreas; they may be called pancreatic islets in some texts.

The Islets of Langerhans

Three structurally and functionally different cells comprise the islets of Langerhans: alpha, beta, and delta cells (Fig. 23–2).

1. Alpha cells are located within the clusters of islet cells. Alpha cells secrete the hormone glucagon, which is often called the hyperglycemic factor. Alpha cells secrete directly into the venous system of the pancreas.
2. Beta cells are located within the clusters of islet cells and are slightly smaller than alpha cells. Beta cells secrete insulin. The insulin molecules are very complex amino acid structures.
3. Delta cells are located within the clusters of the islet cells. Delta cells secrete a recently identified hormone called somatostatin. Somatostatin has an effect upon glucagon and insulin secretion.

PHYSIOLOGY

Glucagon

The alpha cells of the islets of Langerhans secrete the hormone glucagon, which affects many body cells, especially the liver cells. Glucagon is secreted when blood amino acid levels rise and in the presence of a decreased blood glucose level.

The primary action of glucagon is as an antagonist to insulin and its primary functioning site is the liver. The most important aspect of this action is to increase blood glucose levels. Glucose metabolism is altered by two important actions of glucagon.

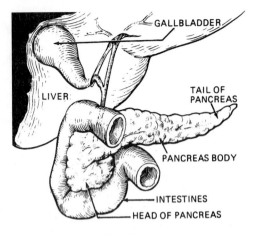

Figure 23–1. The pancreas.

Glycogenolysis (the breakdown of liver glycogen stores) and release of glucose for use in the body. Gluconeogenesis (the formation of glucose from other substances) provides new glucose for the body. There is also an increase in fatty acid oxidation and in urea formation as a natural response to glucagon.

Insulin

Insulin is a small protein of two amino acid chains. If the chains become separated, insulin loses its effectiveness. Once secreted into the circulatory system, insulin is removed by the liver and degraded. Most insulin only circulates for about 10 min before the degradation process occurs. This allows control and rapid initiation or cessation of insulin action when being administered intravenously.

The target cells for insulin action are skeletal muscle, adipose tissue, the heart and certain smooth muscle organs such as the uterus, and especially liver cells. The brain and the erythrocytes do not require insulin. Factors which facilitate secretion of insulin are an increase in blood glucose levels and the growth hormone levels. A decreased insulin level results in hyperglycemia, ketosis, and acidosis.

Insulin action includes transporting glucose across cell membranes, increasing fatty acid storage, enhancing protein synthesis, facilitating the transport of potassium, and decreasing the breakdown of triglycerides in cells.

GLUCOSE METABOLISM DYSFUNCTION

Dysfunction of glucose metabolism treated in critical care areas include diabetic ketoacidosis, hyperosmolar hyperglycemic nonketotic coma, and insulin shock.

Diabetic Ketoacidosis

The digestion of carbohydrates raises the blood glucose level, which stimulates the pancreas to secrete insulin. If insulin cannot be secreted, or secreted in sufficient amounts, hyperglycemia develops.

Pathophysiology

A lack of insulin prevents peripheral cell utilization of available blood glucose. The liver inhibits the production of glycogen, and glycogen which is available is rapidly degraded. This releases free glucose into the blood, further raising the blood sugar level.

Since the cells cannot utilize the free glucose, protein stores release amino acids, and adipose tissue releases fatty acids. The amino acids and free fatty acids are synthesized by the liver, which is

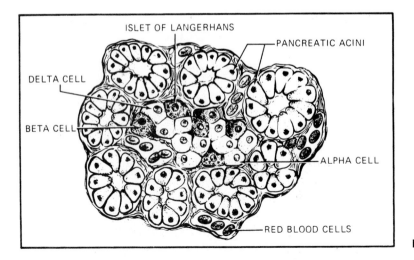

Figure 23–2. Cells of the pancreas.

producing excessive amounts of acetyl-CoA. The acetyl-CoA is rapidly degraded into keto, acetoacetic, and beta hydroxybutyric acids. These acids are produced faster than the kidneys and lungs are able to dispose of them, causing a metabolic acidosis. Ketones (keto acids or ketoanions) are excreted by the kidneys, producing a positive urine acetone test. Acetoacetic acid and beta hydroxybutyric acid are oxidized into acetone. The acetone is exhaled and is responsible for the sweet, fruity smell of the breath. (It is the acetone of the acetoacetic acid that has the odor; beta hydroxybutyric acid is odorless.)

Etiology

The most common causes of diabetic ketoacidosis (DKA) are failure to take insulin, and increased stress due to illness, trauma, surgery, cardiac conditions, and occasionally psychogenic trauma. Pregnancy and pancreatitis may also precipitate a diabetic ketoacidotic state.

Clinical Presentation

The most common symptoms are polydipsia, polyuria, polyphagia (usually with weight loss), dyspnea, and a generalized malaise. Nausea, vomiting, anorexia, and abdominal pain may be present. Signs of dehydration, tachycardia, orthostatic hypotension, and weakness are usually present. Respirations are Kussmaul in character and may have an acetone smell. Mentation ranges from lethargy to coma.

Diagnosis

Serum glucose levels are above 300 mg/dl. Serum ketones are present, as is an anion gap. DKA should be ruled out in any patient who is comatose, dehydrated, and having deep, labored respirations.

Treatment

The objectives of treatment are to correct acidemia, hyperglycemia, hypovolemia, hyperosmolality, potassium deficit, and ketonemia. Underlying conditions responsible for DKA, such as infections, must be treated concurrently.

Resolving DKA is the most effective method of restoring normal acid-base balance.

Hypovolemia is corrected by rapid infusions of 0.9% normal saline or 0.45% normal saline. Isotonic or hypotonic fluids are administered to counter the hyperosmolality which accompanies DKA. When the serum glucose level is decreased to 250 mg/dl, the fluids should be changed from saline to 5% glucose in 0.5% normal saline. This change will help avoid hypoglycemia, hypokalemia, and cerebral edema caused by the glucose diuresis. Correcting the hypovolemia usually corrects the hyperosmolality, and over a period of hours, the ketonemia. Patients may move from DKA coma to insulin shock without regaining consciousness. The addition of glucose by intravenous fluids or, if alert and oriented, feeding the patient helps prevent this.

Hyperglycemia is corrected by insulin administration. Normally, an intravenous bolus of insulin is administered followed by slow continuous intravenous infusion. Insulin may be administered by subcutaneous injections of 10–100 units/hr. Intramuscular and subcutaneous injection is not advocated in the crisis stage of DKA because of poor peripheral absorption. The serum glucose level should fall approximately 100 mg/dl every 1–2 hr. The brain does not require insulin and the blood–brain barrier prevents rapid movement of glucose out of the cerebrospinal fluid. To prevent cerebral edema, a slow decrease in the serum glucose is desired. The glucose is an osmotic particle and pulls fluid to the brain when the serum glucose is rapidly decreased.

Potassium deficits and other electrolyte imbalances may precipitate cardiac and/or neurological disturbances. Potassium is usually added to intravenous fluids as the insulin forces potassium from the plasma back into the cells, producing a hypokalemia. The serum potassium level may appear to be normal or high because of potassium shifting from the cells to the serum. Continuous monitoring and gradual changes to effect a correction over a 24-hr period are safer than massive, rapid changes. The exception to this is the patient whose life is threatened by extremes of hypo-/hyperkalemia.

Complications

Acidosis, electrolyte imbalances, acute renal failure, pulmonary edema, cerebral edema, seizures, cerebrospinal fluid acidosis, shock, and coma are the major complications of DKA.

Nursing Interventions

Maintaining a patent airway and suctioning as required to prevent aspiration are essential. Monitoring respiratory status by observation and arterial blood gases will identify impending hypoxia.

Cardiac monitoring in response to electrolyte imbalances will reveal early dysrhythmias. With hypokalemia, U waves are normally present. In hyperkalemia peaked or tented T waves are present. There may be tachycardia which converts to bradycardia if the hyperkalemia increases.

Monitoring of urinary output and frequent auscultation of lung sounds to identify pulmonary edema, especially in the presence of underlying cardiac diseases, should be performed. Fingerstick glucose should be checked hourly. Once adequate urinary output is present, electrolytes are often added to the intravenous fluids to correct imbalances.

Blood sugar may be monitored hourly by bedside blood glucose monitoring to guide the administration of regular insulin. Long-acting insulin is not used in DKA crisis. Once the serum glucose reaches 250 mg/dl, the patient's intravenous fluids should be changed to 5% or 10% dextrose to prevent hypoglycemia. If the patient is able to eat, food may be given.

Potassium is checked frequently since initially it moves from the cells into the blood and much is excreted in the urine. When insulin is given, potassium shifts back into the cells. In addition to the laboratory results, the cardiac monitor will show whether the patient's serum potassium is low, normal, or high.

Neurological status is assessed hourly. Hyperglycemia does not have a deleterious effect upon brain cells, but other electrolyte imbalances and cerebral edema will affect the cells.

Controversy exists over the use of bicarbonate to correct the acidosis present in DKA. Bicarbonate given intravenously does not cross the blood–brain barrier. It causes a shift in the bicarbonate/carbonic acid ratio which releases carbon dioxide. Carbon dioxide crosses the blood–brain barrier, dissolving in the spinal fluid. This raises the carbonic acid level and increases cerebral acidosis, which may prolong diabetic coma. Bicarbonate may be considered if pH is less than 7.15.

Complications

Complications of DKA are related to treatment. Cerebral edema, hypoglycemia, hypokalemia, and hyperchloremic acidosis are the major concern during the initial treatment of DKA.

Hyperosmolar, Hyperglycemic, Nonketotic Coma

In Hyperosmolar, hyperglycemic, nonketotic (HHNK), coma, there is enough insulin being released in the body to prevent ketosis, but there is not enough insulin to prevent hyperglycemia.

Pathophysiology

Hyperglycemia increases the solutes in the extracellular fluid, causing a hyperosmolality. Cellular dehydration occurs because of the hyperosmolality, which is also the cause of diuresis. Without treatment, an osmotic gradient develops between the brain and the plasma, resulting in dehydration and central nervous system dysfunction. The end result of dehydration is a decreased glomerular filtration rate and the development of azotemia.

Typically, the HHNK coma patient is over 50 years old, becomes ill, and has general malaise. Because of this, the patient is anorexic and eats and drinks poorly, which leads to dehydration. Since the patient is not eating, the body uses protein and fat for energy to maintain body processes. Almost the same pathophysiological pattern of DKA appears in HHNK coma. The difference is that in HHNK coma, a sufficient amount of insulin is released to prevent the development of ketosis. The patient may be stuporous or comatose before being seen by a physician.

Etiology

One of the common causes of HHNK coma is undiagnosed or untreated diabetes. Frequently, a mild diabetic state exists without any problems until the diabetic is under stress. Iatrogenic causes of some cases of HHNK coma include hyperalimentation, the administration of hypertonic intravenous fluids, and the administration of steroids.

Clinical Presentation

Usually the patient is over 50 years old. The patient is lethargic or comatose. Symptoms include polyuria, polydipsia, nausea, vomiting, weight loss. Eventually, the urinary output begins to fall as fluid depletion becomes more severe. Dehydration is apparent, with dry skin and mucous membranes. Tachypnea is present. Tachycardia, hypotension, and glycosuria are present.

Diagnosis

The three most outstanding signs may well be an elevated blood sugar level (commonly over 1000 mg), plasma hyperosmolarity (greater than 350 mOsm/kg), and an extremely elevated hematocrit. Urine and plasma are both negative for acetone. The blood urea nitrogen is usually elevated and there is marked leukocytosis.

Complications

Shock, coma, acute tubular necrosis, and vascular thrombosis are common complications. Death can result with HHNK coma if treatment is not quickly initiated.

Treatment

Correcting the fluid balance is one of the first objectives of treatment. It is essential that fluids be administered in order to correct the hyperosmolality and hypovolemia. If the patient has a cardiac history, slow administration of fluid (300 ml/hr) may be performed. The hypoinsulinemia may be corrected by the use of insulin. Hyperglycemia is not known to have deleterious effects upon the brain, but hyperosmolar dehydration may cause seizures. Return of the anion gap to normal levels may be used as an indication of success in the use of insulin therapy.

If metabolic acidosis is present, it is usually corrected by the administration of sodium bicarbonate. This is controversial for the same reasons as in DKA. Any electrolyte imbalances, such as hypokalemia, should be corrected. Close and continuous monitoring is necessary to identify further changes or deterioration in the patient's electrolyte status. Cardiac monitoring and hourly neurological checks will provide clues to changing status.

Nursing Interventions

The primary nursing responsibility is the administration of intravenous fluids to correct both dehydration and hyperosmolality without putting the patient into pulmonary edema. As much as 20 L of isotonic or hypotonic (controversial) fluids are given over the first 48 hr. The nurse must monitor breath sounds hourly to determine if pulmonary edema is developing.

Cardiac monitoring is continuous to identify dysrhythmias due to electrolyte imbalances—especially hypo-/hyperkalemia. Also, one must monitor the patient to detect early signs of congestive heart failure.

Administration of insulin to correct hyperglycemia is usually accomplished by a loading intravenous dose of insulin followed by repeated doses as indicated by the blood glucose level. Continuous insulin infusion is used with caution. The nurse may monitor the patient's glucose level by blood glucose monitoring hourly.

Neurological status should be evaluated hourly to provide information on the efficacy of treatment. Skin and mouth care are important aspects of preventing infection and keeping the patient comfortable.

Hypoglycemic Reaction (Insulin Shock)

Pathophysiology

A decreased blood level of glucose is the criterion for the diagnosis hypoglycemic reaction or insulin shock. The decrease may be due to a defect in the process of forming glucose, either glyconeogenesis or glycogenolysis, or by the removal of glucose by the use of adipose, muscle, or liver tissues.

Etiology

Causes of hypoglycemia include an intolerance of fructose, galactose, or amino acids. Postgastrectomy patients may have hypoglycemia. A broad range of drugs such as alcohol, insulin, and sulfonylurea drugs may be the origin. Endocrine dysfunctions, liver disease, severe congestive heart failure, and pregnancy may cause hypoglycemia. In diabetic patients, overdoses of insulin and exercising without adjustment of insulin dosage are the common causes of insulin shock.

Clinical Presentation

The early signs and symptoms are restlessness, diaphoresis, tachycardia, and hunger. (Propranolol hydrochloride [Inderal] may hide these signs and symptoms.) If the hypoglycemia progresses to less than 50 mg/dl, the central nervous system is affected and the patient may exhibit behavior ranging from bizarre to a coma. Headache, dizziness, irritability, fatigue, poor judgment, confusion, visual changes, hunger, weakness, tremors, seizures, nausea, and personality changes are common signs and symptoms.

Diagnosis and Treatment

A glucose level of less than 45 mg/dl with blood glucose monitoring is sufficient to require infusion of 50 mg of 50% dextrose intravenously. The patient will usually respond within 1–2 min. A sample of blood should be drawn prior to giving the glucose to confirm the diagnosis by laboratory tests. If hypoglycemia is present in a *non*diabetic, additional tests must be performed to rule out endocrine disorders or tumors. If hypoglycemia is present in a known diabetic, the underlying cause of the insulin shock must be identified and corrected.

Complications

The brain obtains almost all of its energy from glucose metabolism. If the glucose level is maintained below 45–50 mg/dl, cerebral ischemia, edema, and neuronal hyperexcitability occurs. If the blood glucose level drops to 20–40 mg/dl, clonic convulsions may occur. If the blood glucose level drops below 20 mg/dl, coma develops. If not promptly reversed, the low blood glucose levels may cause irreversible brain damage, myocardial ischemia, infarction, and death.

The Somogyi Effect

When too much insulin is administered, hypoglycemia occurs. The hypoglycemia alerts the body's defense systems, which overreact. With hypoglycemia, certain anti-insulin hormones are secreted. These include epinephrine, glucagon, glucocorticoids, and growth hormones. The secretion of these hormones causes hyperglycemia. A cyclical pattern develops: hypoglycemia one day may be followed by one or more days of hyperglycemia. In some patients, the cycle is so short that periods alternate within the same day. Symptoms of hypoglycemia in a hyperglycemic patient may indicate a Somogyi effect. Blood sugar levels may reach dangerously high levels because of this rebound effect.

The Dawn Phenomenon

Early morning increases in blood glucose concentration can occur with no corresponding hypoglycemia during the night. This phenomenon is thought to be secondary to the nocturnal elevations of growth hormone.

Anatomy, Physiology, and Dysfunction of the Adrenal Glands

EDITORS' NOTE

As with thyroid disturbances, adrenal dysfunction is less likely to be addressed on the CCRN exam. If it is present, it usually appears in the context of another system. Consequently, read this chapter to introduce yourself to key concepts and to familiarize yourself with major functions of the adrenal glands.

ANATOMY

The adrenal glands are a pair of glands located on the top of each kidney (Fig. 24–1). Each of the pair of adrenal glands is identical to the other.

The adrenal gland is composed of two separate parts (Fig. 24–2): the adrenal cortex, the outer two-thirds of the gland, and the adrenal medulla, the inner one-third of the gland. A mnemonic for remembering where each part lies in the letter "M". "M" stands for the medulla and the middle.

The Adrenal Cortex

The adrenal cortex is composed of three distinct regions or zones (Fig. 24–3). The outermost zone is the zona glomerulosa. The middle zone is the zona fasciculata. The innermost zone is the zona reticularis. The zona glomerulosa functions by itself. The zona fasciculata and zona reticularis function together as a unit.

The zona glomerulosa is a thin zone located on the outer part of the cortex, directly under the capsular covering. The cells in this zone are arranged in clumps. The regulation of the hormone (aldosterone) secreted in the zona glomerulosa is completely independent of the regulatory controls over the zona fasciculata and the zona reticularis. The regulatory control of the zona glomerulosa is the release of adrenocorticotropic hormone-(ACTH) releasing factors from the hypothalamus and ACTH-stimulating factors from the adenohypophysis.

The zona fasciculata is the largest of the three zones. Its cells are arranged in straight rows. The zona reticularis is composed of an anastomosing network of cells. These two zones function together to regulate cortisol and androgen hormones and are controlled by the same regulatory mechanisms of the adenohypophysis.

The Adrenal Medulla

Cells of the adrenal medulla (Figure 24–2) develop from the same embryological source as the sympathetic neurons. The cells are also called chromaffin cells because of their histological staining characteristics. Because of their origin, the adrenal medulla cells are related functionally to the sympathetic nervous system.

PHYSIOLOGY

Functionally, the adrenal cortex and the adrenal medulla are totally different. Without adrenal cortex hormones or replacement therapy, death occurs in 3–14 days.

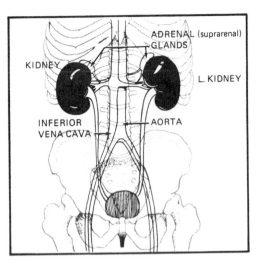

Figure 24–1. Location of the adrenal glands

Adrenal Cortex Hormones

The hormones secreted by the adrenal cortex are classified as corticosteroids since they are synthesized from the steroid cholesterol. As a group, the more than 30 corticosteroids may be referred to as corticoids.

The adrenal cortex secretes three classes of hormones: the glucocorticoids, the mineralocorticoids, and the androgenic hormones.

The Glucocorticoids

Originally, the glucocorticoids were thought to control the blood glucose level in the body. It has since been discovered that glucocorticoids play a major role in utilization of carbohydrates, proteins, and fats.

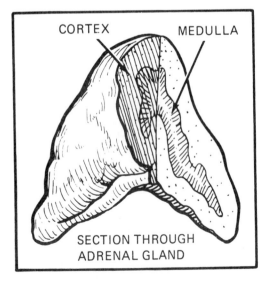

Figure 24–2. Section showing cortex and medulla of the adrenal gland.

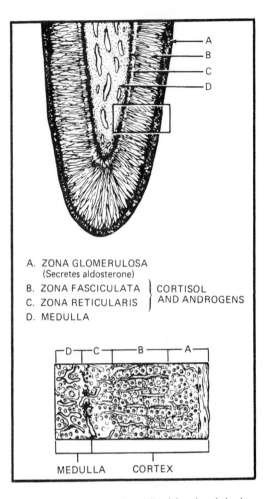

A. ZONA GLOMERULOSA
(Secretes aldosterone)
B. ZONA FASCICULATA } CORTISOL
C. ZONA RETICULARIS } AND ANDROGENS
D. MEDULLA

Figure 24–3. Zones and medulla of the adrenal gland.

Cortisol. This glucocorticoid is responsible for 95% of the adrenocortical secretory actions. Cortisol is the most important hormone of this class of steroid hormones. Cortisol affects all body cells (especially the liver). It is secreted by the zona fasciculata and the zona reticularis in response to stress (both physical and psychogenic), trauma, and infection.

Cortisol is active in all metabolic processes. These include the ability of the body to stimulate gluconeogenesis by the liver up to 10 times its normal rate. (It does this by increasing the migration of amino acids from the extracellular fluids to the liver, by increasing the migration of amino acids from muscles into the liver, and by increasing all of the enzymes needed to convert the amino acids into glucose in the liver.) Cortisol causes a moderate decrease in the rate of glucose utilization by the cells. Both the increased rate of gluconeogenesis and the moderate reduction in rate of glucose utilization by the cells cause the blood glucose concentration to rise. Cortisol decreases protein storage in all body cells except the liver, resulting in muscle weakness and decreased functions of immunity in the lymphoid tissues. The proteins stored in tissues are shifted to the liver (called mobilization of amino acids), and this shift results in decreased protein synthesis.

Cortisol promotes fatty acid mobilization weakly, but that mobilization is sufficient to provide some fat for body energy in the absence of the normal glucose.

Cortisol has a strong anti-inflammatory effect and, in sufficient amounts, may block and/or reverse the inflammatory process.

Secretion of the glucocorticoids is controlled almost entirely by ACTH secreted by the anterior pituitary gland. The hypothalamus provides the negative feedback mechanism responsible for cortisol-releasing factors (CRF) and cortisol-inhibitory factors (such as exogenous intake of corticosteroids).

The Mineralocorticoids

Mineralocorticoids are named as such since their action is chiefly with the extracellular fluid electrolytes (minerals) sodium and potassium. The most important mineralocorticoid is aldosterone, which is secreted in the zona glomerulosa.

Aldosterone. This mineralocorticoids' most important function is regulation of sodium and potassium movement through renal tubule walls. It also plays a minor part in hydrogen ion transport.

Aldosterone exerts its action on the distal convoluted tubules and the collecting ducts. There is a slight effect upon sweat glands (to conserve salt in hot conditions). The primary aldosterone action causes an increase in sodium reabsorption and potassium and hydrogen ion excretion by the kidney. Since water follows sodium, aldosterone secretion tends to change the extracellular fluid volume in proportion to its secretion.

Aldosterone excess may rapidly cause severe hypokalemia and alkalosis, including a muscle weakness, and muscle paralysis if the potassium level is reduced to half its normal value. Hypertension may occur as a result of the increase in the extracellular fluid volume.

The release of aldosterone is stimulated by an increased serum potassium level, the renin-angiotensin cascade, decreased serum sodium levels, and ACTH.

Decreased levels of aldosterone allow the extracellular level of potassium to rise to double the normal potassium level, resulting in severe hyperkalemia and cardiac toxicity as evidenced by weakness of contractions. A concurrent decrease in serum sodium and increase in water loss occurs. A potassium level only slightly higher will cause a cardiac death.

The Androgens

Several androgens are secreted by the adrenal cortex, but their alterations are not usually a primary cause for treatment in a critical care area and will not be covered in this text except to mention that they are secreted by the zona fasciculata and the zona reticularis.

Adrenal Medullary Hormones

The hormones secreted by the adrenal medulla are classified as catecholamines and have very far-reaching effects. Catecholamines are synthesized in the adrenal medulla as well as by sympathetic adrenergic nerve fiber endings, the brain, and some peripheral tissues. Both of the catecholamines secreted by the adrenal medulla have an effect on the adrenergic (sympathetic) receptor sites. There are three sites termed alpha, beta-1 (β_1), and beta-2 (β_2). Table 24–1 lists the adrenergic receptors and their functions.

Ordinarily, the norepinephrine secreted directly in a tissue by adrenergic nerve endings remains active for only a few seconds, illustrating that its reuptake and diffusion away from the tissue is rapid. However, the norepinephrine and epinephrine secreted into the blood by the adrenal medulla remain active until they diffuse into some tissue where they are destroyed by enzymes. This occurs mainly in the liver. Therefore, the effects last about 10 times as long as compared to direct sympathetic stimulation.

Epinephrine (Adrenalin)

Epinephrine (Adrenalin) accounts for 80% of the total catecholamine secreted by the adrenal medulla and excites both alpha and beta adrenergic receptor sites equally.

A major action of epinephrine is the "fear, fight, flight" body response to stress. These actions would include positive effects on the cardiac muscle, shift-

TABLE 24–1. ADRENERGIC RECEPTORS AND THEIR FUNCTIONS

Alpha Receptor	Beta Receptor
Vasoconstriction	Vasodilatation (β_2)
Iris dilatation	Cardioacceleration (β_1)
Intestinal relaxation	Increased myocardial strength (β_1)
Intestinal sphincter contraction	Intestinal relaxation (β_2)
Pilomotor contraction	Uterus relaxation (β_2)
Bladder sphincter contraction	Bronchodilatation (β_2)
	Colorigenesis (β_2)
	Glycogenolysis (β_2)
	Lipolysis (β_1)
	Bladder relaxation (β_2)

ing blood to certain muscles, decreasing gastrointestinal function, bronchiole dilatation accompanied by hyperpnea and tachypnea, and a serum glucose level increase.

Epinephrine is released by sympathetic nervous system stimulation and other hormones such as insulin and histamine.

Norepinephrine

Norepinephrine accounts for 20% of catecholamines secreted by the adrenal medulla. Norepinephrine excites mainly alpha receptors and to a slight degree beta receptors. Norepinephrine action is similar to epinephrine, with two notable exceptions. The effect of norepinephrine is not as intense as epinephrine on cardiac and metabolic functions. Also, norepinephrine has a more intense action than epinephrine on skeletal muscle vasculature. This increases peripheral vascular resistance as a result of the increased vasoconstriction.

The sites of action for norepinephrine are body cells and vascular beds, and releasing factors for norepinephrine are the same as for epinephrine.

DYSFUNCTION

Adrenal insufficiency is a major life-threatening dysfunction of the adrenal cortex. It is also known as hypoadrenalism and/or hypocorticism.

Addison's Disease

Addison's disease is a chronic dysfunction of the adrenal glands, resulting in an inadequate adrenal secretion of cortisol and aldosterone (adrenal insufficiency).

Pathophysiology

The adrenal cortex dysfunction results in a deficiency of mineralocorticoids and glucocorticoids.

Mineralocorticoid decrease results in an aldosterone deficiency. Without aldosterone, there is an increased excretion of sodium chloride and water in the urine. The depletion of sodium leads to dehydration and hypotension. At the same time, there is a retention of potassium. If the potassium concentration increases sufficiently, there is first a flaccidity of the cardiac myocardium followed by cardiac cells paralysis as the potassium level rises. Hemoconcentration, acidosis, decreased cardiac output, shock, and death due to the cardiac paralysis occurs.

A decrease in glucocorticoids results in a cortisol deficiency with normal blood glucose concentration between meals. Anorexia, nausea, vomiting, and abdominal pain result in weight loss. The neurological effects of cortisol deficiency include fatigue, lethargy, apathy, confusion, and psychoses. Cardiovascular effects include an impaired response to the vasoactive catecholamines. Energy-producing mechanisms, for example, decreased glucogenesis (causes hypoglycemia) and fat mobilization, are altered. The decreased cortisol level stimulates the hypophysis to secrete ACTH unrestrained. There is a decreased resistance to both physical and psychogenic stress.

Melanin pigmentation (Fig. 24–4) is increased in most cases of Addison's disease. The increased pigmentation is unevenly distributed and is probably due to increased secretion of melanocyte-stimulating hormone (MSH) and ACTH from the adenohypophysis.

Etiology

The most frequent cause is a primary atrophy of the adrenal cortex. This may be an autoimmune process. Often tubercular destruction of the cortex or a cancerous tumor causes Addison's disease. Stress may be a factor.

Treatment

If untreated, the patient dies within a period of a few days to a few weeks. Replacement therapy of small amounts of mineralocorticoids and glucocorticoids may prolong life for years.

Strict adherence to a diet low in potassium and high in sodium will help prevent complications. If a tumor is the etiological factor, surgery is performed.

Complications

Addisonian crisis may be fatal. A crisis may occur any time there is an increase in stress since the adrenal cortex cannot increase its production of cortisol. Steroids should be increased in patients with Addison's disease who are under stress. Even a slight cold necessitates increased steroid hormone levels. The only successful treatment of addisonian crisis is massive doses of glucocorticoids. Often as much as 10 or more times the normal dose must be used to prevent death.

Acute Adrenal Insufficiency

Adrenal crisis and addisonian crisis are synonyms for acute adrenal insufficiency and may be used interchangeably.

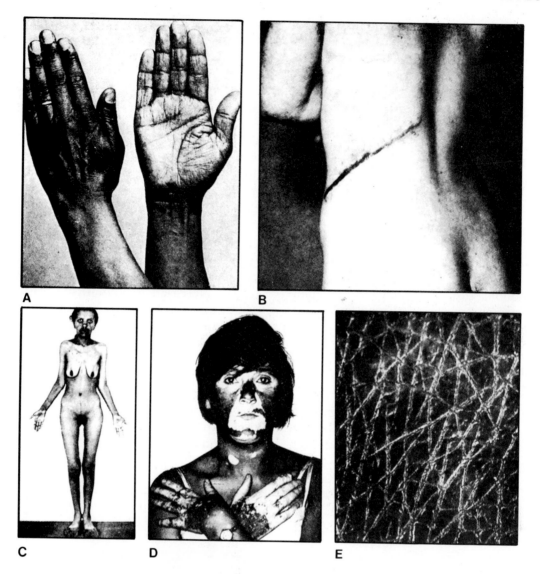

Figure 24–4. Melanin oversecretion in Addison's disease.

Etiology

Usually an underlying chronic condition (Addison's disease) is present before a crisis. In addition to this chronic disease, an infection, trauma, a surgical procedure, or some extra stress occurs and the patient develops acute adrenal insufficiency. Less common causes of acute adrenal insufficiency are adrenalectomy, Waterhouse–Friderichsen syndrome, abrupt cessation of steroid therapy, chemotherapy, and hypothalamic diseases. An autoimmune response may be a factor.

Clinical Presentation

Anorexia, nausea, vomiting, diarrhea, and abdominal pain lead to increased fluid and electrolyte disturbances. Fever may lead to alterations in consciousness. Hypotension precedes shock and coma.

Diagnosis

Patient history, physical examination, and presenting symptoms are usually sufficient to provide a tentative diagnosis and to indicate the need for immediate treatment. Definitive laboratory studies are those evaluating endocrine function and identifying resultant system dysfunction or imbalances in the electrolytes.

Complications

Death is the common complication, although it is usually preceded by dysrhythmias, hypovolemia, shock, and coma.

Treatment

Adequate circulatory volume is vital. Continuous monitoring of vital signs to identify developing dysfunction provides for early intervention. Glucocorticoids must be replaced. An intravenous glucocorticoid such as hydrocortisone should be given. Physical and psychological stress should be avoided.

Nursing Interventions

Continuous monitoring of the respiratory system with a ventilator on standby is indicated. If serial arterial blood gases show deteriorating respiratory status, the patient may be intubated and placed on the respirator. Standard nursing procedures for all artificially ventilated patients should be instituted.

Cardiac and hemodynamic monitoring will reveal early signs of impending dysrhythmias and shock, providing an opportunity for early intervention. Intake and output records will indicate renal function. Emotional support of the patient and family is of utmost importance in an attempt to decrease exogenous stress as much as possible.

Hypercorticism (Cushing's Syndrome)

Hypercorticism is a marked increase in the production of mineralocorticoids, glucocorticoids, and androgen steroids resulting in the condition known as Cushing's syndrome (not to be confused with Cushing's triad).

Etiology

Cushing's syndrome is usually due to adrenal tumors or a pituitary tumor. A pituitary tumor causes increased release of ACTH which results in hyperplasia of the adrenal cortex. An ectopic ACTH-secreting adenoma of the lungs (most common), pancreas, thyroid, or thymus and carcinoma of the gall bladder, cervix, or prostate may also cause hypercorticism.

Clinical Presentation

Increased glucocorticoids (cortisol) causes increased glucogenesis resulting in hyperglycemia. It causes increased protein tissue wasting. It also causes increased fat, resulting in the typical "moon face," and increased trunk fat or "buffalo hump" (Fig. 24–5).

The increased cortisol causes mood swings ranging from euphoria to depression. Changes in mental status, from depression, mood swings and insomnia to severe psychotic paranoia, are seen, as are short-term memory deficits and decreased attention span.

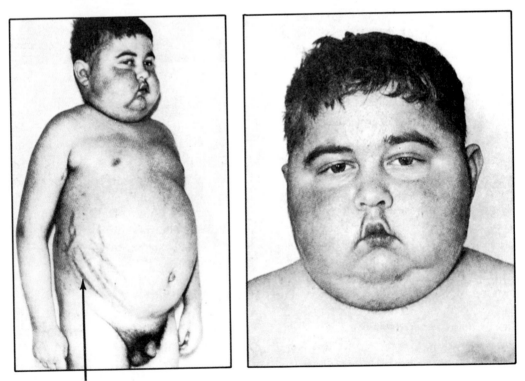

PURPLE STRIAE

Figure 24–5. Cushing's syndrome, showing "moon face," trunk fat, and purple striae.

Increased mineralocorticoids (aldosterone) results in increased potassium excretion, causing dysrhythmias, renal disorders, and muscle weakness. The increased aldosterone causes a decrease in sodium secretion. The increased sodium causes an increase in fluid retention resulting in edema and usually an increase in blood pressure and weight. (Eighty percent of patients with Cushing's syndrome have hypertension.) Increased sex hormones (androgens) cause increased facial hair and acne. Skin thins and becomes fragile and prone to injury secondary to protein wasting. Pink and purplish striae of the abdomen, under arms and on buttocks may be seen. There is easy bruising and hematoma formation.

Diagnosis
Patient history, physical examination, and presenting symptoms are usually sufficient to provide a tentative diagnosis. Definitive laboratory studies are those evaluating endocrine function and identifying resultant system dysfunction or imbalance. Hyperglycemia, acidosis, and increased cortisol levels are present.

Treatment
Treatment consists of removing the tumor, if possible, which will necessitate steroid replacement. A diet low in sodium and high in potassium is required.

Nursing Interventions
Routine postsurgical nursing care is required. In addition, the patient must be assessed for endocrine imbalance, indicating a need for replacement therapy. The patient's immune system will have been depressed because of the increased steroid levels prior to surgery, so signs of infection must be closely monitored. Education relating to diet therapy and medication regimens is essential to prevent endocrine crises in the future.

Note: The increase in mineralocorticoids may also cause Conn's syndrome (increased sodium and blood pressure and decreased potassium levels due to a benign aldosterone secreting tumor).

Hypofunction of the Adrenal Medulla

Hypofunction of the adrenal medulla does not cause systemic problems because the sympathetic nervous system will compensate for decreases in epinephrine and norepinephrine.

Hyperfunction of the Adrenal Medulla

Hyperfunction of the adrenal medulla can be life-threatening primarily because of the severe persistent or paroxysmal hypertension that leads to cerebrovascular accident and congestive heart failure. In hyperfunction, epinephrine increases blood pressure, cardiac output, pulse, and metabolism. Norepinephrine increases the blood pressure more than epinephrine does. Hyperfunction may be precipitated by stress and/or exertion, ingestion of tyrosine-containing foods, increased caffeine intake, external pressure on the tumor, and anesthesia.

Pheochromocytoma

Hyperfunction of the adrenal medulla is the most common cause of pheochromocytoma. Pheochromocytoma is an encapsulated, vascular tumor of chromaffin tissue of the adrenal medulla.

Diagnosis
Signs and symptoms are the major diagnostic clues. However, hyperfunction of the adrenal medulla often resembles other disorders which must be ruled out. These include diabetes mellitus, essential hypertension, and psychoneurosis.

Clinical Presentation
The outstanding symptom is the extremely high blood pressure (diastolic blood pressure greater than 115 mm Hg) secondary to the excessive medullary hormones. Other signs and symptoms include increased sympathetic nervous activity, sweating, headache, palpitations and dysrhythmias, postural hypotension, apprehension, nausea/vomiting, tremor, pallor or flushing of the face, abdominal and/or chest pain, and hyperglycemia.

Treatment
Treatment is surgical removal of the pheochromocytoma. A preoperative diet low in sodium and carbohydrates is usual.

Nursing Interventions
Preoperatively the nurse should promote rest and decrease patient apprehension. Postoperative routine procedures are instituted; in addition, the patient must be closely monitored for shock, hypotension (due to decreased levels of epinephrine and norepinephrine), hypoglycemia, and hemorrhage (the adrenal glands being very vascular).

ENDOCRINE BIBLIOGRAPHY

Agana-Defensor, R., & Proch, M. (1992) Pheochromocytoma: a clinical review. *AACN Clin Issues, 3*(2), 309–318.

Altkinson, A.B. (1991) The treatment of Cushing's syndrome. *Clin Endocrinol, 34*(6), 507–513.

Batcheller, J. (1992) Disorders of antidiuretic hormone secretion. *AACN Clin Issues, 3*(2), 370–378.

Batcheller, J. (1994) Syndrome of inappropriate antidiuretic hormone secretion. *Crit Care Nurs Clin North Am, 6*(4), 687–692.

Becker, K.L., ed. (1995) *Principles and Practice of Endocrinology and Metabolism,* 2nd ed. Philadelphia: J.B. Lippincott.

Bell, T.N. (1994) Diabetes insipidus. *Crit Care Nurs Clin North Am, 6*(4), 675–686.

Clark, A.P. (1994) Complications and management of diabetes: a review of current research. *Crit Care Nurs Clin North Am, 6*(4), 723–734.

Grossman, A. (1992) What is the cause of Cushing's disease? *Clin Endocrinol, 36*(5), 451–452.

Gumowski, J., Proch, M., & Kessler, C.A. (1992) Endocrinopathies of hyperfunction: Cushing's syndrome and aldosteronism. *AACN Clin Issues, 3*(2), 331–349.

Jones, T.L. (1994) From diabetic ketoacidosis to hyperglycemic hyperosmolar nonketotic syndrome: the spectrum of uncontrolled hyperglycemia in diabetes mellitus. *Crit Care Nurs Clin North Am, 6*(4), 703–722.

Jordan, R.M. (1995) Myxedema coma: Pathophysiology, therapy and factors affecting prognosis. *Med Clin North Am, 79*(1), 185–194.

Kitabchi, A.E., & Wall, B.M. (1995) Diabetic Ketoacidosis. *Med Clin North Am, 79*(1), 9–37.

Lorber, D. (1995) Nonketotic hypertonicity in diabetes mellitus. *Med Clin North Am, 9*(1), 39–51.

Lee, L.M., & Gumowski, J. (1992) Adrenocortical insufficiency: A medical emergency. *AACN Clin Issues, 3*(2), 319–331.

Mulcahy, K. (1992) Hypoglycemic emergencies. *AACN Clin Issues, 3*(2), 361–369.

Orth, D. N. (1995) Cushing's syndrome. *New Engl J Med, 332*(12), 791–803.

Sauve, D.O., & Kessler, C.A. (1992) Hyperglycemic emergencies. *AACN Clin Issues, 3*(2), 350–360.

Service, F.J. (1995) Hypoglycemia. *Med Clin North Am, 79*(1), 1–8.

Spittle, L. (1992) Diagnosis in opposition: thyroid storm and myxedema coma. *AACN Clin Issues, 3*(2), 300–308.

Tietgens, S.T., & Leinung, M.C. (1995) Thyroid storm. *Med Clin North Am, 79*(1), 169–184.

Toto, K.H. (1994) Endocrine physiology: a comprehensive review. *Crit Care Nurs Clin North Am, 6*(4), 637–660.

Toto, K.H. (1994) Regulation of plasma osmolality: thirst and vasopressin. *Crit Care Nurs Clin North Am, 6*(4), 661–674.

Werbel, S.S., & Ober, K. P. (1995) Pheochromocytoma: Update on diagnosis, localization and management. *Med Clin North Am, 79*(1), 131–151.

Endocrine Practice Exam

1. An increase in hormone concentration will cause which of the following?
   (A) an inhibition of hormone-releasing factors
   (B) an increase of hormone-releasing factors
   (C) increased production by the pituitary
   (D) increased production by the hypothalamus

2. The hormones of the adrenal medulla are under the control of which structure?
   (A) hypothalamus
   (B) posterior pituitary (neurohypophysis)
   (C) anterior pituitary (adenohypophysis)
   (D) autonomic nervous system

3. All of the adenohypophyseal hormones have an effect on a target gland EXCEPT:
   (A) adrenocorticotropin
   (B) growth hormone
   (C) thyroid-stimulating hormone
   (D) luteinizing hormone

4. The anterior pituitary receives stimulation from the hypothalamus through which of the following?
   (A) vascular system
   (B) sympathetic nervous system
   (C) parasympathetic nervous system
   (D) central nervous system

5. Which of the following is NOT secreted by the anterior pituitary gland:
   (A) ACTH (adrenocorticotropic hormone)
   (B) thyroid-stimulating hormone
   (C) growth hormone
   (D) ADH (antidiuretic hormone)

6. Which of the following is a factor inhibiting the release of growth hormone?
   (A) hypoglycemia
   (B) exercise
   (C) hyperglycemia
   (D) decreased amino acid levels

7. ADH (antidiuretic hormone) release is inhibited by which of the following?
   (A) increased serum osmolality
   (B) decreased serum osmolality
   (C) increased serum sodium
   (D) increased potassium level

Questions 8 and 9 refer to the following scenario.
A 25-year-old male is admitted to the intensive care unit with a diagnosis of brain stem contusion. Two days after admission, the patient is consistently thirsty. You note that the urine output is nearly 2000 ml in 8 hr with an intake of 950 ml. Blood pressure is 140/74, pulse 84, and respiratory rate 22. The following laboratory data are available:

SERUM		URINE	
Na^+	155	Na^+	14
K^+	3.7	Osmolality	312
Cl^-	114	Specific gravity	1.005
HCO_3^-	23		

8. Based on the preceding information, which condition is likely to be developing?
   (A) SIADH (syndrome of inappropriate antidiuretic hormone secretion)
   (B) adult-onset diabetes mellitus
   (C) anterior pituitary stimulation
   (D) diabetes insipidus

9. Which treatment could be expected to be given to this patient?
   (A) Desmopressin acetate (DDAVP, 1-desamino-8-D-arginine vasopressin)
   (B) D_5W in a 200 ml/hr fluid bolus
   (C) diuretics
   (D) fluid restriction

10. A patient is admitted to the intensive care unit with a diagnosis of SIADH (syndrome of inappropriate antidiuretic hormone secretion). Which laboratory data would be expected if this diagnosis is correct?

(Answers cont'd.)

(A) hyponatremia
(B) hypernatremia
(C) increased serum osmolality
(D) hyperkalemia

11. A common clinical finding of SIADH (syndrome of inappropriate antidiuretic hormone secretion) may include which symptom?
    (A) mental status changes
    (B) tachycardia
    (C) polyuria
    (D) polydipsia

12. Which of the following treatment modalities would NOT be an appropriate treatment modality for SIADH (syndrome of inappropriate antidiuretic hormone secretion)?
    (A) fluid restriction
    (B) diuretic administration
    (C) administration of normal saline
    (D) Kayexalate enemas

13. The critical care nurse should recognize that a major complication of diabetes insipidus could include:
    (A) dehydration
    (B) hyponatremia
    (C) hyperkalemia
    (D) bradycardia and hypertension

14. What is the dominant effect of ADH (antidiuretic hormone) on the kidneys?
    (A) It causes them to excrete water and sodium.
    (B) It causes them to reabsorb water and concentrate urine.
    (C) It causes them to reabsorb sodium and excrete potassium.
    (D) It causes them to reabsorb potassium and excrete sodium.

15. Which hormone(s) does the thyroid gland NOT secrete?
    (A) thyroxine
    (B) triiodothyronine
    (C) calcitonin
    (D) ADH (antidiuretic hormone)

16. The release of thyroxine is inhibited by which situation?
    (A) hyperthermia
    (B) hypothermia
    (C) hypokalemia
    (D) hypernatremia

17. Calcitonin is released by which organ?
    (A) pituitary gland
    (B) adrenal gland

(C) parathyroid gland
(D) thyroid gland

18. Which of the following is another name for hyperthyroidism?
    (A) myxedema coma
    (B) Graves' disease
    (C) hirsutism
    (D) Lugol's syndrome

Questions 19 and 20 refer to the following scenario.
A 48-year-old female is admitted to your unit with a possible syncopal episode. She is currently awake although she is nervous and anxious. Vital signs are as follows:

blood pressure	178/108
pulse	129
respiratory rate	28
temperature	39°C

During your initial examination, you note that she has exophthalmos and that her skin is warm and wet.

19. Given the preceding information, which condition could be present?
    (A) myxedema coma
    (B) parathyroid crisis
    (C) thyroid storm
    (D) aldosterone crisis

20. Which of the following would be administered in this situation?
    (A) calcitonin
    (B) propranolol (Inderal)
    (C) normal saline
    (D) parathyroid hormone

21. On which organ does calcitonin exert its major effect?
    (A) kidney
    (B) bone
    (C) parathyroid
    (D) liver

22. Parathormone release is inhibited by which serum situation?
    (A) increased calcium
    (B) decreased magnesium
    (C) increased phosphate
    (D) increased magnesium

23. Parathormone secretion is stimulated by which humoral event?
    (A) decreased calcium
    (B) increased magnesium
    (C) increased phosphate
    (D) all of the above

24. Which of the following is a symptom of hypothyroidism?
    (A) paresthesia of the fingers
    (B) sensitivity to cold
    (C) dry, scaly skin
    (D) all of the above

25. Which of the following is NOT a symptom of myxedema coma?
    (A) hypothermia
    (B) hypoventilation
    (C) hyponatremia
    (D) hyperthermia

Questions 26 and 27 refer to the following scenario.
A 51-year-old female is admitted to your unit with hypotension, bradycardia, and decreased level of consciousness. Her core temperature is 35.5°C. The temperature in her apartment was 25°C (77°F). No history is available regarding prior medical problems. She appears to be overweight, with dry, scaly skin and puffy face and lips. Blood gas analysis reveals the following information:

pH	7.25
$PaCO_2$	56
PaO_2	63

Shortly after admission, she has a grand mal seizure. She is intubated and placed on mechanical ventilation.

26. Based on the preceding information, which condition is likely to be developing?
    (A) acute CHF (congestive heart failure)
    (B) ARDS (adult respiratory distress syndrome)
    (C) thyroid crisis
    (D) myxedema coma

27. Which treatment would be required to correct the condition?
    (A) dobutamine (50 mg/kg/min)
    (B) cooling blanket
    (C) levothyroxine (0.2 mg)
    (D) calcitonin (2 mg/kg/hr)

28. Which of the following is NOT a common precipitating factor of myxedema coma?
    (A) stress
    (B) exposure to heat
    (C) infection
    (D) exposure to cold

29. Which of the following is NOT a common symptom of hyperthyroidism?
    (A) marked fatigue
    (B) cold intolerance

    (C) tachycardia
    (D) weight loss

30. Which of the following is NOT associated as a precipitating factor with thyrotoxic crisis?
    (A) diabetic ketoacidosis
    (B) trauma
    (C) increased intracranial pressure
    (D) infection

31. A deficiency of parathormone causes which clinical sign?
    (A) hypocalcemia
    (B) hypercalcemia
    (C) hyponatremia
    (D) hyperkalemia

32. Appropriate response to treatment of myxedema coma would be illustrated by which of the following changes in physiological parameters?
    (A) increase in $PaCO_2$
    (B) reduction in heart rate
    (C) increase in body temperature
    (D) decrease in pH

33. Which of the following is NOT associated with hypoparathyroidism?
    (A) Trousseau's sign
    (B) thyroidectomy
    (C) hypocalcemia
    (D) gastric ulcers

34. Which part of the endocrine system secretes aldosterone?
    (A) zona glomerulus of the adrenal cortex
    (B) zona fasciculata of the adrenal cortex
    (C) adrenal medulla
    (D) zona reticularis of the adrenal cortex

35. Which category of hormone is NOT secreted by the adrenal cortex?
    (A) glucocorticoids
    (B) mineralocorticoids
    (C) androgenic hormones
    (D) adrenergic hormones

36. Primary adrenal insufficiency is characterized by which of the following?
    (A) hyperpigmentation
    (B) hypertension
    (C) bradycardia
    (D) skeletal tremors

Questions 37 and 38 refer to the following scenario.

A 35-year-old male is admitted to your unit with hypotension and probable dehydration. He is confused and it is difficult to obtain a history regarding past medical problems. He has multiple hyperpigmented areas on his body. He complains of nausea, abdominal pain, and marked fatigue. Laboratory data reveal the following:

Na⁺	154
K⁺	5.9
Cl⁻	109
HCO₃⁻	20
glucose	46

37. Based on the preceding information, which condition is likely to be developing?
    (A) myxedema coma
    (B) adrenal insufficiency
    (C) hyperparathyroid storm
    (D) Cushing's syndrome

38. What treatment would most likely be initiated to reverse all of the above symptoms?
    (A) parathormone administration
    (B) thyronine administration
    (C) glucocorticoids administration
    (D) pituitary extract administration

39. Which of the following is another term for adrenal insufficiency?
    (A) Graves's disease
    (B) myxedema crisis
    (C) Addison's disease
    (D) Cushing's syndrome

40. Aldosterone exerts its action on the distal convoluted tubule to cause which effect?
    (A) potassium reabsorption
    (B) sodium excretion
    (C) sodium reabsorption
    (D) chloride excretion

41. Aldosterone release is stimulated by all of the following EXCEPT:
    (A) decreased potassium level
    (B) renin-angiotensin cascade
    (C) increased potassium level
    (D) decreased sodium level

42. Which of the following stimulates insulin secretion?
    (A) thyroid hormone
    (B) growth hormone
    (C) glucocorticoids
    (D) prolactin

43. Which term best describes gluconeogenesis?
    (A) utilization of oxygen stores due to deficits of serum glucose

(B) breakdown of protein
(C) formation of glucose from other substances
(D) breakdown of glycogen stores in the liver

Questions 44 and 45 refer to the following scenario.

A 67-year-old male is admitted to your unit with a decreased level of consciousness. He was brought to the hospital by the police after being found in a shopping mall "acting strange." He complains of fatigue but is generally disoriented as to time and place. His respiratory rate is deep and rapid. Vital signs and laboratory data are given below:

blood pressure	96/58
pulse	114
respiratory rate	34
glucose	760
osmolality	307
PaO₂	91
PaCO₂	20
pH	7.28
Na⁺	156
K⁺	5.0
HCO₃⁻	14

The blood pressure also decreases when the patient changes from a lying to a sitting position.

44. Based on the preceding information, which condition is likely developing?
    (A) adrenal crisis
    (B) thyroid storm
    (C) HHNK (hyperosmolar, hyperglycemic, non-ketotic) coma
    (D) DKA (diabetic ketoacidosis)

45. Which of the following would most likely be administered to this patient?
    (A) glucocorticoids
    (B) thyroxine
    (C) sodium bicarbonate
    (D) insulin and normal saline

46. Which blood gas change is usually present in DKA (diabetic ketoacidosis)?
    (A) respiratory acidosis alone
    (B) metabolic acidosis alone
    (C) respiratory alkalosis and metabolic acidosis
    (D) respiratory acidosis and metabolic alkalosis

47. Initial insulin therapy for DKA (diabetic ketoacidosis) is usually administered by which route?
    (A) intravenous bolus
    (B) intravenous bolus followed by a continuous infusion

(C) subcutaneously

(D) intramuscularly

48. Presenting signs and symptoms of DKA (diabetic ketoacidosis) could include which of the following?

(A) shallow, slow respirations

(B) decreased urine output

(C) tachycardia and orthostatic hypotension

(D) peripheral edema and dependent pulmonary crackles

49. Insulin therapy brings about which electrolyte change?

(A) increased serum potassium

(B) decreased serum sodium

(C) increased intracellular potassium

(D) decreased intracellular calcium

50. HHNK (hypersosmolar, hyperglycemic, nonketotic) coma is differentiated from DKA (diabetic ketoacidosis) by which of the following?

(A) hyperglycemia

(B) absence of ketosis

(C) serum osmolality

(D) serum potassium levels

Questions 51 and 52 refer to the following scenario.

A 57-year-old female is admitted to the unit following a seizure at home. She has no history of seizures. The family describes the patient as not feeling well for several days and as having not eaten or taken fluids normally during this time. Her vital signs and laboratory data are as follows:

blood pressure	92/54
pulse	108
respiratory rate	31
glucose	1089
osmolality	389
PaO_2	79
$PaCO_2$	30
pH	7.29
Na^+	149
K^+	3.0
HCO_3^-	20

51. Based on the preceding information, which condition is likely to be developing?

(A) adrenal crisis

(B) thyroid storm

(C) HHNK (hyperosmolar, hyperglycemic, nonketotic) coma

(D) DKA (diabetic ketoacidosis)

52. Which treatment would most likely be initially administered to this patient?

(A) glucocorticoids

(B) continuous insulin drip and isotonic volume expanders

(C) sodium bicarbonate

(D) D_{50} bolus and intermittent IM insulin

53. Hyperfunction of the adrenal medulla is referred to as which of the following?

(A) pheochromocytoma

(B) Addison's disease

(C) Graves' disease

(D) Cushing's syndrome

54. Dehydration in HHNK (hyperosmolar, hyperglycemic, nonketotic) coma is primarily due to which event?

(A) lack of ADH (antidiuretic hormone)

(B) inability of the kidney to concentrate urine

(C) nausea and vomiting

(D) osmotic diuresis from the high glucose level

55. HHNK (hyperosmolar, hyperglycemic, nonketotic) coma is partially differentiated from DKA (diabetic ketoacidosis) by which laboratory test?

(A) hyperglycemia

(B) absence of ketosis

(C) hyperkalemia

(D) serum osmolality

Questions 56 and 57 refer to the following scenario.

A 69-year-old, overweight male is in your unit following resection of a perforated bowel. He has a history of adult-onset diabetes and mild hypertension. The patient is alert and oriented with stable vital signs at the beginning of your shift. During your shift he becomes disoriented. His skin is cool and clammy, he has muscle tremors, and he complains of nausea. Serum electrolytes are drawn and the laboratory results are listed below:

Na^+	133
K^+	3.7
Cl^-	100
HCO_3^-	25
glucose	43
osmolality	282

56. Based on the preceding information, which condition is likely to be developing?

(A) hyperosmolar, hyperglycemic, nonketotic acidosis

(B) hypoglycemia

(answers cont'd.)

(C) diabetic ketoacidosis
(D) diabetes insipidus

57. Which treatment would most likely be given to this patient?
(A) insulin bolus followed by infusion
(B) glucose (dextrose) bolus (D_{50})
(C) normal saline bolus with potassium
(D) glucocorticoids

58. The clinical situation of large fluctuations in blood glucose, such as hypoglycemia symptoms in a patient with hyperglycemia, is described by which term?
(A) Somogyi effect
(B) Addison's response
(C) Adams' syndrome
(D) pancreatic flash

59. Which of the following physical signs is more indicative of hypoglycemia rather than hyperglycemia?
(A) cool skin
(B) rapid breathing

(C) warm skin
(D) tachycardia

60. At which blood glucose level does change in mentation begin?
(A) 10 to 20 mg/dl
(B) 20 to 30 mg/dl
(C) 30 to 40 mg/dl
(D) any level below 50 mg/dl

61. High serum glucose levels can directly cause which physical symptom?
(A) increased urine output
(B) decreased urine output
(C) hypotension
(D) decreased respiratory rate

62. Which of the following are symptoms of a pheochromocytoma?
(A) hypertension, tachycardia, and hyperglycemia
(B) hypertension, hypoglycemia, and bradycardia
(C) hyperglycemia, hypotension, and tachycardia
(D) hypotension, headache, and hyperglycemia

PART III

Endocrine Practice Exam

1. _____
2. _____
3. _____
4. _____
5. _____
6. _____
7. _____
8. _____
9. _____
10. _____
11. _____
12. _____
13. _____
14. _____
15. _____
16. _____

17. _____
18. _____
19. _____
20. _____
21. _____
22. _____
23. _____
24. _____
25. _____
26. _____
27. _____
28. _____
29. _____
30. _____
31. _____
32. _____

33. _____
34. _____
35. _____
36. _____
37. _____
38. _____
39. _____
40. _____
41. _____
42. _____
43. _____
44. _____
45. _____
46. _____
47. _____

48. _____
49. _____
50. _____
51. _____
52. _____
53. _____
54. _____
55. _____
56. _____
57. _____
58. _____
59. _____
60. _____
61. _____
62. _____

Answers

1.	A	p 246	17.	D	p 257	33.	D	p 258	48.	C	p 267

1.   A p 246
2.   D p 246
3.   B p 251
4.   A p 249
5.   D p 250–251
6.   C p 251
7.   B p 252
8.   D p 252
9.   A p 252
10.   A p 253
11.   A p 253
12.   D p 253
13.   A p 253
14.   B p 251–252
15.   D p 256–257
16.   A p 256

17.   D p 257
18.   B p 260
19.   C p 260–261
20.   B p 261
21.   B p 257
22.   A p257
23.   D p 257
24.   D p 258
25.   D p 259–260
26.   D p 259–260
27.   C p 260
28.   B p 259
29.   B p 260
30.   C p 261
31.   A p 257–258
32.   C p 260

33.   D p 258
34.   A p 273
35.   D p 273
36.   A p 274
37.   B p 274
38.   C p 276
39.   C p 274
40.   C p 273
41.   A p 273
42.   B p 266
43.   C p 266
44.   D p 267
45.   D p 267
46.   C p 267
47.   B p 267

48.   C p 267
49.   C p 267
50.   B p 268
51.   C p 268
52.   B p 268–269
53.   A p 277
54.   D p 268
55.   B p 268
56.   B p 269
57.   B p 269
58.   A p 269–270
59.   A p 269
60.   D p 269
61.   A p 268
62.   A p 277

IV

IMMUNOLOGY AND HEMATOLOGY

Donna S. McCormick

Physiology of the Immunologic and Hematologic Systems

EDITORS' NOTE

Immunologic and hematologic concepts account for 4% (eight questions) of the CCRN exam. The major content areas covered under immunology and hematology include organ transplantation, disseminated intravascular coagulation (DIC), and immunosuppression. To correctly answer the questions on anaphylactic shock and immunosuppression, one must have a working knowledge of immune response principles. To answer questions on DIC, normal coagulation concepts must be known. The following chapter presents key information normally encountered on the CCRN exam regarding both the four major concepts and the principles necessary to achieve the understanding required for the CCRN exam.

As with most other chapters, concentrate on key principles rather than on details or pure anatomy and physiology points. Nurses often find immunology and hematology to be a difficult area of the CCRN exam because of their lack of clinical familiarity with the concepts. Study this chapter and then try to apply the information during your work. The more you can integrate the information after reading it, the more likely the information will be retained for the test.

IMMUNE SYSTEM

The immune system is a dynamic system, consisting of many cell types and structures. In fact, approximately 1 in every 100 of the body's cells is an immune cell. It is dynamic not only in the sense that it does not necessarily remain in one place as does, say, the heart, but also in the sense that its many components are in a constant state of dynamic interaction.

The mature immune system is capable of performing three general types of functions: defense, homeostasis, and surveillance. In providing defense, resistance to infection is facilitated by both nonspecific innate mechanisms and more specific acquired immune responses that bring about the destruction of foreign antigens (anything recognized by the body as nonself, e.g., microorganisms, proteins, and cells of transplanted organs). Maintaining immunologic homeostasis involves keeping a balance between immune protective and destructive responses and the removal of senescent immune cells from the body. Although the function of the immune system is inherently protective, there are conditions in which natural immune responses become destructive to the host. Examples of such conditions are the numerous autoimmune diseases as well as allergic and anaphylactic reactions. Surveillance involves the recognition of microorganisms or cells bearing foreign antigens on their membranes. Some of the immune cells, lymphocytes in particular, are highly mobile and travel throughout the vascular and lymphatic systems in search of potentially harmful antigens. Some types of cancer cells, in particular, are sought out and destroyed by immune cells in this way.

Immune responses can be classified into two major types: natural or innate responses and acquired responses. Both types of responses play critical roles in host defense.

Innate Immune System

The innate immune system consists of natural or nonspecific mechanisms for the protection of an individual against foreign antigens. These natural defenses are present from birth and do not necessarily require exposure to specific antigens to develop. Natural defenses, the body's first line of defense, consist of anatomical, chemical, and cellular defenses against microbial invasion. Anatomical defenses include the skin, mucous membranes, and ciliated epithelia. Chemical defenses include gastric acid, lysozymes, natural immunoglobulins, and the interferons. Cellular defenses include leukocytes.

Anatomical and Chemical Defenses

The skin provides the initial physical barrier to external environmental antigens. The outermost skin layer, the stratum corneum, is the main barrier to microbial invasion. Certain conditions (pH, humidity, and temperature) influence the growth of potentially pathogenic organisms on the skin. Alterations in normal conditions related to these factors favor the development of infection. The normally acid pH of the skin inhibits the growth of microorganisms. When the acid-base balance of the skin is altered in favor of a higher pH, this protective mechanism is lost. When water loss from epidermal cells exceeds intake, the stratum corneum can dry and crack, predisposing the host to microbial invasion. On the other hand, excessive moisture decreases barrier efficiency.

Skin cells are constantly exfoliating, and in this process organisms are sloughed along with dead skin cells. In addition, the skin is colonized with normal flora (mainly aerobic cocci and diphtheroids), which, through various mechanisms, prevents the colonization of potentially pathogenic organisms. The resident flora maintains the skin's pH in the acidic range and competes effectively for nutrients and binding sites on epidermal cells, making it difficult for nonresident flora to survive. It is when the normal flora is altered, such as occurs with long-term or broad-spectrum antibiotic therapy and with the use of disinfectants or occlusive dressings, that potentially pathogenic organisms become opportunistic. Opportunistic organisms take advantage of the lack of competition for nutrients and epidermal binding sites, and multiply to cause infection.

The sebaceous glands, mammary glands, respiratory epithelium, gastrointestinal mucosa, genitourinary mucosa, and conjunctivae all secrete a protective immunoglobulin (another word for antibody) called secretory IgA. Ciliated respiratory epithelial cells also facilitate the removal of bacteria and other foreign antigens from the respiratory tract; the low pH of the gastric mucosa prevents bacterial growth in the stomach.

Leukocytes

All leukocytes (white blood cells [WBCs]) develop as stem cells in the bone marrow. Leukocytes develop along two major lineages: the myeloid lineage and the lymphoid lineage. The myeloid lineage includes all leukocytes except the lymphocytes. The lymphoid lineage consists of T and B lymphocytes. Myeloid cells make up the backbone of the natural or innate defense system. Myeloid leukocytes can be further classified into two major groups: granulocytes and monocytes. The major function of both is phagocytosis.

Granulocytes. Granulocytes, commonly referred to as polymorphonuclear granulocytes (PMNs) or polymorphs, are produced in the bone marrow at the rate of approximately 80 million per day, and their average life span is about 2–3 days. Sixty to seventy percent of all leukocytes are PMNs. These cells are sometimes called polymorphs because their nuclei are multilobed; they are called granulocytes because they contain intracellular granules. These intracellular granules contain hydrolytic enzymes that are cytotoxic to foreign organisms. Furthermore, granulocytes are classified, according to the histological staining reactions of the granules, into three more distinct types: neutrophils, eosinophils, and basophils. Granulocytes may leave the circulation to become tissue phagocytes (Fig. 25–1).

Neutrophils are the most abundant cells in the bone marrow and blood, comprising about 90% of all granulocytes. Three forms of neutrophils can be

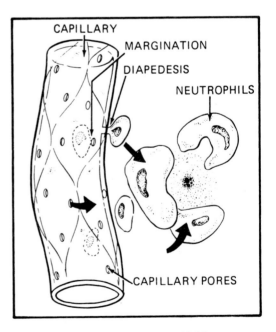

Figure 25–1. Diapedesis of WBCs.

identified in the peripheral blood: segmented neutrophils, bands, and metamyelocytes. Segmented neutrophils are fully mature, bands are slightly immature, and metamyelocytes are completely immature neutrophils. Neutrophils are strongly phagocytic: that is, they ingest microorganisms or other cells and foreign particles, and they digest the ingested material within their phagocytic vacuoles.

In conditions such as infection, there is an increased demand for neutrophils. The bone marrow responds by releasing more neutrophils into the circulation, and in this process immature cells are released along with the mature cells. As a result, the percentage of bands in the peripheral blood is increased. This condition is referred to as a "shift to the left" and indicates acute inflammation or infection. In more serious conditions, metamyelocytes will also appear in increased numbers in the peripheral blood. The normal neutrophil count in the adult is between 1000 and 6000 cells/mm³ blood, or approximately 60% of the differential WBC count. Bands normally number about 600 cells/mm³ blood, or approximately 0 to 5% of the differential WBC count. Metamyelocytes should not be present in the peripheral blood.

Eosinophils are weakly phagocytic cells that are seen in increased numbers in the circulation specifically during parasitic infections and allergic reactions. Eosinophils degranulate (release their cytotoxic granules) upon antigenic stimulation and kill organisms extracellularly. The normal eosinophil count is about 200 cells/mm³ blood, or between 2 and 5% of the differential WBC count.

Basophils are responsible for anaphylactoid reactions to allergens. Like eosinophils, basophils are capable of releasing their cytotoxic granules when stimulated by certain antigens to effect extracellular killing. Basophils are morphologically identical to mast cells but can be differentiated from mast cells in that basophils are bloodborne and mast cells reside in tissues outside of the circulation. In other words, when a basophil migrates out of the circulation to reside in tissue, it becomes a mast cell. The normal basophil count is about 100 cells/mm³ blood, or about 0.2% of the differential WBC count.

Monocytes. PMNs can be differentiated from monocytes by their multilobed nuclei and many intracellular granules. Monocytes are mononuclear cells and do not contain cytotoxic intracellular granules. They do, however, release the prostaglandin PGE_2, which is a mediator of the inflammatory response. The normal monocyte count is about 200 to 1000 cells/mm³ blood, or about 5% of the differential WBC count.

A specific type of monocyte is the antigen-presenting cell (APC). APCs are formed in the epidermis, where they are called Langerhans cells, and in the lymphoid system. APCs play an important role in linking the innate immune system with the acquired immune system. APCs carry foreign antigens that enter the host via the respiratory or gastrointestinal tract, or the skin, through the lymphatic system and present them to lymphocytes in the lymph nodes and spleen, thereby triggering cellular and humoral immune responses.

Phagocytosis. Monocytes, like granulocytes, may leave the circulation to become tissue macrophages. Together, blood and tissue macrophages comprise a highly mobile network of cells for first-line defense called the reticuloendothelial system. These cells are strategically and conveniently located in the liver, spleen, lymph nodes, kidney, lung, peritoneum, brain, and synovia.

Phagocytosis, which means "cell eating," is the first step in host defense. Phagocytes (or macrophages) have surface receptors that allow them to seek out and attack nonspecific foreign organisms, engulf them, and ultimately destroy them (Fig. 25–2). Phagocytosis is the process by which excess antigen and dead cells are removed from the body. Phagocytosis is also essential in the initiation of cellular and humoral immune responses by T and B lymphocytes.

Inflammation. Inflammation is an attempt to restore homeostasis. It is the body's initial reaction to injury and the first step in the healing process. Wound healing cannot occur if the inflammatory response is fully inhibited. During the inflammatory response, a series of cellular and systemic reactions is triggered; these responses serve to localize and destroy the offending antigen, maintain vascular integrity, and limit tissue damage.

Tissue injury provides the initial stimulus for activation of inflammatory mechanisms and results in the cellular release of vasoactive substances such as histamine, bradykinin, and serotonin. The circulatory effects are vasodilatation and increased blood flow to the affected site, increased vascular permeability that facilitates diapedesis of immune cells from the circulation to the tissues, and pain. The clotting system is activated in an attempt to "plug up" the injury. Increased blood flow and capillary permeability lead to local interstitial edema and

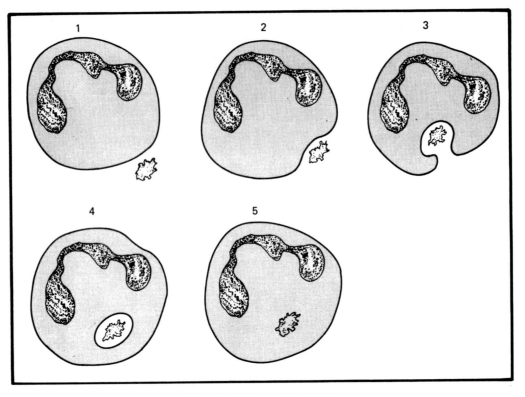

Figure 25–2. Phagocytosis of WBCs.

swelling. Leukocyte migration occurs as phagocytes are attached to the affected site (chemotaxis), and dying leukocytes release pyrogens, which stimulate the hypothalamus to produce a state of fever. Pyrogens also stimulate the bone marrow to release more leukocytes, thus perpetuating the process.

Finally, the complement system is activated. The complement system consists of a complex set of approximately 20 interacting proteolytic enzymes and regulatory proteins found in the plasma and body fluids that attack antigens. The complement system is conceptually similar to the coagulation system in that complement proteins react sequentially in a series of enzymatic reactions in a cascading manner. Several factors are responsible for activation of the complement system: the formation of insoluble antigen-antibody complexes, aggregated immunoglobulin, platelet aggregation, release of endotoxins by gram-negative bacteria, the presence of viruses or bacteria in the circulation, and the release of plasmin and proteases from injured tissues. Complement proteins can mediate the lytic destruction of cells, including (erythrocytes [RBCs]) and WBCs, platelets, bacteria, and viruses.

The inflammatory response can be altered or suppressed in many situations: the administration of corticosteroids or other immunosuppressive drugs,

malnutrition, advanced age, chronic illness, and prolonged stress. Conversely, the inflammatory response can become exaggerated in conditions such as anaphylaxis and septic shock.

The innate immune mechanisms just discussed will be called upon as the first line of defense in ridding the host of foreign antigens. However, if these mechanisms are not entirely successful, a second set of defenses, the acquired immune system, is activated to work in concert with the innate immune system. The acquired immune system is composed of lymphocytes and other lymphoid structures necessary for specific immune responses.

Acquired Immune System

The lymphoid system matures during the fetal and neonatal periods, when lymphoid stem cells differentiate into T and B lymphocytes. At this time, the mechanisms for conferring genetic specificity to lymphocytes develop. This property of specificity is what differentiates the lymphoid cell from the myeloid cell, which can react with any antigen. The process of lymphopoiesis (lymphocyte origination and differentiation into functional effector cells) begins in the yolk sac and then continues later in life in the thymus gland, the liver, the spleen, and finally the bone marrow, which is the primary site of lymphopoiesis in the full-term neonate.

Primary Lymphoid Tissue

Primary lymphoid tissue consists of central organs that serve as major sites of lymphopoiesis. Lymphoid stem cells originate in the bone marrow. These cells give rise to the various components of the acquired immune system.

Secondary Lymphoid Tissue

Secondary lymphoid tissue is peripheral tissue that provides an environment for lymphocytes to encounter antigens and proliferate if necessary. Secondary lymphoid tissue consists of the bone marrow, spleen, lymph nodes, thymus, liver, and mucosal associated lymphoid tissue in the tonsils, respiratory tract, gut, and urogenital tract. Localization of secondary lymphoid tissue is not coincidental, as all of these structures provide major portals for the entry of foreign microorganisms into the body. Once in secondary lymphoid tissue, lymphocytes may migrate from one lymphoid structure to another by vascular and lymphatic channels.

Lymphatics. The lymphatic system consists of (1) a capillary network, which collects lymph (a clear, watery fluid in the interstitial spaces); (2) collecting vessels, which carry lymph from the lymphatic vessels back to the vascular system; (3) lymph nodes; and (4) lymphatic organs, such as the tonsils. Lymphatic channels provide a major transit system for lymphocytes while they carry out specific functions related to immunologic surveillance. Both superficial and deep lymphatics empty into the large thoracic duct, which drains into the left subclavian vein (Fig. 25–3).

Lymph Nodes. Lymph nodes are small, oval-shaped bodies of lymphatic tissue encapsulated by fibrous tissue that are situated in the course of lymphatic vessels. The interior of the lymph nodes resembles a matrix of connective tissue that forms compartments that are densely populated with lymphocytes. Afferent lymphatics carry lymph to the lymph nodes, and efferent lymphatics serve as exit routes for lymphocytes from lymph nodes (Fig. 25–4). Lymph nodes are located at the junctions of lymphatic vessels and form a complete network for the draining and filtering of extravasated lymph from interstitial fluid spaces.

Spleen. The spleen is a soft, purplish, highly vascular, coffee bean-shaped organ in the left upper quadrant. It lies between the fundus of the stomach

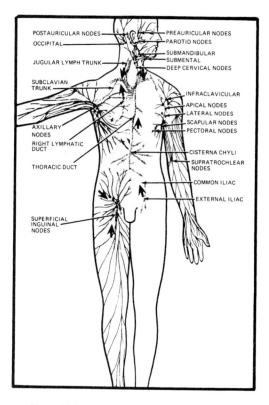

Figure 25–3. Location of lymph nodes in the body.

and the diaphragm. It is covered by a fibroelastic membrane that invests the organ at the hilum to form fibrous bands (trabeculae) that constitute the internal framework of the spleen and contain the splenic pulp.

During fetal and neonatal life, the spleen gives rise to RBCs. The physiological function of the spleen in adult life is not completely understood. However, a major function of the spleen seems to be the removal of particulate matter from the circulation. It is known that it has reticuloendothelial, immunologic, and storage functions. The spleen produces monocytes, lymphocytes, opsonins, and IgM antibody-producing plasma cells.

Blood flow within the spleen is sluggish, which allows phagocytosis to occur. The spleen clears the blood of encapsulated organisms (*Neisseria meningitidis, Haemophilus influenzae, Streptococcus pneumoniae*), and antigens in the rest of the body are phagocytosed and carried to the spleen to be eradicated by antibodies.

Postsplenectomy sepsis syndrome is seen predominantly in young immunosuppressed individuals who have been splenectomized, but this syndrome can occur in the healthy adult after splenectomy. The etiology of this often-fatal syndrome is the loss

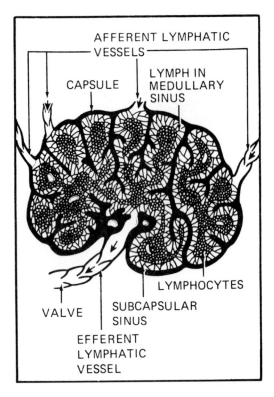

AFFERENT LYMPHATIC
VESSELS

CAPSULE

LYMPH IN
MEDULLARY
SINUS

LYMPHOCYTES

VALVE

SUBCAPSULAR
SINUS

EFFERENT
LYMPHATIC
VESSEL

Figure 25–4. Typical lymph node.

of particulate filtering, coupled with IgM and opsonin production by the spleen.

Normally about 30% of the total platelet population is sequestered in the spleen, but this can increase to 80% with splenomegaly. Increased numbers of red and white blood cells will also be sequestered and destroyed in splenomegaly. Therefore, pancytopenia (anemia, leukopenia, and thrombocytopenia) occurs during splenomegaly.

Thymus. The thymus is a prominent organ in the infant, occupying the ventral superior mediastinum. In the older adult, it may be scarcely visible because of atrophy. The thymus is composed mostly of lymphocytes. Its only known function is the production of lymphocytes.

Lymphocytes

Lymphocytes are the primary defenders of the acquired immune system. Lymphocytes have surface receptors that are specific for surface molecules (antigens) located on the surfaces of foreign proteins and are therefore the only cells that have the intrinsic ability to recognize specific antigens.

There are two major types of lymphocytes: T lymphocytes (T cells) and B lymphocytes (B cells). T cells are involved in immunologic regulation and

mediate what is called the cellular immune response. B cells produce antibodies and mediate what is called the humoral immune response.

T Lymphocytes (T Cells). Under the influence of thymic hormones, immature T cells develop. As mediators of the cellular immune response, T cells defend against viruses, fungi, and some neoplastic conditions, and they destroy transplanted organs by mediating accelerated and acute rejection responses. T-cell function is inhibited by viral and parasitic infections, malnutrition, prolonged general anesthesia, radiation therapy, uremia, Hodgkin's disease, and advanced age.

T cells are divided into four functionally distinct but interactive cell populations or subsets: cytotoxic, helper (T4), suppressor (T8), and memory T cells.

Cytotoxic and memory T cells are referred to as *effector cells* because they have a specific cytotoxic effect on antigen-bearing cells. Cytotoxic T cells bind to target cells and facilitate their destruction via substances known as lymphokines, which stimulate inflammatory cells, and via the production of cytolytic proteins.

Lymphokines are one of the two soluble products of lymphocytes, the other being antibodies. Lymphokines are inflammatory and regulatory hormones of the immune system that serve a variety of functions, such as the recruitment of macrophages to antigen sites (chemotaxis), augmentation of T-cell function in general, and inhibition of viral replication.

Lymphokines carry molecular signals between immunocompetent cells for the purpose of amplification of the immune response. Their role in amplification of the T-cell response is crucial to cellular immunity. Two of the most important lymphokines are interleukin-1 (IL-1) and interleukin-2 (IL-2). IL-1 stimulates T-cell proliferation, induces fever, stimulates the liver to produce acute-phase proteins, and stimulates the release of prostaglandin. IL-2 (T-cell growth factor) also stimulates T-cell proliferation. The reaction of T cells with IL-1 is necessary for the production of IL-2.

Memory T cells are T cells that have been sensitized to a specific antigen and then cloned to remember the antigen. Memory cells remain present in the body for many years and are therefore available for defense upon repeated exposure to an antigen. Repeated exposure to an antigen that the host has been previously sensitized to will result in a more rapid and accelerated immune response than on the first exposure.

Helper and suppressor T cells are *regulatory* in nature. Helper T cells are active in lymphokine-mediated events. They produce multiple lymphokines that promote the proliferation and activation of other lymphocytes and macrophages. Although the B cell can produce antibody by direct interaction with surface antigen on a macrophage, the assistance of helper T cells is required for the majority of antibody production. They recruit cytotoxic T cells to antigen sites and interact with macrophages in the spleen and lymph nodes to facilitate antibody production by B cells. Helper and suppressor T-cell activity is normally balanced to maintain immunologic homeostasis. Too much suppressor T-cell function, for instance, will inhibit helper T-cell function.

B Lymphocytes (B Cells). B cells are effector cells that mediate the humoral immune response through the production of antibodies, which is their major function. B cells are important in defense against pyrogenic bacterial infections and can destroy transplanted organs by mediating hyperacute graft rejection. When a B cell is stimulated by a particular antigen, it differentiates into a lymphoblast. The lymphoblast differentiates into a plasmablast, which further differentiates into a plasma cell. Plasma cells, which are capable of producing and releasing antibody, do so until the antigen is destroyed. Memory of the offending antigen is retained for at least several months.

Antibodies are also referred to as immunoglobulins (see Table 25–1). Immunoglobulins are specifically modified proteins present in serum and tissue fluids that are capable of selectively reacting with inciting antigens. The body produces several million antibodies that are capable of reacting with just as many antigens. However, each is specific and can usually recognize only one antigen. When viruses or bacteria, for instance, enter the body, their structural surface features are recognized by the body as not belonging

to it. Antibodies are then formed and attracted to these foreign structures, for which they have identical matching receptors. In this way, antibodies are able to bind with antigens in a process called antigen–antibody complex formation. Mechanisms of antigen interaction by antibody include agglutination, precipitation, neutralization, and lysis.

Antibodies can be divided into five major classifications: IgM, IgG, IgA, IgD, and IgE. IgM is the principal mediator of the primary immune response. IgM is a natural antibody; i.e., there is no known contact with the antigen that stimulated its production. About 10% of all antibodies are of the IgM type. IgG is the principal mediator of the secondary immune response, which requires repeated exposure to the same antigen. IgG is the major antibody against bacteria and viruses. About 75% of all antibodies are of the IgG type. IgA is the secretory immunoglobulin present in bodily secretions and offers natural protection against nonspecific foreign antigens. About 15% of all antibodies are of the IgA type. The function of IgD is not known, but about 1% of antibodies are of this type. Although only about 0.002% of antibodies are of the IgE type, IgE antibodies present on basophils and mast cells play a significant role in inflammatory and immune reactions.

Lymphocyte Responses

All cells express foreign antigens. Foreign cells, of course, express antigens that are genetically different from those of the host. It is through specific receptors on the surfaces of lymphocytes that B and T cells can be differentiated, and it is also through these receptors that B and T cells are able to recognize foreign antigens. During lymphocyte maturation, each B and T cell acquires specific cell membrane surface receptors that allow the cell to "match up" with certain foreign antigens. This matching between host lymphocytes and foreign antigens is the recognition phase of the acquired immune response. When this occurs, lymphocytes are activated to differentiate, proliferate, and then quickly mount an effective immune response against the offending antigen.

Cellular Immune Response. The cellular immune response is the immune response mediated by T cells. T cells recognize foreign antigens only after they are displayed on the surfaces of macrophages or APCs. The cellular immune response can be summarized as follows:

1. Naturally, the presence of a foreign antigen is necessary to initiate the response.

TABLE 25–1. TYPES AND FUNCTIONS OF IMMUNOGLOBULINS

Type	Function
IgM	First antibody in fetal life
	First antibody after exposure to a new antigen
IgG	Major antibody of adult life
	Produced after repeated exposure to the same antigen
IgA	Found in secretions: tears, saliva, mucous secretions in gastrointestinal and respiratory tracts
	Meets antigen at port of entry
IgE	Mediates allergic reactions
IgD	Function unclear, but may be regulatory in nature

2. Initially, macrophages encounter the antigen and begin to phagocytize it. Antigenic fragments are released and then carried to T cells in the lymph nodes by APCs.

3. Resting virgin or memory T cells are activated when the antigen–APC complex binds with the T-cell surface receptor.

4. APCs are stimulated to produce IL-1, which summons helper T cells.

5. Helper T cells are then responsible for a number of actions, including the release of IL-2, which causes the differentiation and proliferation of T cells. The helper T cells also stimulate antibody production by B cells.

6. Clonal expansion greatly increases the sensitized T-cell population.

7. Ultimately, the antigen-bearing cells are destroyed by the direct cytotoxic effect of effector T cells. Some sensitized T cells are returned to the lymphoid system with the memory of the antigen for future challenge.

Examples of cellular immune responses include tumor cell surveillance, defense against viral and fungal infections, acute organ rejection, graft-versus-host disease, and autoimmune diseases.

Humoral Immune Response. The humoral immune response is mediated by B cells. Antigens trigger B cells by stimulating immunoglobulins on their surfaces. The humoral immune response can be summarized as follows:

1. Naturally, as with the cellular immune response, the presence of a foreign antigen is necessary to initiate the process. Unlike T cells, B cells can recognize an antigen in its native configuration.

2. Initially, macrophages encounter the antigen and begin to phagocytize it. Antigenic fragments are released and then carried to B cells in the lymph nodes and spleen by APCs. Resting virgin or memory B cells are activated when antigen binds to surface immunoglobulin.

3. IL-1 is released by APCs, and helper T cells stimulate the sensitization and clonal proliferation of effector B cells. B cells are activated to differentiate and produce antibody when antigen binds to their receptors.

4. Antigen–antibody complexes form, and ultimately the antigen-bearing cells are destroyed.

5. As in the cellular immune response, some of the plasma cells with specific memory of the antigen are cloned and returned to the lymphoid system.

In addition, B cells can process and present antigen to T cells. Examples of humoral immune responses include resistance to encapsulated pyrogenic bacteria such as pneumococci, streptococci, meningococci, and *H. influenzae*, hemolytic transfusion reactions, and hyperacute organ rejection.

The first exposure of an antigen to an activated lymphocyte evokes a primary immune response. Repeated exposure of the identical antigen to activated lymphocytes evokes an accelerated secondary response. In the secondary immune response, the latent period is shorter and the amount of antigen required to initiate the response is less.

The difference between cell and humoral responses are listed in Table 25–2.

Hypersensitivity Reactions

When an adaptive immune response occurs in an exaggerated or inappropriate form, causing tissue damage, a hypersensitivity reaction is said to occur. Hypersensitivity reactions occur on second exposure to the causative antigen. Four types of hypersensitivity reactions are described.

Type I

Type I hypersensitivity reactions (allergic or anaphylactic) are immediate in nature. This antibody (IgE)-mediated response results in the release of histamine by mast cells, which produces an acute inflammatory reaction. The distinguishing clinical feature of a type I hypersensitivity reaction is an immediate wheal-and-flare reaction.

Type II

Type II hypersensitivity reactions are caused by the presence of preformed circulating cytotoxic antibodies. These antibodies destroy the target cells on contact.

Examples of type II hypersensitivity reactions are transfusion reactions, autoimmune hemolytic anemia, and hemolytic disease of the newborn (HDNB). In a transfusion reaction, antibodies (IgM) to ABO antigens cause agglutination, complement fixation, and intravascular hemolysis. A direct Coombs test will confirm the presence of antibody on the RBCs. An indirect Coombs test measures the degree of hemolytic activity. In autoimmune hemolytic anemia, antibodies against

TABLE 25–2. COMPARISON OF B- AND T-CELL IMMUNITY

Characteristic	B Lymphocyte	T Lymphocyte
Type of immunity	Humoral	Cell-mediated
Immune functions	Antibody formation	Direct cytotoxicity
	Immediate hypersensitivity	Delayed hypersensitivity
		Immune surveillance
		(destruction of cancer cells)
		Graft rejection
		Immune regulation
Organisms	Pyogenic bacteria	Intracellular bacteria
protective against	*Staphylococcus*	*Pseudomonas*
	Haemophilus	*Listeria*
	Neisseria	Mycobacteria
	Viruses	Viruses
	Hepatitis B virus	Herpes simplex virus
	Adenovirus	Herpes varicella-zoster virus
	Enterovirus	Cytomegalovirus
	Echovirus	Epstein-Barr virus
		Retrovirus (excluding HIV)
		Fungi
		Candida
		Cryptococcus
		Aspergillus
		Protozoa
		Pneumocystis carinii
		Toxoplasma gondii

the body's own RBCs are produced. This reaction is provoked by allergic reactions to drugs, when a drug and antibody to the drug form a complex that attacks the RBCs. HDNB occurs during the pregnancy of a mother who has been sensitized to blood group antigens on a previous infant's RBCs and makes IgE antibodies to them. The antibodies cross the placenta and react with the fetal RBCs, causing destruction. Rhesus D (Rh factor) is the most commonly involved antigen.

Type III

Type III hypersensitivity reactions are immune complex-mediated reactions. In this condition, large quantities of antigen–antibody complexes are deposited in the tissues and cannot be cleared from the body by the reticuloendothelial system. This leads to a condition known as serum sickness. Causes are persistent infection, autoimmune disease, and environmental antigens.

Type IV

In type IV (delayed-type) hypersensitivity reactions, when the host comes into contact with a foreign antigen, antigen-sensitized T cells release lymphokines that destroy the antigen. Allergic contact dermatitis, acute allograft rejection, and delayed hypersensitivity skin testing are examples of type IV hypersensitivity reactions.

Anaphylaxis

Anaphylaxis is an acute, generalized, and violent antigen–antibody reaction that may be rapidly fatal even with prompt emergency treatment.

Pathophysiology

Upon first exposure to an antigen, antibodies (of the immunoglobulin IgE) are formed and attach to mast cells in tissues and basophils in the vascular system. Once antibodies have been formed, a second exposure to the antigen results in an immune reaction (releasing histamine) that may vary from mild to fatal. In its severe form, the reaction is called anaphylactic shock.

The reaction of anaphylactic shock is primarily a histamine reaction, setting off a chain of multiple chemical reactions that cause further reactions. The more reactions that occur, the more severe the anaphylaxis and the greater the mortality.

The release of histamine results in vasodilatation of the capillaries (causing hypotension) and a markedly increased cellular permeability. The increase in intracellular fluid alters the cell shape, leaving spaces between the previously compact cells. This promotes movement from the vascular system, thus increasing the colloid osmotic pressure. As more colloids move into interstitial spaces, edema and a decreased circulating volume of blood occur. This has the effect of decreasing cardiac output.

Histamine occurs in two forms, H_1 and H_2. H_1 causes vasoconstriction of the bronchi and intestines. H_2 increases gastric acid secretion and minor cardiac stimulation. Both H_1 and H_2 are responsible for vasodilatation.

The release and action of histamines result in the release of other amines into the bloodstream. Bradykinin, serotonin, slow-reacting substances, a chemotactic factor attracting eosinophils, prostaglandins, and acetylcholine all play a role in the physiological development of anaphylaxis. These chemicals may also activate the complement system. These amines increase arteriolar and venous dilatation, capillary permeability, and abnormal shift of fluid from the vascular tree into the interstitial compartment. This shift decreases circulating blood volume but does not decrease total blood in the body. With blood remaining in the microcirculation, decreased systolic and diastolic pressure occurs. These substances and H_1 and H_2 cause an intense bronchiolar constriction that leads to a general hypoxemia.

Etiology

Drugs, especially antibiotics, are the major allergens in anaphylaxis. Other drugs, iodine-based contrast dye, and blood transfusions are also involved in anaphylaxis.

Aside from medications injected or ingested, bites and stings from insects are the major causes of anaphylaxis. Of these, the stings of bees and yellow jackets are the most common, but wasp and hornet stings may also cause anaphylaxis.

Clinical Presentation

The major symptoms resulting from release of histamine and other chemicals are anxiety, severe dyspnea (the patient may have cyanosis), and angioedema. Angioedema is edema in membranous tissues and is most easily seen in the eyes and mouth. It also occurs in the tongue, hands, feet, and genitalia. There is a diffuse erythema occurring more in the upper body parts than in the lower. Occasionally, abdominal cramps, vomiting, and/or diarrhea may occur. Unconsciousness occurs early in severe anaphylaxis.

As fluid shifts from the capillaries into the interstitial tissue, edema of the uvula and larynx occurs. This edema may produce an acute respiratory obstruction. Laryngeal edema is accompanied by impaired phonation and a barking or high-pitched cough. If the patient is alert, he or she will show signs of increased anxiety and complain of air hunger.

Cardiovascular effects of anaphylaxis are the same as those associated with other types of shock—mainly hypotension, tachycardia, and changes in the electrocardiogram similar to those that occur in myocardial injury. Temporary changes in the ST segment and the T wave suggest coronary ischemia. However, the serum enzymes are normal.

The changes in ventilation (causing hypoxia) and decreased circulating blood may result in convulsions and unconsciousness. Circulatory failure and laryngeal edema are the usual causes of death in anaphylaxis.

Complications

Myocardial infarction secondary to venous dilatation and a decreased blood pressure may occur. With decreased blood pressure, increased tissue hypoxia occurs. Increased tissue hypoxia results in increased tissue anoxia and destruction. Hypoventilation occurs as a result of the decreased venous return of blood to the heart and increased tissue hypoxia.

Pulmonary status, already compromised by bronchiolar constriction, may be further damaged as a result of overadministration of the intravenous fluids that are used to compensate for the decreased vascular volume. Chemical reactions causing further imbalances may lead to central nervous system convulsions and coma. If the pulmonary, cardiac, or vascular system is refractory to treatment, anaphylaxis is fatal.

Treatment

The primary objective of treatment is to dilate the bronchioles, which is accomplished by the administration of epinephrine either subcutaneously or intramuscularly. Antihistamines may help control local edema and itching, but they cannot alter the circulatory failure and bronchoconstriction to a significant degree. After administration of epinephrine, the respiratory system should be supported by mask, intubation, or tracheostomy with the use of a ventilator.

The second goal of therapy is to improve the patient's circulatory status. Promoting the movement of fluid from the interstitial compartment back into the vascular compartment is usually achieved through the use of intravenous fluids. Vasopressors may be used to cause constriction of the blood vessels. However, this can make tissue anoxia more severe, and use of vasopressors is controversial. The third-space loss of fluid is believed to be caused by leakage through the injured capillary walls. Glucocorticoids help to decrease cellular damage, reduce the severity of anaphylaxis, and prevent inflammation of the damaged tissues. Hydrocortisone given intravenously is the drug usually used. Steroids stabilize the membrane of the basophils, reducing the chemical reactions in anaphylaxis.

In addition to maintaining respiratory status, using epinephrine, and administering glucocorticoids (both those formed by the body in response to stress and synthetic forms), intravenous fluid will increase the circulating blood volume. Intravenous fluids may have electrolytes added to control acid-base imbalances.

Nursing Intervention

Assessment of the symptoms in all body systems is extremely important. Research has shown that laryngeal edema and hypotension are major factors causing death.

Anaphylaxis may occur in susceptible patients immediately or as much as an hour after injection of an antigen (drug, blood). Respiratory assessment includes identifying signs of stridor, the use of auxiliary muscles for breathing, and or cynosis; auscultating lung fields for crackles, rhonchi, or wheezes; and measuring arterial blood gases. Mechanical ventilation should be on standby if not already in use. Normal nursing interventions for patients on respirators are applicable for these patients.

Monitoring the patient's cardiac and circulatory status is best achieved by using a pulmonary artery catheter. Death can occur within minutes if there is circulatory failure or pulmonary edema. These parameters must be observed continuously until the patient is stable and then at very frequent intervals (at least every 15 min for four times, then every 30 min for four times, and then every one to 2 hr).

Antihistamines are not usually helpful in altering circulatory failure and bronchoconstriction. The use of antihistamines does not affect the release of histamine but they do occupy receptor sites, thus preventing the attachment of histamine. Administration of these drugs requires close observation because of their depressive effects on the central nervous system. If epinephrine is used intravenously, monitoring for hypertension and cardiac dysrhythmias is essential.

Renal status is monitored by Foley catheter to prevent fluid overload as the extracellular fluid moves back into the vascular system with appropriate drugs. In severe anaphylaxis, the patient is frequently comatose, and establishing the monitoring and support systems may leave little, if any, time for psychosocial support. As the patient's condition stabilizes and his or her level of consciousness returns to normal, emotional support is essential. Explaining to the patient what has happened, what all the monitoring equipment is being used for, and that these monitors will be removed as his or her condition improves will help to alleviate the patient's fear.

HEMATOLOGIC SYSTEM

Red Blood Cell Formation and Anemias

Hematopoiesis

The bone marrow is a spongy substance within the bone where maturation of blood cells occurs. In the adult, bone marrow is primarily located in the long, flat bones (skull, ribs, sternum, pelvis, shoulder girdles, vertebrae, innominates). The mature erythrocyte, leukocyte, and thrombocyte all begin as a primitive cell called a stem cell. In response to specific stimuli, called colony stimulating factors, a stem cell becomes "committed" to a particular cell line and matures to perform the functions of either an RBC, WBC, or platelet. Once the stem cell is committed, it is no longer capable of mitosis. It matures within the bone marrow and is released into the peripheral blood. The following diagram illustrates the relationship of the stem cell to the mature blood cells seen in the peripheral blood (Fig. 25–5). Stem cells increase in number during times of increased demand (hypoxia, infection) in order to increase production of the needed blood cell type.

Red blood cell production is stimulated by the hormone erythropoietin. Erythropoietin is released by the kidney in response to tissue hypoxia. This hormone results in increased erythrocyte production by (1) increasing the number of stem cells placed into the maturational process, (2) decreasing maturational time, (3) increasing hemoglobin synthesis, and (4) causing a premature release of reticulocytes from the bone marrow. Reticulocytes may appear in the peripheral blood within 2 days of increased demand, but an increase in mature erythrocytes is not apparent until 6–8 days. An increase in the peripheral reticulocyte count is an indication of increased RBC production.

The primary function of the RBC is the transportation of oxygen and carbon dioxide. Hemoglobin is the molecule responsible for this function. It is produced throughout most of the maturation of the RBC. Normal hemoglobin production is dependent upon sufficient iron supply, protoporphyrin, and globin.

The life span of the mature RBC in the circulation is approximately 120 days. As the cell

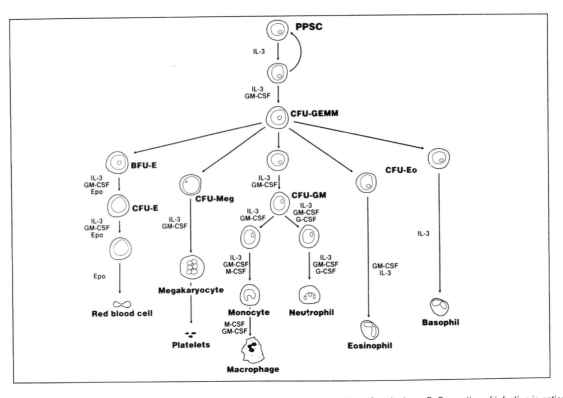

Figure 25–5. Relationship of the stem cell to the mature blood cell. (Reprinted with permission from Cunningham, R. Prevention of infection in patients receiving myelosuppressive chemotherapy. New York: Triclinica Communications, 1992.)

becomes older, it is no longer able to traverse the microvasculature, and then it is phagocytized by the reticuloendothelial tissue.

Platelet Production

Platelet production is thought to be regulated by the hormone thrombopoietin. Platelets mature in the bone marrow and migrate to the spleen. They travel between the spleen and circulatory system in order to maintain a steady state of circulating platelets. Platelets contribute to hemostasis by the formation of a plug over an area of damaged endothelium. Plug formation requires an adequate number of functioning platelets as well as vascular integrity. Platelets are a source of phospholipids, which are necessary in the coagulation process.

Normal Coagulation and Pathologic Hematologic Conditions

EDITORS' NOTE

This section contains supplemental information helpful in answering CCRN questions addressing the concepts of disseminated intravascular coagulation and thrombolytic ther-

apy. Understanding concepts in this chapter will be useful in answering several questions on the exam. Use this chapter to supplement your understanding of clinical conditions requiring thrombolytic treatment and coagulopathies.

Three sequential events occur to aid in preventing bleeding. Vasoconstriction and platelet aggregation are the first two events in hemostasis. The third hemostatic mechanism is coagulation.

Normal Coagulation

Normal coagulation is dependent upon the presence of all clotting factors and the appropriate functioning of other separate, but interrelated components. These components are the extrinsic cascade, the intrinsic cascade, and the common final pathway.

A cascade is similar to a row of dominoes standing on their ends. When the first domino falls, it strikes the next domino, starting a chain reaction that continues until all of the dominoes have been toppled. This necessitates positioning the dominoes so that each will connect with the next. Within the circulating blood, there is a plethora of clotting factors to continue a cascade once initiated. It is interesting to note that there is at least one specific spot in each of the three cascades (extrinsic, intrinsic, and final common pathway) that requires calcium ions (Ca++, factor IV) to continue activation of these cascades. These sites are identified in Fig. 25–6, which shows the normal coagulation process.

Extrinsic Cascade. (Fig. 25–7) is activated by injury to vessels and tissue. The end result of this cascade is the release of thromboplastin into the circulatory system.

A second mechanism for activating clotting factors is the release of phospholipids from platelets

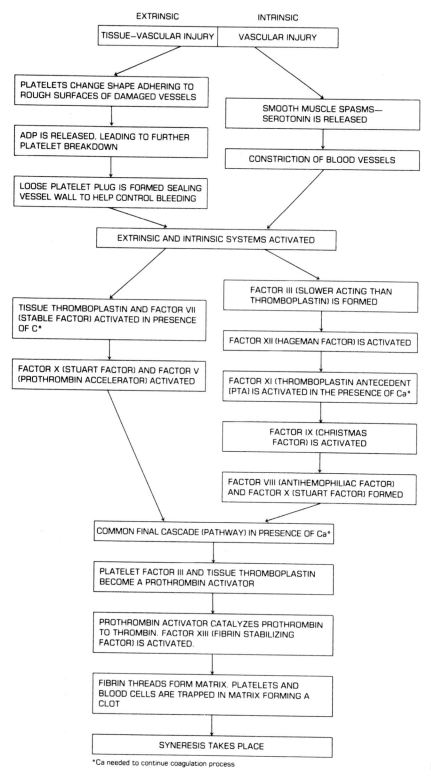

*Ca needed to continue coagulation process

Figure 25–6. Normal coagulation process.

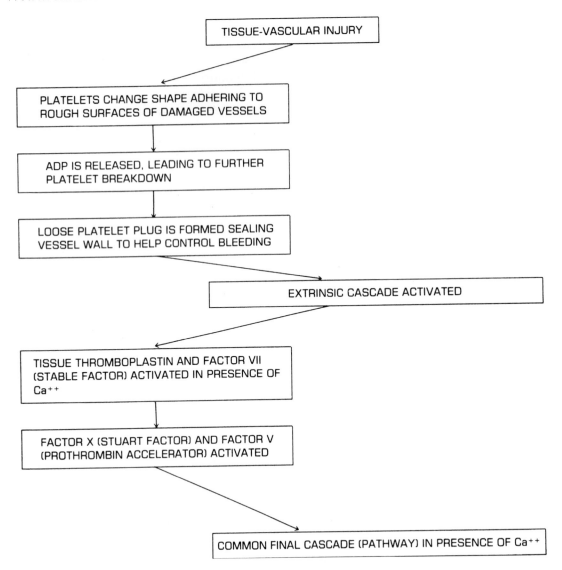

Figure 25–7. Extrinsic cascade segment of the overall normal coagulation process.

and damaged tissue. This is thought to increase the rate of blood coagulation through both extrinsic and intrinsic cascades.

Intrinsic Cascade. (Fig. 25–8) is initiated when factor XII (the Hageman factor, the surface substance) comes into contact with collagen or the basement membrane of the blood vessel's damaged endothelium.

Common Final Pathway Cascade. Both the extrinsic and intrinsic cascades react to completion and, in the presence of calcium ions, join to form the common final pathway (cascade) shown in Fig. 25–9.

Syneresis is the final step in coagulation and the first step in clot stability. Syneresis is the process of particle suspension in a gel that begins to aggregate and form a compact mass—the clot. Clot retraction

occurs soon after syneresis is complete. Platelets contain an enzyme called thromboplastin. This enzyme causes the fibrin strands and cells in the clot to be drawn together, expressing a clear, serous fluid. Clot retraction is responsible for drawing the edges of damaged vessels together, which fosters healing.

Anticoagulation

When the vascular damage has been repaired, dissolution of the clot begins. This is termed fibrinolysis. Up to this point, the various cascades have clotted the injured vessels but have not caused massive intravascular clotting. Massive clotting is avoided because excess thrombin is carried away from the clot site by the circulating blood and antithrombin III is released from mast cells.

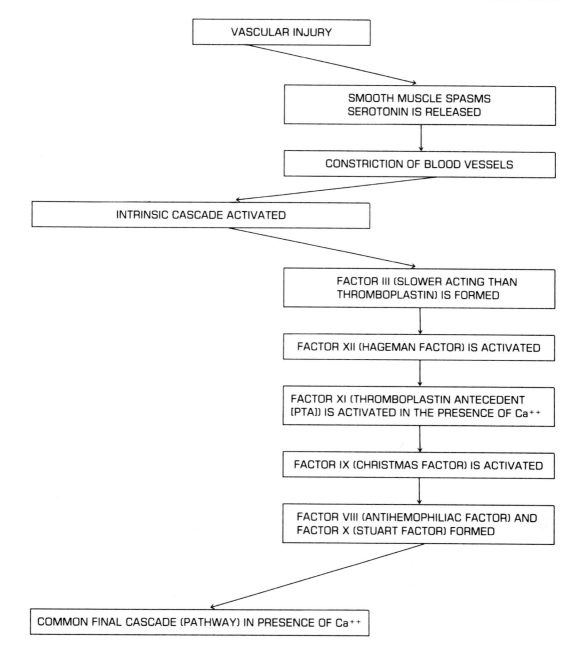

Figure 25–8. Intrinsic cascade segment of the overall normal coagulation process.

There are actually two mechanisms to prevent excessive clotting: the fibrinolytic system and the antithrombin system.

Fibrinolytic System. In this system, plasminogen is converted to plasmin. Plasmin lyses the clot. Clot lysis (fibrinolysis) is accomplished by two mechanisms: clearance of activated clotting factors by the reticuloendothelial system and the actual lysis of the fibrin structure in the clot. Lysis of the clot is initiated by either the internal or external pathway. In the internal pathway, factor XII is activated to XIIa

upon contact with an abnormal or irregular vascular lining. At the same time, XIIa catalyzes prekallikrein to kallikrein (a blood plasminogen activator). The extrinsic system provides tissue plasminogen activators from damaged vascular areas. Both types of plasminogen activators convert plasminogen to plasmin. Plasmin breaks the fibrin structure, causing the mesh holding blood components, such as platelets, to weaken and dissociate as a stable unit. The breakdown of the fibrin structure causes an increase in fibrin degradation products (or fibrin split products). An increase in fibrin degradation products

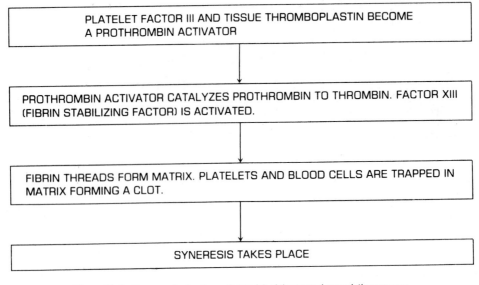

Figure 25–9. Common final pathway (cascade) of the normal coagulation process.

may signal the onset of a coagulopathy such as disseminated intravascular coagulation (DIC).

Fibrinolytic Therapy. Fibrinolytic therapy in the treatment of acute myocardial infarction and pulmonary emboli employs the principles of normal clot lysis. Normally, the fibrinolytic system converts plasminogen to plasmin, which degrades fibrin into soluble fragments. In the presence of large thrombi, this system cannot dissolve the large fibrin mass. However the introduction of exogenous plasminogen activators produces more plasmin, which depletes circulating fibrinogen and promotes lysis. Exogenous plasminogen activator also destroys coagulation factors V and VIII, causing a systemic lytic state that increases the potential risk of bleeding.

The fibrinolytic agents used most frequently include streptokinase (SK), urokinase (UK), and tissue plasminogen activator (tPA). SK is derived from beta hemolytic streptococci and activates the fibrinolytic process by forming an activator complex with plasminogen. SK depletes fibrinogen and other coagulants factors predisposing the patient to systemic bleeding. Allergic, anaphylactic reactions can be induced upon a second exposure to the drug due to its nature as a bacterial protein.

Urokinase is a naturally occurring human enzyme that acts directly on the circulating plasminogen to produce plasmin. tPA is also a naturally occurring human enzyme that activates plasminogen only after plasminogen has bound to fibrin contained in the thrombus. Relatively little circulating plasmin is produced, and clotting factors are not depleted. The risk of systemic bleeding is lessened.

Neither UK nor TPA produces allergic reactions because they are naturally occurring within the human body. TPA is shorter acting (ten minutes) than streptokinase (several hours) or urokinase (approximately 1 hr).

Antithrombin System. This system protects our bodies from excessive intravascular clotting by neutralizing the clotting capability of thrombin. Antithrombin III is the neutralizing agent. Heparin functions as an antithrombin III and inhibits all serine proteases in all cascades. These include Xa, Ha, Vt12, and thrombin. It interrupts the action of thrombin on fibrinogen.

When clot retraction is complete, profibrinolysis is activated by factor XII. This activation results in fibrinolysin (plasmin), which phagocytizes the clot and other clotting factors present in excess of the normal amount. In this way, both intravascular clotting and bleeding are controlled.

Diagnosis and Treatment of Immunologic and Hematologic Problems

EDITORS' NOTE

This chapter is supplemental to other chapters in this section. It provides additional information on diagnostic tests, pharmacology, and treatments for immunologic and hematologic problems. No specific questions will be derived from this chapter, although questions may be derived indirectly from the content of this chapter. Read this chapter to improve your general understanding of diagnostic tests and treatments related to hematology, immunology, and human immunodeficiency virus testing.

COMPLETE BLOOD COUNT

The red blood cell count (RBC) consists of the total number of circulating RBCs, the part of the blood that transports oxygen. See Table 26–1 for normal values. The hemoglobin (Hb) measures the oxygen-carrying capacity of the red blood cell, while the hematocrit (Hct) compares the RBC volume to the plasma volume. Other valuable indices include mean corpuscular volume (MCV), which is the average size of the red blood cell. The mean corpuscular hemoglobin (MCH), which measures the average weight of the Hb per RBC. Finally, the mean corpuscular hemoglobin concentration (MCHC) measures the average percentage of Hb in a RBC. A peripheral smear allows the practitioner to examine the RBC and get composition, size, and shape.

Another useful test when evaluating the hematologic system is the reticulocyte count. This test identifies the bone marrow's ability to produce young erythrocytes.

The white blood cell count (WBC) measures the total number of white cells, or leukocytes. Further breakdown of the WBC count is called the differential. Components of the differential include neutrophils, monocytes, lymphocytes, basophils, and eosinophils. Absolute counts in the differential are more important because they are in direct relation to the WBC count. For abnormal components and causative agents of the differential, see Table 26–2.

The erythrocyte sedimentation rate (ESR) is often used in evaluating infectious diseases. It is a nonspecific test that examines the volume of RBCs that settle in 1 hr. Elevation is usually seen with an acute infectious process.

Other helpful tests include radiographs, scans, and biopsies.

HEMOSTATIC SCREENING TESTS

Normal clotting has three stages: (1) vascular injury activates thromboplastin activity in both the extrinsic and intrinsic pathways, (2) thromboplastin converts prothrombin to thrombin, and (3) thrombin converts fibrinogen in the plasma at the site of injury to form a fibrin plug.

Specific tests can be performed to evaluate blood-clotting activity, to identify abnormalities, and to ascertain patient response to therapy.

TABLE 26–1. NORMAL LABORATORY VALUES FOR THE COMPLETE BLOOD COUNT

Red cell count (RBC)	
Females:	3.8–5.2 × 10/ml
Males:	4.4–5.9 × 10/ml
Hemoglobin (Hb)	
Females:	11.7–15.7 g/dl
Males:	13.3–17.7 g/dl
Hematocrit (Hct)	
Females:	34.9–46.9%
Males:	39.8–52.2%
Platelets (Plt):	150,000–400,000
White cell count (WBC):	3500–11,000/ml
Neutrophils:	39–79%
Lymphocytes:	10–40%
Monocytes:	3–8%
Basophils:	0–2%
Eosinophils:	0–5%
Reticulocyte count:	0.5–1.5%
Erythrocyte sedimentation rate (ESR)	
Females:	1–20 mm/hr
Males:	1–13 mm/hr
Prothrombin time (PT):	11–16 sec
Activated partial thromboplastin time (aPTT):	20–35 sec
Bleeding time:	<4 min

Prothrombin Time

The prothrombin time (PT) measures the activity level and patency of the extrinsic cascade and the common final pathway. The PT measures factors I, II, V, VII, and X. Normal values are the same as control values (should be 11–16 sec). Warfarin (Coumadin) effectiveness is assessed with the PT.

Activated Partial Thromboplastin Time

The activated partial thromboplastin time (aPTT) measures the activity level and patency of the intrinsic cascade and common final pathway. Normal values of 20–35 sec are used to assess all clotting factors except VII and XIII. Heparin effectiveness is assessed with the aPTT.

Bleeding Time

Platelet plug formation time is measured with the bleeding time. Normal values are less than 4 min (Ivy), 1–4 min (Duke), and 1–9 min (Mielke).

Platelet Count

This is a specific count of platelets seen in a blood smear. Normal values are 150,000–450,000 platelets mm². Values below 100,000 platelets/mm² are pathognomonic for thrombocytopenia, the cause of which must be determined. A lower platelet count results in excessive bleeding since there is an insufficient number of platelets to clot. Counts less than 20,000 are associated with spontaneous bleeding.

HUMAN IMMUNODEFICIENCY VIRUS SCREENING TESTS

The enzyme-linked immunosorbent assay (ELISA) is the initial diagnostic test for human immunodeficiency virus (HIV). If it is negative, the patient is considered to be negative unless he or she is in the window period of seroconversion. In that case, the patient should be retested in 6 months. If the ELISA is positive, a confirmation test called the Western Blot is performed. In order for this to be positive, two of the three antigen bands from the virus are required. Another test is a p24 antigen which identifies free viral protein in the plasma. Other diagnostic studies that have proven useful in tracking HIV progression and the response to therapy are CD4 counts and HIV viral load. The CD4 cell is the primary target and binding site of HIV. As the virus progresses, the CD4 count drops, although with the new antiretroviral therapy available today, it is not uncommon to see the CD4 count rise significantly. A new diagnostic marker called HIV viral load is now available. It measures the free virus in the plasma. This test can also show response to new therapy or indicate the need for a treatment change.

TESTS FOR OTHER INFECTIOUS DISEASES

Diagnostic tests that are often ordered for patients with a suspected infectious disease include cultures, susceptibility, and Gram stain. These procedures will be collected by the nurse or physician and sent to the microbiology lab. Sources include blood, sputum, urine, and drainage from wounds. In addition, the nurse should review subjective and objective assessments and be aware of the various signs of hematologic and immunologic disease (Table 26–3).

BLOOD AND COMPONENT THERAPY

The primary reason for transfusing blood is to increase the oxygen available for preventing tissue

TABLE 26–2. INFLUENCE OF DISEASE ON BLOOD CELL COUNT

Cell type	How affected
Neutrophils	Increased by: • Infections: osteomyelitis, otitis media, salpingitis, septicemia, gonorrhea, endocarditis, smallpox, chickenpox, herpes, Rocky Mountain spotted fever • Ischemic necrosis due to myocardial infarction, burns, carcinoma • Metabolic disorders: diabetic acidosis, eclampsia, uremia, thyrotoxicosis • Stress response due to acute hemorrhage, surgery, excessive exercise, emotional distress, third trimester of pregnancy, childbirth • Inflammatory disease: rheumatic fever, rheumatoid arthritis, acute gout, vasculitis and myositis Decreased by: • Bone marrow depression due to radiation or cytotoxic drugs • Infections: typhoid, tularemia, brucellosis, hepatitis, influenza, measles, mumps, rubella, infectious mononucleosis • Hypersplenism: hepatic disease and storage diseases • Collagen vascular disease, such as systemic lupus erythematosus • Deficiency of folic acid or vitamin B_{12}
Eosinophils	Increased by: • Allergic disorders: asthma, hay fever, food or drug sensitivity, serum sickness, angioneurotic edema • Parasitic infections: trichinosis, hookworm, roundworm, amebiasis • Skin diseases: eczema, pemphigus, psoriasis, dermatitis, herpes • Neoplastic diseases: chronic myelocytic leukemia, Hodgkin's disease, metastases and necrosis of solid tumors • Miscellaneous: collagen vascular disease, adrenocortical hypofunction, ulcerative colitis, polyarteritis nodosa, post-splenectomy, pernicious anemia, scarlet fever, excessive exercise Decreased by: • Stress response due to trauma, shock, burns, surgery, mental distress • Cushing's syndrome
Basophils	Increased by: • Chronic myelocytic leukemia, polycythemia vera, some chronic hemolytic anemias, Hodgkin's disease, systemic mastocytosis, myxedema, ulcerative colitis, chronic hypersensitivity states, nephrosis Decreased by: • Hyperthyroidism, ovulation, pregnancy, stress
Lymphocytes	Increased by: • Infections: pertussis, brucellosis, syphilis, tuberculosis, hepatitis, infectious mononucleosis, mumps, German measles, cytomegalovirus • Other: thyrotoxicosis, hypoadrenalism, ulcerative colitis, immune diseases, lymphocytic leukemia Decreased by: • Severe debilitating illness, such as congestive heart failure, renal failure, advanced tuberculosis • Defective lymphatic circulation, high levels of adrenal corticosteroids, immunodeficiency due to immunosuppressives
Monocytes	Increased by: • Infections: subacute bacterial endocarditis, tuberculosis, hepatitis, malaria, Rocky Mountain spotted fever • Collagen vascular disease: systemic lupus erythematosus, rheumatoid arthritis, polyarteritis nodosa • Carcinomas, monocytic leukemia, lymphomas

hypoxia. Blood is administered primarily when the hemoglobin/hematocrit levels are low (generally when hemoglobin levels are below 7 g/dl), when intravascular volume is low, and to replace deficient or utilized substances such as protein, platelets, and clotting factors.

Whole Blood

One unit of whole blood is approximately 500 mL of blood cells, serum, platelets, proteins, and other intravascular nutrients and substances. Whole blood is the best substance to transfuse in hemor-

TABLE 26–3. SIGNS AND SYMPTOMS OF HEMATOLOGIC AND IMMUNOLOGIC DISEASES

Subjective
Fatigue
Dyspnea
Inability to perform activities of daily living

Objective
Altered mental status
Fever
Tachycardia
Hypotension
Tachypnea
Cough
Dysrhythmia
Abnormal lab values
Positive cultures
Skin lesions
Poor urine output
Lymphadenopathy

rhage, since it replaces both volume and elements. Due to shortages whole blood actual transfusion of whole blood is rare. Whole blood can be divided into PRBCs, FFP and cryoprecipitate making it possible for more than one patient to benefit from the donation of 1 unit of whole blood.

Normally, during the administration of a blood transfusion, the cold (due to storage) donor blood is rapidly warmed as it mixes with circulating blood at normal infusion rates. Rapid replacement with cold blood predisposes the patient to cardiac arrest, hypothermia and coagulopathies. When massive, rapid transfusions are necessary, the blood can be passed through a warmer to reach body temperature, thus reducing these dangers.

Red Blood Cells (Packed RBCs)

Packed RBCs provide the advantage of less blood volume (200 to 300 ml) to infuse, thereby decreasing the chance of fluid overload. Packed RBCs are used in severe anemias without blood loss and hemorrhage. PRBCs are given cautiously in patients with congestive heart failure, cardiac disease, or with renal failure related to the increased risk of fluid overload.

Fresh Frozen Plasma

Fresh frozen plasma (FFP) is the fluid portion of blood after centrifugation to remove the RBCs. Due to freezing the plasma, all clotting factors (especially V and VII) are preserved except for platelets.

Administration of plasma is indicated when there is a coagulopathy or hypovolemia with little or no actual blood loss, for example, in burns and crush injuries. In an emergency, FFP may be used as a volume expander in hypovolemic bleeds until fresh whole blood is available.

Cryoprecipitates

Cryoimmunoglobulins are serum proteins that precipitate at temperatures below 20°C. Cryoimmunoglobulins must be obtained and processed at temperatures above 20°C and ideally before refrigeration, which may cause cryoproteins to be caught in the blood clots. Many authorities believe that cryoprecipitates are antigen-antibody protein compounds.

Cryoprecipitates usually compose 20–30 ml/unit of blood and must be infused immediately after thawing. Cryoprecipitates contain factors VIII and XIII, and fibrinogen. It is not uncommon to infuse as many as 30 bags of cryoprecipitates at one time, using a special transfusion administration set.

The administration of cryoprecipitates is indicated in disseminated intravascular coagulation (DIC), hemophilia A, and von Willebrand's disease.

Platelets

Less than 40,000–50,000 platelets/mm^3 is considered inadequate for hemostasis. Prolonged bleeding time is a better index of the need for platelet transfusion than an actual platelet count. There is an approximate increase of 10,000/unit (platelet)/mm^3. A post-platelet transfusion bleeding time is the most accurate index of response to therapy.

In thrombocytopenia, splenomegaly, and DIC, platelet transfusions are useful until more definitive therapy can be instituted. Alloimmunity may require cross-matching to have any value for platelet transfusion. Platelets can be safely kept at room temperatures for up to 3 days and are inactivated if refrigerated.

Volume Expanders

Albumin, hetastarch (Hespan), and, in some institutions, dextran 40 and dextran 70 are used as volume expanders.

Salt-Poor Albumin

This is a concentrate of human serum albumin packaged in 50-ml ampules with a total protein of 12.5 g in 50- to 100-ml amounts. It is not low in sodium content, nor does it supply any clotting factors. Its sole value is its blood volume expansion, increasing colloid osmotic pressure for up to 24 hr (time may be as low as 4 hr).

Hetastarch (Hespan)

Hetastarch is a large, glucose-based colloidal volume expander. It has approximately the same molecular weight as albumin and similar volume expansion properties. Only about 20% of the volume of crystalloid solutions (lactated Ringer's or normal saline) is necessary with hetastarch to achieve similar hemodynamic responses. Normally, hetastarch is administered in a 6% solution. Hetastarch is cleared via renal excretion in about 24–36 hr. While similar to albumin in volume expansion, it has the advantage of costing only about one-third as much as albumin.

Dextran

This is commercially available in two forms: dextran 70 (Macrodex) or dextran 40 (low-molecular-weight dextran [LMWD]).

Dextran 70 is a 6% solution in 0.9 normal saline or D_5W composed of both small and large molecules. It has colloid effects similar to those of plasma.

Dextran's greatest value lies in its expansion properties in addition to its lowering of blood viscosity. The lower blood viscosity is due to a lower hematocrit and reduction of platelet and RBC aggregations, which improve tissue perfusion. LMWD may help prevent a vascular thrombus occlusion of a vessel or graft.

Major complications of dextran use are allergic reactions, impaired coagulation (due to interference with platelet aggregation), and difficulty in future type-matching and cross-matching attempts for whole blood infusions. The allergic reactions may range from urticaria to anaphylaxis, which may occur immediately or after more than 30 min. Nausea, vomiting, and hypotension may occur.

Dextran therapy is not indicated in oliguric patients, CHF patients, and patients with blood-clotting dyscrasias. Its use has markedly decreased over the past years.

Granulocytes

Centers performing leukopheresis have the ability to filter out granulocytes. Each unit is about 200–300 ml, and the recipient must be compatible with the donor. An infusion of granulocytes improves phagocytosis from the marginal cells, not increasing the already circulating white blood cell pool. The marginal cells are those being released from the bone marrow.

It is common for the patient to have fever and chills during granulocyte infusion. Steroids and antihistamines given before the infusion will help control the fever, whereas meperidine hydrochloride (Demerol) will control the chills.

Reactions to Blood and Component Therapy

In spite of meticulous procedures for blood and component therapy, reactions do occur. There are four major reactions.

1. Circulatory overload occurs when too much fluid or too rapid an infusion is administered to patients with underlying cardiac, renal, liver, pulmonary, or hematologic disease. With proper monitoring and assessment, circulatory overload should not occur. If it does occur, prompt and appropriate intervention will remove sufficient fluid to restore the normal fluid status.
2. A bacterial reaction to transfusion therapy is the most common reaction and is characterized by the development of a fever in a previously afebrile patient. If the patient is febrile, a rising temperature may indicate a reaction.
3. Allergic reactions may occur with almost any product transfused. A slight reaction may be manifested by a mild urticaria. A severe allergic reaction is indicated by anaphylaxis that may or may not be reversible.
4. A hemolytic reaction usually occurs within the first 30 min of the transfusion. It results in actual hemolysis of the RBCs, and the transfusion must be stopped. A Coombs' test will diagnose this problem.

Clinical Presentation

The signs and symptoms will differ with the type of reaction, length of transfusion, substance being infused, and intensity of the reaction. Common signs and symptoms may include chills, fever, hives, hypotension, cardiac palpitations, tachycardia, flushing of the skin, headache, loss of consciousness, nausea and vomiting, shortness of breath, back pain, and hemoglobinuria. In some instances, warmth along the vein carrying the infusion may be detected.

Nursing Intervention

The nurse must immediately stop the infusion (saving the substance being transfused) and keep the vein open with 0.9 normal saline. Accurate assessment of patient status must be completed quickly and efficiently for a comparison with pretransfusion baseline data. The physician and the blood bank are notified of the reaction, and physician's orders are carried out. If the reaction is anaphylactic, emergency resuscitative measures are instituted while personnel contact the physician and laboratory and save the substance being transfused.

Nursing support of the patient and family is best achieved by rapid but efficient and professional conduct in instituting all necessary interventions. Education as to the cause of the reaction may prevent a recurrence.

Clotting Factors

Confusion often occurs with the nomenclature assigned to the specific clotting factors. Consequently, an international committee agreed that all clotting factors would be designated by roman numerals for the inactive clotting factors. It was further agreed that once activated, the clotting factors would be identified by the roman numeral and a subscript "a." Table 26–4 lists the clotting factors and their synonyms. There is no designated factor VI.

Most of the clotting factors are found in circulating blood, the blood elements, and tissues surrounding and within the microcirculatory system. Clotting factors I (fibrinogen), II (prothrombin), and V, VII, IX, and X are synthesized in the liver. Factors XI and XIII may also be synthesized in the liver. Factor VIII is most likely synthesized by macrophages in the spleen. Lymphocytes and the bone marrow may work in conjunction with the macrophages to form factor VIII.

Four clotting factors, factors II, VII, IX, and X, are dependent on vitamin K for synthesis by the liver. Research indicates that factor XI may also be vitamin K-dependent. It is known that at least 30 substances may be connected with the clotting process; however, the 17 listed in Table 26–4 are the most significant.

TABLE 26–4. CLOTTING FACTORS AND THEIR SYNONYMS

Factor	Synonym
I	Fibrinogen
Ia	Fibrin
II	Prothrombin
IIa	Thrombin
III	Thromboplastin
IV	Calcium
V	Acglobulin (labile factor, proaccelerin)
VII	Proconvertin (autoprothrombin I)
VIIa	Convertin
VIII	Antihemophiliac globulin
IX	Christmas factor (autoprothrombin II), plasma thromboplastin component
IXa	Activated plasma thromboplastin component
X	Stuart–Prower factor (autoprothrombin III)
XI	Plasma thromboplastin antecedent
XII	Hageman factor
XIIa	Activated Hageman factor
XIII	Fibrin-stabilizing factor

TREATMENTS FOR HEMATOLOGIC AND IMMUNOLOGIC DISORDERS

Neutropenia

Treatment for neutropenia involves administering colony stimulating factors such as neupogen. This medication stimulates granulocyte precursors and must be given intravenously or subcutaneously. The dosage is 5 to 7.5 µg/kg 3–7 times per week.

Anemia

Certain anemias can be treated with epogen injections. This is the erythropoietin hormone produced by recombinant DNA technology. The usual dosage is 100 units/kg 3 times per week. The route must be intravenously or subcutaneously because of poor bioavailability when given orally.

Infection

At the first indication of infection, the patient is pancultured. On an empirical basis, antimicrobial coverage is generally aimed at bacterial infection. Of course, once culture results are obtained, the antimicrobial regimen can be individualized. Refer to Table 26–5 for a list of commonly used antimicrobials. Antimicrobials have potentially serious side effects and require careful monitoring by the nurse. Some of the undesirable side effects possible with these agents include bone marrow suppression, a

TABLE 26–5. ANTIMICROBIALS COMMONLY USED AGAINST INFECTIONS IN THE IMMUNOCOMPROMISED HOST

Type of Infection	Antimicrobial
Bacterial	Penicillin
	Cephalosporin
	Aminoglycoside
	Vancomycin
	Fluroquinolones
Fungal	Nystatin
	Ketoconazole
	5-Flucytosine
	Amphotericin B
	Itraconazole
Viral	Acyclovir
	Ganciclovir
	Foscarnet
Protozoal	Trimethoprim/sulfamethoxazole (Septra)
	Pentamidine

change in the normal body flora allowing colonization by more pathogenic hospital-acquired organisms, development of resistance by the organism, and liver and kidney toxicity.

Often critically ill patients in the intensive care unit require a combination of antimicrobial therapies, thus making benefits versus adverse effects a delicate balance.

When using antibiotic therapy, you must give careful attention to the administration schedule as well as culture results. Organism resistance is becoming more evident. Vancomycin-resistant staphylococcus has been demonstrated in laboratory settings and vancomycin-resistant enterococcus is evident in many hospitals in the United States. These examples are the main reason hospitals have antibiotic restriction policies.

Included in treatment should be appropriate infection control. Isolation should be used according to disease specifications. The goal is to decrease nosocomial infections.

Immunodeficiency

Finally, the treatment for HIV/AIDS is ever changing. New medications are being studied and approved by the Food and Drug Administration quicker than ever before. The drugs will be broken down into the categories of antiretrovirals, prophylaxis, and treatment for this chapter (Table 26–6). Antiretrovirals should be offered to every HIV-infected patient. However, they do require close monitoring because of their side effects, such as bone marrow suppression, peripheral neuropathy, and gastrointestinal upset. Nucleoside analog combination therapy, such as AZT+ D4T+ 3TC, has been proven to be the most beneficial. Recently, protease inhibitors were approved, and are used in combination with the nucleoside analogs. Refer to Chapter 27 for more information on HIV disease. Drugs for prophylaxis and treatment of various opportunistic infections, such as PCP, MAC, toxo, and CMV.

Pneumocystis carinii pneumonia, *Mycobacterium avium* complex, and cytomegalovirus are listed in Table 26–7.

TABLE 26–6. ANTIRETROVIRAL TREATMENTS

Drug	Dosage	Side effects
Nucleoside analogs		
Retrovir AZT	200 mg, PO, tid	Bone marrow suppression, GI upset, peripheral neuropathy
DDI Videx	200 mg, PO, bid	Pancreatitis, elevated LFTs, thrombocytopenia, diarrhea
DDC Hivid	0.75 mg, PO, tid	Peripheral neuropathy, stomatitis
D4T Zerit	30–40 mg, PO, bid	Peripheral neuropathy, pancreatitis
3TC Epivir	150 mg, PO, bid	Minimal
Protease inhibitors		
Saquinavir Indinavir	600 mg, PO, tid	Poor bioavailability
Ritonavir Norvir	600 mg, PO, bid	Large number of drug interactions
Inivase Crixivan	800 mg, PO, tid	Unknown

LFTs, liver function tests

TABLE 26–7. THERAPEUTIC AND PROPHYLACTIC DRUG REGIMENS FOR HIV

Pathogen	Indication	First Choice	Alternatives
			Preventive Regimens
Strongly recommended as standard of care:			
Pneumocystis carinii	CD4+ count of <200/μl *or* unexplained fever for ≥2 w *or* oropharyngeal candidiasis	TMP-SMZ, 1 DS PO qd (AI)	TMP-SMZ, 1 SS PO qd (AI) *or* 1 DS PO tiw (AII); dapsone, 50 mg PO bid *or* 100 mg PO qd (AI); dapsone, 50 mg PO qd, *plus* pyrimethamine, 50 mg PO qw, *plus* leucovorin, 25 mg PO qw (AI): dapsone, 200 mg PO qw, *plus* pyrimethamine, 75 mg PO qw, *plus* leucovorin, 25 mg PO qw (AI): aerosolized pentamidine, 300 mg qm via Respirgard II nebulizer (AI)
Mycobacterium tuberculosis			
Isoniazid-sensitive	TST reaction of ≥5 mm *or* prior positive TST result without treatment *or* contact with case of active tuberculosis	Isoniazid, 300 mg PO, *plus* pyridoxine, 50 mg PO qd × 12 mo (AI); *or* isoniazid, 900 mg PO, *plus* pyridoxine, 50 mg PO biw × 12 mo (BIII)	Rifampin, 600 mg PO qd × 12 mo (BII)
Isoniazid-resistant	Same as above: high probability of exposure to isoniazid-resistant tuberculosis	Rifampin, 600 mg PO qd × 12 mo (BII)	Rifabutin, 300 mg PO qd × 12 mo (CIII)
Multidrug-resistant (isoniazid and rifampin)	Same as above: high probability of exposure to multidrug-resistant tuberculosis	Choice of drugs requires consultation with public health authorities	None
Toxoplasma gondii	IgG antibody to *Toxoplasma* and CD4+ count of <100/μl	TMP-SMZ, 1 DS PO qd (AII)	TMP-SMZ, 1 SS PO qd *or* 1 DS PO tiw (AII); dapsone, 50 mg PO qd, *plus* pyrimethamine, 50 mg PO qw, *plus* leucovorin, 25 mg PO qw (AI)
Recommended for consideration in all patients:			
Streptococcus pneumoniae	All patients	Pneumococcal vaccine, 0.5 ml IM × 1 (BIII)	None
Mycobacterium avium complex	CD4+ count of <75/μl	Rifabutin, 300 mg PO qd (BII)	Clarithromycin, 500 mg PO bid. (CIII); azithromycin, 500 mg PO tiw (CIII)
Not recommended for most patients; indicated for consideration *only* in selected populations or patients:			
Bacteria	Neutropenia	Granulocyte colony stimulating factor, 5–10 μg/kg SC qd × 2–4 w; *or* granulocyte-macrophage colony stimulating factor, 250 μg/m², IV over 2 h qd × 2–4 w (CIII)	None
Candida species	CD4+ count of <50/μl	Fluconazole, 100–200 mg PO qd (CI)	Ketoconazole, 200 mg PO qd (CIII)
Cryptococcus neoformans	CD4+ count of <50/μl	Fluconazole, 200 mg PO qd (BI)	Itraconazole, 200 mg PO qd (CIII)
Histoplasma capsulatum	CD4+ count of <50/μl, endemic geographic region	Itraconazole, 200 mg PO qd (CIII)	Fluconazole, 200 mg PO qd (CIII)
Coccidioides immitis	CD4+ count of <50/μl, endemic geographic region	Fluconazole, 200 mg PO qd (CIII)	Itraconazole, 200 mg PO qd (CIII)

Pathogen	Indication	First choice	Alternatives
Cytomegalovirus	CD4⁻ count of <50/μl and CMV antibody positivity	Oral ganciclovir, 1 g PO tid (CIII: only preliminary data available)	None
Unkown (herpesviruses?)	CD4⁻ count of <200/μl	Acyclovir, 800 mg PO qid (CIII)	Acyclovir, 200 mg PO tid/qid (CIII)
Recommended for consideration:			
Hepatitis B virus	All susceptible (anti-HBc-negative) patients	Energix-B, 20 μg IM × 3 (BII): or Recombivax HB, 10 μg IM × 3 (BII)	None
Influenza virus	All patients (annually, before influenza season)	Whole or split virus, 0.5 ml IM/y (BIII)	Rimantadine, 100 mg PO bid (CIII), or amantadine, 100 mg PO bid (CIII)
Recommended for life as standard of care:			
Pneumocystis carinii	Prior *P. carinii* pneumonia	TMP-SMZ, 1 DS PO qd (AI)	TMP-SMZ, 1 SS PO qd (AI) or 1 DS PO tiw (AII); dapsone, 50 mg PO bid or 100 mg PO qd (AI); dapsone, 50 mg PO qd, *plus* pyrimethamine, 50 mg PO qw, *plus* leucovorin, 25 mg PO qw (AI); dapsone, 200 mg PO qw, *plus* pyrimethamine 75 mg PO qw, *plus* leucovorin, 25 mg PO qw (AI); aerosolized pentamidine, 300 mg qm via Respirgard II nebulizer (AI)
Toxoplasma gondii	Prior toxoplasmic encephalitis	Sulfadiazine, 1.0–1.5 g PO q6h, *plus* pyrimethamine, 25–75 mg PO qd, *plus* leucovorin, 10–25 mg PO qd–qid (AII)	Clindamycin, 300–450 mg PO q6–8h, *plus* pyrimethamine, 25–75 mg PO qd, *plus* leucovorin, 10–25 mg PO qd–qid, (AII)
Mycobacterium avium complex	Documented disseminated disease	Clarithromycin, 500 mg PO bid, *plus* one or more of the following: ethambutol, 15 mg/kg PO qd; clofazimine, 100 mg PO qd; rifabutin, 300 mg PO qd; ciprofloxacin, 500–750 mg PO bid (BIII)	Azithromycin, 500 mg PO qd, *plus* one or more of the following: ethambutol, 15 mg/kg PO qd; clofazimine, 100 mg PO qd; rifabutin, 300 mg PO qd; ciprofloxacin, 500–750 mg PO bid (BIII)
Cytomegalovirus	Prior end-organ disease	Ganciclovir, 5–6 mg/kg IV 5–7 d/w or 1000 mg PO tid (AI); *or* foscarnet, 90–120 mg/kg IV qd (AI)	Sustained-release implants used investigationally
Cryptococcus neoformans	Documented disease	Fluconazole, 200 mg PO qd (AI)	Itraconazole, 200 mg PO qd (BIII); amphotericin B, 0.6–1.0 mg/kg IV qw–tiw (AI)
Histoplasma capsulatum	Documented disease	Itraconazole, 200 mg PO bid (AII)	Amphotericin B, 1.0 mg/kg IV qw (AI); fluconazole, 200–400 mg PO qd (BIII)
Coccidioides immitis	Documented disease	Fluconazole, 200 mg PO qd (AII)	Amphotericin B, 1.0 mg/kg IV qw (AI); itraconazole, 200 mg PO bid§ (AII); ketoconazole, 400–800 mg PO qd (BII)
Salmonella species (non-*typhi*)	Bacteremia	Ciprofloxacin, 500 mg PO bid for several months (BII)	...
Recommended only if subsequent episodes are frequent or severe:			
Herpes simplex virus	Frequent/severe recurrences	Acyclovir, 200 mg PO tid or 400 mg PO bid (AI)	...
Candida species (oral, vaginal, or esophageal)	Frequent/severe recurrences	Fluconazole, 100–200 mg PO qd (AI)	Ketoconazole, 200 mg PO qd (BII); itraconazole, 100 mg PO qd (BII); clotrimazole troche, 10 mg or PO 5 × /d (BII); nystatin, 5 × 10⁵ U PO 5 × /d (CIII)

Hematologic and Immunologic Failure and Its Effects on Other Organ Systems

EDITORS' NOTE

The CCRN exam may contain two to eight questions on disorders of the immune system. Although specifics of different types of diseases, such as cancers, are not likely to be addressed on the exam, it is important to understand the general concepts presented in this chapter. Immunologic concepts are sometimes difficult to apply clinically, but the major concepts are important to the assessment and therapeutic interventions associated with critical-care immunology.

DISORDERS OF THE HEMATOLOGIC SYSTEM

Anemia

Definition and Etiology
Anemia is the most common problem of the erythrocyte (red blood cell; RBC). It is a clinical sign defined as (1) a reduction in the number of RBCs, (2) a reduction in the quantity of hemoglobin, and/or (3) a reduction in the volume of RBCs. There are numerous causes of anemia. Table 27–1 outlines the classification of anemias.

Clinical Presentation
The signs and symptoms of anemia are the result of tissue hypoxia or the compensatory mecha-nisms activated to prevent damage resulting from hypoxia. Persons are symptomatic at varying levels. Someone with mild anemia may be asymptomatic. Anemia may be the first indication of a serious underlying disease such as cancer or renal failure. If it occurs gradually, adaptation allows for minimal signs and symptoms. A person with rapid onset of anemia may be very symptomatic. The signs and symptoms associated with anemia are as follows: increased pulse, respiration, and pulse pressure; decreased blood pressure; palpitations; chest pain; dyspnea on exertion; fatigue; weakness; vertigo; bone tenderness; and delayed wound healing.

Diagnosis
Laboratory findings that are indicative of anemia are (1) decreased hemoglobin and hematocrit, (2) decreased RBC indices, (3) increased reticulocyte count, and (4) decreased erythrocyte count.

Nursing Intervention
Nursing interventions for the patient with anemia are based upon the principles of minimizing complications, conserving energy, and instituting medical therapies. The key interventions include the following:

1. History
   a. Signs of blood loss
   b. Bleeding tendencies
   c. Exposure to marrow toxins (drugs, radiation, chemicals)

d. Previous history of anemia

e. Surgical history (e.g., gastric resection)

f. Changes in nutritional status

2. Physical assessment

a. Oxygenation: Vital signs, lung sounds, tolerance of activity

b. Skin, mucous membranes: Pallor, jaundice, purpura, petechiae, intravenous line sites, wounds, indwelling catheters, stomatitis

c. Gastrointestinal: Ascites, splenomegaly

d. Mobility: Paresthesias, impaired sensation, bone pain (sternum, ribs, vertebrae)

3. Minimize energy expenditure by:

a. Organizing activities according to patient tolerance

b. Planning rest periods

c. Limiting external stimulation

d. Preventing chills

4. Maintain skin integrity

5. Promote a diet adequate in protein, iron, vitamins, and minerals

6. Maintain physical safety (e.g., assist with ambulation if the patient is dizzy)

7. Institute an appropriate oral hygiene program

Thrombocytopenia

Thrombocytopenia is a quantitative decrease in the number of circulating platelets. The risk of bleeding increases as the platelet count decreases. Normal platelet count is 100,000 to 300,000/mm^3. Usually persons are placed on bleeding precautions when the platelet count falls below 50,000/mm^3. The risk of spontaneous bleeding increases at a platelet count of less than 20,000/mm^3. Table 27–2 outlines causes of thrombocytopenia.

Clinical Presentation

Signs and symptoms associated with thrombocytopenia include petechiae, bruising, ecchymosis, hematemesis, hemoptysis, hematuria, vaginal bleeding, rectal bleeding, blood in stools, anemia, and active bleeding from mucous membranes, wounds, indwelling catheters, and sites of invasive procedures.

Treatment

Platelet transfusions are administered to thrombocytopenic patients who are actively bleeding, undergoing invasive procedures, or at increased risk of spontaneous bleeding. Platelet transfusions

can be a random donor pooling or a single-donor human leukocyte antigen (HLA)-matched product. Upon exposure to an increasing number of platelet transfusions, the patient may become refractory to the benefits of the transfusion as a result of antibody formation to platelets. A person with fever usually has increased destruction of platelets. A 1- to 2-hr post-transfusion platelet count is performed to document the effectiveness of the platelet transfusion. Reactions or complica-

TABLE 27–1. CLASSIFICATION OF ANEMIA

I. Blood loss
  A. Acute
  B. Chronic

II. Deficient RBC production
  A. Iron deficiency
  B. Vitamin B$_{12}$ deficiency
  C. Folic acid deficiency
  D. Bone marrow failure or suppression
    1. Myelofibrosis
    2. Aplastic anemia
    3. Marrow toxin (drugs, radiation)
    4. Infectious agents

III. Excessive RBC destruction
  A. Hemolytic anemia
  B. Defective glycolysis (G6PD deficiency)
  C. Membrane abnormalities
  D. Physical causes (prosthetic heart valves)

IV. Defective hemoglobin synthesis
  A. Thalassemias
  B. Sickle cell anemia

V. Anemias of chronic disease
  A. Renal disease
  B. Liver disease
  C. Endocrine disorders
  D. Cancers

TABLE 27–2. CAUSES OF THROMBOCYTOPENIA

Symptom	Cause
Decreased production	Leukemia
	Lymphoma
	Multiple myeloma
	Metastatic cancer
	Chemotherapy
	Radiation therapy
	Drugs (thiazides, estrogen)
	Alcohol
Increased destruction	Autoimmune disorders
	Idiopathic thrombocytopenic as in purpura
	Malignant disorders
	Disseminated intravascular coagulation
	Infectious agents
Abnormal platelet function	Aspirin
Decreased availability	Sequestration in spleen

tions of platelet transfusions are similar to those of whole blood transfusions.

Nursing Intervention

Nursing interventions are based upon (1) protection of the patient from bleeding and associated complications and (2) early detection of bleeding. Most institutions have policies (bleeding precautions, platelet precautions) that are instituted when the platelet count is less than 50,000/mm^3. A sign is placed near the patient to alert all health team members that the patient is at risk of bleeding. Key interventions include:

1. Bleeding precautions for a platelet count of less than 50,000/mm^3
2. Assessment of sites of potential bleeding
   a. Skin
   b. Mucous membranes
   c. Indwelling catheter sites
3. Assessment of bodily excrement for occult and frank bleeding
   a. Urine
   b. Stool
   c. Sputum
   d. Pad count in menstruating females
4. Routine neurological assessment
5. Prevention of trauma
   a. Use soft toothbrushes or toothettes for oral hygiene
   b. Use electric razors
   c. Coordinate blood sampling to avoid multiple venipunctures
   d. Institute bowel routine to prevent constipation
   e. Avoid intramuscular injections
   f. Avoid prolonged use of tourniquets
   g. Avoid use of urinary catheters
   h. Use soft restraints only when absolutely necessary
   i. Use padded siderails when the patient is in bed
   j. Assist the patient with ambulation, if indicated
   k. Institute measures to minimize vomiting
6. Avoid use of aspirin or aspirin-containing compounds
7. Control of temperature elevations
8. Monitoring of pertinent laboratory data
   a. Hemoglobin
   b. Hematocrit
   c. Platelet count
   d. Pre- and postplatelet transfusion counts

Hemophilia and Von Willebrand's Disease

EDITORS' NOTE

It is unlikely that these two conditions will be on the CCRN exam. This section is included simply to provide a more complete description of abnormal coagulation concepts.

Hemophilia is the name given to three inherited disorders that have bleeding in common. The bleeding is due to a lack of or deficiency in a plasma clotting factor. Von Willebrand's disease is included in this section since it also involves a deficient clotting factor.

Etiology

Hemophilia A and B are sex-linked recessive disorders. They affect men mainly, but do occur rarely in women. It is more common that the female is a "carrier" and genetically transmits these diseases to the male. Hemophilia C is an autosomal trait. Von Willebrand's disease is an autosomal dominant mode of inheritance, so it should occur equally among men and women. Von Willebrand's disease is an actual lack of factor VIII. A complete absence of this factor may occur or there may be a reduced amount of structurally normal factor. Hemorrhaging may occur in a muscle mass, forming an extremely painful hematoma. These hematomas (masses) press against nerves, resulting in transient motor and/or sensory loss. Gastrointestinal bleeding is the next most common symptom, in which there is often no evidence of ulceration to account for the bleed. Epistaxis is also common.

Joint deformity with eventual crippling may occur. Hematuria is often present in hemophiliacs and may continue for weeks without a known cause.

Hemorrhage into the central nervous system (CNS) is rare in hemophiliacs but is extremely severe when it does occur. It is not uncommon for these patients to die secondary to hemorrhage into the CNS. This bleeding is often caused by trauma.

Hemophiliacs seem to fluctuate in the frequency and severity of the bleed during the year. Hemophiliacs tend to bleed less with age. The reasons for these two variables are unknown at this time. All of these symptoms except hemarthrosis also occur in von Willebrand's disease also.

Diagnosis

A familial tendency to excessive bleeding is known, and the family frequently reports the diagnosis as "the bleeding disease." The clinical condition can be verified by laboratory tests. The partial thromboplastin time (PTT) is prolonged. Factor assays reveal decreased factor VIII in hemophilia A and normal to decreased factor VII in von Willebrand's disease. Factor IX is decreased in hemophilia B. Platelet aggregation is normal in hemophilia but decreased in von Willebrand's disease.

Treatment

The goal of therapy is to prevent crippling deformities and prolong life expectancy. A cure is not available at this time. Stopping the bleed and increasing the plasma levels of the deficient factors will help prevent the degenerative stages of joint destruction.

In hemophilia A, cryoprecipitated antihemolytic factor (AHF) is administered to raise the factor to 25% of normal to allow coagulation. Surgery requires increasing the AHF to 50% of normal. If the AHF is not available, fresh frozen plasma or plasma fraction, rich in AHF, may be administered.

In hemophilia B, administration of fresh frozen plasma or of factor IX itself will increase the blood level of factor IX.

In von Willebrand's disease, the infusion of cryoprecipitates or blood fractions rich in factor VIII and von Willebrand's factor (VWF) will shorten the bleeding time. Prior to surgery or in bleeding states, an intravenous infusion of cryoprecipitate or fresh frozen plasma is needed to raise the factor VIII level to 50% of normal.

A patient with hemophilia or von Willebrand's disease needs the care of a hematologist for surgical procedures and dental extraction.

Nursing Intervention

During hemophiliac bleeds, administration of the deficient clotting factor or plasma is ordered. AHF is effective for 48–72 hr. This means that repeat transfusions may be required to stop the bleed.

Apply cold compresses to the injured area, raise the injured area if possible, and cleanse any wounds. Thrombin-soaked fibrin or sponge may be utilized for wound care in some institutions. Restrict activity for 48 hr after the bleeding is controlled to prevent recurrence. Control pain with analgesics such as acetaminophen (Tylenol), propoxyphene hydrochloride (Darvon), codeine, or meperidine hydrochloride (Demerol). Avoid intramuscular injections to prevent a hematoma at the injection site. Aspirin is contraindicated because it affects platelet aggrega-

tion. If the patient bleeds into a joint, immediately elevate the joint and immobilize it in a slightly flexed position. Watch for signs of further bleeding such as increased pain and swelling, fever, or possible shock-like symptoms. Monitor the patient's PTT.

In von Willebrand's disease monitor the patient's bleeding time for 24–48 hr after surgery and observe for signs of new bleeding. During a new bleed, elevate the injured part and apply cold compresses and gentle pressure to the bleeding site.

Education as to the causative factors and treatment of minor injuries is indicated, as well as discussion of conditions for which the patient should seek medical attention.

Educate the patient and parents (if the patient is a child) in how to control minor trauma and warn against using aspirin or aspirin-containing drugs. Refer the parents to a genetic counseling service.

The National Hemophilia Society, local hemophiliac groups, genetic evaluation, or psychotherapy may be useful for fostering better acceptance of the disease and forming an association with other patients who are managing successfully.

Sickle Cell Disease

EDITORS' NOTE

Sickle cell disease is not likely to be on the CCRN exam. It is included primarily to give a better picture of abnormal coagulation conditions.

Sickle cell disease is also referred to as sickle cell anemia because of the pathophysiology.

Pathophysiology

With an abnormal hemoglobin molecule known as hemoglobin S, the RBCs become insoluble when hypoxic. Because of this, RBCs become rigid, rough, and elongated. The hemoglobin becomes shaped like a crescent or sickle.

Sickling hemolyzes and altered cells collect in the capillaries and small vessels. This impairs normal circulation and results in pain, swelling, tissue infarctions, and anoxia. This increases blood viscosity, causing further impairment of circulating blood. Blockages extend in the capillaries and small vessels, leading to further sickling obstruction. A vicious cycle has started.

Etiology

This congenital hemolytic anemia occurs most often in blacks. The causative factor is a defect in the hemoglobin S molecule.

There is a homozygous and a heterozygous inheritance. Homozygous inheritance involves the substitution of the amino acid valine for glutamic acid in the beta hemoglobin chain, resulting in the disease itself. In heterozygous inheritance, the patient carries the sickle cell trait but may be asymptomatic.

Clinical Presentation

Several types of crises occur, but common to all are the symptoms and physical findings of tachycardia, cardiomegaly, murmurs, pulmonary infarctions, chronic fatigue, dyspnea (with or without exertion), hematomegaly, jaundice or pallor, aching bones, chest pain, ischemic leg ulcers, and increased susceptibility to infection. Infection, stress, dehydration, and hypoxic states (e.g., strenuous exercise) may induce a crisis.

The most common crisis is the painful crisis. This is a vaso-occlusive or infarctive crisis. It does not usually develop for the first 5 years but then appears sporadically. It is a result of RBCs obstructing blood vessels by rigid, tangled sickle cells. Tissue anoxia and possible necrosis occur, causing severe thoracic, abdominal, muscular, and bone pain. Jaundice may occur along with dark urine and a low-grade fever. After the crisis resolves, infection may occur within 4 days to several weeks secondary to occlusion and necrosis of the blood vessel.

Autosplenectomy occurs with long-standing disease. Autosplenectomy is the process of splenic damage and scarring, inducing shrinkage of the spleen such that it is no longer palpable. After autosplenectomy, the patient is very susceptible to diplococcal pneumonia, which is rapidly fatal without immediate aggressive treatment. Lethargy, sleepiness, fever, and/or apathy occur as signs and symptoms of infection.

Aplastic (megaloblastic) crisis is a result of bone marrow suppression and is often associated with a viral infection. Signs and symptoms include fever, markedly decreased bone marrow activity, pallor, lethargy, dyspnea, possible coma, and RBC hemolysis.

Acute sequestration develops in some children from 8 months to 2 years old. There is a sudden, massive entrapment of RBCs in the liver and spleen. Symptoms of this rare crisis are lethargy and pallor. If not treated, it progresses to hypovolemic shock and death. This is the leading cause of death in sickle cell children under 1 year old.

A hemolytic crisis is rare and is usually confined to those who have a glucose-6-phosphate dehydrogenase (G6PD) deficiency. This crisis usually occurs as an infectious response to complications of sickle cell disease rather than to the disease itself.

Diagnosis

A family history and the clinical picture point toward sickle cell disease. A blood smear shows sickle-celled RBCs rather than normal RBCs. Hemoglobin electrophoresis showing hemoglobin S is pathognomonic.

Treatment

Treatment is palliative, since no cure and no reversible treatment have been established for this disease. Usually home care will suffice, but in a crisis state, hospitalization is needed.

Treatment of aplastic crisis includes transfusion of packed RBCs, oxygen, and supportive therapies. In sequestration crisis, treatment includes whole-blood transfusion, oxygen, and large amounts of oral or intravenous fluids.

Nursing Intervention

Supportive care during exacerbations will help avoid such crises and provide a more normal life. During the crisis, apply warm compresses to painful areas and cover the child with a blanket. Avoid cold compresses, since their use may result in vasoconstriction and prolong the crisis. Encourage bedrest and administer analgesics, antipyretics, and antibiotics as ordered.

Patient and family education will help avoid some crises. Such education would include avoidance of drinking large amounts of cold fluids, swimming in cold water, clothing that restricts circulation, and any activity that would produce hypoxia, such as flying in small (unpressurized) aircraft. A large fluid intake will prevent dehydration and decrease blood viscosity, reducing the chance of another crisis. Stress the importance of childhood immunizations and prompt treatment for infections.

THE IMMUNE SYSTEM

Cells of the Immune System
Infection

The ultimate effect of immunodeficiency is an impaired ability of the body to defend against foreign antigens. This leads to an increased susceptibility to infection and certain other diseases believed to sometimes be linked to an impaired immune status, such as cancer and autoimmune disorders. The incidence of infection, the most common complication of immunosuppression, increases with both the duration and the severity of the immunodeficiency. In fact, the highest risk of infection occurs when the leukocyte (white blood cell; WBC) count is less than 1000 cells/mm^3 and the neutrophils number less than 500 cells/mm^3. The infections that develop are related to the underlying immune defect and the organisms to which the individual is now most susceptible. Most infections associated with immunosuppression are opportunistic or secondary to endogenous organisms that do not cause infection in the presence of a normal functioning immune system. However, many of the organisms colonizing a hospitalized patient are actually acquired during the hospitalization. Also, the infections that develop in immunosuppressed patients tend to be more severe, to be of longer duration, and to have a greater potential for dissemination than those seen in the general population. The lung is the most common site of serious infectious complications. Refer to Table 27–3 for a review of common infections in the immunocompromised host.

Immunosuppression

EDITORS' NOTE

This section provides an overview of immunosuppression and related nursing care. Expect one to three questions based on the content to be on the exam. For specific causes of immunosuppression (i.e., AIDS/HIV and organ transplantation), see the section on disorders of the immune system which follows this section.

The immune system serves many functions, such as surveillance, homeostasis, and defense. Immunosuppression is an alteration in normal immune protective responses, a state of decreased responsiveness of the immune system. The individual who cannot mount an effective immune response is said to be anergic. Anergy can occur as a natural phenomenon in the life cycle, as in the cases of the very young and the elderly, or it can occur as a result of intentional and unintentional immunosuppression, as in organ transplantation and HIV/AIDS.

Opportunistic Infection

Immunosuppressed individuals are vulnerable to opportunistic infections. Opportunistic infections are caused by organisms that are ubiquitous in the environment (internal and external) but rarely cause disease in the immunocompetent host. Organisms responsible for opportunistic infections are listed in Table 27–3. Natural protection from opportunistic infection depends on the presence of normal and intact innate and acquired immune mechanisms.

The three major determinants of nosocomial infection are the hospital environment, microorganisms, and host defense. Hospitalization and the critical care environment alone predisposes an individual to an increased risk of infection. Hospitalization initiates the conversion of normal cutaneous flora to colonization of a new microbial population, that which is prevalent in the hospital. Colonization by itself is not harmful to the individual. However, when the first lines of defense are broken or bypassed, colonization leads the way for infection.

Fifty percent of patients admitted to intensive care units (ICUs) become colonized with gram-negative bacteria within 72 hr. The major vector of these bacteria is the human hand. Nosocomial infections occur in 25–50% of patients admitted to ICUs. Infection is more prevalent in teaching hospitals and on surgical services. The most frequent types of nosocomial infections are urinary tract infections, wound infections, respiratory infections, and septicemia, in that order.

Other factors that predispose critically ill patients to infection include surgery, trauma, endotracheal intubation, shock, malnutrition, renal failure, liver failure, splenectomy, broad-spectrum antibiotic or corticosteroid therapy, and obesity.

Immunosuppressed individuals are usually neutropenic (see Chapter 25 for a discussion of the anatomy and physiology of neutrophils; see Chapter 26 for treatment). The longer the patient is neutropenic, the greater the chance for mortality (Table 27–4). In part, this is due to the fact that signs and symptoms of infection—redness, tenderness, swelling, and erythema—are often absent as a result of the lack of granulocytes. Sometimes, the only sign is fever. The immunosuppressed patient can be infected with bacteria, fungi, viruses, or a combination of these.

Nursing Care

Nursing care of the patient who is immunosuppressed is based on the nursing diagnosis of potential for infection related to specific, and many times

TABLE 27–3. COMMON INFECTIONS IN THE IMMUNOCOMPROMISED HOST

Site of Infection	Bacteria	Viruses	Fungi	Protozoa
Skin	*Staphylococcus aureus* *Staphylococcus epidermidis*	Herpes simplex virus Herpes varicella-zoster virus	*Candida*	
Oropharynx		Herpes simplex virus	*Candida*	
Gastrointestinal tract *histolytica*	Gram-negative rods *Mycobacterium avium-intracellulare*	Herpes simplex virus (esophagitis) Cytomegalovirus	*Candida*	*Ciardia lamblia* *Cryptosporidium* *Entamoeba*
Urinary tract	Gram-negative rods		*Candida*	
Lungs	Gram-negative rods *Mycobacterium tuberculosis* *Mycobacterium avium-intracellulare*	Cytomegalovirus	*Candida* *Aspergillus* *Histoplasma capsulatum*	*Pneumocystis carinii* *Toxoplasma gondii*
CNS	*Listeria monocytogenes* *Streptococcus pneumoniae* *Pseudomonas aeruginosa* *Haemophilus influenzae*	Herpes varicella-zoster virus Herpes simplex virus	*Cryptococcus neoformans* *Aspergillus*	*Toxoplasma gondii*
Blood			Gram-negative rods	*Candida*

TABLE 27–4. CAUSES OF DEATH IN NEUTROPENIC PATIENTS

Complication	% of Patients
Infection	35%
Hemorrhage	27%
Progression of disease	18%

Other
   Renal insufficiency
   Myocardial infarction
   Pulmonary edema
	20%

multiple, immunodeficiencies or a disruption in the natural protective barriers to microorganisms Table 27–5. The patient requires frequent and thorough physical assessments because the signs and symptoms of infection are often subtle in the immunocompromised host. Important points regarding assessment and interventions are the following.

Assessment

1. *History*
   a. Age
   b. Past infections
   c. Medications, noting those which are immunosuppressive
   d. Treatment which can be immunosuppressive (e.g., radiation therapy)
   e. Presenting signs and symptoms
   f. Coexisting systemic symptoms (weight loss, malaise, etc.)
2. *Physical examination*
   a. Inspect skin carefully, particularly noting conditions of skin folds, pressure points, and perirectal area (frequent site of infection in the immunocompromised host). Observe for:
      - localized redness or swelling (may not be present with neutropenia or lymphopenia)
      - excoriation
      - lesions, infections, or Kaposi's sarcoma
      - lymphadenopathy
   b. Closely inspect the mouth and throat, a frequent site of infection in the immunocompromised host. Note:
      - condition of teeth and gums (if infected, can cause sepsis)
      - lesions (candidiasis, herpes simplex, Kaposi's sarcoma)
   c. Monitor temperature and note pattern of elevation.
      - An elevated temperature is the best indication of infection in the immunosuppressed.
      - A temperature over 38°C for 12 or more hours is probably indicative of infection.
      - Fever is also part of the disease process of some disorders associated with immunosuppression (leukemia, lymphona, HIV infection).
   d. Assess breath sounds
      - Adventitious sounds are frequently absent or minimal at the onset of infection in the immunosuppressed patient.
      - Note respiratory rate, presence of cough, and character of sputum.

- Be prepared with ventilator support, since rapid deterioration in respiratory status can occur.
  e. Note complaints of tenderness and localized pain, as they may be indicators of infection.
  - Back pain
  - Burning on urination
  - Rectal discomfort with bowel movements
3. *Laboratory data*
   a. WBC (leukopenia or leukocytosis)
   - WBC differential
   - Absolute granulocyte count, especially if less than 500 cells/mm^3.
   - Lymphocyte count
   b. T4 count; T4:T8 ratio (indicators of immune status in patients with AIDS)

Interventions

1. Meticulous personal hygiene
   a. Prevent skin breakdown by turning the patient and using pressure-relieving devices.
   b. Avoid injury (will provide a port of entry for microorganisms), keep nails trim, use electric razor.
   c. Provide meticulous perirectal care.
   - Avoid taking rectal temperatures and using rectal suppositories and enemas because of fragile rectal mucosa and the possibility of causing a break in the mucosa.
   - Initiate a bowel regimen to avoid constipation or control diarrhea.
2. Good oral hygiene
   a. Brush oral cavity, using a soft toothbrush or toothettes.
   b. Moisturize lips and mucosa with water-soluble lubricant.
   c. If stomatitis is present, rinse mouth with normal saline every 2–4 hr.
   d. Avoid commercial mouthwashes.
   e. Advise patient to avoid smoking and use of alcohol.
   f. Encourage a soft bland diet and cool foods or provide nutritional support.
   g. Control pain.
   - Viscous lidocaine
   - Mixture of sodium bicarbonate (5 ml), Maalox (5 ml), 2% viscous lidocaine (5 ml), and diphenhydramine (5 mg). Swish in mouth for 3 min and swallow every 4 hr.

   h. Obtain order for appropriate antimicrobials if secondary infection is present.
3. Aseptic technique
   a. Minimize invasive procedures.
   b. Use smallest-gauge lumens possible on all invasive devices.
   c. Provide meticulous care of vascular access.
   d. Coordinate blood studies.
   e. Keep all systems closed as much as possible.
   f. Avoid transparent, occlusive dressings over drainage wounds (require the presence of WBCs collecting under the dressing to clean out the wound).
4. Manipulation of the environment to minimize exposure to organisms
   a. Eliminate sources of stagnant water (sources of gram-negative bacteria).
   - Change disposable tubing on ventilators daily.
   - Avoid cold mist humidifiers.
   b. Remove live plants and flowers from the room (sources of *Aspergillus*).
   c. Institute protective isolation when the WBC count is less than 1000 cells/mm^3 or the absolute granulocyte count is less than 500 cells/mm^3.
   d. Restrict exposure to persons with infection.
   e. Evaluate the appropriateness of a low bacterial diet.
   - Eliminate raw, unpeeled fruits and vegetables and uncooked eggs and meat from the diet.
   - Effectiveness in decreasing the incidence of infection is controversial.
5. Adequate nutrition
   a. Nutritional intake may be compromised by anorexia, fatigue, stomatitis, dysphagia, nausea and vomiting, and taste changes caused by some medications, including chemotherapy.
   b. Encourage a high-calorie, high-protein diet.
   c. Enteral feedings are preferable to parenteral nutrition because of decreased risk of infection.
6. Alleviation of stress
   a. Allow rest periods.
   b. Maintain day/night schedule as much as possible.
   c. Minimize environmental noise.
   d. Maximize comfort.
   e. Attend psychosocial needs.

TABLE 27–5. ETIOLOGY OF ACQUIRED IMMUNODEFICIENCY

Etiologic Condition	Immune Defect
Injury/Disease	
Burns	Disruption of natural barrier
	Impaired phagocytosis
	Deficient delayed hypersensitivity
Uremia	Abnormal neutrophil function
	Impaired cell-mediated immunity
Diabetes mellitus	Impaired neutrophil function
Cancer	
Solid tumors	Deficiency in cell-mediated immunity
	Impaired neutrophil function
Leukemias	Deficiency in humoral and cell-mediated immunity
Hodgkin's disease	Impaired cellular immunity
Non-Hodgkin's lymphoma	Impaired humoral or cellular immunity (depends on type of lymphocyte involved)
Multiple myeloma	Impaired humoral immunity
AIDS	Impaired cell-mediated immunity with subsequent deficiency in humoral immunity
Certain infections (influenza, cytomegalovirus, Epstein–Barr virus, mononucleosis, tuberculosis, candidiasis)	Depression of lymphocyte and monocyte function
Treatment/Medication	
Surgery	Disruption of natural barriers
	Lymphopenia
Splenectomy	Impaired humoral immunity
Radiation therapy	Neutropenia
	Lymphopenia
Anesthetic agents	Inhibition of phagocytosis
	Impaired humoral and cell-mediated immunity
Cytotoxic drugs (cancer chemotherapy)	Disruption of natural barriers (mucositis)
	Neutropenia
	Deficiencies in humoral and cell-mediated immunity
Steroids	Anti-inflammatory
	Suppressed functioning of neutrophils
	Deficiencies in humoral and cell-mediated immunity
Immunosuppressive agents (azathioprine, cyclosporine, antilymphocyte globulin)	Impaired cell-mediated immunity
Certain antibiotics (pentamidine gentamicin, Septra)	Leukopenia
	Neutropenia
Miscellaneous	
Extremes of age	Deficiencies in humoral and cell-mediated immunity
Protein-calorie malnutrition	Impaired phagocytosis
	Deficiencies in humoral and cell-mediated immunity
Stress	Exact mechanism of immunodeficiency unknown

DISORDERS OF THE IMMUNE SYSTEM

Acquired Immunodeficiency Syndrome

The acquired immunodeficiency syndrome, or AIDS, is the end point of infection by the human immunodeficiency virus (HIV), a retrovirus found in the body fluids of infected individuals. HIV is transmitted by sexual contact (either heterosexual or homosexual), exchange of bloods and body fluids, and perinatally. The profile of the high-risk groups affected by the disease to date include male homosexuals and bisexuals, intravenous drug users, hemophiliacs, blood transfusion recipients prior to

1985, and sexual partners of any of these individuals. However, since 1994, heterosexual individuals represent the group most infected.

Since recognition of the disease in 1981, much has been learned about the spectrum of HIV infection. Individuals who are infected may range from being asymptomatic to having systemic symptoms such as generalized persistent lymphadenopathy, fever, night sweats, diarrhea, and weight loss. AIDS itself is diagnosed when specific "indicator" diseases (i.e., diseases that indicate an underlying immunodeficiency) are present. The diagnosis, under most circumstances, also requires the person to be HIV seropositive. This is determined by enzyme-linked immunosorbent assay (ELISA) and Western blot laboratory tests, which screen for the antibody to HIV. The antibody develops an average of 6–12 weeks after exposure to the virus. The pattern of disease will vary from person to person. Some people have rapid progression of disease while others are considered long-term survivors.

Clinical Presentation

The immunodeficiency of AIDS is multifaceted. HIV primarily infects the T4 cell, and because of the rule of the T cell as the main coordinator of the immune response, devastating deficiencies occur in both the cell-mediated and humoral immune responses. The viral effects on the immune system include a profound lymphopenia and a reverse T4:T8 ratio (less than 1). As a result, the person with AIDS develops opportunistic infections. The opportunistic infections associated with AIDS tend to be severe and become disseminated, but they also tend to recur upon discontinuation of antimicrobial therapy. Most patients with AIDS die as a result of infection due to an organism normally protected against by T cells.

Some of the infections frequently seen with AIDS include cytomegalovirus retinitis, cryptococcal meningitis, toxoplasmosis, mycobacterial infections and, most commonly, *Pneumocystis carinii* pneumonia (PCP). The onset of PCP is usually insidious, characterized by a gradually increasing shortness of breath, dry cough, fever, and on chest roentgenography, pulmonary infiltrates. The respiratory status of a patient with PCP can deteriorate rapidly and necessitate admission to a critical-care unit. Hypoxemia and dyspnea may require ventilatory support. Drug therapy usually includes administration of a 21-day course of intravenous pentamidine or trimethoprim sulfamethoxazole (Septra). Occasionally, high-dose steroids are given. In many patients, it may take 7–10 days for a clinical response to be seen. It is not unusual for a relapse of PCP to occur; when it does, it is often fulminant in nature and associated with a mortality rate of approximately 40%. For this reason, patients are commonly started on prophylactic therapy, which may consist of maintenance doses of oral Septra or aerosolized pentamidine.

Secondary cancers, namely, Kaposi's sarcoma and non-Hodgkin's lymphoma (NHL), can also occur in association with AIDS. Kaposi's sarcoma, which arises from the endothelium of either the lymphatic vessel or the blood vessel, is characterized by skin and mucosal lesions ranging in color from dark red or purple to nearly black. The lesions also tend to develop in the oropharynx, lymph nodes, gastrointestinal (GI) tract, lungs, and on the skin. NHL is typically high grade, of B-cell origin, and present in extranodal sites. In approximately 20% of those with NHL, the cancer presents as a primary lymphoma of the brain, a very rare occurrence in the general population. Generally, the AIDS-related malignancies are much more aggressive and respond more poorly to therapy than the same cancers in the general population.

Neuropsychiatric manifestations accompany AIDS in over 60% of patients and in some cases are diagnostic for the disease. The most common disorder of this type is AIDS dementia complex, a subcortical dementia manifested by changes in cognition, behavior, and motor functioning. Symptoms initially include memory loss, difficulty in concentrating, and lethargy, and may progress to withdrawal, aphasia, ataxia, paresis, and seizures. The condition is thought to occur secondary to HIV infiltration of the brain. The virus is known to infect macrophages, which themselves are not destroyed by the virus but serve to transport HIV across the blood–brain barrier.

Also identified as part of the clinical picture associated with AIDS is the HIV wasting syndrome. This is defined as loss of over 10% of the usual body weight, accompanied by diarrhea, weakness, or fever of a chronic nature. Multiple factors may contribute to development of the syndrome, including difficulty in maintaining adequate nutrition. However, like the cachexia seen with cancer, muscle wasting seems to exceed what is expected.

Treatment

Treatment is aimed at the secondary diseases that develop with AIDS. Appropriate antimicrobial coverage is initiated for the specific opportunistic infection (see Table 27–6). Systemic NHL, usually widely disseminated at the time of diagnosis, neces-

TABLE 27–6. ANTIMICROBIALS COMMONLY USED AGAINST INFECTIONS IN THE IMMUNOCOMPROMISED HOST

Type of Infection	Antimicrobial
Bacterial	Penicillin
	Cephalosporin
	Aminoglycoside
	Vancomycin
	Fluroquinolones
Fungal	Nystatin (oral candidiasis)
	Ketoconazole
	5-Flucytosine
	Amphotericin B
	Itraconazole
Viral	Acyclovir
	Ganciclovir
	Foscarnet
Protozoal	Trimethoprim/sulfamethoxazole (Septra)
	Pentamidine

sitates treatment with an intensive chemotherapy regimen that is fairly toxic and usually poorly tolerated by the patient with AIDS. Primary lymphoma of the brain usually has a good initial response to cranial radiation, but relapse soon occurs, generally within the CNS. Therapy for Kaposi's sarcoma, commonly initiated when the patient develops pain or lymphatic obstruction or when the lesions are cosmetically disturbing, is palliative and consists of chemotherapy and/or radiation. These cancer therapies, particularly chemotherapy, induce myelosuppression and compound the already existing immunodeficiencies of AIDS, making the patient even more susceptible to the development of infection.

For specific medication treatment see Chapter 26.

Nursing Intervention

In addition to requiring nursing care relevant to immunosuppression, patients with AIDS, especially those with PCP, require aggressive pulmonary care and close monitoring of arterial blood gases. Decisions regarding intubation and ventilation should be made prior to severe respiratory dysfunction. As impaired cognitive functioning can occur secondary to hypoxemia, AIDS dementia, opportunistic infection, or CNS malignancy, a close assessment of mental status is required in order to detect any changes from baseline. If impaired concentration and memory are noted, it is necessary to provide simple explanations and directions as well as a safe environment for the patient. Nutritional support measures must also be addressed. If diarrhea is present, a common problem due to either HIV

enteropathy or opportunistic infection, enteral feedings may not be possible. As is evident, the patient with AIDS presents an array of problems with complex etiologies, requiring advanced nursing skills in assessment and symptom management.

Leukemias

Leukemias are a group of malignancies that occur when immature WBCs proliferate uncontrollably and accumulate in the bone marrow and peripheral blood. Leukemias are classified according to the type of cell that is predominant and whether they are acute or chronic in nature. The four general categories of leukemia are acute lymphocytic or lymphoblastic (ALL), acute nonlymphocytic or myelogenous (ANLL or AML), chronic lymphocytic (CLL), and chronic myelogenous (CML).

The accumulation of leukemic cells, which do not function normally, impedes the adequate production of normal RBCs, WBCs, and platelets. This, along with infiltration of other organs by the leukemic cells, is the rationale for the clinical presentation of leukemia. Refer to Table 27–7 for a summary of the signs and symptoms.

Complications

The patient with leukemia requires a critical-care setting when complications, either due to the disease or to its treatment, arise. Both the disease itself and the intensive chemotherapy used to treat it are associ-

TABLE 27–7. MANIFESTATIONS OF LEUKEMIA

Rationale	Signs and Symptoms
Bone marrow failure	Anemia
	Thrombocytopenia
	Leukocytosis (primarily blast cells)
	Granulocytopenia (if ALL, CLL)
	Lymphopenia (if ALL, CML)
Organ infiltration	Bone pain
	Lymphadenopathy
	Splenomegaly
	Hepatomegaly
	Testicular mass or swelling
	Headache, nausea, vomiting (CNS involvement)
Hyperleukocytosis	Stroke
	Adult respiratory distress syndrome
	Splenic infarction
Hypercatabolism and rapid cell turnover (tumor lysis syndrome)	Disseminated intravascular coagulation
	Hyperuricemia
	Hyperkalemia
	Hypocalcemia
	Weight loss

ated with severe and often prolonged myelosuppression. The total WBC count may be less than $100/mm^3$ for a period of one or more weeks after high-dose chemotherapy. As a result, infection is the major cause of morbidity and mortality in the patient with leukemia. Sepsis is common and must be treated immediately and aggressively.

Also contributing to the likelihood of infection is the disruption that can occur in the natural barriers of the skin and mucous membranes, allowing easy entry by microorganisms. The chemotherapy, depending on the drug and the doses, can cause severe stomatitis and mucositis. In patients who have received bone marrow from a donor, graft-versus-host disease (GVHD) can occur as the transplanted marrow recognizes the host tissue as foreign. One of the tissues that the engrafted T cells attempt to reject is the skin. In acute GVHD, this usually starts as a rash and may progress to desquamation. The treatment for GVHD includes immunosuppressive drugs, thus compounding the already existing immunodeficiencies.

Another reason for admission of a leukemia patient to the critical-care unit is severe bleeding and hemorrhage. This can occur secondary to thrombocytopenia, induced by the disease process and/or the chemotherapy. It is not unusual for the platelet count to be under $20,000/mm^3$ which puts the patient at risk for spontaneous bleeding. Of particular concern is the possibility of an intracranial hemorrhage. Because of the multiple platelet transfusions required, single-donor, leukocyte-poor products are administered.

Bleeding may also be seen in association with disseminated intravascular coagulation (DIC), a complication of leukemia, especially progranulocytic leukemia, a subtype of AML. It is caused by the release of tissue thromboplastin from tumor cells. The clotting cascade is triggered, leading to accelerated coagulation and the formation of excessive thrombin. With the ongoing coagulation, the fibrinolytic system is activated. Thus, clotting and bleeding continue until the cycle is interrupted by treating the cause. Besides hemorrhage, organ dysfunction can occur as a result of thromboemboli. Chemotherapy should be initiated immediately. Heparin, although its use is controversial with other etiologies of DIC, has been found to be an effective supportive therapy in acute progranulocytic leukemia.

Leukostasis can also be life threatening. Leukostasis can occur with a WBC count of over $100,000/mm^3$, consisting mostly of blasts. Leukemia blasts plug capillaries, causing rupture, bleeding, and organ dysfunction. Intracerebral hemorrhage is the most common and most lethal complication. Management includes the administration of fluids and allopurinol to counteract the hyperuricemia associated with cell lysis. Appropriate chemotherapy must be initiated. As an emergency measure, leukapheresis may be necessary.

Treatment

The acute leukemias require immediate treatment with chemotherapy. Treatment is approached in three phases. The initial phase, called induction therapy, consists of a combination of chemotherapy drugs given in high doses in order to achieve remission. Complete remission occurs when the number of leukemic cells is below detection, hematopoiesis is restored, and signs and symptoms of the disease are no longer present. However, since leukemic cells remain, even though they are microscopically undetectable, a consolidation phase of therapy is necessary to further decrease or eliminate these cells. This cycle of chemotherapy, also very intensive, is usually administered 6–8 weeks after induction. The third phase, maintenance therapy, involves the administration of moderate doses of chemotherapy over a prolonged time. Given with the intent of maintaining remission, its effectiveness is controversial.

By comparison, chronic leukemia is treated with oral chemotherapy agents with much less associated toxicity. More aggressive therapy may be initiated as the disease progresses, particularly in patients with CML who undergo an end-stage blast crisis, which resembles an acute leukemia.

The rate of relapse, i.e., the recurrence of detectable leukemic cells, either in the bone marrow, peripheral blood, or extramedullary sites, varies with the type of leukemia. However, once it occurs, it is more difficult to induce a second remission. One treatment alternative that is available to patients with ALL, ANLL, and CML who meet specific criteria is bone marrow transplantation. Bone marrow transplantation involves administration of dosages of chemotherapy and radiation therapy that, though ablative to the bone marrow, are also more cytotoxic to cancer cells. Prior to the cytotoxic therapy, bone marrow cells are harvested from the patient or a matched donor. If the patient is to receive his or her own marrow, special techniques are used in an attempt to completely eliminate all leukemic cells before infusion. The bone marrow is reinfused at the time the blood counts reach their lowest point. Engraftment of the bone marrow and functional immune recovery takes approximately 4 weeks.

Nursing Intervention

In the patient with leukemia, nursing care centers around the diagnosis of potential for infection and potential for injury (bleeding), discussed elsewhere in this chapter. In addition to the assessments previously reviewed, assessment of neurological status is important because of the possibility of CNS complications, including intracranial bleeding or stroke. Fluids and electrolyte balance must also be carefully monitored because of the large volume of fluids given and the possibility of tumor lysis syndrome or septic shock. Multisystem failure can occur secondary to leukemic infiltration, leukostasis, DIC, sepsis, or the toxicity of cancer chemotherapy. In addition to the continual assessments, the nurse will administer the extensive supportive therapy required, including multiple antibiotics, blood and blood product transfusions, and usually total parenteral nutrition. Nursing care of the patient with leukemia is a challenge, particularly in terms of protecting the patient from infection amid all of the critical-care interventions.

Other Malignancies Associated with Immunodeficiency

Lymphomas

Lymphomas, in which the malignant cell is a lymphocyte, are broadly classified as either Hodgkin's disease (HD) or non-Hodgkin's lymphoma (NHL). Though similar in many respects, the distinguishing feature of HD is the presence of Reed–Sternberg cells, whose origin and nature are uncertain. The incidence of HD peaks during the second and third decades and again after the age of 60. NHL occurs primarily in older individuals and is four times more common than HD.

The pathology of lymphomas is the transformation of the lymphocyte into a malignant cell at some stage of its development, which accounts for the different histologic subtypes of both HD and NHL. What triggers this transformation is unknown, although there is evidence linking HD to a viral etiology, particularly when it occurs in the young. In the case of NHL, there is a strong association with a pre-existing immunodeficiency. Regardless of the histology, the lymphocytes proliferate uncontrollably and invade body organs, although the degree of aggressiveness varies.

The disease usually presents as one or more enlarged lymph nodes, usually in the cervical region. Occasionally, the initial site of disease is the gastrointestinal tract. Approximately one-third of patients also exhibit systemic symptoms consisting of fever, night sweats, and loss over 10% of the usual body weight. Staging procedures are done to determine the extent of disease, as this has implications for treatment. HD tends to spread from one lymph node group to an adjacent group, whereas NHL tends to skip to noncontiguous groups. The workup must determine the involvement, if any, of lymph node groups, the bone marrow, liver, and spleen. Sometimes an explanatory laparotomy may be necessary, especially with HD.

If the lymphoma is localized, radiation therapy is initiated. In HD, this consists of total nodal irradiation and radiation to the spleen (if not removed at laparotomy). For early-stage disease, radiation is given with curative intent, although it is generally more effective in HD than in NHL. Chemotherapy is given for more widespread systemic disease, and sometimes in the case of NHL is recommended as the treatment of choice for localized disease. Both chemotherapy and radiation therapy, if given to areas of major bone marrow activity, are myelosuppressive. Another side effect that is sometimes associated with the chemotherapeutic treatment of NHL is tumor lysis syndrome.

Cure is expected in over 50% of patients with lymphoma. However, if the disease recurs, therapy is more poorly tolerated because of the depressed bone marrow reserve as a result of the initial therapy. Potential complications representing oncologic emergencies that can occur with progressive disease are superior vena cava syndrome and spinal cord compression. In superior vena cava syndrome, the vena cava is obstructed by tumor or enlarged nodes. The impaired venous drainage causes cough, dyspnea, neck vein distension, and facial, trunk, and arm edema. Immediate treatment with radiation is required to relieve pressure on the superior vena cava. The other complication treated on an emergency basis is spinal cord compression, usually due to lymph node extension into the epidural space. Paraplegia can result if treatment is not initiated with radiation therapy or, if the neurological deterioration is rapid, a decompression laminectomy.

Multiple Myeloma

Multiple myeloma is a relatively uncommon malignancy of the plasma cell, the antibody-producing form of the B cell. In this disease, excessive amounts of a single type of immunoglobulin are produced. Refer to Table 27–8 for the clinical manifestations of myeloma. The disease, commonly advanced at the time of diagnosis, is treated palliatively with chemotherapy. Infection, usually bacterial in origin, is the most common cause of death due to the impaired production of normal, functional antibodies.

TABLE 27–8. CLINICAL MANIFESTATIONS OF MULTIPLE MYELOMA

Rationale	Signs and Symptoms
Bone marrow involvement by plasmacytomas (plasma cell tumors)	Anemia (common) Leukopenia Thrombocytopenia
Skeletal involvement by plasmacytomas and tumor activation of osteoclasts	Bone pain Osteolytic lesions Pathologic fractures Hypercalcemia
Production of light chains called Bence Jones protein (part of immunoglobulin)	Proteinuria Renal insufficiency due to tubular damage
Hyperviscosity	Occlusion of small vessels Headache Mental status changes Visual disturbances Retinal hemorrhage Intermittent claudication
Hypervolemia	Congestive heart failure

Organ Transplantation

EDITORS' NOTE

It is uncertain how many questions on organ transplantation will be on the CCRN exam. This chapter, along with the others in this section, will help the critical care nurse with general concepts of organ transplantation, immunosuppression, and critical care issues related to the care of these patients.

In order for organ transplantation to occur the declaration of death of the donor must take place. The physician making the declaration of death cannot be a member of the transplant team or a member of the patient's family, and shall not have special interests in the patient's death. Under the Uniform Anatomical Gift Act, the donor can receive treatment (mechanical ventilation, intravenous medications, etc.) until organ harvesting occurs.

The most common organ transplants in the United States are heart, lung, liver, kidney, and pancreas. For a historical overview of transplantation see Table 28–1. Because the post-transplant course is difficult, only candidates who meet strict requirements are transplanted.

Kidney transplants can be from a cadaver or a living related donor. In the majority of the cases, the native kidneys are left in place, and the donor kidney is implanted into either iliac fossa. Finally, the urinary tract is reconstructed. Urine is produced almost immediately.

Heart transplants are one of the most common of all organ transplants. Orthotopic transplantation is the most common. See Table 28–2 for graft termi-

nology. This procedure requires the patient to be placed on cardiopulmonary bypass.

The donor heart is implanted by anastomosis of the left and right atria. Following the surgical procedure, the patient is weaned off cardiopulmonary bypass.

Liver transplants are indicated for individuals with inevitable end-stage liver disease. They are also orthotopic. In this transplant, time is valuable because of the poor viability of the transplanted organ. Correct size matching is also important because a large liver will compress the diaphragm and cause pulmonary complications. Anastomosis of the new liver involves the hepatic artery, inferior and superior vena cava, the portal vein, and the biliary tract.

Pancreas transplantation offers normoglycemic states in type I diabetic patients. In pancreas transplantation, the native pancreas is left in place. The transplanted pancreas consists of a pancreatic segment (tail or body) or the whole pancreas. The donor pancreas is often placed in the right iliac fossas, and venous drainage is anastomosed into the common iliac vein and arterial blood supply comes from the common iliac artery. The exocrine duct is connected to the bladder for urinary excretion of pancreatic enzymes. Finally pancreatic rejection is very difficult to detect, but much research is being done to improve detection.

In addition to the individual transplants discussed, heart–lung and kidney–pancreas transplants are also performed. The kidney–pancreas transplant success rate is nearly 90%. This success is due in part to careful nursing care.

A knowledge base of immunosuppressive therapy and the response of the patient is helpful in caring for the transplant patient. All transplant recipients will have to take immunosuppressive medications to try to prevent rejection of their new

TABLE 28–1. HISTORICAL OVERVIEW OF TRANSPLANTATION

1905	Development of vascular suture techniques
1933	First kidney transplant attempted
1954	First successful kidney transplant
1960	Development of tissue typing
1962	Azathioprine used as single immunosuppressive agent
1963	First liver transplant attempted
1963	Steroids with azathioprine have synergistic effects
1966	First segmental pancreas transplant attempted
1967	First successful liver transplant
1967	First successful orthotopic heart transplant
1968	First human heart–lung transplant attempted
1970	Cyclophosphamide tried as a substitute for azathioprine
1974	First clinical heterotopic heart transplant
1978	Clinical trials of cyclosporine initiated
1982	First successful heart–lung transplant
1983	Cyclosporine approved by the FDA
1983	Clinical trials of OKT3 initiated
1987	OKT3 approved by the FDA
1989	Clinical trials of FK-506 initiated
1990	Clinical trials of RS-61443 initiated

TABLE 28–2. GRAFT TERMINOLOGY

Nomenclature	Definition
Autograft	A transplant of an organ taken from the recipient
Isograft	A transplant of an organ taken from a genetically identical donor
Allograft	A transplant of an organ from a genetically different donor from the same species
Xenograft	A transplant of an organ from a donor of a different species
Heterotopic transplant	The recipient's native organ is left in place and the donor organ is grafted into an ectopic position
Orthotopic transplant	The recipient's native organ is removed and the donor organ is placed with near normal anatomical reconstruction

organ. The ones commonly used today include cyclosporine, azathioprine, steroids, OKT3, FK-506, and mycophenolate. These drugs are not without side effects. Research studies are constantly progressing in the search for new and better drugs.

Corticosteroids were the first immunosuppressive agents used in solid organ transplants. Even today, low-dose prednisone remains a cornerstone in immunosuppressive therapy. The immunosuppressives act to suppress antibody and complement binding as well as reduce the synthesis of important immunomodulating cytokines. Side effects include hypertension, glucose intolerance, hyperlipidemia, and weight gain.

Azathioprine is key in antirejection therapy. Its immunosuppressive therapy comes from the inhibitory effects on the proliferation of T lymphocytes. A decrease in IgU and Igb antibody synthesis also reduces antigen recognition. Side effects include myelosuppression, leukopenia, thrombocytopenia, and anemia. Hepatotoxicity has been reported in several cases.

Cyclosporine is a cyclicendecapeptide with immunosuppressive activity. It primarily affects the T-cell immune response by blocking interleukin-2 production. This drug has significantly reduced solid organ rejection. Side effects include nephrotoxicity, hypertension, glucose intolerance, hyperkalemia, neurotoxicity, and hyperlipidemia. Careful monitoring of cyclosporine drug levels can help to reduce some of the side effects.

OKT3 was the first monoclonal antibody approved for use in organ transplantation. Early studies proved OKT3 to be successful in steroid-resistant rejection in kidney transplants. Further studies have shown similar success in heart, lung, liver, and pancreas transplant recipients. OKT3 binds to the CD3 receptor on T lymphocytes, causing an inactivation of CD3 cells. Side effects reported are fever, chills, nausea, vomiting, pulmonary edema, and hypotension. Anti-OKT3 antibodies have been noted in some patients.

FK-506 is still an investigational treatment for transplant patients. It is a macnolide that is one hundred times more potent than cyclosporine. FK-506 inhibits the production of interleukin-2. Studies show that a 1-year survival rate of 90% in liver transplant patients with rejection and a 1-year graft survival rate in 80% of kidney transplants. Commonly reported side effects included nausea, vomiting, insomnia, tremors, and hyperesthesias of the feet. FK-506 also causes nephrotoxicity and hyperkalemia.

Finally, RS-61443, or mycophenolate, is an investigational drug that is believed to suppress both cellular and antibody-mediated immunity. Side effects include nausea, vomiting, and diarrhea. So far, liver, renal, or bone marrow toxicity has not been reported.

Life-Threatening Coagulopathies

EDITORS' NOTE

Hematology and immunology comprise approximately 8% (eight questions) of the CCRN examination. The exam is likely to focus on life-threatening coagulopathies, so expect one to three questions on this content.

DISSEMINATED INTRAVASCULAR COAGULATION

Disseminated intravascular coagulation (DIC) is a state of hypercoagulability utilizing all of the clotting factors. The exhaustion of these clotting factors results in hemorrhage.

Pathophysiology

Regardless of the cause, specific pathophysiological signs occur in DIC. The common denominator is the release of procoagulants into the circulatory system. Free hemoglobin, cancer tissue fragments, amniotic fluid, and bacterial toxins are some procoagulants that may activate the clotting cascade. Activation of the cascade results in diffuse intravascular fibrin formation. Fibrin is then deposited in the microcirculation.

With the clotting of the capillaries, blood is shunted to the arteriovenous anastomoses. This shunting causes the capillary tissue to use anaerobic metabolism. With the production of lactic and pyruvic waste products and blood stagnation in the microcirculation, acidemia develops.

Three procoagulant factors develop in capillary blood as a result of the DIC disease process. Acidosis acts as a strong procoagulant along with the "normal" procoagulants in the blood. The third factor is the concentration of procoagulants, which increases secondary to the stagnation of blood. All of these processes result in massive sequestration of clotted blood in the capillaries (Fig. 29–1).

Disseminated intravascular coagulation develops rapidly, so coagulating factors are depleted in the microcirculation faster than the clotting factors can be replenished. Without circulating coagulant factors, hemostasis cannot be maintained (Fig. 29–2) and the patient begins to bleed.

Etiology

Many factors may precipitate DIC, including multiple trauma, crush injuries, hemorrhagic shock, malignant hypertension, incompatible blood transfusion, any and all cancers, burns, and coronary bypass surgery. DIC does not occur in isolation; it is always a sequelae of some initiating event.

Clinical Presentation

In most cases of DIC, arterial hypotension occurs secondary to the arteriovenous anastomoses. The anastomoses are caused by arterial vasoconstriction of the precapillary sphincter and vasodilatation of the capillaries.

Bleeding occurs after injections or venipunctures, from incisions, in the mucosa of the mouth, in the respiratory system, in the gastrointestinal system, and in the genitourinary system. It is common for several of these systems to be bleeding simultaneously; rarely is only one system involved.

Despite the complete depletion of circulating fibrinogen, some circulating thrombin still exists, since fibrinogen is not present to convert it to fibrin. Activation of the clotting process produces thrombin

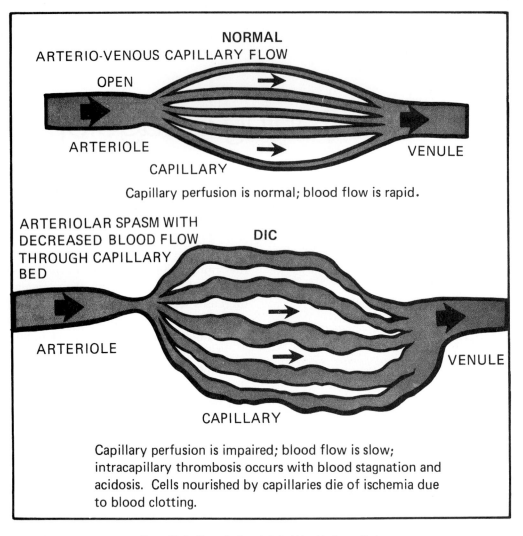

Figure 29–1. Sequestration of clotted blood in the capillaries.

and thereby fibrin. Fibrin and thrombin convert plasminogen to plasmin. Antithrombins (especially antithrombin III) destroy thrombin function. In DIC, thrombin production exceeds antithrombin III production and thereby promotes uncontrolled coagulation.

The initiation of fibrinolysis results in dissolution of clots and degrades fibrin into its fractions, which further adds to the bleeding.

In an attempt to restore hemostasis, the liver produces more fibrinogen or the patient is transfused with blood, plasma, or fibrinogen. This perpetuates the process, making the DIC more severe and intractable.

Pulmonary compromise may require intubation. Following the trend of ABGs and observing for signs and symptoms of hypoxemia will show when suctioning and/or mechanical ventilation is indicated.

Monitor fluid balance especially if the patient receives multiple blood transfusions and other fluids or if the patient has another pre-existing disease.

Skin care to preserve skin integrity is very important. Care must be taken to treat the patient very gently and to maintain good body alignment with adequate support. Sufficient but not excessive pressure is applied to sites of intramuscular injections or venipunctures by laboratory personnel to prevent hematoma formation.

Petechiae are pinpoint flat lesions that appear as reddish purple spots on the skin, buccal mucosa, and conjuctivae. Purpura is characterized by reddish brown spots usually evidencing presence of fluid. Ecchymoses are black and blue bruises.

Psychosocial support is extremely important to decrease the anxiety of the patient who is aware and frightened by all the lost blood and the flurry

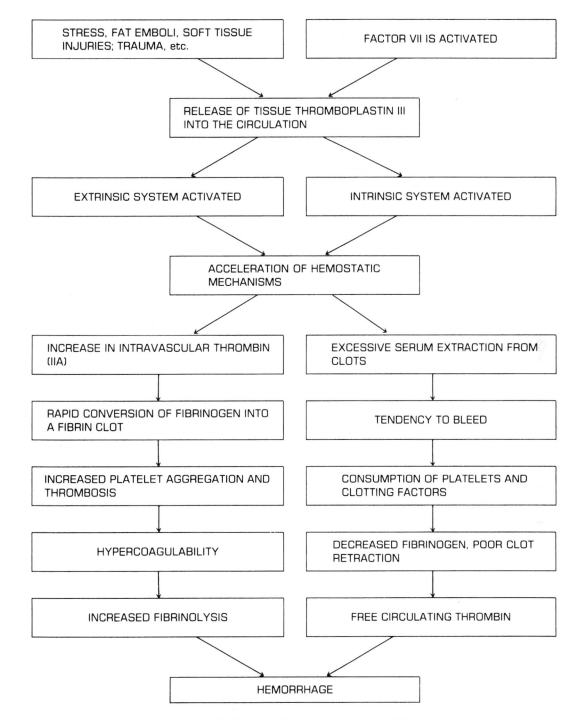

Figure 29–2. Alteration of the coagulation process in DIC.

of activity around him or her. Very brief explanations should be given; for example, "I'm giving you some medicine through the vein to help stop your bleeding."

Being honest with the patient's family as well as with the patient will help to decrease anxiety and foster a positive relationship between all parties involved.

Treatment

The primary treatment of DIC is to treat the underlying disease, which is easier said than done in the face of a patient hemorrhaging.

The second treatment is to halt the DIC. This is accomplished by several concurrent actions. It is necessary to replace the clotting factors so the serum is converted back to plasma. At the same time, the effects of thrombin must be stopped. Also at the same time, correction of acidosis, hypotension, hypovolemia, and hypoxia must be attempted since these four conditions act as procoagulants to continue utilization/depletion of clotting factors. Vitamin K (formation of prothrombin) and folic acid (thrombocytopenia) are administered to correct these deficiencies.

The use of heparin remains controversial since it is difficult to assess its effectiveness. Heparin neutralizes free circulating thrombin by combining with antithrombin III which inactivates the thrombin. Heparin functions as an anticoagulant to prevent further thrombus formation in the microcirculatory system. (It does not alter the thrombi already formed.) Heparin prevents the activation of factor X. Heparin also inhibits platelet aggregation.

Caution: If used, heparin should be given intravenously, not subcutaneously. Factors affecting subcutaneous heparin include the absorption rate, which is dependent on the amount injected, the depth of injection, body temperature, and cardiovascular status. If a hematoma develops at the injection site, absorption is markedly altered. The amount of heparin needed may be too much for subcutaneous administration. The delay in reaching a therapeutic blood level may be too long with subcutaneous administration.

After heparin therapy is started, whole blood, fresh frozen plasma, and/or platelet transfusion are administered.

Complications

Disseminated intravascular coagulation may become an exsanguinating hemorrhage. Death is not uncommon.

Nursing Interventions

Assessment of patients at high risk of DIC include looking for development of petechiae, purpura, and ecchymoses. Oozing of blood from injection sites, intravenous lines, and invasive monitoring lines all may indicate the onset of DIC.

Cardiac status must be monitored for dysrhythmias secondary to acidosis, hypovolemia, hypervolemia, and electrolyte imbalances. Early recognition and treatment of dysrhythmias may prevent progression to more serious dysrhythmias. Renal problems develop as a consequence of fluid overload, fluid depletion, and hypotension. The oliguric or anuric patient cannot eliminate heparin adequately, so the dose must be titrated to match the patient's utilization and excretion of the drug.

Monitor the amount of bleeding and identify the system involved. All drainage should be tested for blood. Observe for frank bleeding.

Watch for signs of thrombus formation. If thrombi develop, the symptoms will vary according to the system involved. The kidneys are most often involved (oliguria or anuria).

Intracranial bleeding may be identified by altered level of consciousness; orientation to person, place, and time; pupil reactions; and extremity movement. These must be checked frequently. Any change will indicate a possible bleed.

Avoid infection. The DIC patient is at high risk for infection, primarily because of all the entry ports for bacteria. Development of a fever is an indication to culture blood, urine, sputum, and any other drainage. If the bacteria is identified, appropriate antibiotics are started.

THROMBOTIC THROMBOCYTOPENIC PURPURA

Thrombotic thrombocytopenic purpura (TTP) can cause multisystem complications requiring critical care during the acute phase. It is a rare disorder with a poor prognosis; however, the survival rate is improving. It is characterized by thromocytopenia, hemolytic anemia, fever, neurological complications, and renal failure. The etiology is unknown. It tends to affect women more often than men, and usually has an onset at about age 40. The pathophysiology of TTP includes widespread deposition of platelet microthromboli that occlude the arteries and capillaries. This is especially evident in the brain, bone marrow, and kidneys. The result is bleeding and petechiae. The complexity and severity of this disease make it a challenge for the critical care nurse.

HEMATOLOGY/IMMUNOLOGY BIBLIOGRAPHY

Anonymous (1994). New trends in immunopharmacology. Symposium Proceedings. *J Allergy Clin Immunol, 94* (3), 565–650.

Anonymous (1995). Hemophilia and von Willebrand's disease: 1. diagnosis, comprehensive care and assessment. *Can Med Assoc J, 153* (1), 19–25.

Anonymous (1995). Hemophilia and von Willebrand's disease: 2. management. *Can Med Assoc J, 153* (2), 147–157.

Barker, L.R., Burton, J.R., & Zieve, P.D. (1995). *Principles of Ambulatory Medicine*, 4th ed. Baltimore: Williams & Wilkins.

Bartlett, J.G. (1995). *The Johns Hopkins Hospital Guide to Medical Care of Patients with HIV Infection*, 5th ed. Baltimore: Williams & Wilkins.

Bartlett, J. (1994). *Medical Management of HIV Infection*. Glenview, IL: Physicians & Scientists Publishing.

Bartlett, J., & Feinberg, J. (1994). Management of opportunistic infections in patients with HIV infection: Update. *Infect Dis Clin Pract, 3* (6), 423–433.

Bartucci, M.R. (1995). Combined kidney and pancreas transplantation. *AACN Clin Issues, 6* (1), 143–152.

Branson, B.M. (1992). The role of CD4 cells in immune system function. *PAAC Notes, 3*, 76–79.

Chaisson, R. (1993). Mycobacterial infections and HIV. *Curr Opin Infect Dis, 6*, 237–243.

Cohen, A.J., & Kessler, C.M. (1995). Treatment of inherited coagulation disorders. *Am J Med, 99* (6), 675–682.

Cunningham, N.H., Boteler, S., & Windham, S. (1992). Renal transplantation. *Crit Care Nurs Clin North Am, 4* (1), 79–88.

Ellenberger, B.J., Haas, L., & Cundiff, L. (1993). Thrombotic thrombocytopenia purpura: Nursing during the acute phase. *Dimens Crit Care Nurs, 12* (2), 58–65.

El-Sadr, N., Oleske, J.M., et al. (1994). Evaluation and management of early HIV infection. Clinical Practice Guideline No. 7. *AHCRP Publication No. 94-0572*. Rockville, MD: Agency for Health Care Policy and Research.

Fischi, M.A. (1992). Treatment of HIV infection. In *The Medical Management of AIDS*, 3rd ed. Philadelphia: W.B. Saunders.

Gallin, J.I., Goldstein, R.M., & Snyerman, R. (1992). *Inflammation: Basic Principles and Clinical Correlates*, 2nd ed. New York: Raven Press.

Gilman, A.G., et al. (1990). *Goodman and Gilman's The Pharmacological Basis of Therapeutics* 8th ed. New York: McGraw-Hill.

Henry, J.B. (ed.) (1990). *Todd-Sanford-Davidsohn Clinical Diagnosis and Management by Laboratory Methods*, 18th ed. Philadelphia: W.B. Saunders.

Herfindal, E.T., Gourley, D.R., & Hart, L.L. (eds.) (1992). *Clinical Pharmacology and Therapeutics*, 5th ed. Baltimore: Williams & Wilkins.

Heron, D. (1992). Leukemia and bone marrow transplant. Talking about a revolution. *Nurs Standards, 7* (6), 52–53.

Huston, C.J. (1994). Disseminated intravascular coagulation. *Am J Nurs, 94* (8), 51.

Kaplan, J.E., Masur, H., et al. (1995). USPHS/IDSA guidelines for the prevention of opportunistic infections in persons infected with human immunodeficiency virus. *Clin Infect Dis, 21* (Suppl 1), 1–43.

Lee, B.L., & Safrin, S. (1992). Drug interactions and toxicities in patients with AIDS. In *The Medical Management of AIDS*, 3rd ed. Philadelphia: W.B. Saunders.

Lee, R.J., et al. (eds.) (1993). *Wintrobe's Clinical Hematology*, 9th ed. Philadelphia: Lea & Febiger.

McIntyre, W.J., & Parr, M.D. (1992). Infections in the immunosuppressed patient. In *Clinical Pharmacology and Therapeutics*, Baltimore: Williams & Wilkins.

Miller, S.B. (1992). Renal diseases. In *Manual of Medical Therapeutics*, 27th ed. Boston: Little, Brown.

Moran, G.J. (1995). Managing the HIV related medical emergency. *Emerg Med, 4*, 18–30.

Murihead, J. (1992). Heart and heart-lung transplantation. *Crit Care Clin North Am, 4* (1), 97–109.

Pallister, C.J. (1992). A 'crisis' that can be overcome: Management of sickle cell disease. *Professional Nurse, 7* (8), 509–513.

Paschall, F.E. (1993). Thrombotic thrombocytopenic purpura: The challenges of a complex disease process. *AACN Clin Issues Crit Care Nurs, 4* (4), 655–663.

Pinching, A.J. (1994). Clinical immunology: A clinical and laboratory discipline. *Neth J Med, 45* (6), 235–237.

Purandare, L. (1995). Caring for patients with chronic leukemia. *Nurs Times, 91* (31), 27–28.

Rossi, J.J., Schroeder, T.J., Hariharan, S., & First, M.R. (1993). Prevention and management of the adverse effects associated with immunosuppressive therapy. *Drug Safety, 9* (2), 104–131.

Saag, M.S. (1992). AIDS testing now and in the future. In *The Medical Management of AIDS*, 3rd ed. Philadelphia: W.B. Saunders.

Sande, M.A., & Volberding, P.A. (1992). *The Medical Management of AIDS*, 3rd ed. Philadelphia: W.B. Saunders.

Sanford, J.P., Gilbert, D.N., & Sande, M.A. (1995). *Guide to Antimicrobial Therapy*. Dallas: Antimicrobial Therapy.

Sanford, J.P., Sande, M.A., & Gilbert, D.N. (1995). *Guide to HIV/AIDS Therapy*. Vienna, VA: Antimicrobial Therapy.

Sequeira, L.A., & Cutler, R.E. (1992). Muromonab CD3 (Orthoclone OKT3). Part 1: Pharmacology. *Dialysis Transplant, 21* (5), 1–4.

Smith, S.L., & Ciferni, M.L. (1992). Liver transplantation. *Crit Care Nurs Clin North Am, 4* (10), 131–148.

Sox, H.C. (ed.) (1990). *Common Diagnostic Tests*. Philadelphia: American College of Physicians.

Virella, G. (1993). *Introduction to Medical Immunology*. New York: Marcel Dekker.

Wade, J.C. (1993). Management of infection in patients with acute leukemia. *Hematol Oncol Clin North Am, 7* (1), 293–315.

Wadhwa, M., Barrowcliffe, T.W., Mire-Sluis, A.R., & Thorpe, R. (1995). Factor VIII concentrates and the immune system—laboratory investigations. *Blood Coagulation Fibrinolysis, 6* (Suppl 2), 65–79.

Warne, I. (1994). Chemotherapy for acute monoblastic leukemia. *Nurs Times, 90* (17), 43–45.

Weber, M.S. (1994). Thrombocytopenia. *Am J Nurs, 94* (11), 46–47.

Williams, B. (1992). A day in the life of a nurse: Cardiac transplant nurse assists patient, family in dynamic process. *Am Nurse, 24* (5), 35.

Williams, W.J., et al. (1990). *Hematology,* 4th ed. New York: McGraw-Hill.

Wilson, J.D., Braunwald, E., Isselbacher, K.J., et al. (eds.) (1991). *Harrison's Principles of Internal Medicine,* 12th ed. New York: McGraw-Hill.

Wormser, G.P. (1992). *AIDS and Other Manifestations of HIV Infection,* 2nd ed. New York: Raven Press.

Wyngaarden, J.B., Smith, L.H., Bennett, J.C. (eds.) (1992). *Cecil Textbook of Medicine,* 19th ed. Philadelphia: W.B. Saunders.

Immunology and Hematology Practice Exam

1. Which cell, known as the "helper cell," is vital in activating the immune response?
   (A) segmented neutrophil
   (B) band neutrophil
   (C) T4 lymphocyte
   (D) T8 lymphocyte

2. Which of the following components of the immune system is referred to as "cell-mediated" in its immune response?
   (A) segmented neutrophils
   (B) band neutrophils
   (C) T lymphocytes
   (D) B lymphocytes

3. Which cell plays an active role in suppressing the immune response once the antigenic stimulus has been eliminated?
   (A) segmented neutrophil
   (B) band neutrophil
   (C) T4 lymphocyte
   (D) T8 lymphocyte

4. Which of the following components of the white blood cell count makes up the largest percent of the differential?
   (A) segmented neutrophils
   (B) band neutrophils
   (C) monocytes
   (D) lymphocytes

5. Which term is used to describe a substance regarded as foreign in terms of the immune response?
   (A) antibody
   (B) antigen
   (C) complement
   (D) cytotoxic

6. Which of the following are NOT considered macrophages?
   (A) segmented neutrophils
   (B) band neutrophils
   (C) monocytes
   (D) lymphocytes

7. A 71-year-old male is admitted to your unit with recurrent pneumonia. Since the pneumonia was present before, which of the following cells would have the ability to remember the *Haemophilus* antigen from a prior infection?
   (A) segmented neutrophils
   (B) band neutrophils
   (C) lymphocytes
   (D) eosinophils

8. A 23-year-old female is in your unit following a motor vehicle accident. During the admission, she develops a urinary tract infection. If this were her first exposure to the bacteria causing the infection, which component of the white blood cell count would be the first to respond to the antigen?
   (A) segmented neutrophils
   (B) eosinophils
   (C) T4 lymphocytes
   (D) T8 lymphocytes

9. Which of the following types of cells produce antibodies?
   (A) segmented neutrophils
   (B) monocytes
   (C) B lymphocytes through plasma cells
   (D) reticuloendothelial cells

10. Which of the following components of the immune system is referred to as "humorally mediated" in its immune response?

(Answers cont'd.)

(A) segmented neutrophils
(B) band neutrophils
(C) T lymphocytes
(D) B lymphocytes

Questions 11 and 12 refer to the following scenario.
A 21-year-old male is in your unit for respiratory distress caused by reaction to chemotherapy for Hodgkin's disease. The following laboratory information is available:

white blood cells	1300/mm^3
segmented neutrophils	25%
banded neutrophils	10%
lymphocytes	25%
platelets	15,000/mm^3
activated partial thromboplastin time	100 sec

11. Based on the preceding information, which complications should you be aware may occur in this situation?
    (A) bleeding and infection
    (B) infection and hypercoagulation
    (C) hypercoagulation
    (D) infection

12. Which of the following measures would potentially be most helpful in this scenario?
    (A) placing the patient on respiratory isolation
    (B) placing the patient on bodily secretion isolation
    (C) drawing blood only from arteries
    (D) placing the patient on reverse isolation

13. Common side effects of antibiotic therapy include which of the following?
    (A) potential bone marrow suppression
    (B) reduction in normal bacterial flora and bleeding tendencies
    (C) development of resistance to antibiotics and reduction in normal bacterial flora
    (D) development of resistance and hypercoagulation

14. Which cell secretes lymphokines (biological response modifiers)?
    (A) segmented neutrophil
    (B) band neutrophil
    (C) T lymphocyte
    (D) B lymphocyte

15. Which of the following is NOT a lymphokine?
    (A) interferon
    (B) interleukin
    (C) GM-CSF (granulocyte-macrophage colony-stimulating factor)
    (D) cyclosporine

16. Which antibody mediates allergic reactions?
    (A) IgD
    (B) IgM
    (C) IgE
    (D) IgG

17. Which is the most dominant antibody in adult life?
    (A) IgA
    (B) IgB
    (C) IgC
    (D) IgG

18. Which of the following would be given to provide passive immunity from accidental puncture with a needle contaminated with hepatitis?
    (A) IgA
    (B) IgB
    (C) IgC
    (D) IgG

19. The human immunodeficiency virus (HIV) works through inhibition of which aspect of the immune system?
    (A) B-cell lymphocytes
    (B) T-cell lymphocytes
    (C) neutrophils
    (D) complement

20. In a patient with pneumococcal pneumonia, which of the following classes of antibiotics may be useful in treatment?
    (A) penicillins and cephalosporins
    (B) aminoglycosides
    (C) cephalosporins and cyclosporine
    (D) amphotericin B

21. Which of the following agents is used to treat *Pneumocystis carinii* pneumonia?
    (A) Septra (Bactrim)
    (B) acyclovir
    (C) amphotericin B
    (D) vancomycin

Questions 22 and 23 refer to the following scenario.
A 64-year-old female is in your unit after a hepatic resection for cancer. During her second postoperative day, she complains of generalized discomfort with no change in incisional pain. She feels warm to the touch and her vital signs indicate the following:

blood pressure	96/56
pulse	115
respiratory rate	28
temperature	39° C

Lung sounds have scattered crackles throughout both lungs. Pulmonary artery catheter readings provide the following information:

cardiac index	5.9
arterial pressure	28/14
PCWP	12
CVP	4
PaO_2	74
$PaCO_2$	35
pH	7.32
FIO_2	0.40

22. Based on the preceding information, which condition is possibly developing?
    (A) sepsis
    (B) CHF (congestive heart failure)
    (C) pneumonia
    (D) ARDS (adult respiratory distress syndrome)

23. Which treatment would most likely be instituted based on the preceding information?
    (A) mechanical ventilation
    (B) amphotericin B and fluid bolus
    (C) fluid bolus and triple antibiotics
    (D) amphotericin B and fluid restriction

24. Bone marrow failure occurring with leukemia can present with which of the following symptoms?
    (A) bleeding, increased risk of infection, and anemia
    (B) increased risk of infection and hypercoagulation
    (C) anemia and hypercoagulation
    (D) decreased risk of infection and anemia

25. In which organ system does much of the development of antibodies take place?
    (A) hepatic
    (B) respiratory
    (C) gastrointestinal
    (D) splenic

26. Which of the following is a/are common clinical presentation(s) of multiple myeloma?
    (A) bone pain
    (B) pathologic fractures and bone pain
    (C) stomatitis and bone pain
    (D) stomatitis and pathologic fractures

27. Which immunologic disorder presents with Bence Jones proteinuria?
    (A) acute myelocytic leukemia
    (B) multiple myeloma
    (C) chronic myelocytic leukemia
    (D) lymphomas

Questions 28 and 29 refer to the following scenario.
A 37-year-old male is admitted to your unit for investigation of the cause of his hypotension. He has a history of weight loss, night sweats, and cervical lymph node enlargement. Laboratory data and vital signs reveal the following information:

blood pressure	88/60
pulse	118
respiratory rate	31
temperature	38.7
white blood cells	6000
platelets	400,000

Reed–Sternberg cells are noted in the laboratory analysis.

28. Based on the preceding information, which condition is likely to be developing?
    (A) sepsis
    (B) multiple myeloma
    (C) Hodgkin's disease
    (D) acute lymphocytic leukemia

29. Which treatment modality or modalities could be employed in this patient?
    (A) splenectomy and chemotherapy
    (B) radiation therapy and chemotherapy
    (C) chemotherapy and splenectomy
    (D) splenectomy, radiation therapy, and chemotherapy

30. Which phase of chronic myelocytic leukemia can resemble an acute leukemia?
    (A) blast crisis
    (B) recombinant phase
    (C) hematoporesis phase
    (D) myelosuppressive phase

Questions 31 and 32 refer to the following scenario.
A 27-year-old male is admitted to your unit with shortness of breath, weight loss, and non productive cough. Current vital signs are:

blood pressure	118/74
pulse	114
respiratory rate	34
temperature	38.4

HIV (human immunodeficiency virus) serum testing is positive.

31. Based on the preceding information, which condition is likely to be present?
    (A) Kaposi's sarcoma
    (B) non-Hodgkin's lymphoma
    (C) *Klebsiella pneumonia*
    (D) *Pneumocystis carinii* pneumonia

32. What is the likely cause for the shortness of breath?
    (A) noncardiogenic pulmonary edema
    (B) lymphocytic infiltration into the bronchi
    (C) V/Q disturbance from pneumonia
    (D) high $PaCO_2$ levels

33. Which side effect of chemotherapy can affect nutritional status?
    (A) loss of serum proteins
    (B) stomatitis
    (C) increased oxygen consumption
    (D) loss of gastrointestinal function

34. Which condition occurs with the graft-versus-host response to transplanted bone marrow?
    (A) The body rejects the transplanted marrow.
    (B) The transplanted cells reject normal cells.
    (C) The donor cells mutate into abnormal host cells.
    (D) Both graft cells and normal cells reject each other.

35. At what point does spontaneous bleeding become a nursing concern in the patient receiving chemotherapy?
    (A) white blood cell count <3000/mm³
    (B) fibrin split product level <400
    (C) platelet count <20,000/mm³
    (D) platelet count >50,000/mm³

36. Which is the first response in coagulation following trauma to a blood vessel?
    (A) vasoconstriction
    (B) platelet aggregation
    (C) fibrin formation
    (D) thrombin formation

37. Which electrolyte is an integral part of the coagulation process?
    (A) sodium
    (B) potassium
    (C) magnesium
    (D) calcium

Questions 38 and 39 refer to the following scenario.
A 41-year-old female is admitted to your unit with an exacerbation of chronic lymphocytic leukemia. She states that she has had small amounts of vaginal bleeding. Ecchymotic areas are noted on her arms and legs. Laboratory data reveal the following:

platelets	15,000/mm³
white blood cells	4000/mm³
granulocytes	50%

38. Which of the following nursing measures should be employed on this patient?
    (A) place on bleeding precautions
    (B) place on reverse isolation and bleeding precautions
    (C) avoid fresh plants and vegetables in the room and place on reverse isolation
    (D) place on reverse isolation

39. Which treatment would most likely be ordered for this patient?
    (A) platelet transfusions
    (B) initiation of aerosolized pentamidine
    (C) low-dose heparin therapy
    (D) amphotericin B

40. Which of the following characterizes disseminated intravascular clotting?
    (A) decreased prothrombin time
    (B) increased levels of fibrinogen degradation products
    (C) antithrombin formation
    (D) platelet proliferation

41. A patient admitted with a diagnosis of pulmonary embolism is to receive a thrombolytic agent. Which of the following is NOT considered a thrombolytic medication?
    (A) tissue plasminogen activator (tPA)
    (B) urokinase
    (C) streptokinase
    (D) heparin

42. Which test is best employed to assess the effectiveness of heparin therapy?
    (A) partial thromboplastin time (PTT)
    (B) prothrombin time (PT)
    (C) platelet levels
    (D) bleeding time

43. The thrombolytic effect of plasmin is due to which action?
    (A) preventing platelet aggregation
    (B) blocking the intrinsic pathway
    (C) breaking down of fibrin
    (D) ionization of calcium

44. Which cell is characteristic of Hodgkin's disease?
    (A) Kaposi
    (B) Reed-Sternberg
    (C) promyelocyte
    (D) Stevens

45. Which lymphoma tends to progress along adjacent groups of lymph nodes, as opposed to skipping to noncontinuous groups?

(A) lymphocytic leukemia
(B) multiple myeloma
(C) non-Hodgkin's lymphoma
(D) Hodgkin's disease

Questions 46 and 47 refer to the following scenario. A 35-year-old male is admitted to your unit with the diagnosis of Hodgkin's disease. He is admitted because of dyspnea, upper trunk edema, jugular venous distention, and cough.

46. Based on the preceding information, which condition is likely to be developing?
(A) right ventricular failure
(B) lymphocytic infiltration into the myocardium
(C) superior vena caval syndrome
(D) venous congestion secondary to splenic enlargement

47. Which treatment would most likely improve the symptoms?
(A) diuretics
(B) radiation therapy
(C) administration of 5-FU (fluorouracil)
(D) surgery to remove lymphatic obstructions

48. An 18-year-old black female is admitted to your unit with complaints of shortness of breath and severe joint pain. She has a history of sickle cell anemia. Measures to reduce patient discomfort should include which of the following?
(A) analgesics
(B) oxygen therapy
(C) normal saline fluid challenge
(D) all of the above

49. Which of the following tests is used to diagnose a hemolytic transfusion reaction?
(A) Coombs' test
(B) PT (prothrombin time)
(C) aPTT (activated partial thromboplastin time)
(D) fibrinogen level

50. What is another name for Factor I?
(A) fibrinogen
(B) thrombin
(C) prothrombin
(D) thromboplastin

51. The extrinsic pathway for coagulation is initiated by which mechanism?
(A) irregularity of the blood vessel wall
(B) presence of atherosclerotic plaques causing increased turbulent blood flow

(C) exposure to interstitial tissue following trauma to the blood vessel
(D) introduction of an extrinsic substance into the blood

52. What is the cause of superior vena caval syndrome?
(A) obstruction of the superior vena cava by thrombi
(B) compression of the vena cava by enlarged lymph nodes
(C) failure of the left and right heart due to lymphocytic infiltration
(D) bronchial obstruction due to tumor growth

53. Advantages of having "normal flora" of bacteria on the skin include which of the following?
(A) They maintain the acidic pH of the skin.
(B) They compete successfully for nutrients with pathologic organisms.
(C) They maintain the skin's acidic pH and compete for nutrients with pathologic organisms.
(D) They produce oxygen for use by superficial cell layers and they compete for nutrients with pathologic organisms

54. Which antibody is naturally present in bodily secretions (e.g., saliva)?
(A) IgG
(B) IgQ
(C) IgA
(D) IgE

55. What is the primary purpose of the complement system?
(A) to aid in the coagulation process
(B) to assist antibodies in destroying antigens
(C) to prevent the development of tumor cells
(D) to act as scavengers to clear antigenic debris

56. The various components of the lymphatic drainage system combine to form a large thoracic duct. Where does the thoracic duct empty?
(A) internal mammary artery
(B) inferior vena cava
(C) right atrium
(D) left subclavian vein

57. What is the first stage in the coagulation process?
(A) conversion of plasminogen to plasmin
(B) conversion of fibrinogen to fibrin
(C) activation of thrombin
(D) activation of thromboplastin

58. Tissue plasminogen activator has potential advantages over streptokinase. What are these potential advantages?
    (A) It is clot-specific as opposed to systemic and is less expensive
    (B) It is clot-specific as opposed to systemic and has a shorter half-life
    (C) It is less expensive and has a shorter half-life
    (D) All of the above

59. Nursing care of the patient receiving thrombolytic therapy includes which of the following?
    (A) Avoiding intramuscular injections and using a soft toothbrush
    (B) Avoiding intramuscular injections and using oximetry rather than blood gas studies for SaO$_2$ determination
    (C) Using a soft toothbrush and using oximetry rather than blood gas studies for SaO$_2$ determination
    (D) All of the above

60. Which component is primarily stored in the spleen?
    (A) platelets
    (B) neutrophils
    (C) lymphocytes
    (D) factor VIII

61. Which hormone is thought to regulate bone marrow production of platelets and red blood cells?
    (A) growth hormone
    (B) erythropoietin
    (C) thyroid-stimulating hormone
    (D) ACTH (adrenocorticotropic hormone)

PART IV

Immunology and Hematology Practice Exam

1. _____
2. _____
3. _____
4. _____
5. _____
6. _____
7. _____
8. _____
9. _____
10. _____
11. _____
12. _____
13. _____
14. _____
15. _____
16. _____

17. _____
18. _____
19. _____
20. _____
21. _____
22. _____
23. _____
24. _____
25. _____
26. _____
27. _____
28. _____
29. _____
30. _____
31. _____

32. _____
33. _____
34. _____
35. _____
36. _____
37. _____
38. _____
39. _____
40. _____
41. _____
42. _____
43. _____
44. _____
45. _____
46. _____

47. _____
48. _____
49. _____
50. _____
51. _____
52. _____
53. _____
54. _____
55. _____
56. _____
57. _____
58. _____
59. _____
60. _____
61. _____

1. ___C___ *p 297*
2. ___C___ *p 297*
3. ___D___ *p 297*
4. ___A___ *p 292*
5. ___B___ *p 291*
6. ___D___ *p 292–293*
7. ___C___ *p 296*
8. ___A___ *p 293*
9. ___C___ *p 297*
10. ___D___ *p 298*
11. ___A___ *p 318, 323*
12. ___D___ *p 324*
13. ___C___ *p 322*
14. ___C___ *p 296*
15. ___D___ *p 296*
16. ___C___ *p 299*

17. ___D___ *p 297*
18. ___D___ *p 297*
19. ___B___ *p 326*
20. ___A___ *p 313*
21. ___A___ *p 314*
22. ___A___ *p 310*
23. ___C___ *p 313*
24. ___A___ *p 323, 324*
25. ___D___ *p 295*
26. ___B___ *p 330*
27. ___B___ *p 330*
28. ___C___ *p 329*
29. ___D___ *p 329*
30. ___A___ *p 328*
31. ___D___ *p 326*

32. ___C___ *p 326*
33. ___B___ *p 323–324*
34. ___B___ *p 328*
35. ___C___ *p 308*
36. ___A___ *p 302*
37. ___D___ *p 303*
38. ___A___ *p 308*
39. ___A___ *p 310*
40. ___B___ *p 334*
41. ___D___ *p 306*
42. ___A___ *p 308*
43. ___C___ *p 305*
44. ___B___ *p 329*
45. ___D___ *p 329*
46. ___C___ *p 329*

47. ___B___ *p 329*
48. ___D___ *p 321*
49. ___A___ *p 311*
50. ___A___ *p 312*
51. ___C___ *p 303*
52. ___B___ *p 329*
53. ___C___ *p 292*
54. ___C___ *p 292*
55. ___B___ *p 294*
56. ___D___ *p 295*
57. ___D___ *p 303*
58. ___B___ *p 68, 306*
59. ___D___ *p 68, 69*
60. ___A___ *p 302*
61. ___B___ *p 301*

V

NEUROLOGY

Karen Sudhoff Allard

Anatomy and Physiology of the Nervous System

Perhaps the questions on the CCRN exam that most often gives nurses problems are those on neurological principles. The difficulty in understanding these concepts can be traced to the complexity of central and autonomic nervous system dysfunction. The neurological aspect of the CCRN exam does not require that you be knowledgeable about every potential disturbance of the nervous system; rather, the primary focus is on problems common in general critical nursing practice. This focus makes preparing for the neurological aspect of the CCRN exam more manageable.

In its present format about 8% (16 questions) of the exam is devoted to neurological concepts. The key aspects covered in the CCRN exam include encephalopathies, head trauma, cerebral bleeding/emboli, aneurysms, space-occupying lesions (brain tumors), neurological infectious diseases, seizure disorders, and acute spinal cord injury. If you are not comfortable with neurological concepts, review the following seven chapters carefully. By studying these chapters, seeking patients with neurological conditions, and practicing neurological assessments and neurological tests during your clinical practice you will be well-prepared for the neurological part of the CCRN exam.

ANATOMY

It is customary to divide the nervous system into three segments to facilitate comprehension of the system and its dysfunctions. The three segments are the central nervous system (composed of the brain and spinal cord), the peripheral nervous system (composed of the cranial, spinal, and peripheral nerves), and the autonomic nervous system (composed of the sympathetic and parasympathetic systems).

Extracerebral Structures

Extracerebral structures include the scalp, skull, and meninges. These structures provide protection to the brain.

Scalp

The letters in the word "SCALP" form a mnemonic for remembering the cranial coverings (Fig. 30–1). "SCA" refers to the single layer of skin and cutaneous and adipose tissue which contains blood vessels. Because these vessels cannot contract, a scalp laceration bleeds more than an identical cut elsewhere on the body. The "L" refers to the dense, fibrous *liga*-ment-like layer called the galea aponeurotica. This layer helps to absorb the forces of external trauma. The "P" represents the *p*ericranium, which contains fewer bone-forming elements than the periosteum.

Skull

The bony calvarium (skull) comprises eight bones fused to form a solid, nondistensible unit. The cranium, which refers to the skull minus the mandible, is hollow and has a volume of 1400–1500 ml. It consists of an outer and an inner layer of regular bone and a middle layer, called the diploë (or diploic space), which is spongy and lightweight. This provides protection to the brain without being heavy.

The bones comprising the cranium are the frontal (single), occipital (single), and pairs of pari-

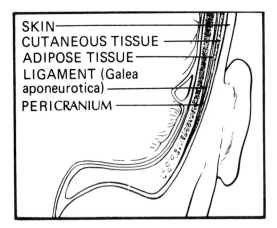

Figure 30–1. Layers of the scalp.

etal, temporal, sphenoid, and ethmoid bones (Fig. 30–2). The main function of the bony calvarium is to protect the brain from external forces. The bones formed during fetal life do not completely fuse until the infant is about 18–24 months of age. The fusion of these bones form three landmarks. The coronal suture is the fusion of the frontal and parietal bones. The sagittal suture is the fusion of the two parietal bones. The lamboidal suture is the fusion of the parietal bones and the occipital bone.

The internal surface of the cranium has three distinct ridges on it that serve to divide the brain into anterior, middle, and posterior segments called fossae (plural; singular is fossa).

Meninges

The three membranes covering the entire brain surface, the spinal cord, and the spinal canal below the cord are the meninges (Fig. 30–3). The mnemonic "PAD" may help you remember the meningeal coverings and their purpose: the *p*ia mater, *a*rachnoid, and *d*ura mater are the meningeal layers and they absorb shocks from sudden movements or trauma—they literally "PAD" the brain.

Starting from the brain itself, the first meningeal layer is the pia mater. The pia mater is contiguous with the brain surface and its convolutions.

The arachnoid layer of the meninges is a delicate, avascular membrane between the dura and pia mater. It looks much like a lacy spiderweb with projections onto the pia mater. The space between the arachnoid layer and pia mater, the subarachnoid space, contains many cerebral arteries and veins which are bathed by cerebrospinal fluid (CSF). The arachnoid membrane also has projections called arachnoid villi which absorb CSF. The subarachnoid space enlarges at the base of the brain to form the subarachnoid cisterns.

The outermost layer of the meninges is the dura mater. The dura mater is actually two layers of tough fibrous membrane that protect the underlying cortical matter. The outermost layer forms the periosteum of the cranial cavity. The inner layer is lined with flat cells, and contains arteries and veins. Between the two layers are clefts, which form the dural venous sinuses. The inner layer also gives rise to several folds that divide the cranial cavity into compartments. Three important folds are the falx cerebri (separating the cerebral hemispheres), the falx cerebelli (separating the right and left cerebellar hemispheres), and the tentorium cerebelli (separating the cerebral hemi-

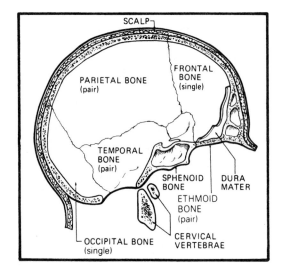

Figure 30–2. Cranium.

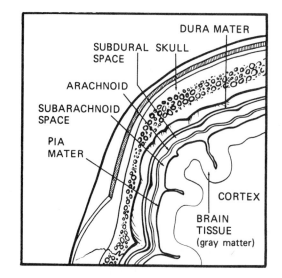

Figure 30–3. Meninges.

spheres from the cerebellum) (Fig. 30–4). These compartmental dividers are significant anatomical landmarks in the brain. The extradural space, also called the epidural space, is a potential space between the inner table of the skull and the outermost meningeal layer, the dura mater. This potential space may become real when an individual experiencing a blow to the head develops an epidural hematoma. Epidural hematomas commonly result from a laceration of the middle meningeal artery in association with a skull fracture at the parietotemporal junction.

Another potential space, the subdural space, lies between the dura mater and the arachnoid. This is the site of subdural hematomas. This type of hematoma is most often venous in origin and results from tearing of the dural veins.

Central Nervous System

The brain is nervous tissue that fills up the cranial vault. It weighs about 3 lb in the adult male. Although it is an integrated unit, for study purposes, it may be divided into six major parts (Fig. 30–5). These parts are the cerebrum (telencephalon), diencephalon, midbrain (mesencephalon), pons, medulla oblongata, and cerebellum.

Cerebrum

The cerebrum is contained in the anterior and middle fossae of the cranium. The left and right cerebral hemispheres are incompletely separated by a deep medial longitudinal fissure formed by the sagittal folds of the dura mater. The fissure is called the falx cerebri. The two cerebral hemispheres are joined by the corpus callosum (Fig. 30–6). The corpus callo-

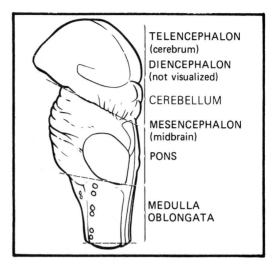

Figure 30–5. Gross anatomical sections of the brain.

sum provides a path for fibers to cross from one hemisphere to the other. Each hemisphere has a lateral ventricle. These two hemispheres together are sometimes referred to as the telencephalon.

The cerebral surface is covered with convolutions which give rise to gyri (raised portions) and sulci or fissures (depressions in the surface). The cerebral surface is about six cells deep and is called the cerebral cortex. It normally appears gray and thus these six layers (Fig. 30–7) are called gray matter. This cortex is estimated to contain 14 billion nerve cells.

Looking at a lateral view of the cerebral hemispheres, we see two fissures dividing the hemisphere (Fig. 30–8). The lateral fissure (also called the fissure of Sylvius) divides the frontal lobe and the temporal lobe (named for the overlying bones). This

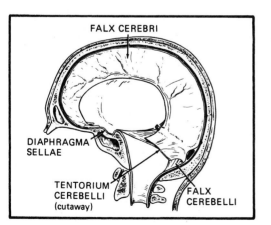

Figure 30–4. Sagittal section showing processes formed by the inner layer of the dura mater.

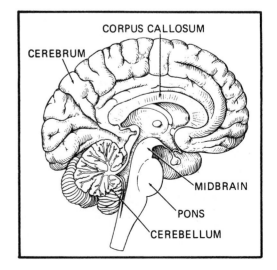

Figure 30–6. Midsagittal section showing the corpus callosum.

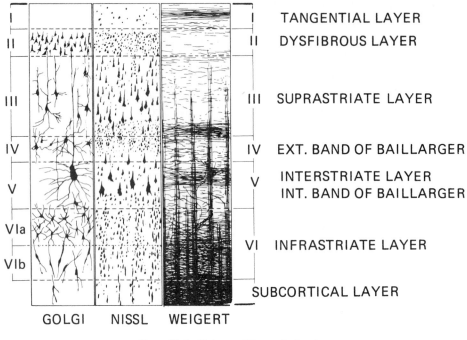

Figure 30–7. Six layers of the cerebral cortex.

area contains the primary auditory center. The central sulcus, also known as the fissure of Rolando, divides the frontal lobe from the parietal lobe. Immediately in front of the central sulcus is the precentral gyrus, which is the primary motor area. Immediately posterior to the central sulcus is the postcentral gyrus, which is the primary sensory cortical area.

When looking at pictures of the brain surface which do not show the cerebellum, imagine the brain as a boxing glove. The thumb of the boxing glove always points toward the frontal area of the

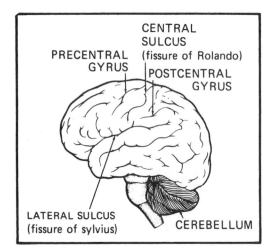

Figure 30–8. Fissures, sulci, and gyri dividing the cerebral hemisphere.

brain. For descriptive purposes, the lateral surface of the hemisphere is divided into four lobes. The frontal lobe (approximately the anterior one-third of the hemisphere) is the portion that is anterior to the central sulcus and above the lateral fissure. The frontal lobe is responsible for voluntary motor function and higher mental functions such as judgment and foresight, affect, and personality. The parietal lobe extends from the central sulcus to the parieto-occipital fissure. This lobe is responsible for sensory function, sensory association, and higher-level processing of general sensory modalities. The occipital lobe is that part lying behind, or caudal to, an arbitrary line drawn from the parieto-occipital fissure to the preoccipital notch. The function of the occipital lobe is visual reception and visual association.

The temporal lobes are located under the lateral fissures of Sylvius. The temporal lobes are each divided into a primary auditory receptive area, a secondary auditory association area, and a tertiary visual association area.

The basal ganglia, or basal nuclei, are also part of the telencephalon. The basal ganglia include the caudate nucleus, putamen, globus pallidus, claustrum, subthalamic nucleus, and substantia nigra (Fig. 30–9).

Specific functions of the brain segments are listed in Table 30–1.

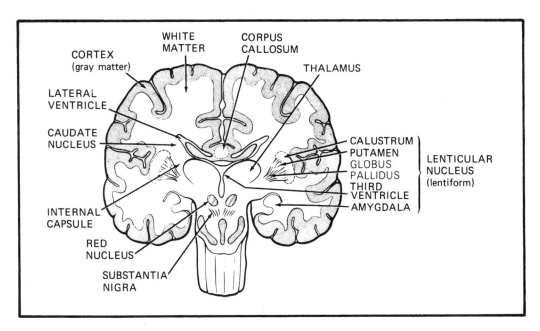

Figure 30–9. Coronal section of the brain showing internal parts of basal ganglia of the telencephalon.

Diencephalon

The diencephalon is the uppermost portion of the brain stem and is covered by the cerebrum (Fig. 30–10). It is a paired structure with a thin fluid space between the two sides. The diencephalon is composed of the thalamus, hypothalamus, and limbic system. The thalamus is the largest structure in the diencephalon; it integrates all body sensations except smell. It is also the major relay area for all neuronal impulses. The hypothalamus connects with the limbic system, thalamus, mesencephalon, and hypophysis (pituitary gland).

Midbrain

The midbrain is also known as the mesencephalon. It is located between the diencephalon and the pons.

TABLE 30–1. FUNCTIONS OF SPECIFIC BRAIN STRUCTURES

Structure	Function
Cerebrum (divided into cerebral hemispheres)	Governs all sensory and motor thought and learning; analyzes, associates, integrates, and stores information
Cerebral cortex (four lobes)	
Frontal lobe	Motor function; motor speech area; controls morals, values, emotions, and judgment
Parietal lobe	Integrates general sensation; governs discrimination; interprets pain, touch, temperature, and pressure
Temporal lobe	Auditory center; sensory speech center
Occipital lobe	Visual area
Basal ganglia	Central motor movement
Thalamus (diencephalon)	Screens and relays sensory impulses to cortex; lowest level of crude conscious awareness
Hypothalamus (diencephalon)	Regulates autonomic nervous system, stress response, sleep, appetite, body temperature, water balance, and emotions
Midbrain (mesencephalon)	Motor condition, conjugate eye movements
Pons	Contains projection tracts between spinal cord, medulla, and brain
Medulla oblongata	Contains all afferent and efferent tracts, most pyramidal tracts, and cardiac, respiratory, vasomotor, and vomiting centers
Cerebellum	Connected by cerebellar peduncles to other parts of CNS; coordinates muscle movement, posture, equilibrium, and muscle tone
Limbic system	Regulation of some visceral activities; some function in emotional personality

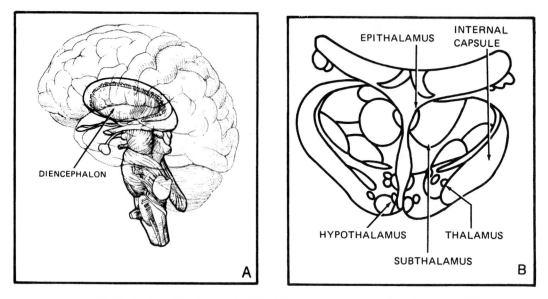

Figure 30–10. Position of the diencephalon **(A)** and the internal components of the diencephalon **(B)**.

It contains the major motor nerves for eye movement, carries impulses down from the cerebrum, and controls the wakefulness of the brain through the reticular activating system (Fig. 30–11). RAS fibers connect with the thalamus, cerebral cortex, cerebellum, and spinal cord. They contain nuclei of the third and fourth cranial nerves.

Pons

The pons is situated between the midbrain and the medulla oblongata. It forms a bridge (thus its name from the Latin word for bridge) between the cerebellar hemispheres and contains the neurons for sensory input and motor output for the face. It contains nuclei of the fifth, sixth, seventh, and eighth cranial nerves. The pons in conjunction with the medulla controls the rate and length of respirations.

Medulla Oblongata

The medulla oblongata is located between the pons and the spinal cord. It is the structure that marks the change between the spinal cord and the brain itself. The corticospinal tracts, which mediate voluntary motor function, descend through the medulla where they decussate in the lower medulla. They are responsible for specific symptoms of dysfunction occurring ipsilaterally (same side as the lesion or injury) or contralaterally (opposite side). Collectively, the mesencephalon, pons, and medulla oblongata are termed the brain stem. Regulation of respiratory rhythm, rate, and strength of heartbeat and blood vessel diameter are controlled by the medulla. The nuclei for

reflex activities such as coughing, sneezing, swallowing, and vomiting and the ninth to twelfth cranial nerves are found here.

Cerebellum

The cerebellum is situated in the posterior fossa of the cranial cavity. It is separated from the cerebrum by dura mater folds forming the tentorium cerebelli. The cerebral hemispheres are above the tentorium cerebelli and are thus supratentorial structures. The two cerebellar hemispheres are connected to each other by a structure called the vermis. They are connected to the brain stem by cerebellar peduncles.

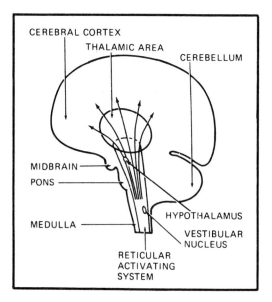

Figure 30–11. Reticular activating system.

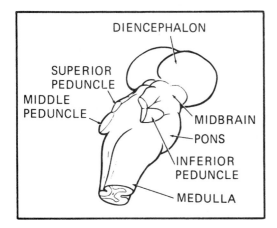

Figure 30–12. Cerebellar peduncles.

There are three cerebellar peduncles (Fig. 30–12). The superior cerebellar peduncles send impulses from the cerebellum to the thalamus. The middle cerebellar peduncles receive cerebral cortex information from nuclei in the pons. The inferior cerebellar peduncles receive impulses that reveal body and extremity positions.

Grey and white matter compose the cerebellum. The cerebellum receives input from the brain stem and spinal cord nuclei, whose axons project to the cerebellar cortex. These tracts carry excitatory impulses to cerebellar cortex.

Equilibrium, posture, muscle tone, and ultimately muscle coordination are mediated by the cerebellum.

Circulation and Formation of Cerebrospinal Fluid

There are four ventricles (cavities) involved in the cerebrospinal fluid (CSF) system (Fig. 30–13). The largest two are the lateral ventricles, which are located in the cerebral hemispheres. The lateral ventricles are connected to the third ventricle via the interventricular foramen, or the foramen of Monro. The cerebral aquaduct of Sylvius exits from the floor of the third ventricle. This channel passes down through the brain stem to the fourth ventricle. The fourth ventricle is continuous with the central canal of the spinal cord. CSF is synthesized by the choroid plexus. This is an area of modified epithelial cells covering tufts of capillaries found in all ventricles but predominating in the anterior segment of the lateral ventricles. CSF is a clear, colorless liquid having a few cells, some protein, glucose, and a large amount of sodium chloride.

The foramen of Monro allows the CSF to leave the lateral ventricles and flow into the third ventri-

cle. Obstruction at this point will produce hydrocephalus. From the third ventricle, CSF flows through the aqueduct of Sylvius into the fourth ventricle. Foramina of Luschka and Magendie direct the CSF from the fourth ventricle into the cisterns and subarachnoid space.

After circulating (in the subarachnoid space) over the entire brain and spinal cord, the CSF is reabsorbed by the arachnoid villi in dural sinuses and by pacchionian bodies found in the superior sagittal sinus.

The CSF "cushions" the brain and spinal cord to protect them from colliding with the cranium and vertebrae in response to moving forces. The CSF also reduces the gravitational weight of the brain. To a limited extent, the CSF adjusts to changes in the intracranial vault's pressure and volume. If the pressure or volume increases in the vault, more CSF will be absorbed and/or pushed into the spinal canal in an attempt to maintain normal pressure. Normally, 125–150 ml of CSF are in the ventricles and the subarachnoid space. An average of 500–800 ml (or approximately 25–35 ml/hr) of CSF is produced in 24 hr. The CSF also participates in the exchange of nutrients and waste material between the blood and the CNS cells.

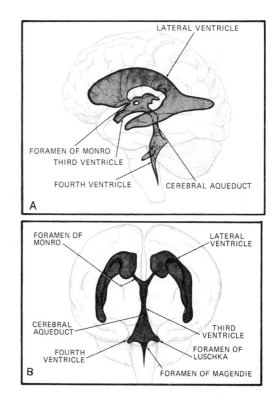

Figure 30–13. Lateral view of the ventricular system of the brain **(A)** and anterior view of the ventricular system of the brain **(B)**.

Cerebral Blood Supply

The brain is supplied with oxygenated blood from two arterial systems: the internal carotid arteries and the vertebral arteries. As a reserve to these two systems, the circle of Willis helps provide adequate circulation through its anastomoses. The circle of Willis anastomoses are between the two vertebral arteries and the two carotid arteries (Fig. 30–14). The internal carotid carries about two thirds of the blood flow to the brain.

External Cerebral Blood Supply. The external carotid arteries bifurcate and form the occipital, temporal, and maxillary arteries. The occipital arteries supply the posterior fossa. The temporal arteries supply the temporal region. The maxillary arteries form the middle meningeal arteries which supply the anterior, middle, and posterior portions of the meninges and the fossae. While not a part of cerebral circulation, the external carotid artery and its branches have been used to supplement cerebral circulation in the individual with cerebrovascular disease.

Internal Cerebral Blood Supply. On entering the skull, the internal carotid artery follows the carotid groove upward through the cavernous sinus and the sphenoid bone and into the circle of Willis at the base of the brain. Before this, smaller vessels originate, one of which is the opthalmic artery to the retina. Temporary blockage of this vessel by microemboli may cause fleeting monocular blindness (amaurosis fugax).

The internal carotid arteries bifurcate to form the anterior cerebral arteries, the anterior communicating arteries, the middle cerebral arteries, the posterior communicating arteries, and the anterior choroidal arteries. The anterior communicating artery connects the left and right anterior cerebral arteries. The posterior communicating artery connects the internal carotid arteries to the basilar artery. These communicating arteries do not supply any part of the brain directly, but some are collateral channels helping to form the circle in the circle of Willis.

The vertebral arteries enter the posterior fossa and join to form the basilar artery. The basilar artery bifurcates to form the superior cerebellar arteries and the posterior cerebral arteries. The superior cerebellar arteries supply the pons and the cerebellum. Posterior cerebral arteries supply the posterior one-third of the cerebrum.

Some of these arteries anastomose with each other to form the circle of Willis. They are the anterior cerebral artery, the anterior communicating artery, the posterior communicating arteries, and the posterior cerebral arteries. All of these arteries are involved in supplying blood to the anterior two-thirds of the cerebrum.

Only about 50% of all people have a "classic" circle of Willis. The most common difference is that the posterior communicating artery is not present and the posterior cerebral artery comes directly from the internal carotid artery.

Veins run parallel with many of the arteries. The middle meningeal arteries are special in that the veins that accompany these arteries are positioned between the arteries and the bones of the cranium. This helps protect the middle meningeal artery, which is frequently torn in skull fractures of the temporal bones.

As there is an internal and external arterial blood supply, there is a corresponding internal and external venous return system. Many of the veins are important in aneurysms and as surgical landmarks. The veins which drain the dura mater and diploë of the skull (external) empty into the venous sinuses which are located between the layers of the dura mater. Internal cerebral veins also empty into venous sinuses.

Venous sinuses are lined with epithelium; they have no valves and no muscle in the walls. The sinuses connect with emissary veins which in turn connect with external cranial veins that empty into the internal jugular veins. The superior sagittal sinus receives

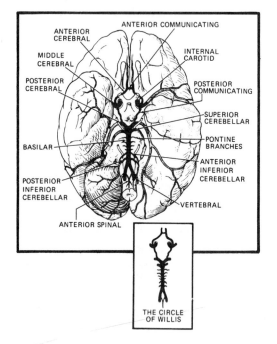

Figure 30–14. Circle of Willis.

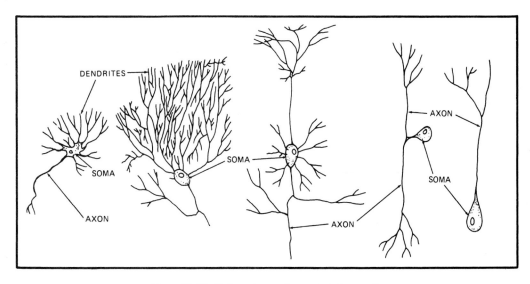

Figure 30–15. Various shapes of neurons and neuroglia.

venous blood from the superior cerebral veins. The inferior sagittal sinus receives venous blood from the medical cerebral hemisphere veins. The straight sinus receives venous blood from the internal cerebral veins. There are many other sinuses that receive venous blood from other areas of the brain.

Components of Nervous Tissue

There are two main types of cells in the brain: neurons (Fig. 30–15) and neuroglia (glial cells). The neuron is the functioning unit of the nervous system and its function is to transmit impulses. There are more than 10 billion neurons in the CNS and three-fourths of them are in the cerebral cortex.

Neurons are categorized in two ways: by the direction of impulse flow and/or by the number of processes emanating from the neuron cell body. Neurons that transmit impulses to the spinal cord or brain are afferent sensory neurons. Those transmitting impulses away from the brain or spinal cord are called efferent motor neurons. Interneurons transmit impulses from sensory neurons to motor neurons. The mnemonic "SAME" helps maintain correct direction and type of neuron, "SA" standing for sensory afferent and "ME" standing for motor efferent.

Neurons will be one of three types according to the number of processes that exist. Unipolar neurons have one process coming from the cell body. After a short distance, this one process will split to form one axon and one dendrite (typical of both cranial and spinal nerves). Bipolar neurons have one axon and one dendrite coming from the cell body (rod and cone cells of the optic system to the CNS).

Multipolar neurons have one axon and multiple dendrites (typical of motor neurons).

Regardless of the category of neurons, they all have certain unique structures common only to neurons (Fig. 30–16), that is, axons, dendrites, neurofibrils, Nissl bodies, myelin, neurilemma, and nodes of Ranvier.

The cell body of a neuron is called a soma or perikaryon. It contains a nucleus and many cytoplasmic organelles. The axon originates from a thickened area of the soma called an axon hillock. The axon transmits impulses away from the soma. There is one axon per neuron. Dendrites are short processes that transmit impulses to the soma. Multipolar neurons have many dendrites. The branching of dendritic processes is termed arborization since the processes look like tree branches. Neurofibrils are thin, threadlike fibers forming a network in the cytoplasm. Nissl bodies specialize in pro-

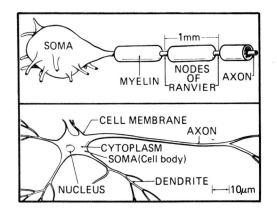

Figure 30–16. Schematic diagram of the structures of the neuron.

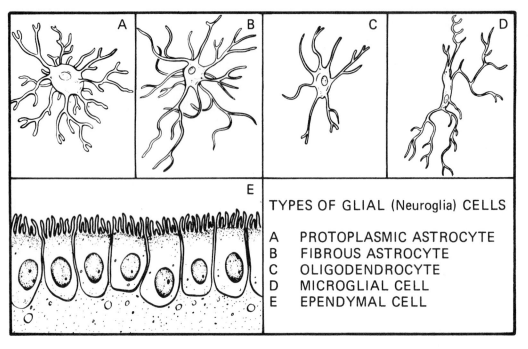

Figure 30–17. Types of glial cells (neuroglia).

tein synthesis with RNA to maintain and regenerate the neuronal processes.

Myelin is a protein–lipid compound that covers some axons. In the CNS, myelin is reduced by oligodendrocytes. In the peripheral nervous system, myelin is produced by Schwann cells. Myelin covers axons of nerve cells in between the nodes of Ranvier. The nodes of Ranvier are bare spots at regular intervals that speed the conduction of impulses.

The neurilemma is an outer coating of the neurons outside of the CNS. The neurilemma encompasses all structures, even myelin. It is the neurilemma that provides for peripheral nerve regeneration. Since the neurilemma is not found on neurons of the brain and spinal cord, these neurons cannot regenerate.

Neurons require an extensive support system to maintain optimal function. The neuroglia are responsible for this support system (Figure 30–17). Neuroglia are composed of glial cells and they outnumber the neurons by 10 to 1. Four types of specific cells compose the glial support system.

1. Astrocytes are star-shaped cells that form the actual tissue support system. Astrocytes, which may be protoplasmic or fibrous tissue, constitute part of the blood–brain barrier by sending foot processes to the blood vessels.
2. Microglia are tiny cells that lie quiescent until nervous tissue is damaged. Because of their origin, microglia are part of the reticuloendothelial cell system. They wander in and out of the CNS in response to need. When damage occurs, the microglia mobile and travel to the damaged tissue. They enlarge and phagocytize the debris.
3. Oligodendroglia help support the nervous tissue, but their primary function is the original formation of myelin in the CNS during fetal, neonatal, and early years. Once the myelin has been formed, the oligodendroglia cannot form it again.
4. Ependyma are special glial cells that are found lining the ventricles of the brain and the central canal in the spinal cord.

The spinal cord is the second part of the central nervous system. It is examined in Chapter 34.

The Peripheral Nervous System

The peripheral nerves, the spinal nerves, and the cranial nerves form the peripheral nervous system. There are 31 pairs of spinal nerves and 12 pairs of cranial nerves.

Instead of being named the 31 pairs of spinal nerves are numbered in relation to the vertebral level at which they emerge from the spinal cord. Spinal nerves do not attach directly to the spinal cord. Instead, the spinal nerves attach to a short anterior (ventral, motor) root and a short posterior (dorsal, sensory) root (Fig. 30–18). The posterior root has a bulge which consists of neuron cell bodies. This bulge is called a spinal ganglia. There are 8 cervical, 12 thoracic, 5 lumbar, 5 sacral, and 1 coccygeal spinal pair of ganglia.

Peripheral nerves often encompass more than one spinal nerve root. The sciatic nerve is a good example. It includes all the spinal nerve roots in the sacrum.

Spinal Nerve Fibers

There are four types of nerve fibers composing the spinal nerves.

1. Motor fibers originate in the ventral (anterior) horn of the spinal cord with efferent fibers relaying motor impulses from the CNS to peripheral skeletal muscles.
2. Sensory fibers originate in the dorsal (posterior) horn of the spinal cord with afferent fibers relaying sensory impulses from organs and muscles to the CNS.
3. Meningeal fibers transmit sensory and vasomotor innervation to the spinal meninges.
4. Autonomic fibers will be considered separately.

Dermatomes

Each spinal nerve dorsal root innervates a specific portion of skin. The skin regions are called dermatomes (Fig. 30–19). These are clinically important in identifying areas of spinal cord injury.

Plexuses

The spinal nerves interweave in three areas that are termed the cervical, brachial, and lumbosacral plexuses (Fig. 30–20). The cervical plexus involves spinal nerves C1 to C4. It sends motor impulses to neck muscles and the diaphragm. It receives sensory impulses from the neck and head. The brachial plexus is composed of spinal nerves C4 to C8 and T1. It innervates the arms. The lumbosacral plexus is formed by spinal nerves L1 to L5 and S1 to S3. This plexus innervates the legs.

Cranial Nerves

Twelve pairs of cranial nerves complete the peripheral nervous system. Three pairs of cranial nerves are totally sensory, five pairs are totally motor, and four pairs are combined sensorimotor. Origin of the nerves is seen in Figure 30–21. By convention the cranial nerves are numbered by roman numerals as well as named.

The cranial nerves are summarized in Table 30–2. The standard mnemonic may help keep them in order: On Old Olympus' Towering Tops, A Finn And German Viewed Some Hops.

The Autonomic Nervous System

The sympathetic nervous system and the parasympathetic nervous system together form the autonomic nervous system. Technically, the autonomic nervous system is part of the peripheral nervous system. However, it seems easier to understand the autonomic nervous system if it is looked at as a separate system.

The sympathetic nervous system releases norepinephrine, which stimulates and prepares our bodies for "fight or flight." Norepinephrine and epinephrine are categorized as adrenergic chemicals (hormones). Fibers originating in the thoracic and lumbar areas form the peripheral sympathetic nervous system division.

The parasympathetic nervous system releases acetylcholine, which is categorized as a cholinergic

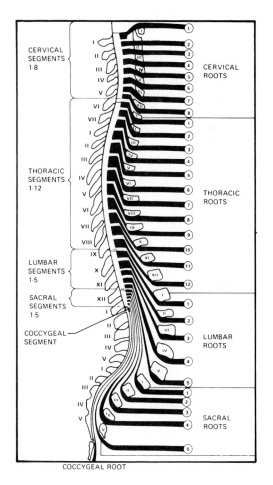

Figure 30–18. Spinal nerve roots and their attachment to the spinal cord.

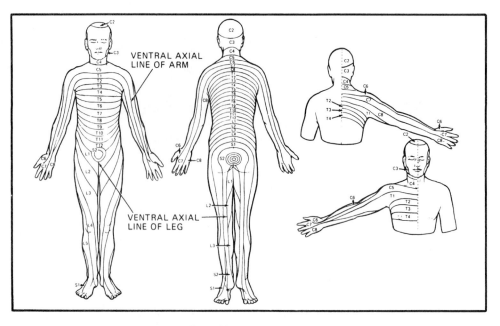

Figure 30–19. Dermatomes.

chemical (hormone). In reality, the parasympathetic system is an antagonist to the sympathetic system and mediates or slows body responses when the "fight, fright, or flight" situation no longer exists. Fibers originating in the cranial and sacral areas form the peripheral parasympathetic nervous system division. Atropine is an example of a parasympatheic stimulant.

Nerve Structures of the Autonomic Nervous System

The sympathetic nervous system has a chain of ganglia situated on both sides of the vertebrae (Fig. 30–22). Nerve fibers between the spinal cord and the ganglia are termed preganglionic fibers (or axons). The nerve fibers between the ganglia and visceral end organ are called postganglionic fibers (or axons). The norepinephrine that is released to maintain body function is not easily nor rapidly neutralized, so the effect is sustained for a period of time. The sympathetic system may be referred to as the thoracolumbar system since major ganglia arise in the thoracic and lumbar regions.

The parasympathetic nervous system does not have a chain of ganglia next to the vertebral column. The preganglionic fibers (or axons) originate in the brain and sacrum (Fig. 30–23). These axons are long to allow them to reach specific organs. Ganglia are found adjacent to or within specific organs. Postganglionic fibers (or axons) are therefore short.

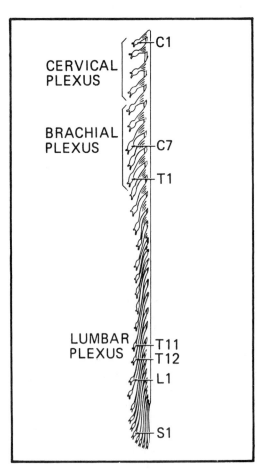

Figure 30–20. The three spinal nerve plexuses.

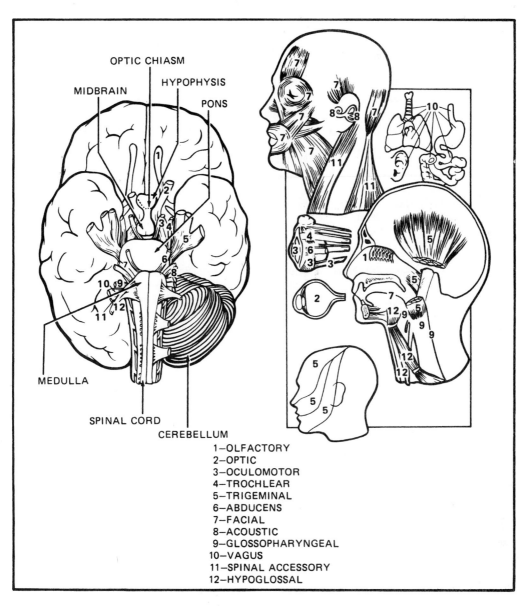

Figure 30–21. Origin of the cranial nerves.

1—OLFACTORY
2—OPTIC
3—OCULOMOTOR
4—TROCHLEAR
5—TRIGEMINAL
6—ABDUCENS
7—FACIAL
8—ACOUSTIC
9—GLOSSOPHARYNGEAL
10—VAGUS
11—SPINAL ACCESSORY
12—HYPOGLOSSAL

The chemical released by the parasympathetic system, acetylcholine, is rapidly neutralized by cholinesterase. Because of this, the parasympathetic effect is brief and must be renewed fairly regularly to counter the sympathetic stimulation. This system may be referred to as the craniosacral system since the preganglionic fibers arise from certain cranial nerves and in the sacral spinal cord.

Neural Cell Depolarization and Repolarization

Depolarization and repolarization of the nerve cell follow the same principles as depolarization and repolarization of the cardiac cell.

Depolarization

The neuron in a resting state (resting membrane potential, or RMP) is positively charged outside the cell membrane and negatively charged on the inner surface of the cell membrane. When the cell is stimulated, sodium rapidly enters the cell and potassium leaves the cell. This produces a positive ionic charge at the entry site and decreases the resting membrane potential. This positive ionic charge is transmitted along the length of the neuron and is termed a wave of depolarization.

Repolarization

As soon as potassium reenters the cell and sodium leaves the cell, the resting state of the cell is re-estab-

TABLE 30–2. SUMMARY OF CRANIAL NERVES

Number	Name	Major Functions
I	Olfactory	Sense of smell
II	Optic	Central and peripheral vision
III	Oculomotor	Eye movement; elevation of upper eyelid; pupil constriction
IV	Trochlear	Downward and inward eye movement
V	Trigeminal	Touch, pain, temperature; jaw and eye muscle proprioception; mastication
VI	Abducens	Abduction of the eye
VII	Facial	Close eyelid, muscles of facial expression; secretion by glands of mouth and eyes; taste (anterior two-thirds of tongue)
VIII	Acoustic Vestibular branch Cochlear branch	Equilibrium Hearing
IX	Glossopharyngeal	Movement of pharyngeal muscles; secretion by parotid glands; pharyngeal and posterior tongue sensation
X	Vagus	Pharyngeal and laryngeal movement; visceral activities; pharyngeal and laryngeal sensation; taste
XI	Spinal accessory	Pharyngeal, sternocleidomastoid, and trapezius movement
XII	Hypoglossal	Tongue movement

lished. This is called repolarization. A specific mechanism exists to force the sodium ions that entered the cell's cytoplasm back into the extracellular fluid. The mechanism is termed the sodium pump. Without the sodium pump, ion homeostasis could not be preserved. At the same time, a potassium pump exists to maintain potassium ion homeostasis by forcing potassium ions back into the cell.

An action potential occurs when an ionic charge on one side of the membrane is different from an ionic charge on the other. Depolarization occurs when a stimulus is strong enough (threshold) to alter the cell membrane permeability to sodium, allowing a change in the ionic charge. (Sodium ions enter and potassium ions leave the cell interior.) Once an action potential exists and a stimulus of threshold-level magnitude occurs, the neuron totally depolarizes. The neuron depolarizes following the all-or-none principle. It depolarizes in its entirety or else it does not depolarize at all. As with the cardiac cell, the neuron has a complete refractory period during which it is repolarizing and cannot be stimulated. Also like the cardiac cell, the neuron has a relative refractory period. During this period, the neuron can be stimulated (or excited), but only when the stimulus is at a threshold level.

Two terms are important in relation to action potentials. Summation refers to repetitive, accumulated discharges that eventually reach threshold level (much like building blocks one on top of the other until the top is reached). Facilitation is an increase in every subsequent neuron stimulus even though the stimulus remains below threshold levels. No action potential occurs in facilitation. Action potential does occur in summation.

The rapid velocity of conduction of the impulse is due in part to the neuron structure (Fig. 30–24) and the size of the nerve fiber. Myelin is a protective, lipid insulation of the neuron that is nonconductive. This prevents an easy flow of ions into the nerve fiber. The myelin sheath is segmented. At specified intervals the myelin sheath is totally absent. These noninsulated points are called nodes of Ranvier. Ions flow easily around the nerve fiber at the nodes of Ranvier. The action potential on myelinated nerve fibers jumps from one node of Ranvier to the next node of Ranvier. This is called saltatory conduction and is far faster than conduction in an unmyelinated fiber. In unmyelinated fibers, the impulse must travel the entire length of the neuron.

Chemical Synapses

A synapse is a point of junction, but not of contact, between one neuron and another neuron, a muscle cell, or a gland cell. Synapses differ in shape and size, but function similarly in transmitting impulses.

The neuron's axon enlarges at its end, forming a synaptic knob. This knob may be called a terminal button or a presynaptic terminal (Fig. 30–25). The synaptic knob contains vesicles which are filled with specific

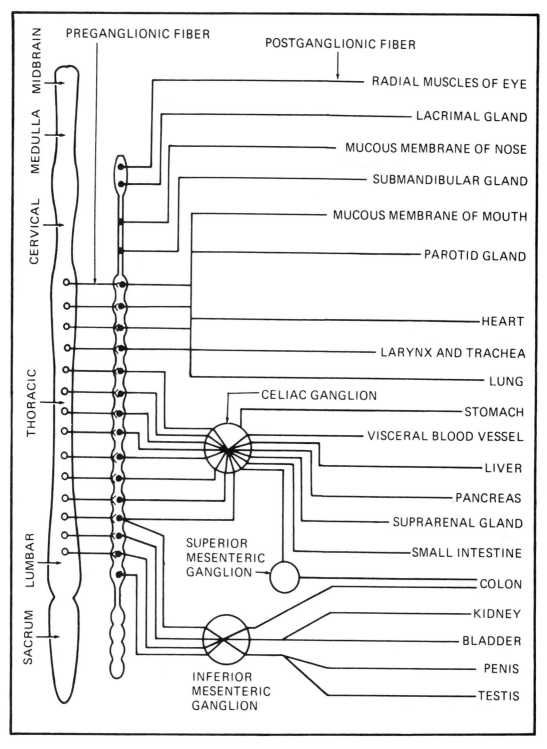

Figure 30–22. Sympathetic nervous system ganglia.

neurotransmitter chemicals. When the axonal knob is stimulated, these chemicals are released from the vesicles. The presynaptic terminal is separated from the postsynaptic side by a minute space termed the synaptic cleft. The postsynaptic membrane is slightly thicker at the synaptic cleft than elsewhere and is termed the subsynaptic membrane. The extra thickness is thought to be due to an increased number of receptor sites for the neurotransmitter.

When the axons of a motor neuron synapse with skeletal muscle, the presynaptic terminal (synaptic knob) is called a neuromuscular junction or a neuromuscular end plate (Fig. 30–26). At this specific synapse, the presynaptic terminal looks like a plate.

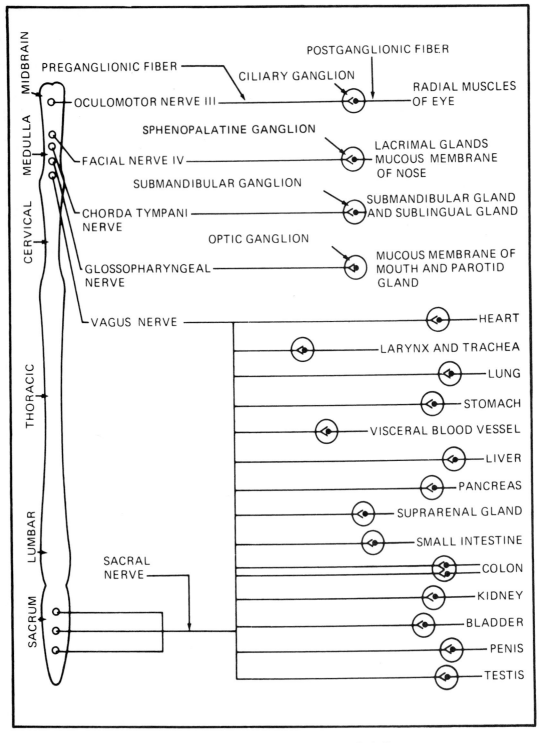

Figure 30–23. Parasympathetic nervous system ganglionic fibers.

The neuromuscular junction is the only synapse specifically named.

Neurotransmitters

Acetylcholine

Acetylcholine is the neurotransmitter chemical found in the vesicles of neuromuscular junctions and in the parasympathetic system. Acetylcholine is the primary neurotransmitter of the peripheral nervous system. As the action potential in the axon reaches the neuromuscular junction, the neuromuscular junction is stimulated to release the chemical in its vesicles. The chemical diffuses across the synaptic cleft, coming in contact with receptors on the postsynaptic membrane. Acetylcholine acts on the postsynaptic mem-

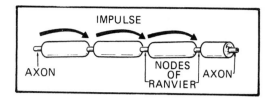

Figure 30–24. Nodes of Ranvier providing saltatory conduction.

brane briefly before it is neutralized by the enzyme acetylcholinesterase (ACH). The milliseconds that acetylcholine is in contact with the postsynaptic membrane are enough to propagate conduction of an impulse. ACH is found in abundance in skeletal muscles and blood, so it very rapidly breaks down acetylcholine into acetic acid and choline. This rapid degradation of acetylcholine ensures that only one action potential occurs at a time at the receptor sites on the postsynaptic membrane. The end products (acetic acid and choline) are resynthesized in the synaptic vesicles for use again.

The end result of the release of acetylcholine at many peripheral synapses is muscular contraction. The amount of acetylcholine released is determined in part by calcium ion diffusion into the presynaptic terminal. Calcium ions are necessary for depolarization at other peripheral synapses, so it is assumed that calcium plays a similar role at all chemical synapses.

Acetylcholine is a cholinergic neurotransmitter. It is thought that more cholinergic synapses exist in the CNS, but they have not been positively identified.

Monoamines

The monoamines that have been identified as neurotransmitters in the CNS include the catechol-

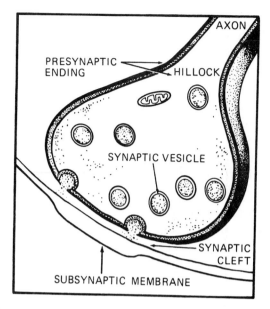

Figure 30–26. Neuromuscular junction or neuromuscular end plate.

amines dopamine, norepinephrine, and epinephrine, and the indolamine serotonin. Catecholamines are produced in the brain and in the sympathetic ganglia from their amino-acid precursor tyrosine. Serotonin is produced in the brain and other tissues by the body from the amino acid tryptophan. The activity of the monoamine neurotransmitters in the synaptic cleft is limited by their reuptake into the presynaptic ending, where they are recycled into vesicles for future release.

Dopamine

Dopamine is a precursor of epinephrine and norepinephrine. Dopamine acts as an inhibitory chemical transmitter and is one of the most important chemicals involved in basal ganglionic functions (acetylcholine is the other important transmitter in basal ganglionic functions). Dopamine is decreased in the brains of patients with parkinsonism. It may play a role in eating, drinking, and sexual behavior.

Epinephrine and Norepinephrine

Epinephrine and norepinephrine are found in adrenergic fibers of the sympathetic nervous system. In the CNS, norepinephrine cell bodies are confined to the brain stem, but their axons extend to all parts of the CNS. Epinephrine neurons are restricted to the lower brain stem.

Like dopamine, norepinephrine has been found to have inhibitory influences on postsynaptic neurons. Little is known of the action of epinephrine as a central neurotransmitter. Within the sympathetic nervous system epinephrine and norepinephrine are found in adrenergic fibers. They exert

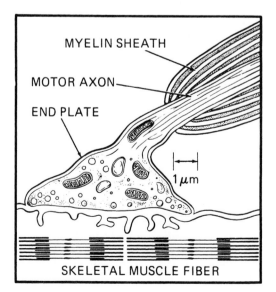

Figure 30–25. Chemical synapse.

a generalized "fight, flight, or fright" response in the body.

Serotonin

Serotonin is also a monoamine chemical. It is an inhibitory transmitter and is linked to slow-wave sleep patterns. Although serotonin has been implicated in a physiological role with sleep, psychotic states, pain transmission and response to hallucinogenic drugs, there is little known about its specific function.

Gaba-aminobutyric Acid

Gamma-aminobutyric acid (GABA) is a neutral amino acid that has an inhibitory effect on synaptic function. It is found in the CNS.

Reflexes

A reflex is a stereotypical reaction of the CNS to specific sensory stimuli. There are two types of reflexes: the monosynaptic reflex and the polysynaptic reflex.

Monosynaptic Reflex Arc

This constitutes the simplest reflex in the body and is depicted in Figure 30–27. Inside every group of muscles is a structure called a muscle spindle. The muscle spindle is made of small fibers that are bound together by afferent sensory fibers (Fig. 30–28). As a muscle spindle is stretched, an action potential develops and a sensory impulse travels to the dorsal root

ganglion. From the ganglion the impulse enters the spinal cord. In the gray matter (unmyelinated) of the spinal cord, the impulse synapses with interneurons in the anterior portion of the cord. These interneurons have efferent (motor) fibers that leave the spinal cord through the anterior (ventral) root. The efferent fibers carry an impulse back to the original muscle. The muscle contracts upon receiving this impulse.

The monosynaptic reflex arc is more important in research than in practice. However, the muscle stretch reflex (knee jerk) is the most commonly tested reflex.

Polysynaptic Reflex Arcs

The withdrawal reflex is a common example of the polysynaptic reflex (Fig. 30–29). Afferent nerve fibers in the peripheral muscles are excited, producing an impulse. This impulse enters the spinal cord via a dorsal root ganglion. This excited neuron will synapse with appropriate interneurons within the gray matter of the spinal cord.

The interneurons in the anterior (ventral) horn emerge from the spinal cord through efferent (motor) fibers. These fibers transmit the motor impulse to the original muscle that produced the sensory impulse. The muscle then contracts. There are literally hundreds of interneurons with which the impulse could and does snyapse, thus the name polysynaptic reflex arc.

When impulses effect a muscular contraction, other impulses must negate the function of opposing muscle groups. For the knee to bend, extensor

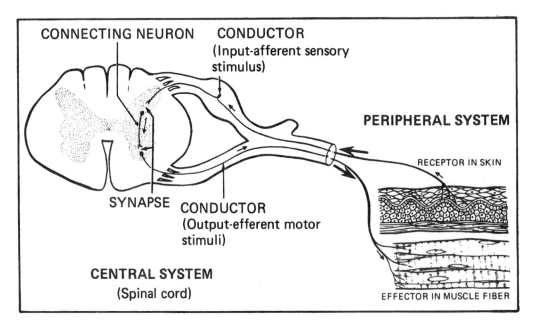

Figure 30–27. Monosynaptic reflex arc.

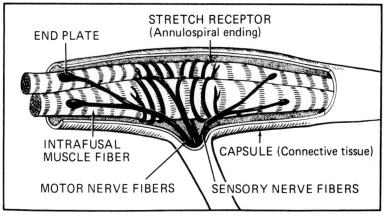

Figure 30–28. Muscle spindle.

muscles are inhibited and concurrently flexor muscles are excited. This is termed the law of reciprocal innervation.

Metabolism in the Brain

Both white matter (myelinated) and gray matter (unmyelinated) have the same metabolic needs.

The cerebral need for oxygen does not decrease in a resting state. Even though it weighs only about 3 lb (2% of the body weight), brain tissue requires about 20% of the body's oxygen supply. The brain needs a constant supply of oxygen and is unable to store oxygen for future use. The energy necessary for metabolic functions of the brain is obtained from the oxidation of glucose. All oxidative reactions require

oxygen. Hypoxia may occur without irreversible anoxic injury to brain cells. If the anoxic state lasts 4 or more minutes at normal body temperature, cerebral neurons are destroyed. Once destroyed, cerebral neurons cannot regenerate. The area of the brain most sensitive to hypoxia is the telencephalon, particularly the hippocampus, which is most likely to be damaged by small amounts of decreased oxygen. Since the cerebral cortex is only six layers (cells) deep (see Fig. 30–7), the entire cerebral cortex, especially layer four, is very sensitive to decreases in oxygen. Damage here results in a condition termed laminar cortical necrosis.

The brain stem is the area most resistant to hypoxic damage. If hypoxia occurs in this area beyond the 4–5-min limit, irreversible coma or a persistent vegetative state usually develops.

Nutritional Needs

The extensive, continuous activity of the brain results in very high metabolic energy needs. Glucose, a carbohydrate, is the main source of energy (adenosine triphosphate, or ATP) for cellular activity. Glucose and oxygen are essential for re-establishing electrochemical gradients for impulse transmission, for the synthesis of neurotransmitters, and for maintaining cellular integrity. If the cerebral glucose level is less than 70 mg/100 ml, confusion results. With a glucose level of less than 20 mg/100 ml, coma develops followed by death (without treatment). Whereas hypoglycemia causes confusion, coma, and death, hyperglycemia does not appear to have a direct influence on nervous system functions. Certain vitamins are essential in adequate amounts to ensure normal central nervous system functions.

Vitamin B_1 (thiamine) is important in the Krebs cycle of energy production. Insufficient B_1, common in alcoholics, causes Wernicke–Korsakoff's syn-

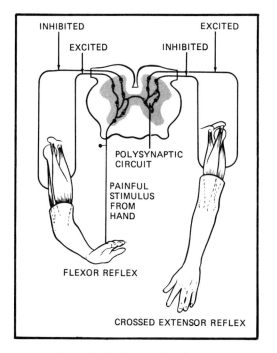

Figure 30–29. Polysynaptic reflex arc.

drome, which in late stages causes cerebellar degeneration.

Vitamin B_{12} function is not understood. However, insufficient B_{12} results in a gradual degeneration of the brain, optic nerves, spinal cord (especially posterior and lateral columns), and dorsal root entry zone of the peripheral nerves. Degeneration often starts with the spinal cord. Pernicious anemia is the dominant systemic disease of vitamin B_{12} deficiency. A deficiency is also present in alcoholism and other malnutritional states.

Pyridoxine is a coenzyme and participates in many enzymatic reactions in the CNS. Pyridoxine deficiencies produce polyneuropathies, seborrheic dermatitis, glossitis, and conjunctivitis.

Nicotinic acid is needed for synthesis of coenzymes. Insufficient nicotinic acid results in altered mentation, leading to coma, extrapyramidal rigidity, and tremors of the extremities. This form of encephalopathy seems to be becoming nonexistent in the United States. There may be a relationship between inadequate nicotinic acid and pellagra.

Circulatory Needs

The brain needs a more continuous supply of oxygenated blood, even during sleep, than any other organ because the brain's needs are never decreased. The cerebral blood flow (CBF) is determined in part by the cerebral perfusion pressure (CPP). This pressure is the difference between mean arterial (systemic) pressure (MAP) and intracranial pressure (ICP) (CPP = MAP − ICP). The size of the cerebrovascular system, activity, disease, fever, injury, and other factors determine the actual amount of blood needed at any given time.

Hypercapnia ($PaCO_2$ greater than 45 mm Hg) and to a lesser extent hypoxia (PaO_2 less than 60 mm Hg) will cause an arteriolar dilatation of the cerebral arteries, increasing the amount of blood flowing into the brain regardless of the actual amount needed. This may cause an increase in ICP that the healthy brain could accommodate but that an injured or diseased brain may not be able to accommodate.

Increases in ICP will result in a decrease in blood perfusion to the brain because of compression of the arteries, veins, and brain mass as a whole. The brain has its own autoregulatory mechanism which functions mainly by increasing (constricting arteries) resistance to blood flow or by decreasing (dilatation of arteries) resistance to blood flow, thus altering the diameter of the vessels. Autoregulation maintains constant blood flow over a range of perfusion pressures. The limits of autoregulation are generally thought to be a MAP between 50 and 150 mm Hg. This system works well until the ICP increases beyond a certain unknown point when compensatory mechanisms fail.

Blood–Brain Barrier

A barrier is known to exist between the blood and brain which controls the diffusion of substances from the blood into the extracellular fluid or the CSF of the brain. The location and structure of this carrier is thought to be related to the "tight junctions" of cerebral endothelial cells. The permeability of cerebral capillaries and the choroid plexus controls the movement of specific substances.

Water, oxygen, glucose, and carbon dioxide move quickly through the blood–brain barrier. Other substances either move slowly or not at all across the barrier. This control determines the level of metabolism, ionic composition, and the homeostasis of cerebral tissue.

In addition to a blood–brain barrier, there is a blood–CSF barrier. This barrier functions like the blood–brain barrier in controlling the composition of the CSF. This is a vitally important function because substances in the CSF are rapidly absorbed into the interstitial brain fluid.

Intracranial Pressure

In this chapter, the concepts of intracranial pressure are covered. Expect one to three questions on the CCRN exam to refer to the contents of this chapter.

PHYSIOLOGY OF INTRACRANIAL PRESSURE

The volume of the cranial vault is about 80% brain tissue, 10% cerebrospinal fluid (CSF), and 10% intravascular fluid (blood). Together these three components almost completely fill the cranial vault.

In the adult the cranial vault is nondistensible (it is bone) and the components of the vault are essentially noncompressible. Based on these tenets, a relationship between the vault and its contents can be construed. This is known as the Munro–Kellie hypothesis, and is the basis for changes in intracranial pressure.

Within a very narrow range, the contents of the cranial vault can adjust to increases in ICP. When the limits of range and time are exceeded, the ICP rises precipitously.

An increase in one component of the vault contents necessitates a reciprocal decrease in either one or both of the other components. If the reciprocal decrease does not occur, there is a rise in ICP. Normal ICP is less than 10 mm Hg. Most practitioners treat a sustained ICP above 15–20 mm Hg. Intracranial hypertension is considered an ICP above 20 mm Hg.

Compensatory Mechanisms for Increasing Intracranial Pressure

Initial increases in the volume of the cranium are compensated for by two mechanisms, compression of the low-pressure venous system and the displacement of CSF.

1. A decrease in intravascular fluid (blood) occurs by compression of the low-pressure venous system. Intravascular volume is the most alterable of the three component of cranium (brain tissue, CSF, and blood). There is a specific limit to the extent of compressibility. When this limit is exceeded, ICP rises.
2. Displacement of CSF is the second compensatory mechanism for increasing ICP. As the ICP rises, CSF is displaced from the cranial vault into the spinal canal. When maximum displacement of CSF has occurred, there is probably an increase in CSF absorption which aids compensatory mechanisms.

These mechanisms function to keep the ICP constant. They function well when the ICP increases slowly. Even then, the mechanisms will lose their compensatory function at a certain point (variable with the individual). If the ICP rises rapidly, the compensatory mechanisms are unable to function.

Intracranial Compliance

The relationship of change in pressure to change in volume is termed compliance. When intracranial compliance is low, a small increase in volume causes a large rise in pressure. The ICP provides information about intracranial compliance. Cerebral perfusion pressure (CPP), the difference between the mean arterial pressure (MAP) and the mean ICP (CPP = MAP − ICP), is equally as important as compliance. It reflects the pressure in the cerebral vascular system. This pressure approximates cerebral blood flow (CBF). Decreases in the CPP reduce CBF. The CBF affects delivery of both oxygen and glucose to the brain tissue. The normal brain has an extremely good autoregulatory system that maintains normal blood flow with a CPP as low as 50 mm Hg. In the injured brain, activity of the autoregulatory system is not known. Thus, many authorities consider a CPP of greater than 80 mm Hg ideal and a CPP of 60 mm Hg to be the least acceptable pressure. If the patient is neurologically unstable, CPP is extremely important when the MAP is low or when the ICP is high. If the MAP is low or the ICP is high, the brain is *not* being adequately perfused with oxygenated blood.

INTRACRANIAL PRESSURE MONITORING

Indications

The outcome of many neurological conditions can be mediated by early recognition of and intervention in increasing ICP. Six areas are identified:

1. Head injuries. A Glasgow Coma Scale of 8 or less indicates significant neurological impairment. The parameters and scoring for the Glasgow Coma Scale are shown in Chapter 32, Table 32–1. With ICP monitoring, intracranial problems can be identified and treatment initiated *before* clinical signs and symptoms develop.
2. Treatment of increasing ICP can be evaluated for effectiveness. Treatment includes fluid balance, osmotic diuretic therapy, and hyperventilation.
3. Postoperative cerebral edema. Certain brain tumors grow slowly, allowing the cranial contents to compensate for the increasing mass volume. After the tumor is removed, cerebral edema may be severe and life-threatening. ICP monitoring will allow early intervention.
4. Reye–Johnson syndrome. The mortality of Reye–Johnson syndrome may be due to cerebral hypoglycemia and ischemia. This could be the result of poor cerebral perfusion and

increasing ICP. By monitoring the ICP, therapies can be used to maintain a good CPP.
5. Infections are not usually associated with increasing ICP. However, if coma (and/or brain stem involvement) is present, cerebral edema is a potential problem.
6. Preoperative and postoperative monitoring is common in intracerebral hemorrhage. The removal of a tumor, treatment of an underlying lesion, or evacuation of the hemorrhagic hematoma may result in cerebral edema and increasing ICP.

Measurement Sites

The ICP can be measured in many loci: the lumbar sac, cisterna magna, fontanelles in newborns, cerebral ventricles, cranial subdural space, parenchyma, and cranial epidural space. The ICP values will depend on (1) the site selected for monitoring, and (2) the patient's position. The ICP is usually measured supratentorially by an intraventricular cannula or by a subdural catheter or bolt or intraparenchymal sensor.

Monitoring System Components

The monitoring system has three parts: a sensor, a transducer, and a recording instrument. It is like an arterial pressure monitoring system *except* that the ICP monitoring system is *closed* with no heparinized continuous-flush system and no interflow.

Monitoring sensors are of four types: epidural, subarachnoid/subdural, intraparenchymal, and intraventricular. The exact placement and the advantages and disadvantages of ICP monitoring devices are given in Table 31–1. There are three types of ICP monitoring systems: fluid-filled transducers, fiberoptic catheters (Camino), and microsensors (Codman) (Fig. 31–1).

Techniques

When using a fluid-filled system, the transducer is positioned at the level of the foramen of Monro. A fiberoptic system is zeroed upon insertion with the transducer located at the tip of the catheter. The microsensor is zeroed at time of insertion and one must use the same interface box during use. Both the fiberoptic sensor and the microsensor have factory-set calibrations. Two types of noninvasive ICP monitors are being investigated:

TABLE 31–1. ADVANTAGES AND DISADVANTAGES OF ICP MONITORING SENSORS AND THEIR PLACEMENT

Type of Sensor	Placement of Sensor	Advantage of Sensor	Disadvantage of Sensor
Epidural	Between the skull and dura	Less invasive Fiberoptic sensor does not require recalibration Intact dura	Easily obstructed or diaphragm can rupture, fragile catheter affected by heat or fevers Inaccurate because of dampened waveform Inserted postoperatively Requires special equipment Unable to drain CSF
Subdural	Below the dura and above the subarachnoid space	No penetration of brain Easy placement—often after surgery completed	Poor waveform, trend data only Unable to drain CSF Brain tissue may migrate into device with high pressure/unreliable at high pressures
Subarachnoid	In subarachnoid space via a bolt device	No penetration of brain Easy placement	Unable to drain CSF Brain tissue may migrate into device with high pressure/unreliable at high pressures
Intraparenchymal	Placed approximately 1 cm below the subarachnoid space in parenchymal tissue via a bolt device	Easy placement Accurate reading of ICP and waveform Lower risk of infection than intraventricular	Unable to drain CSF Requires separate monitoring system
Intraventricular	Inserted in the frontal horn of the lateral ventricle of the non-dominant hemisphere	The gold standard-more reflective of whole brain pressure Excellent waveform New catheters with fiberoptics or microsensors allow accuracy with fiberoptic transducer monitor with second port for drainage of CSF. Access for: —determination of volume pressure curve —CSF for drainage and sampling	If ventricles small, difficulty locating ventricles Requires separate monitoring system and drainage system Increased risk of infection Penetrates tissue and may cause additional injury especially with cerebral trauma, edema or increased ICP

tympanic monitors, which measure the perilymph pressure, and Gardner–Wells tongs, which measure pressure-induced changes in the bitemperal skull diameter.

Waveforms

Pulse Waveforms

The ICP pulse waveform corresponds to each heartbeat. The waveform arises primarily from pulsations of the intracranial arteries and retrograde venous pulsation. Three defined peaks compose the ICP pulse waveform. The first peak is the percussion wave. The choroid plexus pulsations create a sharp peak which is consistent in amplitude. This peak is known as the P1. The tidal wave forms the P2. The P2 peak varies in size and shape and ends with the dicrotic notch. The P3 wave, also called the dicrotic

wave, begins the final tapering of the waveform. Normally a descending sawtooth waveform appears. As the ICP increases, the amplitude of all the waves increases. As the ICP continues to increase, the changes in P2 signal a decrease in brain compliance and the P2 wave becomes greater in amplitude than the P1.

Occlusion of the monitoring tip causes a flatline tracing. The flat line may be high or low. As long as a tracing is scalloped in phase with arterial pulsation, the readings are acceptable.

Trend Waveforms

Three trend waveforms (A, B, and C) are seen in ICP monitoring (Fig. 31–2). The shape of the waves is affected by both cardiac pulsations and the respiratory cycle.

A waves, or plateau waves, occur when there is a sudden, sustained rise in ICP. A waves may be pres-

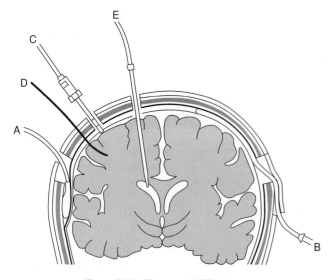

Figure 31–1. Placement of ICP devices.

ent for 5–20 min. A waves are not normally present and occur if the ICP rises to 50–100 mm Hg and is sustained. A waves reflect cerebral ischemia secondary to a decreased arterial blood pressure and intracranial hypertension.

B waves are evident when the ICP is elevated to 20–40 mm Hg but may rise to approximately 50 mm Hg. These waves are variable in shape and size and usually last for 0.5–2 min. They can occur with changes in cerebrovascular resistance or pressure and respiratory variations.

C waves occur every 4–8 min and raise ICP up to 20 mm Hg. Their significance has not been established.

With intraventricular monitoring, sharp-peaked waveforms occur. Systolic and diastolic portions of the wave cycle are "dampened." A dampened waveform is

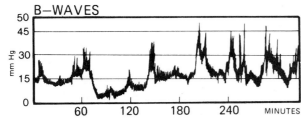

NORMAL ICP WAVEFORM

1. Normal waveform has steep upward systolic slope, followed by downward diastolic slope with dicrotic notch. Ordinarily, this waveform occurs continuously and indicates an ICP measurement between 4 and 15 mm Hg.

A–WAVES

2. The A–waves (sometimes called plateau waves) typically reach elevations of 50 to 100 mm Hg and then drop sharply. If they're recurring or are sustained for several minutes, A–waves indicate a rapid, dangerous rise in ICP and a decreased ability to compensate. Consider such waves ominous. Sustained A–waves may indicate irreversible brain damage.

B–WAVES

3. The B–waves are sharp and rhythmic, with a sawtooth pattern. They occur every 1½ to 2 minutes and may reach elevations of 50 mm Hg. But high elevations aren't sustained. They seem to occur more frequently with decreasing compensation. Sometimes they precede A-waves. Watch them closely.

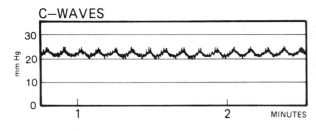

C–WAVES

4. C–waves are rapid and rhythmic, less sharp in appearance than B–waves, and may fluctuate with respirations or changing systemic blood pressure. C–waves aren't clinically significant.

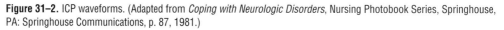

Figure 31–2. ICP waveforms. (Adapted from *Coping with Neurologic Disorders*, Nursing Photobook Series, Springhouse, PA: Springhouse Communications, p. 87, 1981.)

acceptable in ICP monitoring because the ICP mean is the measurement of significance. *Caution:* Do *not* confuse this with pulmonary artery monitoring, where dampened waveforms are *not* acceptable!

IMPLICATIONS AND INTERVENTIONS

Intracranial pressure monitoring is useful in early intervention (stages 1 and 2) to control the ICP.

1. Cellular hypoxia is most likely to occur during A waves (plateau waves). A waves indicate sustained pressure peaks up to 100 mm Hg (roughly 136 cm H_2O). These waves frequently coincide with headache, decreasing level of consciousness (LOC), and generalized neurological deterioration. If the patient is on a respirator, hyperventilation is utilized to maintain the $PaCO_2$ between 28 and 35 mm Hg. This will cause vasoconstriction, which may help control ICP.
2. With increasing ICP, the LOC decreases and the reticular activating system (RAS), or "alerting system," fails. Medications such as mannitol and loop diuretics may help decrease the ICP.
3. Motor responses such as hemiparesis or decorticate or decerebrate positioning occur as a result of cortical and midbrain compression of motor tracts. In some centers, barbiturate coma therapy may be tried.
4. Changes in vital signs and the respiratory pattern are late changes indicating compression of the brain stem (the pons and medulla oblongata). Interventions will include those listed above. Prognosis is poor.

Nursing Interventions

Most nursing procedures have an effect on the ICP. Turning the patient may increase the ICP. The increase is lessened if the patient is log-rolled with the head in alignment. If the patient can cooperate, having him or her exhale while turning prevents a Valsalva maneuver (Valsalva maneuvers increase ICP). If two nursing actions both increase ICP, space the nursing actions to allow the ICP to diminish after the first action before starting the second action.

Suctioning is imperative if the patient cannot clear his or her secretions. The increase in ICP may be decreased by preoxygenating with 100% oxygen, limiting suctioning to a maximum of 10 sec and one or two passes, use of an appropriate-sized suction catheter, use of less than 120 mm Hg negative pressure suction, and cautious hyperventilation of the patient before and after the procedure. Preventing thick, tenacious secretions limits the increase in the ICP with this procedure.

Dehydration and electrolyte imbalances may occur rapidly in conditions precipitating increased ICP. Careful monitoring of the electrolytes and serum osmolality will allow early interventions to regulate ICP responses.

Infections are a major threat in intraventricular and subdural monitoring. If irrigation is performed by the physician, an antibiotic solution may be used. Fever increases cerebral metabolism and may increase the ICP. Hypothermia blankets may be used to help control febrile states. The most important step in preventing infection is maintaining a "closed" system.

Glucocorticoids may be used to decrease cerebral edema, particularly with brain tumors. The use of glucocorticoid in head injury is controversial. Maintaining an elevated head (up to 30° in midline position in alignment with the body) is thought to help cerebral edema by promoting venous return from the cranium.

Nurses play a major role in monitoring for early signs and symptoms of increased ICP. Baseline neurological assessment followed by routine and ongoing assessments are essential to early identification of increased ICP. Transient increases in ICP may be seen with activity and in the presence of symptoms such as confusion, difficulty in arousal, sluggishness, slight pupillary dilatation, monoplegia or hemiparesis, headache, aphasia, Cheyne–Stokes respirations, or a change in vital signs. These transient changes may reverse in 5–20 min.

As cerebral compliance decreases further, the changes become consistent. Early signs include a decreased LOC, pupillary dysfunction, motor weakness, sensory deficits, cranial nerve palsy, possible headache, and seizures. Late findings include continuous decreased LOC, possible vomiting, headache, hemiplegia, decortication or decerebration, alteration in vital signs, respiratory irregularities, and impaired brain stem reflexes (corneal and gag reflexes).

It has become obvious through ICP monitoring that the physical signs of decreasing LOC, Cushing's triad (hypertension, widened pulse pressure, and bradycardia), and pupillary changes occur late in the course of increasing ICP. Reliance on only these physical parameters may result in irreversible brain damage and/or death.

Acute Head Injuries and Craniotomies

The primary focus of the chapter is head injury and space-occupying lesions (brain tumors). The CCRN exam may have one to three questions on content covered in this chapter.

Acute head injuries are almost always the result of violent assault or automobile accidents. A history is often very difficult to obtain, but it can be vital in establishing potential damage done by acceleration/deceleration forces. Acceleration injuries may be called coup (pronounced *coo*) and deceleration forces, contrecoup.

EXAMINATION OF THE PATIENT

ABCs: Airway, Breathing, and Circulation

Always establish a patent airway using extra care until the cross-table lateral roentgenograms confirm no neck fracture. An emergency tracheostomy or cricoidotomy is preferable to manipulating the neck for insertion of an endotracheal tube if the films have not been made. Continually monitor the respiratory and cardiac systems to ensure early intervention in cases of dysfunction. Inadequate function of either system may result in extension of neurologic impairment. Level of consciousness is a key initial assessment in any neurologically impaired patient.

Shock

Monitor for signs of impending shock. Be prepared to intervene by establishing an intravenous line while awaiting specific physician instructions. Treatment of shock should include determination of cause and maintenance of the mean arterial pressure (MAP) to prevent a precipitous drop in the central perfusion pressure (CPP) in the patient with increased intracranial pressure (ICP). If shock occurs, it is not due to intracranial bleeding if the cranium is intact. There is insufficient room in the cranium to contain the volume of blood necessary to cause hypovolemic shock.

Abdomen

Palpate for involuntary guarding and increasing girth, which may indicate an intra-abdominal hemorrhage leading to shock.

Long Bones

Long bones such as the femur and other extremity bones need to be checked for fractures. Such fractures may lead to fat emboli, shock, and other complications.

Neurological Exam
Scalp
Check for tears and/or swelling, which may indicate a subgaleal hematoma.

Face
Palpate the eye orbits, nose, teeth, maxilla, and mandible for facial fractures. Some facial fractures may provide for leakage of cerebrospinal fluid (CSF), and this would be an entry port for infection.

Ears
Blood in the external canal usually indicates a basal skull fracture.

Carotid Arteries

Palpate each carotid artery by itself to check for cerebral hemorrhage. If the carotids cannot be palpated, check for palpation of the superficial temporal arteries, which are a branch of the external carotids.

Mentation

There are five possible states or levels of consciousness (LOC). The definition and/or progression may differ in various institutions.

1. Alert: The patient is oriented to person, place, and time.
2. Lethargic: The patient prefers to sleep and when aroused, the degree of alertness or confusion is variable.
3. Obtunded: The patient can be aroused with minimal stimulation, but will drift off to sleep quickly.
4. Stuporous: The patient is aroused only by constant, deep, and usually painful stimuli. The patient may respond by some attempt to withdraw, moaning, or exhibiting decerebrate or decorticate positioning.
5. Coma: The patient cannot be aroused.

The Glasgow Coma Scale (Table 32–1) is one of the standards for use in identifying levels of consciousness (mentation) and for prognosis of the outcome of the injury. The Glasgow Coma Scale measures both arousal and awareness. Eye opening is a measure of arousal. Verbal and best motor response is a measure of awareness. A score of less than 15 is considered a decrease in LOC. Twelve to 14 may indicate a mild head injury. Nine to 12 indicates moderate head injury and 8 or less a severe head injury.

Cranial Nerves

Some of the 12 cranial nerves can be checked during routine patent care and during neurologic checks:

II: Optic nerve. (This will be covered in detail at the end of the chapter.) The most common result of injury to the optic tract is homonymous hemianopsia. When looking at the optic disc, it usually has a sharp, clear outline. If pulsations in the veins of the optic disc are visible, there is usually *no* increased ICP. Papilledema is present when the head of the optic nerve appears raised or increased (bulging) instead of flat.

III: Oculomotor nerve. This controls four of the six eye muscles (all but the lateral rectus and superior oblique). The parasympathetic

TABLE 32–1. GLASGOW COMA SCALE

Eye Opening (E)	Best Motor Response (M)	Verbal Response (V)
Spontaneous = 4	Obeys = 6	Oriented = 5
To speech = 3	Localizes = 5	Confused conversation = 4
To pain = 2	Withdraws = 4	Inappropriate words = 3
No response = 1	Abnormal	Incomprehensible sounds = 2
	Flexion = 3	No response = 1
	Extension = 2	
	No response = 1	

The lowest score received has the worst prognosis.

nerves cause pupil constriction. The sympathetic nerves cause pupil dilatation.

IV: Trochlear nerve. This controls the superior oblique muscle. It turns the eye down and out.

V: Trigeminal nerve. Corneal sensation provides the sensory side of arc for corneal reflex. The seventh nerve (facial) provides the motor side of arc.

VI: Abducens nerve. This controls the lateral rectus muscle. It turns the eye out. This is the longest unprotected nerve in the brain (some physicians think the trochlear nerve is the longest).

VII: Facial nerve. This exits the skull through the bone in the mastoid area. It controls the muscles of facial expression and plays a part in the production of tears.

X: Vagus nerve. This controls palate deviation. If the nerve is damaged, the uvula deviates away from the side of the paralysis. In vagal nerve paralysis, there is ipsilateral paralysis of the palate, pharynx, and larynx muscles. The soft palate at rest is usually lower on the affected side and if the patient says "ah," it elevates on the intact side.

XI: (Spinal) Accessory nerve. It turns the head by use of sternocleidomastoid muscles. It has some function with the upper trapezius muscles.

XII: Hypoglossal nerve. This controls tongue movement. If it is damaged, the patient cannot move the tongue from side to side, and tongue protrusion results in deviation toward the side of nerve damage.

Motor Function

Check to see if the patient moves all extremities voluntarily *and* equally. Note a one-sided weakness. If muscle weakness is suspected, have patient close eyes and extend arms directly in front. If there is a muscle weakness, there will be a drifting downward of the weakened extremity. Usually, there is no spasticity immediately after an injury. Flaccidity is usually present for about 10 days.

Sensation

In trauma, patients may respond only to pain. The response to sensation may include withdrawal of the appropriate limb from noxious stimuli, purposeless movement, or decorticate or decerebrate positioning in the unconscious patient.

CLASSIFICATION OF INJURY

Closed Head Injuries

In a closed head injury, the scalp is intact. The injury can be concussion, contusion, diffuse axonal injury, and/or skull fracture.

Concussion

Blunt trauma to the head by an accelerative or decelerative force causes a concussion. The two types of concussions are mild and classic concussion. Clinically, duration of unconsciousness may alter terminology of the injury, but the primary consideration is that of neurological deficit. Cortical dysfunction (attention span and memory) occurs with mild concussion and results from a temporary axonal disturbance. There is no loss of consciousness. Momentary confusion and disorientation may be seen with post-traumatic amnesia (antegrade and ret-

rograde). The patient with classic concussion will have recovered consciousness within about 6 hr. The duration of unconsciousness is an indication of the severity of the concussion. It may be 2 or 3 days before the patient can recall correctly all the factors leading to the concussion.

Although the patient appears to have recovered, postconcussive syndrome can develop. Postconcussive syndrome presents within 1 week to 1 year later. The symptoms are headache, dizziness, irritability, emotional lability, fatigue, poor concentration, decreased attention span, memory difficulties, and intellectual dysfunction.

Contusion

As with concussion, there is an immediate elimination of consciousness due to accelerative or decelerative blunt trauma forces to the head. These forces propel the brain against the rigid cranium (the coup force). With initial impact, the brain is then rotated or thrown back in the opposite direction (the contrecoup force). This is shown in Figure 32–1. This trauma invariably results in cerebral bruising and edema. If the forces are strong enough, lacerations and scattered intracerebral hemorrhages may occur. These usually occur along the axis line of the coup and contrecoup forces. In severe contusion, subarachnoid hemorrhage may occur, resulting in coma. Mild contusions will clear as the bruising and edema resolve, leaving no neurological deficit. Temporal lobe contusions carry a great risk for swelling and brain herniation. Some patients present with a period of lucidity which is followed by rapid deterioration and death without surgical interven-

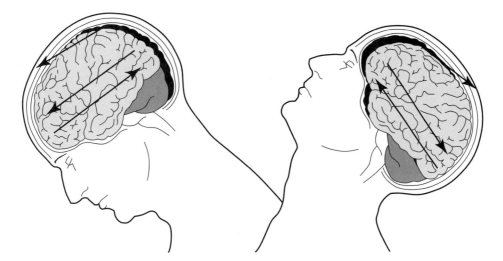

Figure 32–1. Coup and contracoup forces.

tion. Severe contusions that do not resolve, as indicated by the patients remaining comatose, indicate that the original bruising and/or lacerations caused a necrosis of brain tissue (possibly secondary to prolonged cerebral hypoxia at the injury sites).

Brain Stem Injury

Brain stem injury is associated with other diffuse cerebral injury. An immediate loss of consciousness with pupillary changes and posturing will be seen. On exam, cranial nerve deficits and changes in vital functions such as respiratory rate and rhythm are present. These injuries are classified as diffuse axonal injuries.

Diffuse Axonal Injury

Diffuse axonal injury (DAI) is also known as diffuse neuronal injury or shearing injury. Damage to nerve fibers are produced by linear and rotational shear strains following high-speed deceleration injuries. The injury disconnects the cerebral hemispheres from the reticular activating system. DAI is characterized by immediate coma. Mild DAI has loss of consciousness lasting 6–24 hr. Basal skull fractures are associated with moderate DAI. Severe DAI is seen with primary brain stem injuries. The patient presents with prolonged coma, increased ICP, hypertension, and fever. Prognosis is poor.

Skull Fractures

Skull fractures are usually classified as linear, depressed, or basilar. A linear skull fracture that does not tear the dura mater will heal without treatment. If the linear fracture occurs over the temporal lobe and tears the dura (Fig. 32–2), there is a chance that the middle meningeal artery will also be torn. Such an injury constitutes a medical emergency since the bleeding is arterial; this is commonly known as an acute epidural hematoma. The fracture may tear the dura mater over a venous sinus, resulting in slow bleeding that causes a chronic (nonacute) epidural hematoma. A depressed skull fracture that is *not* depressed more than the thickness of the skull is usually just monitored. However, a depressed skull fracture greater than the thickness of the skull (usually more than 5–7 mm) requires surgery to relieve the compression. Assessment of the extent of brain injury is essential. If the dura is torn, bone fragments may have entered brain tissue, requiring removal within 24 hr, and the chance of infection is greatly increased.

With a basilar skull fracture there is a high risk of injury to cranial nerves, infection, and residual

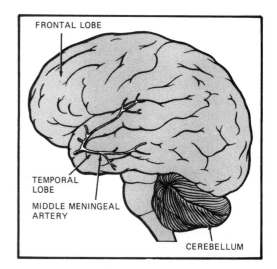

Figure 32–2. Linear skull fracture over the middle meningeal artery.

neurological deficits due to coup and contrecoup forces (Fig. 32–3). Basilar fractures may occur in the anterior or posterior fossa. CSF draining from the nose (rhinorrhea) or the ear canal (otorrhea) is a sign of basilar fracture. A temporal or basilar fracture in the posterior fossa is indicated by Battle's sign, an area of ecchymosis over the mastoid projection. "Raccoon eyes" is a sign of bleeding into the paranasal sinuses and refers ecchymosis developing around the eyes. This indicates a basilar fracture in the anterior fossa. Other symptoms of basilar fracture include tinnitus, facial paralysis, hearing difficulty, nystagmus, and conjugate deviation gaze. Patients with rhinorrhea will complain of a salty taste as the CSF drains into the pharynx. Caution the patient against blowing the nose, and avoid suctioning or nasal packing if rhinorrhea is present. Otorrhea can be tested for glucose. (Laboratory testing is more accurate than glucose testing sticks.) If glucose is present, the drainage is CSF. The "halo sign," a yellow ring that appears around bloody drainage on a nasal or ear pad, is another indication of CSF leakage. The goal is early detection of intracranial fluid leakage and prevention of infection. Severe neurological deficits are common with basilar fractures.

Compound Injuries

Compound injuries involve a laceration of the scalp with a head injury or skull fracture. If there is a laceration with a head injury (depressed fracture), surgery is usually performed immediately because of the threat of infection.

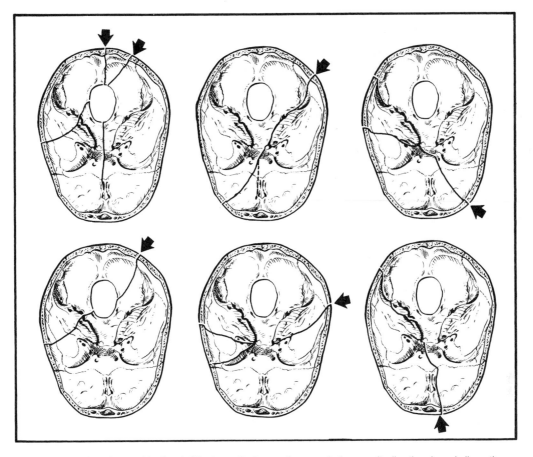

Figure 32–3. Coup forces of basilar skull fractures. Contracoup forces go in the opposite direction along similar paths.

Intracranial Mass Lesions

Acute Epidural Hematoma

Epidural hematomas are a true neurosurgical emergency. They occur at the time of the injury (Fig. 32–4) and are usually associated with a temporal or parietal skull fracture with laceration of the middle meningeal artery (and often vein). There is usually a loss of consciousness which may be followed by a brief period (up to 4–6 hr) of lucidity, followed by increasing restlessness, agitation, and confusion progressing to coma in one-third of patients. During the lucid period, nausea and vomiting often occur. Other signs may include ipsilateral oculomotor paralysis and seizures, contralateral hemiparesis/hemiplegia, and positive Babinski reflexes. As the hematoma increases in size, uncal herniation is the most common type to occur.

In one type of epidural hematoma, the linear fracture occurs across the sagittal sinus or the transverse sinus. In this instance, venous blood oozes into the area above the dura mater, producing a chronic epidural hematoma. Symptoms may be delayed for several days.

Subdural Hematomas

Subdural hematomas are the most common type and have the highest mortality rate. There are three types of subdural hematomas: acute, subacute, and

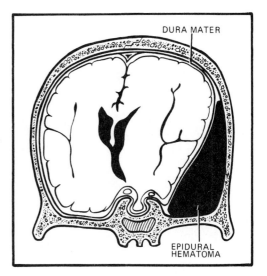

Figure 32–4. Epidural hematoma.

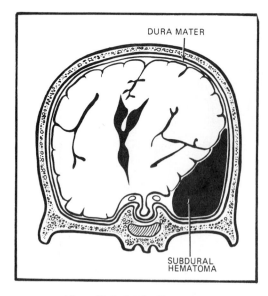

Figure 32–5. Subdural hematoma.

chronic forms. Subdural hematomas develop from bleeding in the subdural space between the dura mater and the arachnoid. The hematoma consists of some gel and some xanthochromic liquid.

In the acute subdural hematoma (Fig. 32–5), symptoms may occur from the first 2 or 3 days usually following cortical or brain stem injury. Acute subdural hematomas usually present with signs of increasing ICP, decreasing LOC, and ipsilateral oculomotor paralysis with contralateral hemiparesis. The signs and symptoms are those of a rapidly expanding mass lesion.

From 48 hr to 2 weeks after the initial injury a subacute subdural hematoma may develop, requiring surgery. A steady decline in level of responsiveness indicates a potential subacute hematoma. Symptoms include headaches, slowness in thinking, confusion, and sometimes agitation. These symptoms progressively worsen.

In the chronic subdural hematoma, a period of weeks may follow the low-impact injury before symptoms occur. These symptoms include giddiness, exaggeration of certain personality traits, confusion, occasionally headaches, and rarely a seizure. The CSF may be clear, bloody, or xanthochromic. ICP may be normal, elevated, or decreased. If symptoms do not occur for several weeks, a membrane forms around the subdural hematoma, walling it off from the rest of the brain. (In some cases, this walled-off section will calcify.)

Subdural hematoma may occur spontaneously without any form of injury in patients on anticoagulant therapy or in those with clotting dysfunction. Computed tomography will provide a diagnosis. Surgery is the treatment of choice in subdural hematomas.

Intracerebral Hemorrhage

Many intracerebral hemorrhages occur as hypertensive strokes (Fig. 32–6). Other causes include skull fracture, penetrating trauma (bullets), contrecoup decelerative forces, and systemic disease such as leukemia and aplastic anemia. If the hemorrhage occurs in the internal capsule of the brain, paralysis results. If the hemorrhage occurs in the dominant hemisphere, dysfunction is variable, dependent upon the location of hemorrhage. Signs and symptoms include nausea, vomiting, dizziness, headache, signs of increasing intracranial pressure, and a contralateral hemiplegia. A delayed intracerebral hemorrhage may occur hours to days after a closed head injury.

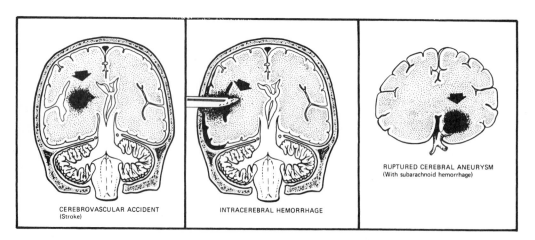

Figure 32–6. Examples of intracerebral hemorrhages.

Subarachnoid Hemorrhage

This may occur after trauma in the presence of hypertension with atherosclerosis or a congenital aneurysm or arteriovenous malformation. Symptoms usually include headache, dizziness, tinnitus, facial pain (pressure on the fifth cranial nerve), ptosis, a unilaterally dilated pupil, nuchal rigidity, and hemiparesis or hemiplegia. Areas and function affected by a subarachnoid hemorrhage on the dominant hemisphere are shown in Figure 32–7.

COMPLICATIONS OF HEAD INJURY

Closed Head Injuries

Complications include cerebral edema (vasogenic and cytotoxic), hydrocephalus, seizures, increased ICP, diabetes insipidus, and residual neurological deficits. Metabolic complications include respiratory insufficiency, infection, and systemic dysfunction as a result of associated trauma.

Intracranial Hemorrhage

Respiratory hypoxia, secondary to the intracranial hemorrhage, causes hypoxemia and hypercapnia. This results in an increased cerebral blood flow increasing ICP. The increased pressure results in neurological dysfunctions. Subarachnoid hemorrhage may occur because of the increased pressure or trauma and a hydrocephalus may result. If the hypothalamus and/or pituitary gland are affected, diabetes insipidus will most likely occur. Biochemical stress ulcers are common and are frequently associated with electrolyte disturbances. Depending on the site and degree of injury, seizures may develop. Infections, both cerebrospinal and respiratory, are continuous threats.

Intraventricular Hemorrhage

These patients usually die. A frequent complication is acute hydrocephalus with increased ICP. A long-term complication is a communicating hydrocephalus. A drain may be placed. If the $PaCO_2$ falls below 65 mm Hg, hypoxic brain damage may occur. A rising $PaCO_2$ will dilate cerebral vessels, increasing blood flow and pressure. For these reasons, the $PaCO_2$ is maintained between 30 and 35 mm Hg. In the past, hyperventilation to a $PaCO_2$ level of 25–28 was considered ideal. Cerebral vessels become refractory to $PaCO_2$ of 25–28 and the risk of hyperventilation is currently being evaluated. Use of jugular bulb S_vO_2 monitoring and cerebral blood flow studies are being done to assess the effects of hyperventilation.

NURSING INTERVENTIONS

The primary nursing intervention after assurance of a patent airway and the prevention of hypoxia is the frequent neurological assessment. Signs of increasing ICP may be treated with osmotic diuretics, hyperventilation, diuretics, drainage of CSF via intraventricu-

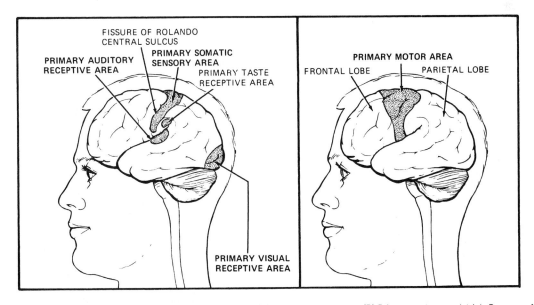

Figure 32–7. Areas and functions affected by subarachnoid hemorrhage. **(A)** Somatic sensory areas. **(B)** Primary motor area (strip). Because of rapidly increased ICPs of the subarachnoid hemorrhage, the entire brain can be affected.

lar cannulas. Nursing interventions include facilitating venous drainage by elevating head of bed 15°–30° and maintaining head in neutral position, avoiding hypoxemia or hypercarbia with suctioning procedures, preventing hyperthermia and shivering, and avoiding Valsalva maneuvers. ICP monitoring may be instituted. In some centers, barbiturate coma therapy may be utilized.

Monitoring vital signs and maintaining fluid balance and accurate intake and output records will help in evaluating treatment modalities aimed at stabilizing the patient. Assessment for dysphagia is helpful in prevention of aspiration. Standard procedures to prevent infections are employed.

DIAGNOSTIC TESTS AND FINDINGS

Computerized tomography (CT) is the number one diagnostic test in head injuries. It will reveal if:

1. Air has entered the brain from fractures of the eye, mastoid, or sinuses.
2. Blood is present in brain tissue or in the ventricular system.
3. Blood is on the surface of the brain or in the basal cisterns.
4. Ventricles are of normal size and in normal position.
5. The pineal gland has calcified and is in normal position.

Lumbar puncture is contraindicated in increased ICP and is rarely done in the diagnosis of head injuries.

Arterial blood gas determinations in intracranial hematoma reveal respiratory alkalosis (due to hyperventilation). Metabolic acidosis may occur if the patient is in shock, is hypoxic, or has a high level of physical activity (combativeness will produce lactic acidosis as does decerebrate posturing).

In closed head injuries, skull roentgenography, brain scan, and angiography may be essentially normal. The CT scan may show cerebral edema and areas of petechial hemorrhage in severe contusions. Hydrocephalus may be present. The echoencephalogram has a high percentage of false-positive results.

In intracranial hematomas, a CT scan will show increased density that indicates the presence, location, and extent of the hematoma. Skull films may show fractures or increased ICP, a calcified pineal gland, or a choroid plexus shifted from midline. Cerebral angiography may reveal an avascular mantle with displacement or stretching of vessels. Cervical

spine films may show injury. Brain scan may show increased uptake of isotope in the area of hematoma or tumor. Echoencephalography may reveal a shift of midline structures and is reserved for use in diagnosing the cause of coma in patients where other tests have failed to reveal the cause.

VISUAL PATHWAY DEFECTS

Visual field defects may occur as a result of cranial trauma, various other pathologies, and/or craniotomies. Figure 32–8 demonstrates the most com-

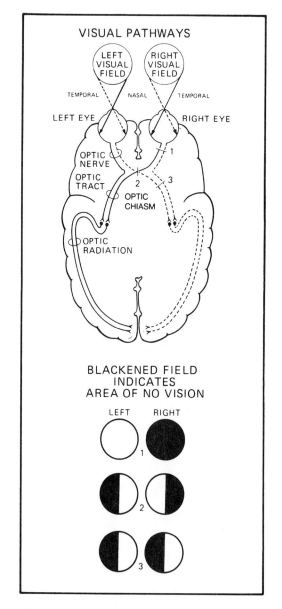

Figure 32–8. Visual field defects. (Adapted from B. Bates, *A Guide to Physical Examination*, Philadelphia: J. B. Lippincott, p. 49, 1974. Reprinted with permission of J. B. Lippincott.)

mon visual field defects. The key to interpreting the visual field defects depicted in Figure 32–8 is to recognize that the left eye is on the left and the right eye is on the right in the figure. The image is not reversed as with heart drawings.

Visual images from the peripheral field (temporal) hit on the nasal side of each retina. Fibers from the nasal side of each retina carry the visual impulses along the optic nerve toward the optic tract. Just prior to the optic tract, these fibers cross (at the optic chiasm). They then continue on the inside of the optic tract through the optic radiation to the end of the optic tract.

Visual images from the central (nasal) field of vision hit on the outer, temporal side of each retina. Fibers from the outer side of each retina carry the impulses to the optic nerve and follow the optic nerve tract on the outside, through the optic radiation to the end of the tract. Lesions between the eye and the point where nerve fibers cross cause a blind eye. Lesions of the eye itself will also cause unilateral blindness.

A lesion at the point where the optic nerve fibers cross (the optic chiasm) will result in bitemporal blindness. Images from the periphery of both eyes are blocked, resulting in bitemporal blindness.

A lesion of the fibers of the right optic tract blocks visual images on the same side of each eye. This is a left homonymous (same side) hemianopsia (one-half the visual field).

In the same way, a lesion of fibers of the left optic tract blocks visual images on the same side of each eye. In this case, a right homonymous (same side) hemianopsia (one-half the visual field) exists. These are the two most common visual defects associated with optic tract injuries.

A lesion may occur in the optic radiation. If the lesion is completely across the optic radiation, a homonymous hemianopsia develops. However, if the lesion affects only the outer fibers, a homonymous quadratic defect occurs.

CRANIOTOMIES

Craniotomies are performed for many reasons. Postoperative care includes routine postoperative care plus:

1. Neurological monitoring, to compare pre- and postoperative functions, right side to left side function, and hour-to-hour functions.
2. Pain control, which may be achieved with codeine and/or fentanyl. Careful neurological monitoring is necessary.
3. Monitoring of ICP, which must be maintained within normal range. This is achieved by the administration of osmotic and diuretic therapy, by elevating the head of the bed 15°–30°, and by keeping $PaCO_2$ between 30 and 35 mm Hg. Use of glucocorticoids is controversial; they are primarily used to treat the expected cerebral edema following tumor removal.
4. Installation of a patent CSF drainage system, which may be used for 24–48 hr, to help control ICP and monitor type and amount of drainage.
5. Observation for clear drainage through dressings, which may be CSF and should be reported to the physician immediately.
6. Monitoring for stress ulcers (also known as Cushing's ulcers), which are a common occurrence. They may be treated and/or prevented with use of H_2 antagonists and/or antacids.
7. Monitoring of cardiovascular status, since certain head injuries cause bradycardia. Bradycardia may be a precursor to other dysrhythmias and cardiac failure. Intravenous fluid needs are calculated daily to prevent fluid overload and to maintain electrolyte balance.

Diabetes insipidus occurs with some head injuries and with other cerebral pathologies. This condition is covered in Chapter 23.

Intracranial Aneurysms and Cerebrovascular Accident (Stroke)

EDITORS' NOTE

In this chapter, the concepts of intracranial aneurysms and stroke are presented. Expect one to three questions covering the content in this chapter.

INTRACRANIAL ANEURYSMS

An aneurysm is a congenital, developmental, or traumatic defect in the muscle layer of arteries, normally occurring at points of bifurcation. (Recall that there are three layers in the arterial wall: the inner endothelial layer (the intima), a middle smooth muscle layer (the media), and an outer layer of connective tissue (the adventitia).

Pathophysiology

The congenital weakness of the arterial wall results in a gradual "ballooning out" of that segment of the artery over a period of years. When an increase in vascular pressure rises to a sufficient (unknown) pressure, the weakened ballooning segment of the artery bursts.

Location, Incidence, and Etiology

Most cerebral aneurysms develop in the anterior arteries of the circle of Willis. Aneurysms are the fourth leading cause of cerebrovascular problems. Aneurysms are rare in children and teenagers and most common in middle-aged persons. Slightly more females than males develop aneurysms. Some 10–20% of patients with aneurysms have more than one (may be found on same or opposite side).

One etiological factor is hypertension (present in a majority of cases). No specific precipitating factors are present in all patients. Congenital anomalies account for some aneurysms and others occur for unknown reasons.

Clinical Presentation

Aneurysms are commonly asymptomatic until a bleed occurs. The exception is a very large aneurysm, which may cause symptoms related to pressure against surrounding tissues. Severe headache (unlike any other headaches) occurs as the aneurysm starts to bleed. Unconsciousness may occur and be transient or sustained secondary to ischemia and/or necrosis of brain tissue. Nausea and vomiting are common. Transient neurological deficits include numbness, aphasia, and paresis.

Nuchal rigidity, photophobia, diplopia, Kernig's sign (inability to fully extend leg when thigh is flexed at a 90° angle to the abdomen), Brudzinski's sign (involuntary adduction and flexion of legs when neck is flexed), and headache are common because of meningeal irritation. All these signs except diplopia are sometimes grouped together under the term meningismus.

Diagnosis

A lumbar puncture is usually performed. Elevated cerebrospinal fluid (CSF) pressure, elevated protein levels, elevated red blood cells and oxyhemoglobin, decreased glucose, and grossly bloody CSF indicate hemorrhage in the subarachnoid space. Computed tomography and magnetic resonance imaging will reveal areas of intracerebral bleed.

Note: In the adult, an intracerebral bleed is *never* the cause of a hypovolemic shock state if the cranium is intact. The intact cranium does not have sufficient space to accommodate the quantity of blood required to cause a hypovolemic shock state.

Carotid and vertebral angiography may reveal the presence of other small aneurysms. Angiography may determine the patient's suitability for preventative measures such as hypotensive drugs or intracranial–extracranial bypass anastomosis, clipping/ligating, or reinforcing the artery.

Classification of Clinical State Following Aneurysmal Rupture

Aneurysms may be placed in one of five categories (grades). These grades are summarized in Table 33–1. If patients can be stabilized in grade I or II, they may be candidates for surgical intervention.

Prognosis

The prognosis depends on the site and severity of the bleed. Persistent coma beyond 2 days is a poor sign. Bleeding may recur as the original clot that formed around the bleed is absorbed (or lysed). This usually occurs between the seventh and eleventh days after the original bleed and carries a poor prognosis. Increasing and/or persistent vasospasm results in increasing cerebral ischemia. Vasospasm is commonly seen about the fourth day postbleed. Marked cerebral edema and/or the development of hydrocephalus indicate a poor prognosis.

Nursing Interventions

Stabilization of the patient is the primary objective of treatment. Once the patient is stabilized and the condition approaches grade I or II, surgical intervention is usually successful.

1. Complete bed rest in a quiet, dark environment promotes stabilization.
2. The head of the bed may be elevated up to 30° in an attempt to promote cerebral venous return by gravity. A bedside commode may be used.
3. Fluid intake is recommended up to 3 L/day to prevent vasospasm. (Maintenance or mean arterial pressure above 100 mm Hg and cardiac output at 6.5–8 L/min, and prevention of congestive heart failure are common goals in therapy.)
4. If alert, the patient should avoid Valsalva manuevers and any other action that produces straining, such as forced coughing to clear secretions. These actions will increase intracranial pressure (ICP) and may start a rebleed.
5. Sedating drugs may be used to decrease stress, anxiety, or restlessness of the patient and may have the additional side effect of lowering the blood pressure in a hypertensive patient. Antihypertensive drugs may be used to prevent increases in pressure rather than to bring hypertension down to normal levels.
6. Anticonvulsants (e.g., phenytoin) may be used to prevent or control seizure activity.
7. Calcium channel blockers, such as nimodipine, which cross the blood–brain barrier may be utilized to treat vasospasm.
8. Control of ICP may be done with ventriculostomy.

TABLE 33–1. GRADES OF ANEURYSMS

Symptom	Grade I	Grade II	Grade III	Grade IV	Grade V
Level of consciousness	Alert	Decreased	Confused	Unresponsive	Moribund
Headache	Slight	Mild to severe	—	—	—
Nuchal rigidity	Slight	×	×	×	—
Vasospasm	—	—	—	May be present	May be present
Decerebrate posturing	—	—	—	—	×

× = present; dash = absent.

Surgical Intervention and Nursing Implications

If an aneurysm is diagnosed prior to a bleed, surgery may be performed to prevent a bleed, depending on the size and location of the aneurysm. If an aneurysmal bleed has occurred and the patient has stabilized in grade I or II, surgery may be performed.

Surgery may consist of one of several procedures:

1. Clipping the aneurysm is probably the oldest and the most frequent surgical treatment (Fig. 33–1). If the aneurysm is extremely large, clipping may not be possible.
2. Reinforcing the arterial wall at the site of the aneurysm by wrapping some of the new mesh materials (strips of muscle, gauze, or plastic) around it may prevent further enlargement or rupture (Fig. 33–1). Caution must be taken not to decrease the arterial lumen, especially if atherosclerotic disease is present.
3. Trapping the aneurysm by ligating proximal and distal to the aneurysm may be the procedure of choice if the aneurysm is large (Fig. 33–1).
4. Embolization of the aneurysmal clot may be performed once the patient is stabilized, especially if the aneurysmal clot is impinging upon important structures (Fig. 33–1).

If the aneurysm cannot be reached and/or surgical risk of one of the above procedures is extremely high, the common carotid artery may be clamped. Prior to this procedure, angiography must demonstrate that vascular perfusion of the involved hemisphere is adequate from the opposite side.

The nursing responsibilities include assessment of neurological status for signs of increasing ICP, prevention of and monitoring for cerebral vasospasm, and hypertensive–hypervolemic therapy to maintain the mean arterial pressure above 100 mm Hg and cardiac output above 6.5–8 L/min, prevention of CHF fluid overload and rebleed, observing for signs of impending seizures and hydrocephalus, dysphagia screening, and performing the routine postoperative and postcraniotomy care.

CEREBRAL VASCULAR ACCIDENT (STROKE)

EDITORS' NOTE

In this section the concept of cerebrovascular disturbance will be covered. Common interruptions in cerebrovascular blood flow may be the result of thrombosis, embolus, or hemorrhage. The CCRN exam will most likely have one to three questions on this content.

A stroke is a sudden focal or global neurological deficit due to cerebrovascular disease. A stroke is the most common cause of cerebral dysfunction in this country.

ETIOLOGY

The end result of any interruption of oxygen to brain tissue for more than a few minutes is the death of

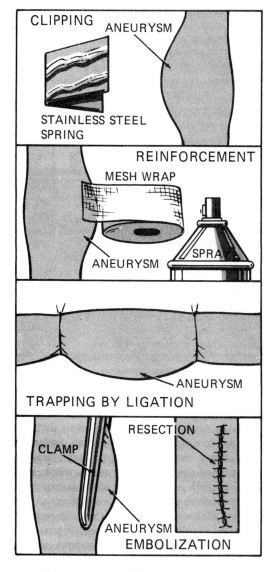

Figure 33–1. Surgical treatment of aneurysms.

those neurons not being oxygenated. The decrease in oxygen may be partial or complete. Vascular origin of a stroke is from (1) a thrombotic or embolic occlusion of the cerebral vascular resulting in an infarction or (2) a spontaneous rupture or a vessel leading to intracerebral or subarachnoid hemorrhage. Other causes are tumor and compression or spasm of cerebral arteries.

CLINICAL PRESENTATION

The common symptom in stroke regardless of the cause is the sudden onset of symptoms. Specific symptomology depends on location of the injury and the hemispheric dominance of the patient. Homonymous hemianopsia, hemiparesis, and/or hemiplegia are common symptoms.

If the right cerebral hemisphere is involved, left sided motor functions are involved, as well as spatial-perceptual deficits resulting in apraxia. Apraxia may be constructional or dressing. Constructional apraxia is the inability to complete the left half of figures one is drawing or arranging words in an incorrect manner, superimposing words and such. Usually a constructional apraxia will include an inability to complete the drawing of a picture (e.g., a clock). Dressing apraxia is the inability to dress oneself properly. Both constructional apraxia and dressing apraxia are common in right cerebral strokes. Neglect of the paralyzed side, impulsive quick behavior, and poor judgment of abilities and limitations occur with right cerebral strokes.

Left cerebral hemispheric strokes have right-sided motor impairment plus astereognosis and autotopagnosia. Astereognosis is an inability to identify a common object placed in the hand with one's eyes closed. Autotopagnosia is an inability to determine the position of parts of the body in relation to the rest of the body.

In addition, these strokes tend to cause a finger agnosia (inability to identify a finger being touched) and a right–left disorientation. Behavior is slow, cautious, and disorganized. Aphasia, both expressive and receptive, is common. Expressive aphasia is the inability to express oneself verbally and understandably. Receptive aphasia is the loss of the ability to understand spoken or written word.

Regardless of which hemisphere is involved in a stroke, the patients tend to have a reduced memory span, are emotionally labile, and have spasticity of the affected extremities. Some patients will have an anosognosia, which is the denial of a neurological deficit such as hemiplegia. Anosognosia is different than a psychological denial stage. Deviation of the head and eyes is toward the cerebral hemisphere involved in the stroke of pontine lesions. Frontal lobe lesions produce the opposite signs.

Diagnosis

The diagnosis of stroke is usually made on the basis of history and clinical symptoms. The history frequently reveals transient ischemic attacks (TIAs), reversible ischemic neurological deficits (RIND), and possibly "small" strokes in the past. CT scan will reveal decreased density in ischemic and infarcted areas. It will reveal increased density in hemorrhage areas. Angiography may show spasms, arteriovenous malformations, and aneurysms.

Treatment

In most centers, treatment is supportive. Thrombolytic therapy (tPA) has been FDA approved for use within 3 hours after ischemic stroke. Anticoagulant therapy (heparin, aspirin or ticlid) may be considered if embolic etiology is suspected. Research is continuing and looks promising for extracranial and intracranial bypass anastomoses in reversible ischemic neurological deficits (RIND). Carotid endarterectomy and bypass patients are seen in critical care areas more than the uncomplicated stroke patient.

Nursing Interventions

To some extent nursing interventions (and patient complications) depend on the site of a stroke, the patient's age, general health, and the extent of neurologic deficit.

Communication with the patient is achieved in any way possible—through writing, pictures, gestures, and so on. Different aphasias make this task difficult.

Accurate systematic monitoring and assessing neurological status will identify extensions of deficit which may be treatable. Nursing assessment should include the LOC and pupil size and reactivity; signs and symptoms of increased ICP; arterial blood gas levels; cranial nerve function; signs of meningeal irritation, seizure, or hydrocephalus; and change in motor function, sensation, perception, and ability to detect temperature and pain. Early dysphagia screening (decreased or absent gag) decreases the risk of aspiration and resultant pneumonia. Some centers utilize the National Institutes of Health Stroke Scale for assessment of the stroke patient.

The goal of care is to maintain or restore cerebral perfusion, maintain life support, prevent further injury or escalation of the life-threatening problem, and preserve motor function, speech, and cognition to the greatest possible extent.

Supportive "comfort" measures are important and include training, positioning, skin care, fluid and nutritional intake, emotional support, and early implementation of rehabilitation.

34

The Vertebrae and Spinal Cord

EDITORS' NOTE

In this chapter, anatomy, physiology, and concepts of spinal cord dysfunction are reviewed. The CCRN exam usually has one to three questions on dysfunction or trauma associated with the spinal cord. This chapter should provide you with the essential information necessary to address content from the exam on the spinal cord. Again, keep in mind that anatomy and physiology questions are usually not directly asked on the CCRN exam. Focus your studying on the function of the cord and clinical conditions which are altered by cord injury/dysfunction.

VERTEBRAL COLUMN

The spinal cord is protected by and housed by the vertebrae. The vertebral column comprises a total of 33 vertebrae. There are eight cervical vertebrae. Some texts state that there are seven cervical vertebrae. These texts apparently count the atlas and axis as one since they articulate directly with each other. There are 12 thoracic vertebrae, 5 lumbar, 5 sacral, and 3–5 fused as the coccygeal segment.

The body of a typical vertebra (Fig. 34–1) is the solid portion which lies anteriorly. Opposite the vertebral body is the spinous process (the bony segment felt down the back). Projecting laterally from each side of the vertebra are the transverse processes. The lamina is the curved portion of bone joining the transverse processes to the spinous process. The lamina is the most frequently fractured portion of the vertebra. The vertebrae may be fractured in the same way that other bones in the body are. Between the vertebral body and the spinous process is the spinal foramen, the cavity through which the spinal cord passes.

The Cervical Vertebrae

The cervical vertebrae are the smallest. Figure 34–2 shows the atlas (C-1), which articulates with the occipital bone and the axis (C-2). The axis has an odontoid process (the only one) which permits the atlas to articulate directly and provides rotation of the head. Trauma to the odontoid process is sometimes called the "hangman's" fracture, as when this process is broken the head is no longer stabilized by articulation with the atlas. If the axis is fractured, the force sustained is so great that the vertebra bursts like a star. This causes multiple bone fragments, which may penetrate the spinal cord nerves and vascular structures too.

The Thoracic Vertebrae

The 12 thoracic vertebrae (Fig. 34–3) have points of attachment for the ribs to help support the chest musculature.

The Lumbar Vertebrae

The five lumbar vertebrae (Fig. 34–4) are the largest, and they support the back muscles. These vertebral discs are the most frequently herniated.

The Sacral Vertebrae

The five sacral vertebrae (Fig. 34–5) are fused to form the sacrum, a frequent point of low back pain.

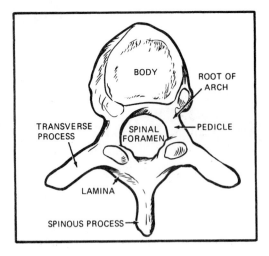

Figure 34–1. Typical vertebra.

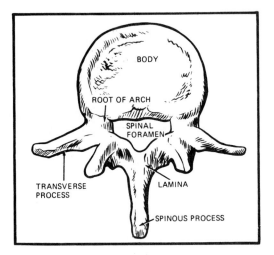

Figure 34–3. Thoracic vertebra.

The Coccygeal Vertebrae

Depending on the individual, three to five vertebrae are fused to form the coccyx (Fig. 34–5).

INTERVERTEBRAL DISCS

Between each of the lumbar, thoracic, and cervical vertebrae, excluding the atlas and axis, is an intervertebral disc. These fibrocartilaginous discs absorb shock and reduce the pressure between one vertebra and another. The center portion of the disc is a gelatinous material called the nucleus pulposus. Unexpected movement and/or force may "rupture" the disc, forcing the nucleus pulposus out of position—the so-called slipped disc. When out of position, the disc may impinge upon the spinal canal, the spinal cord, or the emerging spinal nerves.

Unfortunately, it is very common for the spinal cord to be damaged by extreme hyperextension or

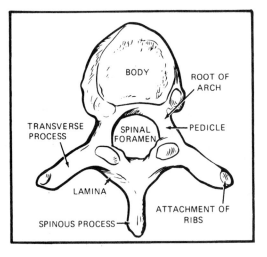

Figure 34–4. Lumbar vertebra.

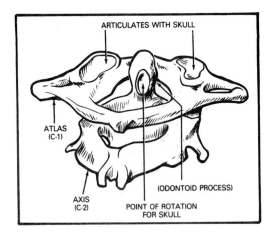

Figure 34–2. Articulation of C-1 and C-2 vertebrae.

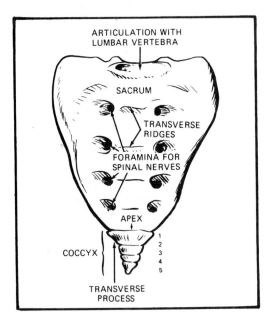

Figure 34–5. Sacral vertebrae and coccyx.

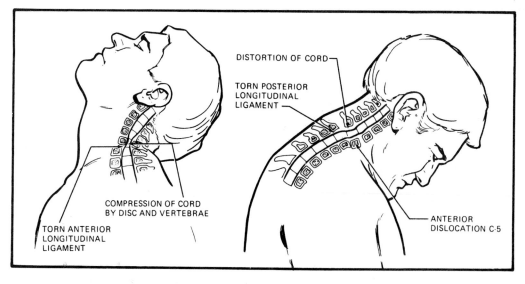

Figure 34–6. Hyperextension and hyperflexion of the spinal cord.

hyperflexion forces (Fig. 34–6). Damage may occur with or without fracture of the vertebrae.

THE SPINAL CORD

The spinal cord is the second major component of the central nervous system (the brain is the other), and is vital for life.

The spinal cord (Fig. 34–7) is continuous with the medulla oblongata in the brain stem. It is located in the spinal canal and is protected by the vertebral column. The cord is some 25 cm shorter than the vertebral column. Within the vertebral column, the spinal cord extends from the foramen magnum to the first lumbar vertebra. Its tapered end is called the conus medullaris. The filum terminale is a group of fibers extending from the conus medullaris at the L-1 level to the first coccygeal vertebra.

Structure of the Spinal Cord

The spinal cord is oval and is surrounded by the meninges, which also encase the brain. Between the L-1 and S-2 vertebrae, the arachnoid membrane enlarges somewhat to form the space known as the lumbar cistern used for lumbar punctures. The spinal cord has a minute cavity in its center known as the central canal. This canal is an extension of the fourth ventricle and contains cerebrospinal fluid (CSF).

The spinal cord is composed of both white (myelinated) and gray (unmyelinated) tissue. The gray matter appears (with a little imagination) to be shaped like an H which is surrounded by white matter

(Fig. 34–8). The amount of gray matter varies with its location in the vertebral column. A mnemonic may help distinguish white/gray matter and myeli-

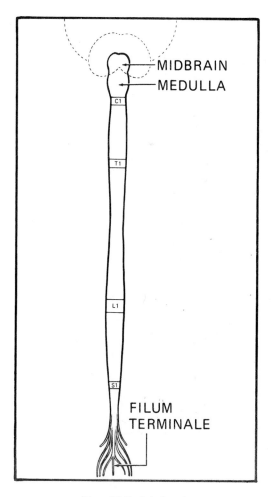

Figure 34–7. Spinal cord.

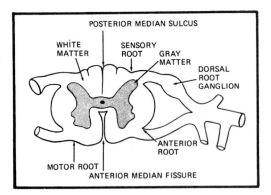

Figure 34–8. Gray and white matter of the spinal cord (cross section).

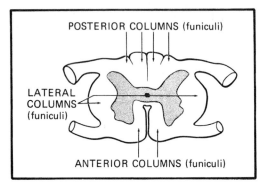

Figure 34–10. Funiculi of white matter in the spinal cord.

nated/unmyelinated fibers. The fourth letter of gray is "y" as is the fourth letter of unmyelinated. So gray matter is unmyelinated fibers.

Gray matter is composed of nerve cells and unmyelinated fibers arranged in three columns (Fig. 34–9). The anterior gray columns are also known as the anterior horns. They contain cell bodies of efferent (motor) fibers. The middle gray columns, known as the lateral columns, contain preganglionic fibers of the autonomic nervous system. The lateral columns are largest in the upper cervical, thoracic, and midsacral regions. The posterior columns, also known as the posterior horns, contain cell bodies of afferent (sensory) fibers.

The white matter (myelinated) is arranged in three columns called the anterior, lateral, and posterior funiculi (Fig. 34–10). Within these columns are ascending (sensory) and descending (motor) tracts termed fasciculi (Fig. 34–11).

The significant ascending tracts are the fasciculus gracilis, fasciculus cuneatus, lateral spinothalamic tract, anterior spinothalamic tract, dorsal and ventral spinocerebellar tracts, and spinotectal tract. These tracts carry sensory impulses.

The significant descending tracts (Fig. 34–11)

are the rubrospinal tract, ventral and lateral corticospinal tracts, and the tectospinal tract. These carry motor impulses.

Lower motor neurons are spinal and cranial motor neurons that directly innervate muscles. Lesions cause flaccid paralysis, muscular atrophy, and absence of reflex responses. Upper motor neurons in the brain and spinal cord activate lower motor neurons. Lesions cause spastic paralysis and hyperactive reflexes.

SPINAL CORD INJURIES

Spinal cord injuries are more and more common and are mainly a result of auto accidents, diving accidents, contact sport accidents, falls, and gunshot wounds.

Spinal injuries may be classified according to many criteria.

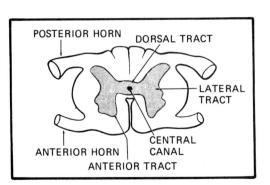

Figure 34–9. Columns (tracts) of gray matter in the spinal cord (cross section).

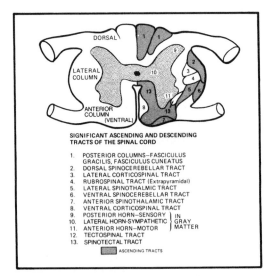

Figure 34–11. Significant ascending and descending tracts of the spinal cord. The left half of the picture is a mirror image of the right half.

Classification of Spinal Cord Injuries

1. The level of injury may be cervical, thoracic, or lumbar. The cervical injury is the most common.
2. The degree of spinal cord involvement may be either complete or incomplete. Complete cord involvement by lesion (or transection) results in total loss of sensory and motor function below the level of the lesion. This loss is a result of irreversible damage to the spinal cord. If the cervical cord is involved, quadriplegia is the common result. If the thoracic or lumbar cord is involved, paraplegia is the common result. Incomplete cord lesion involvement (or partial transection) leaves some tracts intact. The degree of sensory/motor loss is variable depending on the level of lesion. Three syndromes are commonly the result of incomplete lesions.
   a. When the damage is in the cervical central cord, it is termed central cord syndrome. The central cord syndrome is characterized by microscopic hemorrhage and edema of the central cord (Fig. 34–12). There is motor weakness in both the upper and lower extremities, but the weakness is much greater in the upper extremities than in the lower ones.

      Sensory dysfunction varies according to the site of injury or lesion, but is generally more pronounced in the upper extremities. Reflexes in the lower extremities may be hyperactive temporarily. Bladder dysfunction is common. This syndrome is frequently due to hyperextension of an osteoarthritic spine. It is the most common type of cord injury when there is no overt fracture or dislocation. The extent of recovery depends on the resolution of edema and the intactness of the spinal cord tracts. As improvement occurs, it proceeds from proximal to distal parts.
   b. Anterior cord syndrome is characterized by injury resulting in an acute compression of the anterior portion of the spinal cord, often a flexion injury (Fig. 34–13). Compression is usually caused by a disc or bony fragment. It may also be caused by the actual destruction of the anterior cord by an anterior spinal artery occlusion (thrombus). Symptoms include immediate anterior paralysis which is complete from the injury or compression down. Hypesthesia (decreased sensation) and hypalgesia (decreased pain sensation) occur below the level of injury. Since the posterior cord tracts are not injured, there are sensations of touch, position, vibration, and motion. If the syndrome is caused by the compression of the anterior cord from bony fragments, surgical decompression is indicated.
   c. Brown–Séquard syndrome is due to transection or lesion of one-half of the spinal cord (Fig. 34–14). There is loss of motor function (paralysis) and position and vibratory sense, as well as vasomotor paralysis on the same side (ipsilateral) and below the hemisection. On the opposite (contralateral) side of the hemisection, there is loss of pain and temperature sensation below the level of the lesion or hemisection.
3. Spinal cord injuries may be categorized as stable (vertebral column is aligned) or unstable (vertebral column is not aligned).
4. Injuries may be classified according to the injury to the vertebral column. Such injuries include simple fracture, compression fracture, comminuted fracture, teardrop fracture, dislocation, subluxation, and fracture-dislocation.
5. Injuries may be classified in relation to the specific level of injury. These injuries are summarized in Table 34–1.
6. The final classification of spinal cord injuries is in relation to the mechanism involved. This is either hyperextension or hyperflexion. Rarely, rotational injuries may occur.

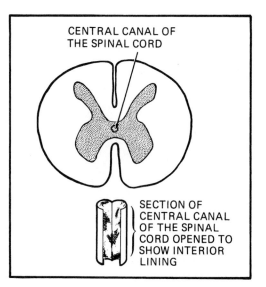

Figure 34–12. Central cord syndrome.

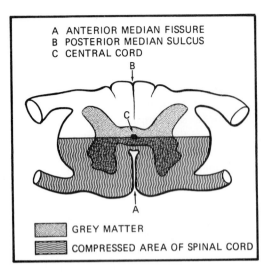

Figure 34–13. Anterior cord syndrome.

Spinal cord injuries are frequently associated with head or other systems trauma.

Disease states may relate specifically to the spinal cord, for example, tumor, arteriovenous malformations, and infections. In these instances, treating the underlying condition may result in improvement in spinal cord function.

Spinal Shock

Spinal shock is a state that exists when irreversible damage has occurred to the spinal cord, resulting in areflexia and flaccid paralysis below the level of injury.

Spinal shock may affect any and all body systems and is more severe in cervical vertebral injuries than other vertebral injuries. Spinal shock may appear from the time of injury to the end of the first week

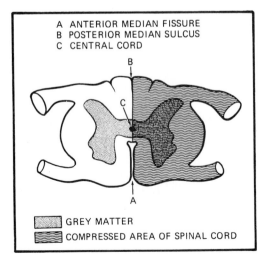

Figure 34–14. The Brown-Séquard syndrome.

postinjury. The duration of spinal shock is 7–10 days. One knows that spinal shock is resolving when flaccid paralysis becomes spastic paralysis and reflexes return.

Neurogenic Shock

Distributive shock, known as neurogenic shock, can occur following cervical and upper thoracic cord injury. Neurogenic shock occurs secondary to the loss of brain stem and higher control of the sympathetic nervous system. Peripheral vasodilation occurs, resulting in hypotension and bradycardia. The loss of cardiac acceleration reflex prevents vasoconstriction and tachycardia. There is no sweating below the level of injury and hypothermia may present. Management of the decreased systemic vascular resistance and decreased cardiac output includes administration of fluids, vasopressors, and other sympathomimetic agents. Atropine should be at the bedside if profound bradycardia occurs.

Treatment

Treatment includes the stabilization of the vertebral column, prevention of further injury with movement, and monitoring for evidence of spinal or neurologic shock, autonomic dysreflexia and complications related to the effects of the spinal injury. Early treatment in the initial 60–90 min is thought to limit or reverse neurological deficit. Treatment consists of Methylprednisolone (8 mg/kg followed by a 23-hr drip) and vertebral stabilization. The goal is prevention of secondary injury from the release of endogenous factors stimulated from the hypoxic and ischemic cord. Vertebral stabilization includes traction and open management if traction is unsuccessful or for exploration of pressure-inducing foreign body or bone fragments. The spine is stabilized by fusion or placement of a halo brace after approximately 1 week. Close monitoring of motorsensory return or increased dysfunction is essential.

Complications

Immediate postinjury problems are (1) maintaining a patent airway, (2) maintaining adequate ventilation, (3) maintaining an adequate circulating blood volume, and (4) prevention of extension of cord damage.

Respiratory System
Cervical injury or fracture above C-4 presents special problems in that total respiratory function is lost.

TABLE 34–1. CLASSIFICATION OF INJURY ACCORDING TO SPECIFIC VERTEBRAL LEVEL

Injury Level	Intact Function	Lost Function
Below L-2	Mixed motor/sensory, depending on intact nerve fibers	Mixed motor/sensory; possibly bladder, bowels, and sexual functioning
T-1 to L-1 or L-2	Arm function	Leg functions; bladder, bowels, and sexual functioning
C-7, C-8	Triceps muscle, head rotation, respiration	No intrinsic muscles of hand; no other function retained
C-6, C-7	Biceps muscle, head rotation, respiration	No triceps; no other function retained
C-5, C-6	Gross arm movement, head rotation, diaphragmatic respiration	No other function retained
C-4, C-5	Head rotation, diaphragmatic respiration	No other function intact
C-3, C-4	Head rotation	No other function intact (many die)
C-1, C-2	None	Most die

Artificial ventilation will be required to keep the patient alive; however, most of these patients will die. Injury or fracture of C-4 or the lower cervical vertebrae will result in diaphragmatic breathing if the phrenic nerve is functioning. Hypoventilation almost always occurs with diaphragmatic respirations because there is a decrease in vital capacity and tidal volume.

Since cervical fractures or severe injuries cause paralysis of abdominal musculature and frequently intercostal musculature, the patient is unable to cough effectively enough to remove secretions; this leads to atelectasis and pneumonia. Artificial airways provide direct access for pathogens, so bronchial hygiene and chest physiotherapy become extremely important. If multiple trauma is involved, neurogenic pulmonary edema may result from the sudden changes in thoracic pressures at the time of the injury. The occurrence of pulmonary edema (as opposed to neurogenic pulmonary edema) is probably due to fluid overload. Respiratory failure is the leading cause of death in the patient with spinal cord injury.

Cardiovascular System

Any cord transection above the level of T-5 abolishes the influence of the sympathetic nervous system. Consequently, immediate problems are bradycardia and hypotension. If the bradycardia is only slight, close cardiac monitoring may reveal a stable cardiac condition. Junctional escape beats may be observed and a junctional rhythm may become established. If the bradycardia is marked, appropriate medications (atropine) to increase the heart rate and avoid hypoxia will be necessary.

With the abolition of the influence of the sympathetic nervous system, vasodilatation occurs, decreasing venous return of blood to the heart. This decreases cardiac output, and hypotension results. Intravenous fluids may resolve the problem, otherwise vasopressor drugs may be required.

Renal System

Urinary retention is a common development in acute spinal injuries and spinal shock. The bladder is hyperirritable. There is a loss of inhibition of reflex from the brain. Consequently, the patient will void small amounts of urine frequently. In spite of this, the bladder becomes distended since this is actually urinary retention with overflow. Urinary retention increases the chance of infection. In addition, urinary calculi are likely to develop in a distended bladder retaining urine. Catheterization is indicated.

Gastrointestinal System

If the cord transection has occurred above T-5, the loss of sympathetic innervation may lead to the development of an ileus or gastric distention. Intermittent suctioning by means of a nasogastric tube may relieve the gastric distention, and standard treatment may be used for an ileus. A common occurrence in the past has been the development of biochemical stress ulcers due to excessive release of hydrochloric acid in the stomach. An H_2 antagonist is frequently used to prevent the occurrence of these ulcers during the initial extreme body stress. Because of the absence of clinical signs, any intra-abdominal bleeding that occurs will be difficult to diagnose. There will be no pain, tenderness, guarding, or other signs or symptoms. Continued hypotension in spite of vigorous treatment is suspicious. Expanding girth of the abdomen may be ascertainable, but not always. If the rectum is not emptied on a regular basis, the patient may develop fecal impaction.

Musculoskeletal System
The integrity of the patient's skin is of primary importance. The deterioration of denervated skin can occur very quickly, leading to major, life-threatening infection. The use of a Roto-Bed (Fig. 34–15) and its variations help to prevent the breakdown of the skin. A certain degree of muscle atrophy will occur during the flaccid paralysis state, while contractures tend to occur during the spastic paralysis stage.

Poikilothermism is the adjustment of the body temperature toward room temperature. This occurs in these injuries because the interruption of the sympathetic nervous system prevents its temperature-controlling fibers from sending impulses that will reach the hypothalamus.

Metabolic Needs
Correcting an existing acid–base disturbance and maintaining acid–base balance will promote the function of other body systems. Recall that nasogastric suctioning may lead to alkalosis, and decreased perfusion may lead to acidosis. Electrolytes must be monitored until a normal diet is resumed and suctioning has been discontinued. A positive nitrogen balance and a high-protein diet will help prevent skin breakdown and infections, and will help decrease the rate of muscle atrophy.

Nursing Interventions

The goal of nursing care is to prevent secondary injury and complication postinjury and to begin planning for return to home.

The primary nursing intervention is ensuring a patent airway at *all* times to provide for adequate ventilation. Most patients with cervical fractures will have an endotracheal tube or a tracheostomy. Frequent, gentle suctioning of the nasopharynx, oropharynx, and endotracheal tube or tracheostomy is imperative to help prevent hypoxia secondary to retained secretions. *However,* suctioning must not exceed 10–15 sec, and the patient should be hyperventilated before and after the procedure to prevent a cardiac arrest, which may occur if hypoxia develops

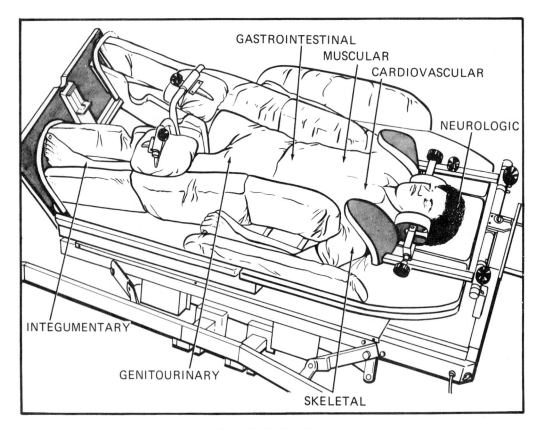

Figure 34–15. Roto-Bed.

and the patient has a bradycardia or junctional rhythm. It is recommended that PaO₂ be kept above 80 mm Hg to help prevent the effect of hypoxia on the ischemic cord surrounding the injury.

The "quad-assist" cough should be done frequently to assist in maintaining airway clearance. The nurse places a fist or heel of the hand between the umbilicus and the xiphoid process and presses inward and upward when the patient coughs. After patient instruction, the patient is asked to take several slow, deep breaths. On the next deep breath, a quad-assist cough is done. Aggressive chest physiotherapy protocols should be followed according to neurological and cardiovascular parameters. The patient's vital capacity, tidal volume, and arterial blood gas levels should be carefully and frequently monitored until the patient is stable and ventilatory support is no longer needed.

Cardiovascular monitoring of dysrhythmias and hypotension is essential. The dysrhythmias which occur may require standard treatment or only continued close monitoring. Hypotension is often controlled with intravenous administration of fluids, which requires that the nurse monitor the patient for the development of pulmonary edema.

The prevention of extension of cord injury is the next major nursing responsibility. If traction is employed, the rope knots should be taped, weights hanging freely, and traction lines kept straight or as positioned by the physician. Motorsensory assessment should be done with vital signs.

Renal status is usually monitored hourly in the first few days following injury. The amount of intravenous fluids necessary to prevent hypotension is usually sufficient to prevent renal complications of oliguria or anuria unless there is multiple trauma involving the kidneys. The common renal problem after vertebral and cord injury above the sacral level is urinary retention. A Foley catheter is often used in the early stages of the injury. If a Foley catheter is not inserted, intermittent catheterization is needed to ensure that an excessive urinary volume is not retained in the bladder, leading to further problems.

Gastrointestinal interventions include initial drainage of the stomach contents followed by intermittent suction by nasogastric tube since gastric distention occurs and acid secretions are increased in the first few days. Contents suctioned should be routinely monitored for blood since biochemical stress ulcers may occur.

Musculoskeletal needs of the patient include proper body alignment, support of bony prominences to prevent skin breakdown, and frequent turning (unless a Roto-bed is used) to promote circulation and induce comfort. During the flaccid paralysis stage, extremities should be maintained in a functional position. During the spastic stage of the paralysis, medications and some physiotherapy may help control the spasms. Assessment should include motor testing every 4 hrs (0 = no movement, 5 = having movement with resistance). Prevention of thrombus formation is important and may include passive range of motion or use of antithrombic devices.

Metabolic needs of the patient are initially met with intravenous fluids. As soon as the patient is stabilized, tube feedings are often started. Depending on the site of the injury and the residual deficits, the patient may be able to start oral feedings relatively soon after the injury. Rarely is hyperalimentation used unless protracted treatment of multiple trauma is required. The patient should be weighed on admission and then at least weekly.

Autonomic Dysreflexia

Autonomic dysreflexia, or autonomic hyperreflexia, is usually seen within the first year after a spinal cord injury at the level of T-6 or higher. The condition is a life-threatening situation requiring immediate attention.

The most common precipitating causes are a distended bladder or a full rectum. Contraction of the bladder or rectum, stimulation of the skin, stimulation of the pain receptors, or sudden change in environmental temperature may also cause autonomic hyperreflexia.

Symptoms include hypertension, blurred vision, severe throbbing headache, unusual apprehension, marked diaphoresis, and flushing above the level of the lesion with pallor and coolness below, bradycardia, piloerection (body hair erect) due to pilomotor spasm, nasal congestion, and nausea. The hypertension may be so severe that the patient may suffer a stroke or myocardial infarction.

Pathophysiology of this condition involves the stimulation of sensory receptors below the level of cord lesion. The intact autonomic system reacts with a reflex arteriolar spasm which increases blood pressure. Baroreceptors in the cerebral vessels, carotid sinus, and aorta sense the hypertension and stimulate the parasympathetic system. The heart rate decreases, but the visceral and peripheral vessels do not dilate because efferent impulses cannot pass through the cord lesion. The hypertension continues until it is blocked by medication. Ganglionic blocking agents are used to interrupt the hyperreflexia state. Drugs used include hydralazine hydrochloride and diazoxide.

Nursing interventions in this very serious emergency include notification of the physician, assessment to determine the cause, and elevation of the head of the bed or putting the patient into a sitting position if possible. Blood pressure should be monitored every 3–5 min. Abdominal palpation for a distended bladder is done very gently to avoid increasing the stimulus. The urinary catheter should be checked for a kink or irrigation performed very slowly and gently to open a plugged catheter. A digital rectal exam should be done only after application of a local anesthetic ointment (Nupercainal) to decrease rectal stimulation and to prevent an increase of symptoms. If signs and symptoms persist after the bladder and bowel have been thoroughly checked, the next step is to check the skin for irritation. Assess the room temperature for sudden change and apply appropriate intervention (blankets or cooling modalities) if necessary. The patient and family need education as to how to monitor for, prevent, and treat autonomic dysreflexia.

Encephalopathies, Coma, and Brain Herniation

EDITORS' NOTE

In this chapter, concepts are covered which address the CCRN test areas of encephalopathies coma and brain herniation. Expect one to three questions from the exam to cover content in this chapter.

ENCEPHALOPATHIES

The primary effects of encephalopathies are behavioral changes and alterations in level of consciousness (LOC). Changes in LOC occur for three reasons:

1. Reduction in oxygen delivery.
2. Reduction in blood glucose.
3. Reduction in cerebral perfusion pressure.

In addition, the accumulation of various metabolites of renal and hepatic failure can cause a change in LOC and behavior.

In any situation in which a patient does not respond appropriately, the above parameters should be assessed. Specific alterations in behavior and LOC from renal and hepatic failure are addressed in later chapters.

COMA (AROUSAL DEFICIT)

Two general types of pathologic processes lead to coma: (1) conditions which widely and directly depress function of the cerebral hemispheres; and (2) conditions which depress or destroy brain stem activating mechanisms. Common to all impairments is a reduction in either cerebral metabolism or cerebral blood flow.

Three categories of disease are important in the aforementioned pathologic processes that lead to coma:

1. A supratentorial mass lesion will encroach on deep diencephalic structures, compressing or destroying the ascending reticular activating system.
2. A subtentorial mass or destructive lesion may directly damage the brain stem central core.
3. Metabolic disorders may result in generalized interruption of brain function.

Coma does not occur as a result of focal injury or ischemia in a specific lobe; it occurs only when both cerebral hemispheres or brain stem divisions are dysfunctional. The major catastrophe of coma is death due to brain herniation.

HERNIATION SYNDROMES

Herniation is the result of increased intracranial pressure (ICP) beyond compensatory levels. The rapid increase in size of a hematoma, tumor or cerebral edema may cause the movement of brain tissue from an area of the cranium where it normally is located. The brain tissue is not evenly distributed and unless the change is corrected rapidly the impingment on blood flow and compression of brain tissue will cause ischemia and permanent damage. This shift of tissue or protrusion through an abnormal opening is called herniation; it occurs from an area of greater pressure into an area of lower pressure.

Frequent neuro assessment and ICP monitoring are important parameters in monitoring for herniation syndrome. *NOTE:* Herniation can occur without fixed or dilated pupils and increases ICP may be localized and not reflected by ICP monitoring.

Herniation

The tentorium cerebelli divides the supratentorial structures (the cerebral hemispheres) from the infratentorial structures (the cerebellum). The tentorium cerebelli has an opening, the incisura or tentorial notch through which the midbrain passes. As the ICP increases, movement of the brain tissue can occurs and forces the brain tissue from the area of higher pressure to an area of lower pressure. Herniation can occur above or supratentorial and/or below, infratentorial herniaition. Four types of supratentorial herniation can occur: cingulate, central, uncal and transcalvarial. Two types of infratentorial herniation can occur: tonsillar or downward cerebellar herniation and upward transtentorial herniation. The symptoms differ with the type and location of the herniation.

Supratentorial Herniation

Cingulate herniation or subfalcine herniation is a space occupying lesion which causes lateral movement of the frontal lobe or unilateral hemisphere and forces the cingulate gyrus under the falx cerebri. The lesion may be a tumor, infarct, hemorrhage, or abscess and may present with accompanying edema. On CAT scan and MRI a midline shift is noted; contralateral swelling may occur secondary to CSF outflow tract obstruction.

Central herniation: increasing ICP forces the cerebral hemispheres and the basal nuclei through the tentorial notch, compressing the diencephalon, mesencephalon (midbrain), and pons. Divisions of the basilar artery are also displaced, causing ischemia and brain stem deterioration. The displacement also blocks the aqueduct of Sylvius effectively preventing the downward displacement of CSF (a compensatory mechanism of increasing ICP). This further increases ICP. Effect of central herniation usually

progress in a head-to-tail direction. Thus, an alteration in LOC is often a subtle first sign of impending herniation.

Uncal herniation occurs when the uncus (medial part of the temporal lobe) impacts upon the tentorial notch. An expanding temporal lobe lesion and/or increasing middle fossa pressure may force the uncus over the edge of the incisura. The movement of the uncus compresses the mesencephalon (midbrain) against the opposite edge of the incisura. Uncal herniation often presses the oculomotor nerve and posterior cerebral artery against the incisura. The earliest consistent sign in uncal herniation is a unilaterally dilating pupil accompanied by a change in the LOC.

Transcalvarial herniation is movement of the brain tissue which is swollen after cranial trauma or penetrating brain injury with skull fracture through the cranium. The bone flap can be removed in anticipation of additional swelling; this is not normal practice.

Infratentorial Herniation

Tonsillar herniation occurs when there is downward displacement of the cerebellar peduncles or tonsils through the foramen magnum. The earliest sign is nuchal rigidity. Changes in heart rate and blood pressure, small pupils and ataxic respirations. Coma and death follow the compression of the brainstem and medulla.

Upward transtentorial herniation is rare. Presenting signs are nuchal rigidity, loss of upward gaze and loss of consciousness. Cranial nerve deficits increase and posturing begins. Drainage of CSF from the ventricle can worsen the hernaition syndrome.

Stages of Herniation

There are four distinct stages of central herniation: (1) the early diencephalic stage; (2) the late diencephalic stage; (3) the mesencephalon–upper pons stage; and (4) the lower pons–upper medulla stage.

There are three stages in uncal herniation: (1) the uncal syndrome–early third cranial nerve stage; (2) the uncal syndrome–late third cranial nerve stage; (3) the lower pons–upper medulla stage.

Monitoring Parameters

Specific parameters can be monitored which indicate impending or active herniation. Serial CAT scan

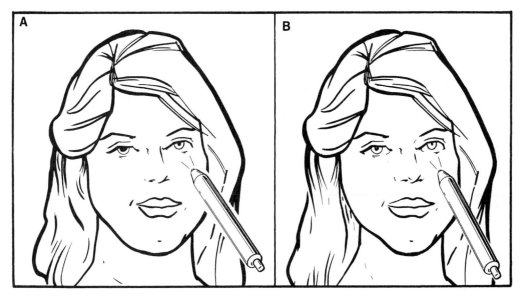

Figure 35–1. Pupillary light reflex **(A)** and consensual light reflex **(B)**.

or MRI can identify pathophysiology; management consists of prevention and control of ICP.

In central herniation, the parameters are LOC, pupillary function (size and reaction to light), respiratory pattern, oculocephalic and oculovestibular responses (doll's eyes and the ice water caloric test, respectively), motor responses, and the ciliospinal reflex.

In uncal herniation, unequal pupillary response and unilateral third cranial nerve palsy are early important signs. Then LOC (both content and degree of alertness) or delirium or lethargy suggest impending herniation. Respiratory, oculocephalic, and oculovestibular responses do not come into play until LOC has declined.

Parameter Norms and Testing Methods

1. Level of consciousness was explained in Chapter 32 and will not be discussed again here.
2. Pupillary function is controlled by both sympathetic and parasympathetic tracts. These tracts are not easily affected by metabolic states. Therefore, the presence or absence of an equal pupillary light reflex is the single most important factor in differentiating metabolic from structural (neurological) coma.

   The pupillary light reflex (Fig. 35–1) is best tested in a darkened room. In a normal state, the pupil will constrict when a light beam is directed into it. Normally, there is also a consensual response; that is, the pupil *not* having a light beam directed into it will constrict with the eye being tested.

3. The ciliospinal reflex is tested by pinching the skin on the back edge of the neck (Fig. 35–2). Normally, this action causes ipsilateral pupillary dilatation.

4. The key eye movements observed in the comatose patient are (1) the spontaneous motion of each eye; (2) the resting position of each eye; and (3) responses of the eyes to the oculocephalic and oculovestibular tests.

   The resting position of the eyes may be conjugate, disconjugate, or skewed. A conjugate position is any resting position with both eyes in the same position. A disconjugate position is a resting position with the eyes in different positions. Right eye midline, midposition and left eye midline, fixed to the right side is an example of a disconjugate position. Skewedness refers to any vertical disconjugate positioning. Skewing indicates a brain stem lesion.

   The oculocephalic response (Fig. 35–3) is often called doll's eyes. Doll's eyes can be tested only in the unconscious patient and is normally recorded as present or absent. To test the oculocephalic response, hold the

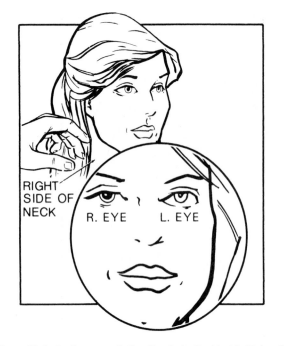

Figure 35–2. Pupil response in the ciliospinal reflex (depicted in inset).

patient's eyelids open and quickly—but gently—turn the head to one side. The normal response is for the eyes to conjugately deviate in the contraversive direction of the head turning. Repeat by flexing and extending the head. Again, the normal response is conjugate (parallel) contraversive movement of the eyes in relation to the direction of head movement. This is recorded using the phrase "doll's eyes present." Abnormal responses are recorded using the phrase "doll's eyes absent." If the eyes move in the same direction as the head is turned (i.e., when the head is flexed, the eyes go down, or when the head is turned right, eyes go right or no further than midline), the test is abnormal (Doll's eyes absent). This means that cranial nerves III, IV, and VI, which are responsible for ocular movements are not intact. Turning the head to both the right and the left will test each pair of these nerves. The oculocephalic reflex must *never* be tested unless cervical spinal cord and vertebral injuries have been ruled out.

The ice water caloric test, in which the oculovestibular reflex is examined, is more powerful in eliciting eye movements. An intact tympanic membrane is essential in order for the test to be accurate. The head of the bed is elevated about 30°. The physician slowly injects ice water until nystagmus (eye deviation) occurs (or until 200 ml of ice water has been used). In the unconscious

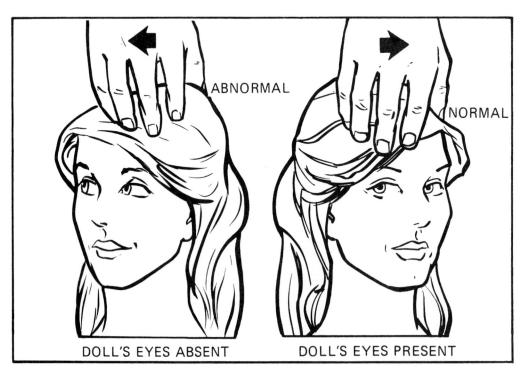

Figure 35–3. Oculocephalic response (doll's eyes phenomenon).

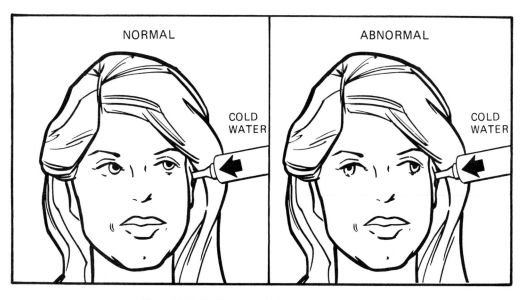

Figure 35–4. Pupil response in the oculovestibular reflex.

patient, the eyes move slowly toward the irrigated ear and remain there 2–3 min (Fig. 35–4). This indicates a supratentorial lesion or a metabolic condition. An extremely abnormal movement (skewing, jerky rotation) usually indicates a cerebellar or brain stem lesion.

5. Motor responses are not dependent on LOC. They usually correlate with LOC. Motor responses are important sources of information concerning the geographical spread of neurological dysfunction.

   Cerebral hemisphere frontal lobe dysfunction is characterized by paraplegia in flexion, tonic grasping, and exaggerated snout reflexes.

   Decorticate posture (Fig. 35–5) is characterized by flexion of the arm, wrist, and fingers. Adduction of arms and extension and internal rotation with plantar flexion of the lower extremities complete the motor responses. Abnormal flexion response is synonymous with decorticate posturing.

   Decerebrate posture is characterized by opisthotonos (arching of the back so that the head and heels remain on the surface and the remainder of the back is raised), with the arms slightly extended, adducted, and hyperpronated (Fig. 35–6). The legs are stiffly extended and the feet are flexed in a plantar position. Abnormal extension response is synonymous with decerebrate posture.

6. Respiratory patterns were discussed in the pulmonary section and will not be discussed again here.

Table 35–1 identifies the stages and parameter responses in central herniation. Table 35–2 identifies the stages and parameter responses in uncal herniation.

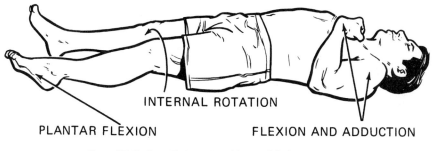

INTERNAL ROTATION

PLANTAR FLEXION   FLEXION AND ADDUCTION

Figure 35–6. Decorticate posture (abnormal flexion response).

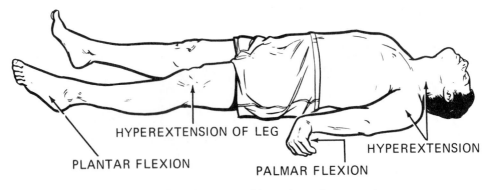

Figure 35–5. Decerebrate posture (abnormal extension response).

Herniation through the Foramen Magnum

If the ICP rises precipitously, the pressure may be sufficient to compress the cerebellum and medulla oblongata through the foramen magnum. A lumbar puncture performed in the presence of high ICP may result in brain stem herniation through the foramen magnum as the counterpressure in the spinal canal is lost. Herniation through the foramen magnum results in death secondary to cardiopulmonary arrest. This form of herniation is not clinically separable from central and uncal herniation.

TABLE 35–1. STAGES AND PARAMETERS OF CENTRAL HERNIATION

	Central—Early Diencephalic	Central—Late Diencephalic	Mesencephalon Upper Pons	Lower Pons—Upper Medulla
Respirations				
Pupillary response				
Consensual light response				
Ciliospinal reflex				
Oculovestibular response				
Doll's eye response				
Babinski response				
Body position response	Rest Stimulus			

TABLE 35–2. STAGES AND PARAMETERS OF UNCAL HERNIATION

	Uncal–Early Third Cranial Nerve	Uncal Mesencephalon–Late Third Cranial Nerve	Lower Pons–Upper Medulla
Respirations		OR	OR
Pupillary response			
Consensual light response			
Ciliospinal reflex			
Oculovestibular response			
Doll's eye response			
Babinski response			
Body position response	Rest Stimulus		

Meningitis, Guillain–Barré, and Myasthenia Gravis

EDITORS' NOTE

In this chapter, we address the syndrome, concepts of infectious diseases of the neurological system that will most likely be covered on the CCRN exam. Meningitis is more likely to be addressed than Guillain–Barré syndrome and myasthenia gravis. As you read this chapter, focus on infectious processes affecting the neurological system. It will be useful to have a basic understanding of the other conditions, although it is unlikely they will appear on the CCRN test. Expect one to three questions on the test to be based on content in this chapter.

MENINGITIS

Meningitis is an acute infection of the pia and arachnoid membrane surrounding the brain and the spinal cord. Because the pia and arachnoid space are communicating structures, meningitis is always a cerebrospinal infection.

Pathophysiology

A pathogenic organism gains access to the pia-subarachnoid space and causes an inflammatory reaction in the pia and arachnoid, in the cerebrospinal fluid (CSF), and in the ventricles of the brain, since these are all communicating structures. The first response is hyperemia of the meningeal vessels, followed by the infiltration of neutrophils into the subarachnoid space. An exudate forms and very quickly enlarges, covering the base of the brain and extending through the subarachnoid space and into the sheaths of cranial and spinal nerves. Polymorphonuclear leukocytes (PMNs) attempt to control the invading pathogen. Within a few days, leukocytes and histiocytes increase in number in an attempt to "wall off" the exudate from the pathogen or its toxins. Toward the end of the second week, the cellular exudate has formed two layers. The outer layer directly under the arachnoid membrane is composed of PMNs and fibrin. The inner layer is composed of lymphocytes, plasma cells, and macrophages, and is next to the pia.

With appropriate drug therapy to destroy the pathogen, these two layers begin to resolve. The outer cellular layer against the arachnoid disappears. If the infection is arrested quickly enough, the inner layer will also disappear. However, if the infection lasts for several weeks, the inner layer, which contains fibrin, forms a permanent fibrous structure over the meninges. This produces a thickened, often cloudy, arachnoid membrane and causes adhesions between the pia and arachnoid membranes.

The adhesions and prior inflammation result in congestion of tissues and blood vessels. A degeneration of nerve cells follows, eventually resulting in congestion of adjacent brain tissue. This congestion causes cortical irritation and increased intracranial pressure (ICP). Cerebral edema may lead to hydrocephalus. If uninterrupted, a progression of vasculitis with cortical necrosis, petechial hemorrhage within the brain, hydrocephalus, and cranial nerve damage occurs.

Etiology

Organisms obtain access to the subarachnoid space through penetrating head injuries, basal skull fractures with a torn dura mater, ICP monitoring, cranial surgery, mastoiditis, acute otitis media, lumbar punctures, injury to the paranasal sinuses, and sepsis. The organism may be viral or bacterial. The most common bacteria is *Haemophilus influenza*. Gram-positive bacteria include *Neisseria meningitidis* (meningococcus) and *Diplococcus pneumoniae*. Gram-negative bacteria include *Haemophilus influenzae, Klebsiella, Escherichia coli*, and *Pseudomonas*. After neurological surgery, *Staphylococcus aureus* or *S. epidermidis* are common bacterial contaminants. In children, it is *H. influenzae*. Other bacteria include *Streptococcus, Pneumococcus*, and occasionally *Mycobacterium tuberculosis*. The outcome of bacterial meningitis is dependent on early and aggressive treatment.

Clinical Signs and Symptoms

Suspect meningitis if a fever, severe headache, and nuchal rigidity (resistance to flexion of the neck) exist. Positive Kernig's and Brudzinski's signs, photophobia, decreased sensorium, and signs of increased intracranial pressure are common. Kernig's sign is the inability to fully extend the leg at the knee when the leg is flexed at the hip. Brudzinski's sign is the involuntary adduction and flexion of the legs with attempts to flex the neck. With meningitis, a headache becomes progressively worse and is accompanied by nausea, vomiting, irritability, confusion, and seizures. Dysfunction of cranial nerves VII and VIII is present. Increased ICP is secondary to purulent exudate, cerebral edema, and hydrocephalus. Papilledema is more likely with brain abscess, subdural empyema, and venous sinus occlusion. Vital sign changes occur with brain stem pressure. If the causative organism is the meningococcus, a skin rash is common.

Diagnosis

A major diagnostic tool is examination of the CSF. Variations in the CSF depend on the causative organism. CSF protein levels are usually elevated, higher in bacterial than in viral cases. A decreased CSF glucose level is common in bacterial meningitis but may be normal in viral meningitis. Appearance of the CSF is purulent and turbid in bacterial meningitis. It may be the same or clear in viral meningitis. The most predominant cell in the CSF is the PMN.

Cultures of blood, sputum, and nasopharyngeal secretions are performed to identify the causative organism.

Roentgenograms of the skull may demonstrate infected sinuses. Computed tomography (CT) scans are usually normal in uncomplicated meningitis. In other cases, CT may reveal evidence of increased intracranial pressure.

Complications

The most common complication of meningitis is residual neurological dysfunction. Dysfunction of cranial nerve III, IV, VI, or VII often occurs in bacterial meningitis. Usually the dysfunction disappears within a few weeks. Hearing loss may be permanent after bacterial meningitis but is not a complication of viral meningitis.

Cranial nerve irritation can have serious sequelae. When cranial nerve II is compressed by increased ICP, papilledema is often present and blindness may occur. When cranial nerves III, IV, and VI are irritated, ocular movements are affected. Ptosis, unequal pupils, and diplopia are common. Irritation of cranial nerve V is evidenced by sensory and corneal changes, and irritation of cranial nerve VII results in facial paresis. Irritation of cranial nerve VIII causes tinnitus, vertigo, and deafness.

Hemiparesis, dysphasia, and hemianopsia may occur. These signs usually resolve within several hours. If resolution does not occur, a cerebral abscess, subdural empyema, subdural effusion, or cortical venous thrombophlebitis is suggested.

Acute cerebral edema may occur with bacterial meningitis, causing seizures, third nerve palsy, bradycardia, hypertension, coma, and death.

A noncommunicating hydrocephalus may occur if the inner layer of the exudate has caused adhesions which prevent the normal flow of CSF from the ventricles. Surgical implantation of a shunt is the only treatment.

Endocrine dysfunction resulting in hyponatremia and excessive release of antidiuretic hormone may increase cerebral edema.

Nursing Interventions

Administration of antibiotics at scheduled times maintains a therapeutic blood level. Respiratory isolation precautions will protect the staff and visitors but need not be continued past 24–48 hr after the institution of antibiotic therapy.

Body temperature can be controlled by administration of antipyretic drugs as indicated, by use of a hypothermia blanket, and by environmental temperature change.

Headache is usually treated with analgesics. A darkened, quiet room will help both the headache and photophobia. Avoid sudden quick movements.

Seizure precautions should be initiated. If seizures occur, anticonvulsant medication is indicated. Documentation of progression, limb involvement, and duration of the seizures will help determine an effective medication regimen.

Dyspnea and respiratory distress require standard treatment. A central venous pressure line or a pulmonary artery catheter may be inserted to monitor fluid balance and the cardiovascular status. Monitoring of electrolyte levels, especially sodium, is essential. Standard nursing procedures for these types of complications are followed.

GUILLAIN–BARRÉ SYNDROME

EDITORS' NOTE

It is possible that a question or two will address Guillain–Barré syndrome, particularly relating to the acute respiratory failure which develops in the advanced stages of this condition. Review this section to understand the critical implications of this condition.

Guillain–Barré syndrome is an acute inflammatory disease, thought to be autoimmune or viral, that affects peripheral nerves, spinal nerves, and sometimes cranial nerves, first with edema and then demyelination. Synonyms for Guillain–Barré syndrome include Landry–Guillain–Barré disease, acute inflammatory polyradiculoneuropathy, and infectious polyneuritis.

Pathophysiology

In the normal course of the disease, the patient usually has had an upper respiratory or gastrointestinal infection 1–2 weeks prior to the development of Guillain–Barré syndrome. The predominant pattern is weakness starting in the lower extremities and advancing (often very rapidly) to motor paralysis as it progresses up the body. The progression may stop at any point. The first pathologic sign of the syndrome is a perivascular lymphocytic infiltration. Following this, characteristic infiltration occurs in the myelin, breaking it down but not damaging the axon. This is called segmental demyelination. If the syndrome progresses, the infiltration becomes more intense and affects the axon, resulting in muscle denervation and atrophy. If the infiltration occurs in the distal segment of the axon, regeneration will occur because the nerve cell body has been spared. If the infiltration occurs at the proximal end of the axon, the nerve cell body may die and regeneration cannot occur. This is known as Wallerian degeneration. Collateral motor fibers may reinnervate the destroyed muscle, restoring the lost function partially or completely. As the infiltration process ends, recovery of motor function begins proximally and progresses distally. In the anterior horn cells and the neurons in the dorsal root ganglia, destruction of the Nissl bodies, which synthesize protein essential for cellular repair and growth, prevents recovery of function.

Diagnosis

Examination of the CSF is done to determine if the CSF protein is elevated (up to 700 mg %) with only a few cells present. This represents albuminocytologic dissociation (high protein/few cells), which is specific for Guillain–Barré syndrome. Increased antibody titers, especially IgM, in serum occurs. Electrical studies indicate a slowing or conduction block in motor or sensory nerve conduction velocity.

Etiology

Specific etiologic agents are unknown. The most popular theory is that a slow-acting measles virus is the causative agent. Guillain–Barré syndrome occurs at any age, with a peak incidence between 30 and 40 years. Both sexes are equally affected.

Clinical Presentation

Symptoms usually develop 1–3 weeks after an upper respiratory infection and occasionally after a gastrointestinal infection. Infrequently, polyneuritis may occur after surgery, after lymphomatous disease, or with immunizations such as those for rabies and swine flu.

Weakness of the lower extremities evolving more or less symmetrically occurs over a period of hours to days to weeks, usually peaking by the fourteenth day. Distal muscles are the more severely affected. Paresthesia (numbness and tingling) is frequent but pain is rare. Paralysis usually follows paresthesia in the extremities. Hypotonia and areflexia are common, persistent symptoms. Objective sensory loss is variable, with deep sensibility more affected than superficial sensations. A "pins and needles" sensation in the hands and feet is described.

Autonomic nervous function is rarely altered. Sinus tachycardia, postural hypotension, hypertension, heart block, and anhydrosis (absence of sweating) are uncommon findings. Urinary retention occurs occasionally, but catheterization is seldom needed for more than a few days.

If cranial nerve involvement occurs, it is most frequent in cranial nerve VII, followed by cranial nerves VI, III, XII, V, and X (most to least frequent). Facial nerve dysfunction includes an inability to smile, frown, whistle, or drink through a straw. Consequently, dysphasia and laryngeal paralysis is common if the paresthesia and paralysis extend to the cranial nerves.

Variations in Clinical Presentation

Ascending paralysis moves from legs to trunk to arms to head. It usually peaks in 10–14 days. Fisher's variant is complete ophthalmoplegia (paralysis of the eye muscles), ataxia, and areflexia.

Cases with a steady or stepwise progression over weeks or months may be asymmetrical. Some body parts will be recovering while others are getting worse. There may be relapses, but these are uncommon.

Complications

The most serious complication is respiratory failure as the paralysis advances upward. Constant monitoring will provide for immediate intervention if failure occurs. Respiratory monitoring is typically provided by measuring forced vital capacities (FVC) and peak (or negative) inspiratory efforts. Arterial blood gas levels (ABGs) may be employed to detect the development of a respiratory acidosis.

Infection, either respiratory or urinary, may occur and intervention begun if fever develops. Due to muscle atony and immobility, ileus, venous thrombophlebitis, and pulmonary emboli may occur.

Treatment and Nursing Interventions

The objective of therapy is to support body systems until recovery occurs. Respiratory failure and infec-

tion are serious threats to recovery. Monitoring the vital capacity and ABGs is essential. If the vital capacity drops to less than 12–15 ml/kg body weight, the peak negative pressure is below –20 cm H_2O the respiratory rate is above 30, there is paradoxical movement of the chest and abdomen (paradox alternans), or if the ABGs reflect development of a respiratory acidosis, intubation or tracheostomy may be done so that the patient can be mechanically ventilated. Strict sterile suctioning is needed to prevent infection whether the patient has an endotracheal tube or a tracheostomy. Excellent bronchial hygiene and chest physiotherapy will help clear secretions and prevent respiratory deterioration. If fever develops, sputum cultures should be obtained to identify a specific pathogen (if one is present in the respiratory tract) so that appropriate antibiotic therapy may be instituted.

A communication system must be established with the patient using whatever muscle action is possible. This is extremely difficult if the disease progresses to involvement of the cranial nerves. At the peak of a severe syndrome, communication from the patient may be impossible. The nurse must explain all procedures before doing them and reassure the patient that muscle function will eventually return to some part of the body, allowing the communication of needs and desires to the nurses. The patient and family need assistance in developing positive coping skills and education regarding the disease process.

Monitoring blood pressure, cardiac rate, and cardiac rhythm is important since some transient cardiac dysrhythmias have been reported. Hypotension, secondary to the muscular atony, may occur in severe cases or at the peak of the attack. Vasopressor agents may be required.

Urinary retention is not uncommon for a few days. Intermittent catheterization may be preferred to an indwelling catheter in an effort to avoid urinary tract infection.

Physiotherapy is indicated very early to help counter the hazards of immobility. Passive range of motion and attention to body extremity position help maintain function and prevent contractures. Splints and a continuous passive motion machine may be used for selected joints.

Nutritional needs must be met with consideration of gastric dilatation, ileus development, and aspiration potential if the gag reflex is lost. Initially, tube feedings may be used to ensure adequate caloric intake or, in some centers, hyperalimentation may be started. Head of bed elevation to 30° may prevent aspiration. Antacids, sucralfate, and H_2

inhibitors may be used to decrease risk of gastro-intestinal bleeding.

Eye care to prevent drying and mouth care to protect the mucous membrane are essential.

Fluid and electrolytes are monitored carefully to prevent electrolyte imbalances and the possible occurrence of dysfunctional antidiuretic hormone secretion.

Intravenous immune globulin is given over 4–5 days. Steroid therapy is controversial as is anticoagulant therapy unless signs of phlebitis or pulmonary embolism develop.

Plasmapheresis

Plasmapheresis is the process of separating blood components in order to remove specific components of the blood. In Guillain-Barré syndrome, plasmapheresis is used to remove autoantibodies in the plasma which are believed to cause the disease. While the role of plasmapheresis is unclear in certain diseases, there is an apparent benefit to its use in diseases such as myasthenia gravis and Guillain–Barré syndrome.

Prognosis

Provided complications from respiratory failure can be avoided, good recovery can be expected with minimal permanent neurological dysfunction. With critical care medical treatment and nursing, specifically the management of respiratory failure, morbidity and mortality will decrease.

MYASTHENIA GRAVIS AND CRISIS

EDITORS' NOTE

....

Remember, it is unlikely that the CCRN exam will cover myasthenia in any detail, if at all. Focus on the critical care aspects of this condition and do not try to remember all the components of the disease.

....

Myasthenia gravis is considered to be an autoimmune disease affecting postsynaptic receptor sites. It is a chronic disorder of neuromuscular transmission resulting in weakness with exercise and improving strength with rest.

Pathophysiology

Three theories have been proposed with regard to the pathophysiology of myasthenia gravis. Acetylcholine is released at nerve terminals and combines at the postsynaptic muscle membrane, producing an electrochemical reaction. The electrochemical reaction results in muscle contraction. In myasthenia gravis, there are either too few postsynaptic receptor sites for the amount of acetylcholine released to bind with to provide for a full muscular contraction, or not enough acetylcholine is released to cause full muscle contraction, or acetylcholinesterase degrades the acetylcholine before sufficient amounts can cause a full muscle contraction.

Etiology

The most prevalent hypothesis is that myasthenia gravis is an autoimmune process that damages the postsynaptic membrane. A statistically significant number of cases are associated with thymoma and thymic hyperplasia. This is substantiated by the finding of serum antibodies produced by sensitized lymphocytes or thymocytes that block the action of acetylcholine and the production of immune bodies by the thymus.

Occurrence

Myasthenia gravis occurs in from 1:10,000 to 1:50,000 people. It may occur at any age, but it rarely occurs in those under age 10 or over 70. Peak occurrence is in the 20–30-year age range. Under the age of 40, the ratio of occurrence in women to men is 3:1; after 40, it is 1:1.

Clinical Signs, Symptoms, and Course

Myasthenia gravis is characterized by fatigability of voluntary muscle groups with repeated use. Pathognomonic signs of myasthenia gravis include uneven drooping of the eyelids, a smile that resembles a snarl, a drooping lower jaw that must be supported by the hand, and a partially immobile mouth with the corners turned downward. However, few patients are first seen with these signs. In more than 90% of the cases, eyebrow and extraocular muscles are involved, accompanied by weakness in eye closure. Ptosis and diplopia are common. The next most commonly affected muscles exhibiting symptoms are those of facial expression, mastication, swallowing, and speaking (dysarthria). Hoarseness occurs after only a few minutes of talking. Neck flexor and extensor muscles, the shoulder girdle, and hip flexors are less frequently involved. There usually is no sensory disturbance.

The course of myasthenia gravis is variable. Remission may occur for no discernible reason in fewer than half the cases and usually does not last longer than 1–2 months. The disease then becomes progressive. Frequently, the disease is slow but progressive from the onset. The greatest danger of death is during the first year, and again during years 4 through 7 in progressive cases. Stabilization of the disease occurs after this time and severe recurrence is rare. Infection of any kind, but especially respiratory infection, trauma of any kind, and emotional stress make the disease worse.

Associated Conditions

Approximately 15% of cases have a tumor of the thymus. There is an increasing incidence of tumors in older males. Thyroiditis, thyrotoxicosis, lupus erythematosus, and rheumatoid arthritis occur more often than statistically expected. A pregnancy may make the disease worse, better, or may have no effect. Close to 15% of babies born to myasthenic mothers exhibit symptoms of the disease. The symptoms are usually transient and resolve within 1–12 weeks.

Diagnosis

A history of an increasing muscular fatigability which improves with rest is a common characteristic of myasthenia gravis. Various laboratory tests can be used to aid in a diagnosis, including fatigue on repetitive electrical stimulation, single-fiber electromyographic testing, elevated serum acetylcholine-R antibody titers, and radiographic evidence of thymus enlargement on CT or magnetic resonance imaging. However, anticholinesterase tests are considered conclusive.

Edrophonium chloride (Tensilon) is injected intravenously after the patient's muscle strength has been assessed. Ten milligrams, given in 2–5-mg doses, is the limit used to test for myasthenia gravis. The duration of action for edrophonium chloride is about 5 min.

Edrophonium chloride is an anticholinesterase agent. When injected, it increases the level of acetylcholine at the myoneural junction by blocking cholinesterase (which breaks down acetylcholine). A clinical increase in muscle strength is positive for myasthenia gravis. No improvement or a deterioration in muscle strength is negative for myasthenia gravis.

If edrophonium chloride testing is not conclusive, neostigmine bromide 0.5 mg intravenously or 1.5 mg intramuscularly may be used. Atropine sulfate (0.6 mg) should be given prior to intravenous neostigmine and may be needed with intramuscular injection of neostigmine to counter nausea, vomiting, increased salivation, and sweating. Intravenous neostigmine may cause ventricular fibrillation or cardiac arrest. After intramuscular injection, maximum effect will be apparent within 30 min, but effects may last 2–3 hr. Curare is seldom used because of its paralytic action, but if properly administered, is definitive.

Treatment

The major objective of therapy is to improve neuromuscular transmission and to prevent complications. Early thymectomy may be employed.

Neuromuscular transmission is improved by administration of anticholinesterase drugs. Pyridostigmine bromide (Mestinon) is a popular choice. If pyridostigmine bromide is not adequate to establish control of neuromuscular transmission, neostigmine (Prostigmin) is used. Prednisone has become an adjunctive drug of choice. It is extremely important to medicate the patient on schedule and to document carefully the patient's muscular response. The medication should be taken with a snack to prevent abdominal cramps and diarrhea. The major difference between pyridostigmine bromide and neostigmine is their duration of action. Mestinon has a 4-hr effect; neostigmine, 2 hr. Fasciculation and increased weakness occurring 50 min after administration of drug is a sign of toxicity and should be reported immediately. Steroids may decrease the amount of anticholinesterase drug required to control myasthenic symptoms. Ephedrine and xanthenes improve the presynaptic release of acetylcholine. The use of steroids results in suppression of immune responses and the resultant problem of infection and biochemical stress. Potassium supplementation may be required secondary to steroid use. Other immunosuppressive agents have been considered, including azathioprine and cyclophosphamide (Cytoxan), cyclosporine A, and intravenous immunoglobulin. With use of azathioprine in the young female, the risk of teratogenicity mandates family planning and birth control education. Birth defects are increased in infants born to a myasthenic gravis mother.

Thymectomy produces an improvement in or remission of symptoms in many patients. An improvement may be gradual over several years (up to 10). Frequently, steroid and anticholinesterase drugs are needed in smaller dosages following thymectomy. New treatments include thoracic duct drainage and plasmapheresis.

Nursing Interventions

A major nursing intervention is to maintain adequate ventilation in spite of a weak cough, an inability to clear secretions, and an increased likelihood of aspiration. Vital capacity is checked every 2–4 hr. Ventilators often are set up and kept available.

Prevention of aspiration, infection from any source, and emotional support of the patient are very important. If the patient is on a respirator, a communication system should be established. If the patient has had a thymectomy, the monitoring and nursing treatment as for any patient with a thoracotomy must be followed.

Specific drugs that impair neuromuscular transmission must be avoided. The aminoglycoside antibiotics and true mycin drugs are contraindicated. Such drugs include aureomycin, kanamycin, polymyxin, neomycin, streptomycin, and gentamicin.

Quinidine, procainamide, morphine sulfate, and sedatives will aggravate muscle weakness.

Nursing education concerning the importance of taking prescribed medications on schedule is extremely important since an early or late dosage may immediately affect muscle strength. Regulation of daily living habits to avoid fatigue and provide rest must be tailored to the patient's life style as much as possible. The patient should understand that minor infection or illness may precipitate an acute attack.

Post-Thymectomy Nursing Interventions

Routine postsurgical care is needed, as are the following:

1. Post-thoracic surgery procedures (e.g., chest tubes).
2. Ventilatory support with frequent suctioning.
3. Anticholinesterase and steroid drugs started slowly.
4. Reassurance that positive effects of a thymectomy occur over long periods (even years).
5. Protection from infections (i.e., sterile technique for suctioning, intermittent urinary catheterization rather than an indwelling catheter, etc.)

Complications: Myasthenic or Cholinergic Crisis?

Myasthenic and cholinergic crises both have extreme weakness as the predominant symptom. Myasthenic crisis is caused by insufficient drug dose. Cholinergic crisis is due to an overdose of drugs and is signalled by increased salivation and sweating. An impending cholinergic crisis can be detected by constricting pupils. Two millimeters is the maximum constriction that should be allowed before intervention. To distinguish between these crises, an edrophonium bromide test is performed with a ventilator on standby. If the patient becomes weaker, a cholinergic (overdose) crisis exists. Treatment is to discontinue anticholinesterase drugs. After 72 hr, drug therapy is usually restarted in small increments. Atropine (an anticholinergic drug) may control symptoms but may also block important symptoms of anticholinesterase overdose. Monitoring ventilatory function with ABGs is imperative.

Myasthenic crisis is established by muscular improvement with the edrophonium bromide test. Anticholinesterase drugs are given and repeated as needed. Steroids are usually avoided during a crisis. Monitoring, assessing, and documenting muscular strength and ABGs are continued throughout the crisis. Muscle assessment may include presence of the gag reflex, voice quality, swallowing difficulty, ptosis on upward gaze, diplopia on lateral gaze, and the ability to do deep knee bends, raise arms above head, rise from chair, or lift head off bed. Identification of the precipitating cause is important to treat and/or correct the cause. Causes of myasthenic crises include infections, heat, emotional upset, surgery, thyroid disease, pregnancy, menses, hypokalemia, and drugs which block the neuromuscular junction. Communication with the patient throughout treatment, by whatever means possible, facilitates rest and trust in the nurse.

Seizures and Status Epilepticus

EDITORS' NOTE

In this chapter, concepts are covered which address the CCRN exam items of seizures and status epilepticus. You can expect anywhere between one and three questions from the test on this content.

SEIZURES

A seizure is a symptom of paroxysmal electrical discharges in the brain resulting in autonomic, sensory, and/or motor dysfunction. Seizures may be associated with infection, trauma, tumors, cerebrovascular disease, genetic or congenital defects, or metabolic dysfunction. If seizures are recurrent and transient, the condition is classified as epilepsy. The term convulsion refers to the musculoskeletal contractions accompanying a seizure.

Classification

There are three types of seizures: partial seizures, general seizures, and unclassified seizures. Table 37–1 gives a classification of seizures.

Partial Seizures

Partial seizures are of three types: simple, complex, and partial secondarily generalizing to generalized tonic–clonic seizure. Simple partial seizures are not associated with a loss of consciousness. The hyperactivity is focused in one area of the brain and does not spread to the other hemisphere. Seizures which initiate in one area and spread to a larger area of the same hemisphere are known as complex partial seizures. In complex partial seizures, loss of consciousness may initiate or be a sequelae of the seizure. Both simple partial and complex partial seizures may evolve into tonic–clonic seizures.

Generalized Seizures

Generalized seizures are characterized by loss of consciousness with involvement of both cerebral hemispheres. They include absence, myoclonic, clonic, tonic, tonic–clonic, and atonic seizures.

Unclassified Seizures

Unclassified epileptic seizures include all seizures for which there are insufficient data as to cause or effect to classify them as partial or generalized seizures. Neonatal seizures are an example of this type of seizure.

Pathophysiology

It is unknown whether seizures occur as a result of increased neuronal excitability or a decreased neuronal inhibitory force. Focal neurons appear to be unusually sensitive to acetylcholine and possibly to deficits in specific neurotransmitters. Altered cell permeability and/or alteration in electrolytes may have a role in seizure activity. It is logical to assume that an electrical threshold for seizures exists in all persons. Factors thought to lower the electrical threshold of neurons include fever, fatigue, altered electrolyte–fluid balance, stress, emotional distress, and/or pregnancy. Regardless of these factors, the hyperexcited neurons become hyperactive. As these localized neuronal discharges become more intense, the hyperirritability spreads synaptically to adjacent neurons. In many instances the entire brain is involved. When only one hemisphere is involved,

TABLE 37–1. CLASSIFICATION OF SEIZURES

Partial seizures
  Simple partial seizure
  Complex partial seizure
  Partial seizure secondarily generalizing to generalized
    tonic–clonic seizure
Generalized seizures
  Absence seizure
  Myoclonic seizure
  Clonic seizure
  Tonic seizure
  Tonic–clonic seizure
  Atonic seizure
Unclassified epileptic seizures

consciousness is preserved. When both cerebral hemispheres are involved, there is usually a loss of consciousness. There are exceptions, however. In the case of bilateral simple partial seizures, loss of consciousness does not occur. Also, in complex partial seizures, consciousness may be altered but is not lost since the seizures occur in the limbic system (even though it is bilateral).

Clinical Presentations

Simple Partial (Focal) Motor Seizures

These seizures were previously known as Jacksonian seizures. The focal point is in the motor strip (the prerolandic gyrus). The typical seizure starts with a twitching of the fingers or toes or around the lips on one side of the body. The muscle movement becomes more severe and spreads (marches) by involving more muscle groups until one side of the body is totally involved. Consciousness is maintained unless the motor seizure becomes generalized and spreads to the remainder of the body.

Simple Partial (Focal) Sensory Seizures

These seizures may be described by the patient as a numbness, tingling, or "pins and needles" sensation. If the causative lesion is in the sensory strip between the frontal and parietal lobes (the postrolandic gyrus), the seizure may progress like a motor seizure. Visual sensations usually indicate an occipital lobe lesion. Auditory sensations are most commonly a buzzing or ringing in the ears. Auditory sensations are often accompanied by olfactory symptoms and dizziness. This indicates a temporal lobe lesion.

Complex Partial Psychomotor Seizures

An aura often precedes a seizure. The aura includes complex visceral and/or perceptual hallucinations. The patient appears to be awake but is in a nonresponsive state. Simple or elaborate behavior patterns known as automatisms may be carried out during the seizure. These robot-like behavior patterns can include such behaviors as lip smacking. The average seizure lasts about 5 min. Attempts to interrupt the behavior pattern often precipitate violence. The seizure may end abruptly with the patient having complete amnesia, or the patient may have a period of headache, confusion, or sleepiness.

Tonic–Clonic (Grand Mal) Seizures

A peculiar sensation or feeling known as an aura (prodroma) may occur at the beginning of a seizure. An aura also accompanies complex partial seizures. For those who do experience an aura, it is almost always the same sensation or feeling. As consciousness is lost, the patient falls (if upright). The body becomes rigid. As air is forced from the lungs, the patient may emit a high-pitched, loud cry. The jaws become locked and the tongue is often caught between clenched teeth. Pupils dilate and are nonreactive. Apnea results in cyanosis. Bladder incontinence is common. This tonic phase of the grand mal seizure lasts 10–20 sec.

The clonic phase of the grand mal seizure is a period of violent, rhythmic, symmetrical, alternating contraction and relaxation involving the entire body. Increased salivation, mixed with blood if the tongue has been bitten, results in "frothing" at the mouth. The patient is tachycardic, is profusely diaphoretic, and remains apneic. The tonic and clonic phases last 1–5 min.

In the postictal phase, the seizure subsides, the patient resumes breathing, cyanosis clears, and the pupils react. The patient should be bagged with a high volume of oxygen during this stage to help compensate for the period of apnea. The patient is fatigued, has a headache, is sleepy and confused, and may have amnesia of the entire seizure excepting the aura. A residual neurological deficit (Todd's paralysis) may continue for several hours.

Absence (Petit Mal) Seizures

These are generalized seizures that consist of frequent episodes of loss of consciousness termed absences. The absences last 10–15 sec and are characterized by the cessation of motor activity, stopping speech in mid-sentence, and/or staring into space. During the seizure, the child (it is rarely seen after age 12) may twitch his or her lips or the lips may droop. The eyes may roll upward. There is no change in muscle tone. The patient may stagger or stumble, but rarely falls. Absence seizures are benign neurologically, however, they may interfere with classroom learning.

Bilateral Myoclonus (Myoclonic Seizures)

These seizures are characterized by sudden, violent contractions of muscle groups. They may be generalized or focal, and symmetrical (both sides) or asymmetrical (one side). Loss of consciousness is unusual in certain types of myoclonic seizure activity. The seizures may consist of a single jerking movement or intermittent periods of active seizure, or be present in varying degrees all of the waking time. The seizures are absent during sleep, being precipitated by stimulation and intensified with intentional movement.

Atonic (Akinetic) Seizures

These may occur by themselves or in cases of absence seizures. There is a sudden, brief loss of muscle tone with or without a loss of consciousness. The child with such seizures falls often and may be labelled clumsy or awkward. Akinetic seizures may cloud the picture of absence seizures. These seizures often result from serious neurological disease which cannot be treated.

Etiology of Epilepsy

Multiple causes of epilepsy are known. The most common is the abrupt cessation of antiepileptic drugs or other chronic sedative medications. Other causes include trauma, tumor, injuries (both perinatal and postnatal), central nervous system (CNS) infections, and cerebral vascular disease, including arteriovenous malformations. Metabolic and toxic disorders may cause seizures. The role of genetics and heredity is controversial at this time. In a large number of cases, the cause is unknown. These cases are termed idiopathic epilepsy.

Diagnosis of Epilepsy

The patient's history of seizure activity (duration, frequency, intensity, and progression) is one of the most useful tools in establishing a diagnosis. The family should be asked for their observations and their knowledge of participating factors if the patient is unable to provide them. Past medical history should be closely examined for previous seizures, head injury, or other illness. Physical examination, laboratory studies, radiologic studies, and electroencephalograms (EEGs) may reveal factors supporting a diagnosis of epilepsy or the studies may all be within normal limits.

Nursing Interventions and Complications

There are five major areas of nursing interventions for the patient having seizures.

1. Protecting the patient from injury is a priority. Remove objects from the immediate environment that might cause injury. Stay with the patient during the seizure. Bedrails should be up and padded and the bed placed in low position. The patient should not be restrained but efforts to protect the patient's head from injury are appropriate (e.g., if a seizure occurs with the patient out of bed, a pillow may be placed under the head or a nurse may cradle—**not** restrain—the patient's head to protect it). **Nothing** should ever be used to pry open the patient's mouth or be forced into the mouth during a seizure. Damage to the mouth and tongue occurs at the start of a seizure and only more damage will result by forcing objects into the mouth.

2. Observing and recording seizure patterns with a video camera may help identify the seizure focus. When surface EEG electrodes are insufficient, then use of an implanted grid for EEG monitoring may be used to locate the lesion. Data collected include precipitating factors, presence and type of aura, duration of unconsciousness, the pattern and progression of seizure activity, body parts involved (generalized or one-sided), incontinence, postictal activity, and if monitored ictally, EEG data.

3. Assessment of the respiratory system is extremely important. The danger in a tonic–clonic seizure is that the patient's respiratory status will be compromised during the tonic phase. The respiratory status may be further compromised by aspiration. Oxygen and suction should be at the bedside. The patient should be turned to the side to protect the airway after the seizure and be allowed to sleep.

4. Administration of medication on a regular basis and the evaluation of its effectiveness in

controlling seizures as well as the psychological effects on the patient are important actions and assessments. Teaching the patient the beneficial effects of following the prescribed medication regimen and identifying and overcoming patient objections may result in better patient adherence in the future.

5. Promoting physical and mental health may sharply curtail the number of seizures. Regular routines for eating, sleeping, and physical activity should be established. Alcohol, stress, and fatigue tend to precipitate seizure activity. Modifying these factors will alter the seizure pattern.

Treatment of Epilepsy

If seizures are the result of tumor, infection, or metabolic dysfunction, correcting the underlying cause is the goal of therapy. In a majority of cases, an underlying cause may not be identifiable or be amenable to curative therapy. These cases are treated with antiepilepsy drugs. It is preferable to use a single drug to achieve control of seizure activity. The most common drugs include phenytoin sodium (Dilantin), phenobarbital, primidone (Mysoline), ethosuximide (Zarontin), clonazepam (Klonopin), carbamazepine (Tegretol), and valproic acid (Depakene). Recently introduced drugs are gabapentin (Neuritin) and lamotrigine (Lamictal). For the therapeutic serum level of these drugs, their affinity for specific types of seizures, and their side effects, the reader is referred to any standard pharmacology text.

If drug therapy is ineffective and seizures are intractable and deny the patient a normal life style, surgery may be performed. After identifying the specific epileptic focus and the patient's dominant hemisphere, a temporal lobectomy, extratemporal resection, or hemispherectomy may be done. Seizures may continue for a period after the surgery, and so the patient's medication is continued for approximately 1 year. Palliative surgery to restrict seizure spread includes partial or complete callosotomy. The patient must continue on antiepiletic medication following palliative surgery.

STATUS EPILEPTICUS

The state of status epilepticus is present when seizures follow each other so closely that a state of consciousness is not recovered between seizures. Status epilepticus may be partial or generalized in origin. EEG is necessary to determine the type or, in the patient in coma, the presence of seizures.

Etiology

Inadequate dosage of antiepileptic medication in a known epileptic is a common precipitating factor. Other factors include sudden withdrawal of antiepileptic drugs and other sedative drugs, hyponatremia, fever, intercurrent infection (commonly in the CNS), cerebral vascular disease, and cerebral hypoxia, anoxia, and edema. Progressive neurological diseases such as brain tumors and subdural hematoma may cause the status epilepticus. A common triad of causes consists of alcohol abuse, drug abuse, and sleep deprivation. Head trauma or pregnancy (pre-eclamptic state) may precipitate status epilepticus. Metabolic causes include hypoglycemia, hyponatremia, hypocalcemia, uremia, and electrolyte imbalances.

Incidence and Prognosis

Approximately 6% of known epileptics will develop status epilepticus. Almost 50% of the cases of status epilepticus occur in known epileptics. Approximately 10% of patients in status epilepticus will die. Death is commonly due to respiratory and metabolic acidosis, hypoxemia, hypoglycemia, hyperthermia, electrolyte disturbances, and/or renal failure.

Pathophysiology

The pathophysiology is the same as that of epilepsy; however, in status epilepticus the seizures are almost continuous. The rapidly repeating tonic–clonic seizures lead to hypoxemia (patients are apneic during such seizures) and cerebral anoxia. The increased metabolic activity of the brain causes hypoglycemia and hyperthermia. Hypoxemia, hypoglycemia, and hyperthermia may themselves precipitate seizure activity, resulting in a vicious cycle.

Clinical Presentation

There are three variants in the clinical picture of status epilepticus.

1. Generalized tonic–clonic status epilepticus is a life-threatening emergency. These seizures are the most common and occur without a period of consciousness between seizures.

2. The second most common presentation is partial status epilepticus, termed epilepsia partialis continua. Focal motor seizures occur continuously or regularly. Consciousness is usually maintained unless generalization occurs. Complex partial status epilepticus presents as a prolonged confusional state followed by postictal confusion and sleepiness.

3. Absence status epilepticus patients may exhibit as many as 200–300 "absences" per day. This nonconvulsive state is difficult to differentiate from complex partial status epilepticus.

Electrical status occurs in every type of status and is not a distinct type. It is always associated with some clinical abnormality. EEG shows continuous epileptic activity.

Treatment

The goal of therapy is to restore physiological homeostasis and to stop the seizures by correcting the underlying cause. The first step in treatment is to ensure a patent airway and to maintain breathing and circulation. The second step is to draw blood for antiepileptic drug levels, toxicology screen, glucose, electrolytes, calcium, magnesium, creatinine, blood urea nitrogen, complete blood count with differential, liver profile, arterial blood gas levels, and creatine phosphokinase and to establish an intravenous line. (This is often achieved as a one-step process with Jelcos or Angiocaths.) Thiamine 100 mg intravenously is administered prior to 50% glucose 50 ml intravenously if alcoholism or hypoglycemia is suspected. The third step is to administer medications to stop seizure activity.

Benzodiazepines, diazepam (Valium) and lorazepam (Ativan) intravenously are often the drugs of choice in spite of their potential for suppressing respirations. Fast-acting antiepilepsy drugs very quickly enter and quickly leave the brain. But these very properties often make benzodiazepines a poor drug for long-term management of status.

Phenytoin is given intravenously. It must be injected slowly (50 mg/min) and cardiac monitoring is essential for early intervention in the event that a dysrhythmia develops. Bradycardia and hypotension are especially common in patients over 40. Phenytoin requires 15–20 min to peak in brain tissue and it remains in brain tissue over a long period.

If seizures persist after 30 min, there is a high probability that acute CNS disease is causing the seizures. Phenobarbital may be tried. A slow intravenous injection is recommended (50–100 mg/min). Respiratory depression and hypotension may develop. Phenobarbital and diazepam should not be administered concurrently. If benzodiazepines are used to stop seizures, phenytoin is given simultaneously to block recurrence of the seizures. A combination of benzodiazepines and barbiturate may cause respiratory depression and hypotension.

Lidocaine as a 20% solution in normal saline may be tried. In some medical centers general anesthesia (barbiturate coma) is administered to a depth of EEG silence when other drugs have failed. Pharmacological neuromuscular blockade will not stop brain electrical activity but will stop movement.

Nursing Interventions

Maintaining a patent airway and providing adequate oxygenation are extremely important. An intravenous line should be maintained. Cardiac drugs should be available as cardiac monitoring may reveal dysrhythmias. Hyperthermia is treated frequently with a hypothermia blanket. Fluid and electrolyte balance is monitored. Neurological status is monitored closely.

NEUROLOGY BIBLIOGRAPHY

Awad, I.A., Carter, L.P., Spetzler, R.F., et al. (1987). Clinical vasospasm after subarachnoid hemorrhage: Response to hypervolemic hemodilution and arterial hypertension. *Stroke, 18,* 2, 365–372.

Barker, E. (1994). *Neuroscience Nursing.* St. Louis: CV Mosby.

Clochesy, J.M., et al. (1993). *Critical Care Nursing.* Philadelphia: W.B. Saunders.

Crosby, L.J., & Parsons, L.C. (1992). Cerebrovascular response of closed head injured patients to a standardized endotracheal tube suctioning and manual hyperventilation procedure. *J Neurosci Nurs, 24,* 1, 40–49.

Dolomon, R., Fink, M.E., & Lennihan, L. (1988). Early aneurysm surgery and prophylactic hypervolemic hypertensive therapy for the treatment of aneurysmal subarachnoid hemorrhage. *Neurosurgery, 23,* 6, 699–703.

Frank, J.I. (1993). Management of intracranial hypertension, *Med Clin North Am, 77,* 1, 61–76.

Germon, K. (1994). Intracranial pressure monitoring in the 1990s. *Crit Care Nurs Quart, 17,* 1, 21–32.

Guyton, A.C., & Hall, J.E. (1991). *Textbook of Medical Physiology,* 8th ed. Philadelphia: W.B. Saunders.

Haley, E.C., Kassel, N.F., & Torner, J.C. (1993). A randomized controlled trial of high-dose intravenous nicardipine in aneurysmal subarachnoid hemorrhage. *J Neurosurg, 78,* 537–547.

Hickey, J. (1992). *The Clinical Practice of Neurological and Neurosurgical Nursing*, 3rd ed. Philadelphia: J.B. Lippincott.

Hodges, K., & Root, L. (1991). Surgical management of intractable seizure disorders. *J Neurosci Nurs, 23*, 2, 93–100.

Inagawa, T. (1993). Management outcome in the elderly patient following subarachnoid hemorrhage. *J Neurosurg, 78*, 554–561.

Juvela, S., Porras, M., & Heiskanen, O. (1993). Natural history of unruptured intracranial aneurysms: a long term follow-up study. *J Neurosurg, 79*, 174–182.

Kerr, M.E., Rudy, E.B., et al. (1993). Head-injured adults: recommendations for endotracheal suctioning. *J Neurosci Nurs, 25*, 2, 86–91.

Levy, M.L., Rabb, C.H., Zelman, V., & Giannotta, S.L. (1993). Cardiac performance enhancement from dobutamine in patients refractory to hypervolemic therapy for cerebral vasospasm. *J Neurosurg, 79*, 494–499.

Marks, M.P., Steinber, G.K., & Lane, B. (1993). Intraarterial papaverine for the treatment of vasospasm. *Am J Neuroradiol, July/August*, 822–826.

Murray, D.P. (1993). Impaired Mobility: Guillain-Barré Syndrome. *J Neurosci Nurs, 25*, 2, 100–105.

Origitano, R.C., Wascher, T.M., Reichman, H., & Anderson, D.E. (1990). Sustained increased cerebral blood flow with prophylactic hypertensive hypervolemic hemodilution ("triple-H" therapy) after subarachnoid hemorrhage. *Neurosurgery, 27*, 5, 729–740.

Parobeck, V. Burnham, S., & Laukhuf, G.A. (1992). An unusual nursing challenge: Guillain–Barré Syndrome following cranial surgery. *J Neurosci Nurs, 24*, 5, 251–255.

Richmond, T.S. (1993). Intracranial pressure monitoring. *AACN Clin Issues, 4*, 1, 148–160.

Rising, C.J. (1993). The relationship of selected nursing activities to ICP, *J Neurosci Nurs, 25*, 5, 302–308.

So, E.L. (1993). Update on epilepsy. *Med Clin North Am, 77*, 1, 203–214.

Neurology Practice Exam

1. Which meningeal layer lies closest to the brain?
   (A) pia mater
   (B) dura mater
   (C) arachnoid
   (D) subarachnoid

2. Which cerebral component is responsible for reabsorbing CSF (cerebrospinal fluid)?
   (A) lateral ventricle
   (B) dura mater
   (C) arachnoid villi
   (D) subarachnoid cisterns

3. Which meningeal layer lies closest to the skull?
   (A) pia mater
   (B) dura mater
   (C) arachnoid
   (D) subarachnoid

4. Which structure separates the left and right cerebral hemispheres?
   (A) dura mater
   (B) subarachnoid space
   (C) fissure of Rolando
   (D) falx cerebri

5. Crossing of impulses between the two hemispheres is made possible by which structure?
   (A) corpus callosum
   (B) lateral ventricle
   (C) postcentral gyrus
   (D) falx cerebri

6. An injury to the temporal lobe would cause disturbances in which sensory component?
   (A) sight
   (B) hearing
   (C) spatial orientation
   (D) taste

7. A patient in your unit has suffered frontal head injuries from a motor vehicle accident. Which type of impairment may result from injury to the frontal lobe?
   (A) loss of sensation
   (B) loss of vision
   (C) alterations in hearing
   (D) alterations in personality

8. Maintenance of an awake and alert status is dependent on the proper functioning of which two cerebral structures?
   (A) reticular activating system and both cerebral hemispheres
   (B) parietal and occiptal lobes
   (C) pons and basal ganglia
   (D) thalamus and hypothalamus

9. The thalamus is responsible for integrating all of the following body sensations except one. Which sense does the thalamus NOT integrate?
   (A) smell
   (B) sight
   (C) hearing
   (D) touch

10. Neurohumoral control of respiration is located in which structure(s)?
    (A) pons and medulla
    (B) diencephalon
    (C) reticular activating system
    (D) basal ganglia

11. The primary function of the cerebellum includes which of the following?
    (A) thought integration
    (B) maintenance of personality characteristics
    (C) sight
    (D) maintenance of equilibrium and muscle coordination

12. The lateral ventricles are connected to the third ventricle via which structure?

(Answers cont'd.)

(A) cerebral aqueduct of Sylvius
(B) choroid plexus
(C) foramen of Monro
(D) foramen of Magendie

13. Obstruction of the foramen of Monro would produce which condition?
(A) ipsilateral dilatation of the pupils
(B) hydrocephalus
(C) hemiparesis
(D) compression of the third cranial nerve

14. CSF (cerebrospinal fluid) is synthesized by which structure?
(A) corticospinal tract
(B) subarachnoid villi
(C) lateral ventricle
(D) choroid plexus

15. Which of the following corresponds most closely to the primary purpose of the CSF (cerebrospinal fluid)?
(A) transport of oxygen to the brain
(B) manufacture of neurotransmitters
(C) cushioning the brain and spinal column
(D) maintenance of cerebral perfusion pressures

16. Which area of the brain is responsible for voluntary motor function?
(A) parietal lobe
(B) frontal lobe
(C) occipital lobe
(D) temporal lobe

17. The parietal lobe is responsible for which function?
(A) temperature regulation
(B) sensory integration
(C) motor function
(D) vision

18. Which artery is responsible for anterior circulation to the brain?
(A) external carotid
(B) internal carotid
(C) basilar
(D) vertebral

19. Adrenergic fibers of the sympathetic nervous system release which of the following neurotransmitters?
(A) serotonin and dopamine
(B) dopamine and acetycholine
(C) epinephrine and norepinephrine
(D) acetycholine and GABA (γ-aminobutyric acid)

20. Autoregulation of the cerebral circulatory system is most sensitive to changes in which of the following parameters?
(A) mean arterial pressure
(B) PaO_2
(C) pH
(D) glucose level

21. Which area of the brain is most sensitive to hypoxia?
(A) brain stem
(B) cerebral cortex
(C) cerebellum
(D) subarachnoid villi

22. Which statement most accurately describes the circle of Willis?
(A) It is located in the cerebrum.
(B) It helps provide adequate circulation through its anastomosis.
(C) It is responsible for sleep and wakefulness.
(D) It is part of the brain stem.

23. Hypothalamic disorders would be manifested by disturbances in which function?
(A) water balance and temperature control
(B) sensory processing
(C) vision
(D) sensory organization

24. The gray matter of the spinal cord represents which type of tissue?
(A) dendrite
(B) axon
(C) unmyelinated tissue
(D) myelinated tissue

25. How are the descending tracts within the spinal cord best described?
(A) columns
(B) funiculi
(C) sensory
(D) motor

Questions 26 and 27 refer to the following scenario.

A patient is admitted to the intensive care unit after sustaining a knife wound to the back. Assessment findings include loss of pain and temperature on the right side and loss of motor function on the left. Vital signs are stable and he is alert and oriented. No other injuries are noted.

26. Based on the preceding information, which type of neurological syndrome is likely to be developing?
(A) central cord
(B) Brown–Séquard

(C) anterior cord

(D) Horner

27. Which type of treatment would be best advised for this syndrome?
(A) insertion of spinal rods
(B) spinal stabilization
(C) insertion of cervical halo rings
(D) administration of endogenous neurotransmitters

28. Which of the following is a necessary immediate assessment for a C-3–4 injury?
(A) heart rate
(B) motor ability
(C) temperature
(D) ventilation

29. Which vital sign changes (due to loss of sympathetic nervous stimulation) would occur after a spinal cord lesion above T-5?
(A) bradycardia and hypotension
(B) hyperthermia and tachycardia
(C) tachycardia and hypotension
(D) hypertension and bradycardia

30. Which symptoms are present in cases of autonomic hyperreflexia?
(A) bradycardia and hypertension
(B) hyperthermia and tachycardia
(C) tachycardia and hypotension
(D) hypertension and hyperthermia

31. The presence of an ICP of 50 with A waves (Babinski) indicates which situation?
(A) a lower motor neuron lesion
(B) cerebral ischemia
(C) peripheral nerve damage
(D) an intact spinal arc

32. All of the following are symptoms of a basilar skull fracture but one. Which symptom is NOT indicative of a basilar skull fracture?
(A) rhinorrhea and otorrhea
(B) Battle's sign, raccoon eyes
(C) tinnitus, nystagmus, and hearing difficulty
(D) loss of consciousness and dilated pupils

33. Which of the following corresponds most closely to the range of adequate cerebral perfusion pressures?
(A) >30 mm Hg
(B) <60 mm Hg
(C) >60 mm Hg
(D) any value less than the intracranial pressure

34. Which of the following can cause an epidural hematoma?

(A) skull fracture lacerating the middle meningeal artery
(B) rupture of an intracranial aneurysm
(C) infectious meningitis
(D) cerebral edema

35. Where are intracranial aneurysms most commonly found?
(A) external carotid arteries
(B) circle of Willis
(C) internal carotid arteries
(D) vertebral arteries

36. A 28-year-old male is admitted to the intensive care unit with a diagnosis of closed head injury. The nurse should be aware of which potential complications?
(A) hypotension
(B) respiratory alkalosis
(C) tremors
(D) cerebral edema

37. Hyperventilation, as a treatment modality for cerebral edema, should be maintained at which range for maximum effect?
(A) 30–35 mm Hg
(B) 35–40 mm Hg
(C) 40–45 mm Hg
(D) 50–55 mm Hg

38. Which of the following is a common factor associated with aneurysms of intracerebral hemorrhage?
(A) cerebral edema
(B) hypertension
(C) prolonged hypotensive episodes
(D) Valsalva maneuvers

39. Cerebral perfusion pressure is calculated according to which of the following formulas?
(A) MAP (mean arterial pressure) – ICP (intracranial pressure)
(B) systolic blood pressure – ICP
(C) ICP + cerebral blood flow
(D) MAP + ICP

Questions 40 and 41 refer to the following scenario.

A 45-year-old male is admitted to your unit with a diagnosis of intracranial hypertension due to subarachnoid hemorrhage. The current vital signs include a blood pressure of 180/90, ICP (intracranial pressure) 15, pulse 140, respiratory rate 20.

40. Based on the preceding information, what is the cerebral perfusion pressure?

(Answers cont'd.)

(A) 90

(B) 105

(C) 120

(D) It cannot be calculated.

41. Which of the following are measures that would improve the cerebral perfusion pressure?
    (A) decrease the ICP (intracranial pressure)
    (B) decrease the MAP (mean arterial pressure)
    (C) decrease the heart rate
    (D) all of the above

42. Which of the following corresponds most closely to the range of minimum cerebral perfusion pressures?
    (A) 30–40 mm Hg
    (B) 40–50 mm Hg
    (C) 50–60 mm Hg
    (D) >60 mm Hg

43. What is an acceptable normal ICP (intracranial pressure)?
    (A) –5 to +5 mm Hg
    (B) <10 mm Hg
    (C) 10–20 mm Hg
    (D) >20 mm Hg

44. Nursing interventions for the patient with an ICP (intracranial pressure) monitoring device include which of the following?
    (A) routine flushing of the system with heparinized saline
    (B) maintaining the transducer at the level of the heart
    (C) administration of prophylactic antibiotics
    (D) monitoring the patient for signs and symptoms of infection

45. The hypothalamus secretes which hormone to regulate water balance?
    (A) aldosterone
    (B) renin
    (C) ADH (antidiuretic hormone)
    (D) oxytocin

46. Approximately two-thirds of the brain's blood supply is transported through which artery?
    (A) internal carotid
    (B) anterior communicating
    (C) vertebral
    (D) middle meningeal

47. What percent of total body oxygen consumption is accounted for by the brain?
    (A) 2–5%
    (B) 5–10%

(C) 10–15%

(D) 20%

48. How much of a reserve of oxygen exists in the brain?
    (A) 100 ml
    (B) 225 ml
    (C) 450 ml
    (D) No reserve exists.

49. Of the following factors, which does NOT play a role in maintaining consciousness?
    (A) cerebral perfusion pressure
    (B) oxygen transport level
    (C) adequate blood glucose level
    (D) normal serum potassium level

50. The reticular activating system is responsible for which of the following functions?
    (A) motor control of skeletal muscle
    (B) relay of sensory impulses to the parietal lobe
    (C) sleep and wakefulness
    (D) secretion of all neurotransmitters

Questions 51 and 52 refer to the following scenario.

A 56-year-old factory worker is admitted to your unit following a 20-foot fall from a scaffold. He is unresponsive on admission to the emergency room and is taken to the operating room for a craniotomy. Upon return to the intensive care unit, he has had an evacuation of an epidural hematoma from a depressed skull fracture. He has an ICP (intracranial pressure) monitor (subarachnoid screw) in place. During the first postoperative day, you note on the ICP waveform pressures of approximately 12 mm Hg. C waves are evident. His level of consciousness is variable, with a Glasgow Coma Score of 12 upon stimulation.

51. Based on the preceding information, which condition is likely to be developing?
    (A) increased ICP (intracranial pressure)
    (B) possible rebleeding, as indicated by the lack of an A wave presence
    (C) an obstruction of the catheter due to the presence of C waves
    (D) A normal postoperative situation exists.

52. Which treatment should be undertaken for this condition?
    (A) apply a closed CSF (cerebrospinal fluid) drainage system
    (B) increase the frequency of ICP (intracranial pressure) monitoring
    (C) flush the ICP catheter with normal saline
    (D) No treatment is necessary.

53. Neurogenic hyperventilation is associated with damage to which structure?
    (A) cerebral cortex
    (B) cerebellum
    (C) thalamus
    (D) brain stem

54. Initial assessment of the neurologically impaired patient should include measurement of which of the following?
    (A) level of consciousness
    (B) pupillary eye movement
    (C) deep tendon reflexes
    (D) brain stem reflexes

55. A fixed and dilated pupil indicates compression of which cranial nerve?
    (A) I
    (B) II
    (C) III
    (D) IV

Questions 56 through 58 refer to the following scenario.

A 79-year-old female is in the intensive care unit following a head injury from a fall down a series of steps. Currently she is unresponsive, opens her eyes with painful stimuli, withdraws to pain in a decerebrate manner, and makes groaning noises when she is given a painful stimulus. During your examination at the start of your shift, you notice that the left pupil is larger than the right, whereas previous examinations noted pupillary equality.

56. Based on the preceding information, what is the Glasgow Coma Score?
    (A) 3
    (B) 6
    (C) 9
    (D) 15

57. What does the change in pupillary size potentially indicate?
    (A) decrease in cerebral perfusion pressure
    (B) loss of upper motor neuron function
    (C) loss of cerebellar function
    (D) increased ICP (intracranial pressure)

58. Treatment for this condition could include which of the following measures?
    (A) cervical support
    (B) spinal tap to relieve increased ICP (intracranial pressure)
    (C) mechanical ventilation to augment MAP (mean arterial pressure)
    (D) osmotic diuretics and hyperventilation (Paco$_2$ goal of 30 mm Hg)

59. Which waveform is considered pathologic in monitoring ICP (intracranial pressure)?
    (A) A wave
    (B) B wave
    (C) C wave
    (D) D wave

60. Which structure(s) is/are a part of the supratentorial space?
    (A) cerebellum
    (B) pons
    (C) cerebral hemispheres
    (D) cranial nerves

61. Which of the following is a common complication of a ruptured intracranial aneurysm?
    (A) hypotension due to hypovolemia
    (B) cardiac dysrhythmias
    (C) acid-base disturbances
    (D) vasospasm of cerebral arteries

62. The risk of rebleeding after the initial rupture of an intracranial aneurysm is greatest during which time period?
    (A) within the first 3 days after initial bleeding
    (B) between the 7th and 11th days after initial bleeding
    (C) after surgical clipping of the aneurysm
    (D) within the first 24 hr after initial bleeding

63. Signs and symptoms of meningeal irritation include all of the following EXCEPT:
    (A) nuchal rigidity and headache
    (B) Kernig's and Brudzinski's signs
    (C) aphasia and paresis
    (D) photophobia

64. Which of the following is an early sign of herniation syndrome?
    (A) dilated pupils
    (B) respiratory depression
    (C) papilledema
    (D) depressed level of consciousness

65. Which of the following reflexes indicate third cranial nerve involvement?
    (A) pupillary light reflexes
    (B) oculocephalic responses
    (C) oculovestibular responses
    (D) spinal reflexes

66. Decerebrate posturing is characterized by which of the following?
    (A) abnormal extension response
    (B) abnormal flexion response
    (C) hyperflexion of the lower extremities
    (D) absent motor response

67. Diagnostic procedures usually performed when intracranial hypertension is suspected may include all of the following but one. Which of the following procedures is NOT performed?
    (A) CT (computed tomographic) scan
    (B) lumbar puncture
    (C) ventriculostomy
    (D) cranial nerve examination

68. Nursing interventions for the patient having seizures include all of the following EXCEPT:
    (A) protecting the patient from injury
    (B) observing and recording seizure patterns
    (C) administering anticonvulsive drugs such as dilantin
    (D) restraining the patient

69. The nurse should be aware of the characteristics of psychomotor seizures. Which of the following statements regarding psychomotor seizures is true?
    (A) They are psychological in origin.
    (B) The patient usually becomes unconscious.
    (C) They involve repetitive behavioral patterns.
    (D) They involve acts of random violence.

70. The most important treatment for the patient in status epilepticus is:
    (A) maintenance of ventilation or respiratory support
    (B) administration of diazepam
    (C) administration of glucose
    (D) administration of phenytoin

71. Pathophysiological consequences of status epilepticus include all of the following except one. Which of the following consequences is NOT associated with status epilepticus?
    (A) hypoxemia
    (B) hypoglycemia
    (C) hyperthermia
    (D) hypothermia

Questions 72 and 73 refer to the following scenario.

A 71-year-old female is admitted to your unit with a possible CVA (cerebrovascular accident). She is currently responsive to painful stimuli and has a Glasgow Coma Score of 8. Her blood pressure is 180/110, pulse 64, respiratory rate 12. Her pupils are equal and reactive. During your shift, you note that her level of consciousness suddenly decreases. Upon examining her eyes, you note that the left pupil is large and unreactive to light. Vital signs are blood pressure 192/114, pulse 56, respiratory rate 10. Blood glucose level is 70.

72. Based on the preceding information, what has most likely occurred?
    (A) Decreasing ICP (intracranial pressure) has caused negative-pressure dysfunction of the second (optic) cranial nerve.
    (B) Hypoglycemia has occured.
    (C) Increasing MAP (mean arterial pressure) has decreased cerebral perfusion.
    (D) Increasing ICP has compressed the third (oculomotor) cranial nerve.

73. What is the prognostic implication of herniation through the foramen magnum?
    (A) With aggressive treatment, neurological function can be recovered.
    (B) Neurological function is unlikely to be recovered.
    (C) Visual defects are likely to be permanent but other neurological functions will recover.
    (D) No implications regarding neurological recovery can be drawn.

74. Myasthenia gravis is characterized by which of the following?
    (A) ascending paralysis
    (B) neuromuscular weakness with exercise and improvement with rest
    (C) uncoordinated motor control
    (D) peripheral sensory deficits

75. Which of the following is the major objective of therapy in myasthenia gravis?
    (A) stimulate synaptic terminals to produce ACTH (adrenocorticotropic hormone)
    (B) supportive care for the patient; the disease is self-limiting
    (C) administration of anticholinesterase medications
    (D) administration of ACTH

Questions 76 and 77 refer to the following scenario.

A 56-year-old male is admitted to your unit with a decreasing level of consciousness. His primary diagnosis is adenocarcinoma of the lung with possible metastatic spread to the brain. The family wants "everything done," which is why he has been admitted to the unit. His pupils are small but reactive. Respiration is cyclic, increasing in depth and rate and then characterized by short periods of apnea. Later in your shift, the level of consciousness decreases further, the pupils become dilated (3–4 mm) and unresponsive to light, and respiration increases in frequency and depth.

76. Based on the preceding information, which condition is likely to be developing?
    (A) central herniation syndrome
    (B) uncal herniation syndrome
    (C) unilateral hemispheric compression
    (D) pontine angle compression

77. Which of the following treatments would NOT be indicated in this situation?
    (A) hyperventilation via mechanical ventilation
    (B) osmotic diuretics
    (C) corticosteroids
    (D) spinal tap

78. Nursing interventions for myasthenia gravis include all of the following EXCEPT:
    (A) monitoring ventilation status due to muscle weakness
    (B) administration of aminoglycosides
    (C) administration of anticholinesterase medications
    (D) timing activities to avoid fatigue

79. Cholinergic crisis in myasthenia gravis is due to which of the following events?
    (A) insufficient dose of medication
    (B) overdose of medication
    (C) fatigue, stress, or infection
    (D) worsening of the disease process

80. Guillain–Barré syndrome affects which neurological component?
    (A) peripheral nervous system
    (B) central nervous system
    (C) autonomic nervous system
    (D) Schwann cells

Questions 81 and 82 refer to the following scenario.

A patient of yours has been in a motor vehicle accident and has received cervical and spinal stabilization. He is alert and oriented with no evidence of head injury. He develops lower extremity paralysis on the same side as the wound and loses pain and temperature sensation on the side opposite the injury.

81. Based on the preceding information, this type of spinal injury response would be referred to as:
    (A) total transection
    (B) anterior cord syndrome
    (C) central cord syndrome
    (D) Brown–Séquard syndrome

82. Treatment for this condition would most likely include:
    (A) spinal tap for decompression

    (B) laminectomy
    (C) spinal traction
    (D) spinal fusion

83. A patient is admitted to the intensive care unit with signs and symptoms of ascending paralysis and respiratory failure. The critical care nurse would investigate for a past history of:
    (A) trauma to the spinal cord
    (B) trauma to the head
    (C) postviral, respiratory, or gastrointestinal infection
    (D) aspiration

84. Which of the following organisms is the most common cause of bacterial meningitis in adults?
    (A) *Meningococcus*
    (B) *Haemophilus influenzae*
    (C) *Staphylococcus*
    (D) *Pneumonococcus*

85. Clinical signs and symptoms of meningitis include all of the following EXCEPT:
    (A) positive Kernig's and Brudzinki's signs
    (B) headache and photophobia
    (C) hemiparesis and atrophy of muscles
    (D) photophobia and seizures

86. Which of the following are treatments for myasthenia gravis?
    (A) pyridostigmine (Mestinon)
    (B) neostigmine (Prostigmin)
    (C) prednisone
    (D) all of the above

87. Which of the following surgical treatments may be useful in myasthenia gravis?
    (A) splenectomy
    (B) thymectomy
    (C) nerve transplants
    (D) pineal transplants

88. What is the reason that even a nonmalignant brain tumor may have dangerous consequences?
    (A) Nonmalignant brain tumors can convert into malignant tumors.
    (B) Brain tumors can secrete exogenous catecholamines.
    (C) The mass in the brain can distort the ability to sense normal balance.
    (D) Any mass will increase the ICP (intracranial pressure) because of the cranial structure's lack of distensibility.

89. Which of the following is NOT considered a neurotransmitter?
    (A) dopamine

(Answers cont'd.)

(B) dobutamine
(C) acetylcholine
(D) norepinephrine

90. Which of the following is the precursor to both epinephrine and norepinephrine?
    (A) dopamine
    (B) dobutamine
    (C) acetylcholine
    (D) norepinephrine

91. Which substrate does the brain depend most heavily on for nutritional needs?
    (A) fats
    (B) proteins
    (C) carbohydrates
    (D) neurotransmitters

92. Anterior gray columns in the spinal cord contain cell bodies of which fiber type?
    (A) afferent (sensory)
    (B) efferent (motor)
    (C) parasympathetic
    (D) sympathetic synaptic

93. Fracture of which vertebra is termed the "hangman's fracture" because of the loss of spinal stabilization of the head?
    (A) C-2
    (B) C-3
    (C) C-7
    (D) T-1

94. Lesions of the cerebellum cause which type of response?
    (A) spastic muscle activity
    (B) changes in level of consciousness
    (C) changes in behavior
    (D) equilibrium disturbances

95. Lesions of the medulla cause which type of response?
    (A) disturbances in heart and respiratory rate or pattern
    (B) changes in level of consciousness
    (C) changes in behavior
    (D) flaccid paralysis

Questions 96 and 97 refer to the following scenario.

A 19-year-old male is admitted to your unit following a motor vehicle accident. He currently is responsive but has no sensation below the upper chest area. Lateral cervical films reveal a possible C-6 fracture. A CT scan reveals transection of the cord at C-6.

96. Based on the preceding information, what is the likelihood of the patient's recovering the ability to walk?

(A) good likelihood with rehabilitation
(B) good likelihood with surgery
(C) possible only if stabilization of the injury allows new spinal growth
(D) unlikely

97. Treatment of this condition would most likely include which of the following measures?
    (A) supportive care since no treatment is effective
    (B) surgical decompression
    (C) bed rest on a spinal board
    (D) cervical traction

98. Which condition characterizes upper and lower extremity weakness with more pronounced upper extremity weakness?
    (A) Guillain–Barré syndrome
    (B) Brown–Séquard syndrome
    (C) central cord syndrome
    (D) anterior cord syndrome

Questions 99 through 100 refer to the following scenario.

A 39-year-old construction worker is admitted to your unit after being crushed between two metal sheets. No head injury occurred and he is alert and oriented. He is able to sense pain and touch although the sensations are faint. He has no ability to move his legs or abdomen.

99. Based on the preceding information, which condition is likely to be present?
    (A) C-6 transection
    (B) Brown–Séquard syndrome
    (C) central cord syndrome
    (D) anterior cord syndrome

100. Which treatment would most likely be indicated for this condition?
    (A) supportive care since no treatment is effective
    (B) surgical decompression
    (C) bed rest on a spinal board
    (D) cervical traction

101. A patient sustains a spinal cord injury at C-6. He is conscious and alert. Barring complications, he should be able to perform all of the following actions EXCEPT one. Which action will he have difficulty performing?
    (A) diaphagmatic breathing
    (B) picking up objects with his fingers
    (C) reaching forward
    (D) sitting upright with support

102. A patient with cerebrospinal rhinorrhea would benefit most from which of the following?

(A) assistance with nasal packing to tamponade the leak

(B) insertion of a nasogastric tube to aspirate swallowed CSF (cerebrospinal fluid)

(C) testing the CSF with litmus paper to determine the origin of the fluid

(D) administration of prophylactic antibiotics

103. Which of the following is an example of a disturbance of the reticular activating system?
(A) poliomyelitis
(B) spinal cord injury below the level of L-1
(C) amyotrophic lateral sclerosis
(D) cerebrovascular accident of the midbrain

104. Which reflex is indicative of an intact VII (cranial) nerve?
(A) spinal reflex
(B) corneal reflex
(C) anal wink
(D) Hering–Breuer reflex

105. A normal consensual light reflex indicates proper functioning of which two cranial nerves?
(A) abducens and acoustic
(B) ophthalmic and hypoglossal
(C) optic and oculomotor
(D) trochlear and vagal

106. What is the highest score on the Glasgow Coma Scale?
(A) 3
(B) 8
(C) 15
(D) 18

107. Which of the following would NOT cause a decrease in level of consciousness?
(A) right-sided cerebral infarct without cerebral edema
(B) glucose level less than 30
(C) cerebral perfusion pressure of 40
(D) oxygen transport of 400 ml/min

108. Given the following information, what is the cerebral perfusion pressure in this patient?

blood pressure	90/60
ICP	15
CVP	12
$PaCO_2$	35
PaO_2	88
pH	7.34

(A) 15
(B) 35

(C) 55
(D) 75

109. Which of the following would be least likely to produce a decreased level of consciousness?
(A) acute blunt head trauma
(B) acute CVA (cerebrovascular accident)
(C) old CVA
(D) diminished cerebral perfusion pressure

Questions 110 and 111 refer to the following scenario.

A 42-year-old female is in the unit following an assault. She suffered head lacerations although her CT scan revealed no major cerebral injuries. She also received several stab wounds to the chest. The chest wounds have been treated but she remains hypoxemic. She has the following parameters:

blood pressure	100/700
pulse	90
cardiac output	5 L/min
PCWP	12 mm Hg
CVP	5 mm Hg
PaO_2	50
FIO_2	0.70

The physician decides to add PEEP (positive end expiratory pressure) to this therapy in order to address the hypoxemia. Following are the new parameters:

blood pressure	90/60
pulse	110
cardiac output	4 L/min
PCWP	13
CVP	15
PaO_2	98
FIO_2	0.70
PEEP	10

110. Based on the preceding information, what is your assessment of the change in oxygenation to the brain based on the addition of the PEEP?
(A) Oxygenation is worse based on the loss of cerebral perfusion pressure.
(B) Oxygenation is better based on improved PaO_2 and little change in cerebral perfusion.
(C) Oxygenation is unaffected since the ICP (intracranial pressure) is unchanged.
(D) Oxygenation cannot be approximated from these parameters.

111. What should be done from a treatment point of view based on the preceding information?
(A) No adjustment in treatment is necessary.
(B) Increase the PEEP to 12 cm as long as the ICP (intracranial pressure) is unchanged.

(Answers cont'd.)

(C) Reduce the PEEP based on cerebral perfusion pressure.

(D) Administer a blood transfusion to improve oxygen transport.

112. Assume that a patient has a severe head injury and does not respond to verbal stimuli. Which of the following supports a potential injury to the brainstem?

(A) hearing deficits

(B) motor responses impairment

(C) hemiparesis

(D) cranial nerve deficits and changes in respiratory rate and rhythm

113. Impending central herniation is indicated by which of the following?

(A) decreased level of consciousness

(B) positive doll's eyes

(C) unilateral pupil dilation

(D) bilateral pupil dilation

114. Which of the following are signs of increasing ICP (intracranial pressure)?

(A) bradycardia and hypertension

(B) bradycardia and hypotension

(C) tachycardia and hypertension

(D) tachycardia and hypotension

115. Which of the following best describes the abnormal doll's eyes response?

(A) movement of the eyes in opposition to the movement of the head

(B) disconjugate eye movements

(C) movement of the eyes in the same direction as movement of the head

(D) eyes remaining stationary, midline, mid-position

Questions 116 and 117 refer to the following scenario.

A patient is admitted after a motor vehicle accident with head and chest trauma. He requires a craniotomy with the insertion of an ICP (intracranial pressure) monitor. On the second postoperative day, he is responsive to stimuli and follows commands. Later in your shift, he becomes responsive only to painful stimuli. The following information is available:

blood pressure	90/58
pulse	107
ICP	24
CVP	13
serum glucose	92
PaO_2	68
$PaCO_2$	36

116. Based on the preceding information, what is the likely reason for the loss of responsiveness?

(A) decreased substrate (i.e., glucose) availability

(B) decreased PaO_2 levels

(C) reduced ICP (intracranial pressure)

(D) decreased cerebral perfusion pressure

117. Which structure primarily regulates the autonomic nervous system?

(A) cerebellum

(B) thalamus

(C) hypothalamus

(D) frontal lobe of the cerebral cortex

118. Which function is primarily regulated by the cerebellum?

(A) speech

(B) vision

(C) coordination

(D) respiration

119. Meningeal irritation is indicated by which of the following signs?

(A) nuchal rigidity

(B) Homans sign

(C) positive extensor plantar (Babinski) reflex

(D) flaccid paralysis

Questions 120 and 121 refer to the following scenario.

A 72-year-old female is admitted to the unit following a fall at home. Her daughter explains that her mother attempted to stand after dinner and immediately fell. Currently she is awake but unable to move her left side. She is able to talk and is alert and oriented. Admission vital signs are as follows:

blood pressure	176/110
pulse	62
respiratory rate	16
temperature	36.8°C

Pupils are equal and reactive; eye movements are normal. The patient states that she has been healthy and has never needed to "see a doctor."

120. Based on the preceding information, which condition is likely to be developing?

(A) left-sided CVA (cerebrovascular accident)

(B) internal carotid vasospasm

(C) right-sided CVA

(D) external carotid obstruction

121. Which neurologic test would be most helpful in establishing the diagnosis in this patient?

(A) CT scan

(B) cold water caloric test

(C) oculocephalic testing

(D) EEG (electroencephalogram)

122. Which neurotransmitter is most important for synaptic transmission?

(A) serotonin

(B) acetylcholine

(C) dobutamine

(D) glucose

123. Contracoup head injuries manifest from which of the following mechanisms?

(A) injury to the side opposite the trauma

(B) injury to the side of the trauma

(C) cranial vault fracture due to high torque forces

(D) epidural tears from superficial scalp pressures

Questions 124 and 125 refer to the following scenario.

A 24-year-old female is admitted to your unit following a fall from a horse. After the fall, the horse kicked her in the temporal region of the head. She is admitted to the unit directly from the emergency room. She is unresponsive except to deep, painful stimuli. Head CT scans reveal a temporal skull fracture. The following data are available:

blood pressure	84/52
pulse	112
respiratory rate	10

124. Based on the preceding information, which condition is likely to be developing?

(A) epidural hematoma

(B) subdural hematoma

(C) obstructive hydrocephalus

(D) contracoup head injury

125. Which treatment would be indicated based on the preceding data?

(A) increasing the ventilator rate

(B) placement of an ICP (intracranial pressure) monitor

(C) immediate craniotomy

(D) mannitol infusion

126. Which of the following is an indication of a basilar skull fracture?

(A) raccoon eyes

(B) decreasing pulse pressure

(C) spastic paralysis

(D) flaccid paralysis

127. Which of the following is the best description for Battle's sign?

(A) generalized petechial development

(B) bleeding from the paranasal sinus

(C) hyperreflexia

(D) ecchymosis over the mastoid projection

128. Which type of head injury typically produces rapid clinical deterioration?

(A) subdural hematoma

(B) depressed skull fracture without displacement

(C) epidural hematoma

(D) subarachnoid hematoma

129. Which test is the most diagnostic for identifying head injuries?

(A) cranial roentgenograms

(B) lumbar puncture

(C) CT scan

(D) PET (positron emission tomographic) scan

Questions 130 and 131 refer to the following scenario.

An 81-year-old male in your unit has a cerebral mass that has compressed the right optic tract. He is alert and oriented with no complaints except for visual disturbances. The physician has described the visual defect as left homonymous hemianopsia.

130. Which visual symptoms would be seen with this lesion?

(A) loss of vision in the right eye

(B) loss of vision in the left eye

(C) loss of peripheral vision on the left and central vision on the right

(D) loss of peripheral vision on the right and central vision on the left

131. What should the nurse do with regard to placing items that might be needed by the patient?

(A) Instruct the patient not to reach for any items without assistance.

(B) No precautions are needed.

(C) Keep objects toward the right.

(D) Keep objects toward the left.

132. Myasthenia gravis is thought to occur due to which mechanism?

(A) loss of myelinated tissue

(B) disturbances in the reticular activating system

(C) deficient production of phenylephrine

(D) disturbance of acetylcholine utilization

Questions 133 and 134 refer to the following scenario.

A 37-year-old female is admitted to your unit with possible aspiration pneumonia. She has complained of a gradual increase in difficulty swallowing, which she believes is what precipitated her respiratory difficulties. During the examination, you note that she has ptosis of both eyes and has weak eye closure strength. Muscle weakness is generalized. No sensory deficits exist. She states that she fatigues easily although she recovers some strength after rest.

133. Based on the preceding information, which condition could be developing?
    (A) multiple sclerosis
    (B) Guillain–Barré syndrome
    (C) temporal lobe tumor
    (D) myasthenia gravis

134. Which test would be performed to help identify the disease?
    (A) administration of edrophonium chloride (Tensilon)
    (B) a 6-min walk
    (C) administration of epinephrine
    (D) CT scan

135. Which of the following is NOT a treatment for myasthenia gravis?
    (A) thymectomy
    (B) Mestinon
    (C) plasmapheresis
    (D) Neo-Synephrine

136. A 69-year-old male has a cardiopulmonary arrest on the floor and is brought to your unit. Which of the following medications, if given previously, would interfere with an assessment of pupillary response?
    (A) atropine and procainamide
    (B) Bretylium
    (C) lidocaine
    (D) atropine and epinephrine

Questions 137 and 138 refer to the following scenario.

A 43-year-old male is admitted to your unit with complaints of severe headache, pain in the neck on flexion, and light sensitivity. He has no specific muscle weakness or sensory deficits. He has a positive Kernig's sign. Vital signs are as follows:

blood pressure	142/84
pulse	118
respiratory rate	30
temperature	40°C

137. Based on the preceding information, which condition is likely to be developing?

    (A) meningitis
    (B) intracerebral bleeding
    (C) myasthenia gravis
    (D) subarachnoid bleeding

138. Which treatment would most likely be instituted?
    (A) craniotomy
    (B) administration of anticholinesterase agents
    (C) insertion of a ventricular drain to reduce the increased ICP (intracranial pressure)
    (D) administration of antibiotics

Questions 139 and 140 refer to the following scenario.

A 36-year-old male is admitted to your unit with rapidly increasing symptoms of generalized weakness following an episode of "flu." He noticed that the weakness started in his arms and legs and has progressed to his upper legs, abdomen, and chest. He has difficulty taking a deep breath. Vital signs are normal and he has some complaints of shortness of breath.

139. Based on the preceding symptoms, which condition is likely to be developing?
    (A) Guillain–Barré syndrome
    (B) myasthenia gravis
    (C) multiple sclerosis
    (D) amyotrophic lateral sclerosis

140. Which treatment is likely to be administered for this condition?
    (A) administration of anticholinesterase agents
    (B) supportive treatments, particularly of the respiratory system
    (C) administration of antibiotics
    (D) administration of sympathetic stimulation agents, such as norepinephrine

141. Which of the following best describes Kernig's sign?
    (A) muscle spasms in the arm upon occlusion with a blood pressure cuff
    (B) twitching of the face upon tapping the cheek
    (C) inability to flex the neck
    (D) inability to extend the leg when the thigh is flexed to the abdomen

142. Brudzinski's sign is best described by which of the following definitions?

(A) adduction and flexion of the legs with neck flexion

(B) pain in the neck upon raising the arms above shoulder level

(C) temporary flaccid paralysis after neck compression

(D) development of superficial muscle tremors after repetitive reflex testing

143. If a patient develops a grand mal (tonic–clonic) seizure, which initial nursing action should take place?

(A) forcing an airway into the mouth

(B) protecting the patient from injury

(C) starting oxygen therapy

(D) placing a padded tongue blade into the mouth

PART V

Neurology Practice Exam

1. _____
2. _____
3. _____
4. _____
5. _____
6. _____
7. _____
8. _____
9. _____
10. _____
11. _____
12. _____
13. _____
14. _____
15. _____
16. _____
17. _____
18. _____
19. _____
20. _____
21. _____
22. _____
23. _____
24. _____
25. _____
26. _____
27. _____

28. _____
29. _____
30. _____
31. _____
32. _____
33. _____
34. _____
35. _____
36. _____
37. _____
38. _____
39. _____
40. _____
41. _____
42. _____
43. _____
44. _____
45. _____
46. _____
47. _____
48. _____
49. _____
50. _____
51. _____
52. _____
53. _____
54. _____

55. _____
56. _____
57. _____
58. _____
59. _____
60. _____
61. _____
62. _____
63. _____
64. _____
65. _____
66. _____
67. _____
68. _____
69. _____
70. _____
71. _____
72. _____
73. _____
74. _____
75. _____
76. _____
77. _____
78. _____
79. _____
80. _____
81. _____

82. _____
83. _____
84. _____
85. _____
86. _____
87. _____
88. _____
89. _____
90. _____
91. _____
92. _____
93. _____
94. _____
95. _____
96. _____
97. _____
98. _____
99. _____
100. _____
101. _____
102. _____
103. _____
104. _____
105. _____
106. _____
107. _____
108. _____

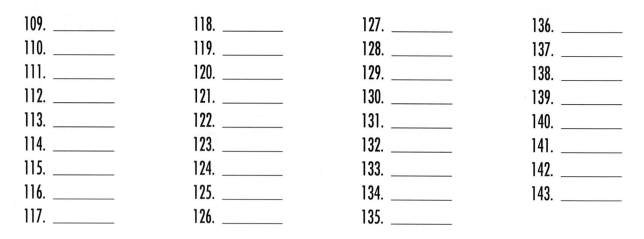

109. _____
110. _____
111. _____
112. _____
113. _____
114. _____
115. _____
116. _____
117. _____

118. _____
119. _____
120. _____
121. _____
122. _____
123. _____
124. _____
125. _____
126. _____

127. _____
128. _____
129. _____
130. _____
131. _____
132. _____
133. _____
134. _____
135. _____

136. _____
137. _____
138. _____
139. _____
140. _____
141. _____
142. _____
143. _____

1. A p 352	28. D p 398	55. C p 364	82. C p 398
2. C p 357	29. A p 399	56. B p 378	83. C p 413
3. B p 352	30. A p 401	57. D p 375	84. B p 412
4. D p 353	31. B p 374	58. D p 375	85. C p 412
5. A p 353	32. D p 380	59. A p 374	86. D p 416
6. B p 355	33. C p 370	60. C p 404	87. B p 412
7. D p 355	34. A p 381	61. D p 388	88. D p 371, 404
8. A p 356	35. B p 387	62. B p 388	89. B p 366–368
9. A p 355	36. D p 379	63. C p 387	90. A p 367
10. A p 356	37. A p 383	64. D p 405	91. C p 369
11. D p 357	38. B p 387	65. A p 404	92. B p 396
12. C p 357	39. A p 370	66. A p 407	93. A p 393
13. B p 357	40. B p 370	67. B p 408	94. D p 357
14. D p 357	41. A p 370	68. D p 421	95. A p 356
15. C p 357	42. D p 372	69. C p 420	96. D p 399
16. B p 354	43. B p 371	70. A p 423	97. D p 398
17. B p 354	44. D p 375	71. D p 422	98. C p 397
18. B p 358	45. C p 245	72. D p 404, 405	99. D p 397
19. C p 367	46. A p 358	73. B p 408	100. B p 397
20. A p 370	47. D p 369	74. B p 415	101. B p 399
21. B p 369	48. D p 369	75. C p 416	102. D p 377–380
22. B p 358	49. D p 403	76. A p 404, 405	103. D p 356
23. A p 355	50. C p 356	77. D p 375	104. B p 364, 378
24. C p 395	51. D p 371, 374	78. B p 417	105. C p 364, 405
25. D p 396	52. D p 371, 374	79. B p 417	106. C p 378
26. B p 397	53. D p 356	80. A p 413	107. A p 403
27. B p 398	54. A p 377	81. D p 397	108. C p 370

109. ___C___ p 403
110. ___A___ p 370, 372
111. ___C___ p 370, 372
112. ___D___ p 380
113. ___A___ p 404
114. ___A___ p 375
115. ___C___ p 406
116. ___D___ p 370, 403
117. ___C___ p 355

118. ___C___ p 355
119. ___A___ p 412
120. ___C___ p 390
121. ___A___ p 390
122. ___B___ p 366
123. ___A___ p 379
124. ___A___ p 379, 381
125. ___C___ p 380
126. ___A___ p 380

127. ___D___ p 380
128. ___C___ p 381
129. ___C___ p 384
130. ___C___ p 385
131. ___C___ p 385
132. ___D___ p 415
133. ___D___ p 415, 416
134. ___A___ p 416
135. ___D___ p 416

136. ___D___ p 361, 362
137. ___A___ p 412
138. ___D___ p 412
139. ___A___ p 413
140. ___B___ p 414
141. ___D___ p 387
142. ___A___ p 387
143. ___B___ p 421

VI

GASTROENTEROLOGY

Lynn Schallom

38

Anatomy and Physiology of the Gastrointestinal System

EDITORS' NOTE

This chapter provides a good review of the general anatomy and physiology of gastrointestinal function. Few if any questions from this chapter will be included on the CCRN exam. Use this chapter to strengthen your overall understanding of gastrointestinal anatomy and physiology.

The process of digestion and absorption of nutrients requires an intact and healthy gastrointestinal tract epithelial lining that is able to resist the effects of its own digestive secretions. It involves the movement of materials through the gastrointestinal tract at a rate that facilitates absorption, and it requires the presence of enzymes that are needed for digestion and absorption of nutrients.

In this system, enzymes and hormones are produced, vitamins are synthesized and stored, and food is dismantled and then reassembled. Nutrients, vitamins, minerals, electrolytes, and water enter the body through the gastrointestinal tract. Catalysts and reactants play a role, and some are recycled and used again. Finally, wastes are collected and eliminated.

UPPER GASTROINTESTINAL SYSTEM

Oral Cavity (Mouth)

The oral cavity consists of the lips, cheeks, teeth, gums, tongue, palate, and salivary glands. Its main functions include ingestion, mastication, salivation, and the first phase of swallowing (deglutition).

The salivary glands' total daily secretion is between 1 and 1.5 L of saliva. Saliva is secreted in the mouth. The salivary glands consist of the parotid, submaxillary, sublingual, and buccal glands. Saliva has three functions. The first of these is protection and lubrication. Saliva is rich in mucus, which serves to protect the oral mucosa and to coat the food as it passes through the mouth, pharynx, and esophagus. The sublingual and buccal glands produce only mucous types of secretions. The second function is its protective antimicrobial action. The saliva not only cleanses the mouth but contains the enzyme lysosome, which has an antibacterial action. Third, saliva contains ptyalin and amylase, which initiate the digestion of dietary starches.

Secretions from the salivary glands are primarily regulated by the autonomic nervous system. Parasympathetic stimulation decreases flow. These nuclei are controlled mainly by taste impulses and tactile sensory impulses from the mouth.

Tongue

The tongue is a mass of striated and skeletal muscles that is covered by a mucous membrane. It is a highly mobile, muscular, and tactile organ, and it plays an important part in articulate speech. It is also necessary to the digestive tract, being involved in mastication and swallowing as well as being the chief organ of taste. The surface of the tongue and its side edges are covered with papillae. The papillae contain the taste buds, which are highly specialized nerve endings. A perfectly dry tongue cannot taste, and the sense itself is limited to four discriminations: bitter, sweet, salty, and sour. Many of the finer sensations attributed to taste are actually received by the organ of smell.

Swallowing is initiated when a bolus of food is pushed backward by the tongue into the pharynx, a voluntary act. The bolus stimulates swallowing receptor areas located in the pharynx, transmitting impulses to the medulla oblongata via the trigeminal nerve. The autonomic nervous system is activated, and a series of pharyngeal, laryngeal, and esophageal contractions result from transmission via the glossopharyngeal and vagus nerves.

Pharynx

The pharynx connects the oral cavity to the esophagus. The pharyngeal walls are composed of longitudinal and circular striated muscle fibers that surround the fibrous tissues involved in deglutition. The pharynx is divided into three sections: nasopharynx, oropharynx, and laryngeal pharynx.

Esophagus

The pharynx ends at the level of the sixth cervical vertebra to become the esophagus. The total length of the esophagus is about 25 cm (10 inches). The upper one-fifth lies in the neck; the lower four-fifths lie in the thorax. It is located posterior to the trachea and is capable of altering its own size.

Three cellular layers compose the wall of the esophagus. The innermost layer of cells is the mucosal layer made up of squamous epithelium. The middle layer is muscle arranged circularly around the lumen. The upper one-third of this middle layer is skeletal (striated) muscle controlled directly by nerves from the brain; the remainder is smooth muscle that is only indirectly controlled by the central nervous system through the effects of the autonomic nervous system on the intramural plexus. The outermost layer of cells is longitudinal muscle fibers.

When food is pushed from the pharynx through the hypopharyngeal sphincter into the esophagus, the propulsion continues throughout the length of the esophagus and is known as peristaltic waves controlled by vagal response. These peristaltic waves often exert as much as 50–70 cm H_2O of pressure. The peristaltic waves move the food bolus down the esophagus, through the gastroesophageal sphincter, and into the stomach. Food normally passes from the mouth through the esophagus and into the stomach in about 7 sec.

Two sphincters keep food boluses from moving in and out of the esophagus. The hypopharyngeal sphincter, the superior end of the esophagus, opens to allow food to enter the esophagus from the pharynx. When the hypopharyngeal sphincter is relaxed, it is closed as a result of passive elastic tension. When the skeletal muscles contract, the sphincter opens and a bolus of food may enter the esophagus, creating a peristaltic wave that advances the food through the esophagus. The sphincter may also open during vomiting to allow the food to be regurgitated.

The gastroesophageal sphincter, also known as the cardiac sphincter, functions in the same way as the hypopharyngeal sphincter. The gastroesophageal sphincter controls food boluses leaving the esophagus and entering the stomach. It opens as peristaltic waves travel along the esophagus to allow the bolus of food to enter and closes to prevent a reflux of food and acid. If the sphincter cannot close, a condition known as achalasia exists. Achalasia is damage of the myenteric level of nerves that innervate the sphincter and prevent it from closing.

A condition known as reflux may occur as a result of inappropriate relaxation of the gastroesophageal sphincter. It may occur in a variety of conditions, such as pregnancy, obesity, excess caffeine and tobacco intake, hiatal hernia, and some medication ingestions. Treatment of the problem may help relieve the sensation of chest pain. Diet change may also relieve discomfort.

The opening in the diaphragm that allows passage of the esophagus is the esophageal hiatus. As soon as the esophagus passes through the opening, it almost immediately enters the stomach. If this opening becomes enlarged, the stomach usually bulges into the opening. This condition is termed a hiatal hernia.

No enzymes are secreted in the esophagus. The esophagus secretes only mucus. The mucus protects the mucosa from excoriation from food that is in its most abrasive form.

Stomach

The stomach is the most dilated portion of the digestive tract and has an average capacity of about 1 L. It is located in the epigastric, umbilical, and left hypochondriac regions of the abdomen. It is subject to considerable variation in shape and size, but an average stomach is J shaped in general outline and has a maximum length of about 25 cm (10 inches) and a maximum breadth of about 14 cm.

The stomach is generally described as having three sections: the fundus, the body, and the pylorus (Fig. 38–1). The upper lateral border of the stomach

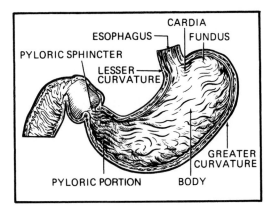

Figure 38–1. Divisions and curvatures of the stomach.

is called the lesser curvature. The lesser curvature carries downward the line of the right border of the esophagus and throughout most of its extent is nearly vertical. The lower lateral border is called the greater curvature. The greater curvature is subject to considerable variation in length and position, depending on the condition of the stomach at the time of examination.

Openings of the Stomach

As the esophagus nears the stomach, it thickens; circular muscles ring the distal end just as it passes into the stomach. These thickened circular muscles form the cardiac sphincter.

The pyloric sphincter has the same anatomical structure and the same physiologic function as the cardiac sphincter. The pyloric sphincter controls the opening at the distal end of the stomach into the duodenum. It lies 3 cm to the right of the midline and about 5 cm below the tip of the sternum. The sphincter is slightly open most of the time, permitting fluids to be squirted out but preventing escape of solids.

Layers

The stomach wall is composed of three muscular layers. The outer layer consists of longitudinal muscle fibers. The middle layer consists of circular fibers. The innermost third layer consists of transverse (oblique) fibers (Fig. 38–2).

The gastric mucosa lines the interior of the stomach. The mucous membrane is thick and velvety, with the appearance of a honeycomb. In the body and the pyloric end, the muscularis mucosa is thrown into folds or ridges called rugae. These rugae allow for distension.

The interior mucosa of the stomach has a layer called the submucosa. The layer is composed of blood and lymph vessels and connective and fibrous tissue.

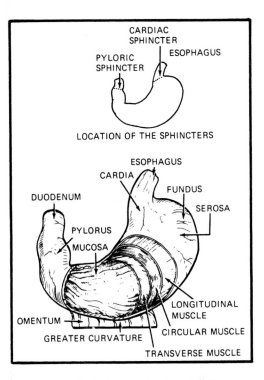

Figure 38–2. Layers of the stomach wall.

Visceral peritoneum covers the exterior of the stomach and consists of tissue which "hangs" in a double layer from the greater curvature of the stomach to cover the anterior side of abdominal viscera. This is the greater omentum (Fig. 38–3).

Gastric Glands

Glands are present throughout the gastrointestinal tract to secrete chemicals that mix with the food and digest it. These secretions are of two types:

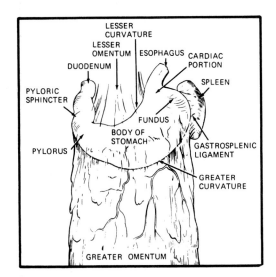

Figure 38–3. Greater omentum.

(1) mucus, which protects the wall of the gastrointestinal tract and liquefies the stomach contents, and (2) enzymes and allied substances that break the large chemical compounds of the food into simple compounds.

Mucus is secreted by every portion of the gastrointestinal tract. It contains a large amount of mucoprotein that is resistant to almost all digestive juices. Mucus also lubricates the passage of food along the mucosa, and it forms a thin film everywhere to prevent the food and hydrochloric acid from excoriating the mucosa. It is amphoteric, which means that it is capable of neutralizing either acids or bases. All of these properties make mucus an excellent substance for protecting the mucosa from physical damage and preventing digestion of the wall of the gut by the digestive juices.

A number of substances, such as aspirin, bile salts, ethyl alcohol, and acetic acid, have been shown to alter ion influxes and potential differences across gastric mucosa, and these changes have been interpreted as a reflection of damage to the gastric mucosa. How these substances disrupt the gastric mucosa is not known. Possibly, active ion transport is inhibited or metabolic processes are altered, thus leading to changes in the permeability of the mucosa, predisposing a person to destruction of mucosa cells (ulcer formation).

The proximal portion of the stomach, the cardia, receives the bolus of food from the esophagus. This stimulates gastric glands to secrete lipase, pepsin, the intrinsic factor, mucus, hydrochloric acid, and gastrone (inhibits secretion of the acids), collectively known as gastric juice. The mucosa of the stomach contains few gastric glands at the fundus, many glands in the body, and fewer glands at the antral (pyloric) portion of the body.

Gastric glands are tubular. The narrow neck of each gland opens into the stomach. Chief cells in the gastric gland's neck have two functions: to secrete mucus and to regenerate cells both for the glands themselves and for the intestinal surface epithelial tissue. Argentaffin cells are present in the tissues of the gastric glands. These cells contain granules which are thought to be the origin of serotonin.

The fundus (blind end of the gland) has parietal (oxyntic) cells that secrete hydrochloric acid, water, and the intrinsic factor. Hydrochloric acid is an enzyme involved in the digestion of proteins. It also activates other enzymes in the stomach for digestion and kills bacteria. Hydrochloric acid secretion may be increased by four endogenous substances: histamine, gastrin, calcium, and acetylcholine.

Atropine, a muscarinic antagonist, may block hydrochloric acid secretion caused by acetylcholine. Cimetidine, ranitidine, nizatidime, and famotidine, which are histamine H_2 receptor antagonists, block histamine-induced hydrochloric acid secretion.

The intrinsic factor from the parietal cell is a mucoprotein that is essential for absorption of vitamin B_{12}. Once released from the parietal cells, the intrinsic factor adheres to epithelial cells in the ileum. If the ileum is surgically resected, exogenous B_{12} must be taken for life.

Zymogenic (chief) cells found in the body of a gastric gland secrete pepsinogen, an inactive proteolytic enzyme. The hydrochloric acid activates the pepsinogen to form pepsin, which is an enzyme that begins the digestion of proteins by splitting amino acid bonds.

The pyloric (antral) portion of the stomach has increased depth, size, and muscle and secretes mucus and pepsinogen. The hormone gastrin, a large polypeptide, is secreted from G cells in the antral mucosa and is absorbed into the bloodstream. This hormone then passes by way of the blood to the fundic glands of the stomach and causes them to secrete a strongly acidic gastric juice. The acid, in turn, greatly aids in the digestion of the meats that first initiated the gastrin mechanism. In this way, the stomach helps to tailor-make the secretion to fit the particular type of food eaten.

Gastric Motility

The rugae allow for a great distention of the stomach without increasing pressure (Laplace's law), which may be termed a receptive relaxation phenomenon. This may allow for stomach contents to approach 6–7 L before peristaltic contractions are initiated.

Factors affecting gastric motility include quantity of contents, pH of contents, degree of mixing and peristalsis that has occurred, and the capacity of the duodenum to accept chyme from the stomach.

Usually, the fundus of the stomach is stimulated to initiate oscillations (mild "mixing waves") when about 1 L of food is in the stomach, but there may be considerably more food present. These mixing waves occur approximately once every 20 sec. When the food (bolus) is digested to the chyme state, it is ready for passage into the duodenum.

However, mixing waves alone are unable to achieve this. If no other influences are functional, malabsorption states will occur. To help the conversion of food boluses to chyme, the mixing waves assist the hormones and acids to mix with the food. As the peristaltic contractions move toward the antral (pyloric) portion of the stomach, they become very strong in order to force the chyme into the duodenum. A pH of 1 to 3 is obtained by the hormone gastrin stimulating the release of hydrochloric acid into the chyme and also stimulating peristaltic contractions, which will occur at a rate of about three per minute.

The enterogastric reflex (which causes lower gastrin and acid secretion) will delay the progression of chyme. This reflex is under vagal influence. It is stimulated by the degree of distension of the duodenum, by the presence of any degree of irritation of the duodenal mucosa, by the osmolality, acidity, and degree of emulsification of the chyme.

Chyme must be of the proper consistency and acidity, and the duodenum must be receptive for the strong antral peristaltic contractions to force the chyme through the pyloric valve. The small size of the pyloric sphincter opening results in little chyme entering the duodenum. Most of the chyme is squirted back toward the body of the stomach as the pyloric valve relaxes and closes. This is an important action in the mixing of the chyme.

Gastric Emptying

The stomach empties at a rate proportional to the volume of its contents. Chemical composition of the chyme in the duodenum determines the rate and quantity of additional chyme entering the duodenum. The duodenum contains osmoreceptors, chemoreceptors, and baroreceptors (stretch receptors for volume distension) that influence duodenal activity. If the chyme has a high fat content upon entering the duodenum, a release of cholecystokinin occurs, inhibiting further release of chyme. High fat content is the factor most known for inhibiting gastric emptying. Secretin may also be released to inhibit gastric emptying by inhibiting the gastrin mechanism.

Other factors such as emotional depression, sadness, and pain (both physical and psychological) inhibit emptying of the stomach. An inadequate fluid intake will retard emptying of the stomach because a large quantity of liquid is necessary to turn fat, protein, and carbohydrates into chyme.

Normally about 2 L of gastric juices (primarily hydrochloric acid) are secreted per day. The pH is 1 to 3. This acidity and its resultant irritation affect gastric emptying by decreasing it. Inadequate protein breakdown and hypertonicity of the chyme will also slow gastric emptying.

Factors increasing gastric motility include aggression, increased volume of chyme, and fluids. The more liquid the stomach chyme is, the greater will be the ease of emptying.

Control of Gastric Secretions

Gastric secretions may be controlled through autonomic nervous system functions, by hormonal alterations, and/or through baroreceptors.

The control of the gastric secretions, specifically hydrochloric acid, may be broken down into three phases: the cephalic, the gastric, and the intestinal phases. These three phases follow the path of food and then chyme through the alimentary tract. When the stomach is at rest, normal secretion occurs at a rate of about 0.5 ml/min. This is known as the basal rate. With food in the stomach, the rate of secretion increases to about 3.0 ml/minute.

Cephalic Phase. The parasympathetic nervous system controls the first phase of regulation of gastric secretion via the vagus nerve. The sight, smell, taste, or thought of food is sufficient to stimulate the release of hydrochloric acid in preparation for the expected arrival of food boluses. In addition to pleasant thoughts of food, hunger, hypoglycemia, and anger will also stimulate secretion of hydrochloric acid.

Vagal control is decreased by certain drugs (especially the anticholinergic drugs), hyperglycemia, and duodenal distension. A vagotomy may eliminate the cephalic phase.

Gastric Phase. This second phase of control over gastric secretion begins when food actually enters the stomach. The predominant regulatory mechanism in this phase is hormonal. Gastrin is the major hormone and it increases acid secretion from the oxyntic cells. It is stimulated by antral distention, secretion of pepsinogen, and an alkaline pH in the stomach. This phase has a negative feedback effect— as hydrochloric acid is released in response to gastrin, the stomach contents eventually become acid. When the number of hydrogen ions (acidity; pH of 2) is adequately high, gastrin secretion decreases.

Intestinal Phase. This phase begins when chyme enters the duodenum. Chyme entering the duodenum is more acid than that in the body of the stomach because as polypeptide fragments move from the body of the stomach to the antrum, they stimulate acid secretion by an unknown mechanism (but to a lesser extent than in the stomach).

When the chyme has a pH below 2.5, it is accepted more slowly into the duodenum. In the gastric phase, the chyme becomes more alkaline so that it will move into the duodenum in the intestinal phase.

Fat in the duodenum stimulates the secretion of cholecystokinin, which directly decreases gastric motility. Of the food types leaving the stomach, carbohydrates are the most rapid, followed by protein and then fat.

Gastric Digestion

Gastric digestion includes carbohydrates, proteins, and fats. The stomach is a poor absorptive area of the gastrointestinal tract. Only a few highly lipid-soluble substances, such as alcohol, can be absorbed in small quantities.

Carbohydrates. Digestion of starches really begins in the mouth with action of ptyalin and continues in the stomach by hydrolyzing carbohydrates into oligosaccharides.

Protein. The first stage of protein breakdown by proteolytic enzymes occurs in the stomach.

Fats. Digestion of fats in the stomach is minimal. The only action the stomach has on fats is by gastric peristalsis, which reduces the size of triglyceride droplets and facilitates contact with a lipase secreted by von Ebner's glands.

LOWER GASTROINTESTINAL SYSTEM

The Small Intestine

The small intestine extends from the pyloric sphincter to the cecum. This 18- to 20-foot tube is divided into three segments. The first segment is the duodenum, which arises at the pyloric sphincter. It is a C-shaped segment about 10 inches long and ends at the ligament of Treitz. The middle segment, the jejunum, extends about 8 feet from the ligament of Treitz and has an alkaline pH (7.8). The third segment is the ileum, which is about 12 feet long. There is no distinct change from the jejunum to the ileum.

Layers of the Small Intestine Wall

The small intestinal wall has the same layering as does the stomach. The wall of the intestine consists of a secreting and absorbing mucous membrane called the mucosa. It is composed of epithelial and columnar cells, smaller blood vessels, nerve fibers, plasma, and blood cells. The next layer is the muscularis mucosa. The muscularis mucosa is lined with areolar tissue (the submucosa). The submucosa contains larger blood vessels, connective tissue, nerves, ganglia, and lymphoid elements. The submucosa is covered with two smooth muscular coats, an outer

longitudinal one and an inner circular one. The intestine also possesses still another coat, since it is closely invested by peritoneum; this coat is the serous membrane (serosa) lining the walls of those cavities and reflected onto the walls of the tube.

The activity of gastrointestinal smooth muscle is controlled by local, humoral, and neural influences. The rhythmic movements are integrated by an intramural network that lies between the two muscular layers of the intestine. This network has two layers of nerve fibers, a submucosal network (Meissner's plexus) and a second layer that lies between the circular and longitudinal layers of smooth muscle (the myenteric or Auerbach's plexus). The intramural network is responsible for many of the locally controlled movements that occur in the digestive tract. The afferent fibers of this system are located largely within the submucosal network, and the motor fibers are within the myenteric plexus.

The intrinsic tone and rhythmic activity of the digestive tract can be modified by the autonomic nervous system. Generally, the parasympathetic nervous system increases gastrointestinal activity, while the sympathetic nervous system slows its activity.

Ileocecal Valve

At the junction of the ileum and the cecum is the ileocecal valve. This valve controls the flow of contents into the cecum and allows no regurgitation of cecal contents into the ileum.

Villi

Villi (singular villus) are the distinguishing characteristics of the small intestine (Fig. 38–4). These fingerlike projections into the lumen provide an extensive surface area. The villi and microvilli increase in absorptive capacity 600-fold for a total surface area of about 250 m². An extraordinary number of villi project from the mucosa into the lumen of the small intestine. Each villus contains microvilli to actively absorb nutrients from the intestinal tract. Each villus also contains a lymph vessel and a dense capillary bed to aid in the absorption process. This lymph vessel is called a lacteal. Carbohydrates, fats, proteins, vitamins, and minerals are absorbed into the small bowel through the villi.

Glands of the Small Intestine

The intestinal lumen is lined with simple, cuboidal, and columnar epithelial cells interspersed with goblet cells. The many goblet cells secrete mucus to protect the mucosa. The goblet cells decrease in numbers markedly toward the end of the ileum. Crypts of

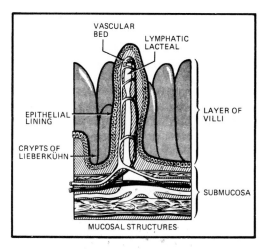

Figure 38–4. Structure of villi (a lacteal).

Lieberkühn (Fig. 38–5) are tubular glands found between the villi in the submucosa of the duodenum.

Absorptive and secreting cells have been identified but not differentiated in function. It is known that the crypts of Lieberkühn are extremely mitotic and replace villous cells. The entire intestinal epithelial surface is replaced every 32 hours.

Crypts of Lieberkühn are small pits found on the entire intestinal surface except in the area of Brunner's glands. The crypts of Lieberkühn secrete a watery fluid immediately absorbed by the villi. This supplies a carrier substance for absorption by villi as chyme contacts them. This secretion is controlled principally by local nervous reflexes.

Brunner's glands are mucus-secreting glands that are concentrated in the first portion of the duo-

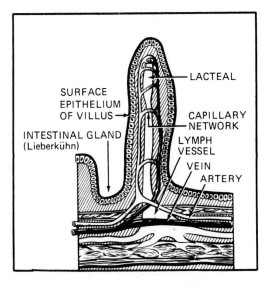

Figure 38–5. Crypts of Lieberkühn.

denum, between the pylorus and the ampulla of Vater. The function of Brunner's glands is inhibited by the sympathetic nervous system. Lack of sufficient mucus may be related to the development site of peptic ulcers. Brunner's glands are thought to protect the duodenum from digestion by the gastric juices.

Peyer's patches are lymphoid follicles that lie in the mucosa and submucosa of the ileum. They participate in antibody synthesis and the body's immune responses.

The small bowel also secretes several hormones that enter the bloodstream and stimulate the pancreas to release its digestive secretions.

Movements of the Small Intestine

The presence of chyme in the small intestine stimulates baroreceptors that initiate a type of concentric contraction called segmentation. When the small intestine becomes distended, many constrictions occur either regularly or irregularly along the distended area. The constrictions then relax, but others occur at different points a few seconds later. Each contraction results in a segmentation of the chyme and moves the chyme forward about 1–2 cm. These segmenting contractions normally occur 7 to 12 times per minute. This helps to mix secretions of the small intestine with the chyme particles.

Propulsive contractions are called peristaltic contractions. They are elicited by distension of the intestine. Peristaltic contractions should be regularly spaced. The peristaltic waves (contractions) push the chyme slowly toward the colon. These waves are short and found predominantly in the first portions of the duodenum and jejunum.

Distension of the small intestine activates the nerves to continue the contraction sequence, known as the myenteric reflex. As the chyme nears the large intestine, contractions in the ileum increase. As chyme reaches the end of the ileum and is ready to enter the colon, a gastroileal reflex is stimulated. The gastroileal reflex regulates the movement of chyme from the small intestine into the large intestine. Between the ileum and the cecum is the ileocecal valve, which is normally closed. The tissue immediately before the ileocecal valve is highly muscular, forming the ileocecal sphincter, and the flaps of the ileocecal valve (Fig. 38–6) extend into the cecum. The sphincter is normally contracted except after a meal, when it relaxes and allows chyme to move from the ileum into the cecum. Chyme is prevented from returning to the ileum during colonic contraction by the valve leaflets being floated out to

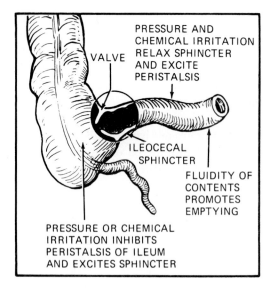

Figure 38–6. Gastroilial reflex.

close the ileocecal valve (in much the same way as the heart valves).

Absorption Mechanisms in the Small Intestine

Normally, absorption from the small intestine each day consists of several hundred grams of carbohydrates, 100 or more grams of fat, 50–100 g of amino acids, 50–100 g of ions, and 8 or 9 L of water. Its absorptive capacity is much greater than this. There are five basic mechanisms for absorption in the small intestine: hydrolysis, nonionic movement, passive diffusion, facilitated diffusion, and active transport.

Hydrolysis. Hydrolysis is the chemical action of uniting compounds with water to split the compounds into simpler compounds. Enzymes and hormones act as catalysts in the process of hydrolysis. Catalysts speed up the process of hydrolysis. (Catalysts speed up a chemical reaction without entering into the reaction.)

Nonionic Movement. Nonionic transport allows substances to move freely in and out of cells with no energy or carrier substances needed. Such molecules include drugs and unconjugated bile salts.

Passive Diffusion. In passive diffusion, there is free movement of molecules based on a concentration gradient, primarily from an area of high concentration to an area of low concentration. Free fatty acids and water are molecules that move by passive diffusion.

Facilitated Diffusion. Facilitated diffusion may be defined as a process by which a carrier picks up an ion, crosses the cell membrane, liberates the ion inside the cell, and then returns outside to pick up another molecule (ion). This diffusion does not require energy, and ions cannot move alone against an electrochemical gradient.

Active Transport. For nutrients to be absorbed by active transport, energy (ATP) is required. Ions such as Na^+ and K^+ and molecules such as proteins and glucose require active transport.

Nutrient Digestion and Absorption

Ninety percent of nutrients and 50% of water and electrolytes are absorbed in the jejunum. Meticulous nutritional counseling and follow-up are important for patients with small bowel resections.

Carbohydrates. Carbohydrates enter the duodenum in the forms of starch, polysaccharides (complex sugars), disaccharides, and monosaccharides. The starch and polysaccharides are hydrolyzed under the influence of amylase to form maltose. Maltose and directly ingested disaccharides such as sucrose, lactose, and maltose are hydrolyzed by intestinal enzymes into simple sugars of monosaccharides, which are then absorbed into the bloodstream via the intestinal mucosa.

Approximately 350 g of carbohydrates are absorbed daily (60% starch, 30% sucrose, and 10% lactose). The three basic sugars are fructose, glucose, and galactose. Each of these basic sugars yields 4 kcal/g. Glucose and galactose are actively transported across the small intestine wall into the blood. Fructose is transported by facilitated diffusion.

Proteins. Dietary proteins are first acted upon by enzymes called proteases. The principal proteases are pepsin (in the gastric secretion) and trypsin (in the pancreatic secretion). These enzymes catalyze the hydrolysis of the very large protein molecules into intermediate compounds (proteoses and peptones) and subsequently into amino acids. In the digestive sequence, protein is broken down into proteoses and peptones in the stomach. These simpler compounds are next broken down into polypeptides and thence into amino acids in the small intestine.

Approximately 70–90 g of protein are absorbed daily, yielding 4 kcal/g. Of the amino acids, eight (isoleucine, leucine, lysine, methionine, phenylalanine, threonine, tryptophan, and valine) are essential. Amino acids are absorbed (primarily from the duodenum and jejunum) by active transport into the blood of the intestinal villi. The transport is carrier mediated and requires an expenditure of energy.

Fats. Before fats can be digested, they must be emulsified. This function is performed in the small intestine by bile, which is secreted by the liver and stored in the gallbladder.

The bile salts aggregate to form micelles. These micelles have a fatty core but are still stable in the intestines because the surfaces of the micelles are ionized, which is a property that promotes water solubility. The fatty acids and the glycerides become absorbed in the fatty portions of these micelles as they are split away from fat globules and are then carried from the fat globules to the intestinal epithelium, where absorption occurs.

The emulsification of ingested fat globules provides a greater contact area between the fat molecules and pancreatic lipase, which is the principal fat-digestive enzyme. The end products of fat digestion are glycerides, fatty acids, and glycerol. Some fatty acids and glycerol may be absorbed into the blood via the blood vessels found in the villi of the intestinal mucosa. However, most fatty acids and glycerides are absorbed into the lymphatic system via the lacteals of the intestinal villi.

Approximately 60–100 g of fat are absorbed daily, providing 9 kcal/g.

Electrolytes. Electrolytes are absorbed in all parts of the intestine by active transport.

Water. Approximately 8–9 L of water per day are absorbed from the intestine. Water is absorbed by diffusion and osmosis.

Water-Soluble Vitamins. The water-soluble vitamins, vitamin C and B complex, are absorbed in all parts of the intestine through passive diffusion directly into the blood.

Fat-Soluble Vitamins. The fat-soluble vitamins, A, D, E, and K, are absorbed from the gastrointestinal tract (mainly the jejunum) in the same way as lipids are. Once in the bloodstream, these vitamins are escorted by protein carriers because they are insoluble in water.

Calcium. The top portion of the duodenum is specialized for the absorption of calcium.

Iron. In the intestines, only about 10% of dietary iron is normally absorbed, but if the body's supply is diminished or if the need increases for any reason, absorption increases. This regulation is provided by a blood protein, transferrin, which captures iron from food and carries it to tissues throughout the body by active transport.

Large Intestine

The large intestine (colon) is 5–6 feet long and extends from the ileum to the anus. It is significantly different from the small intestine in that it contains no villi. The colon is 2.5 inches in diameter (larger than the small intestine) and has many sacculations (saclike segmentations) called haustra.

There are three segments of the colon: cecum, colon, and rectum. The colon is further subdivided into four sections: the ascending, transverse, descending, and sigmoid colons. The large intestine, or colon, is mainly responsible for the absorption of water and some electrolytes and the elimination of waste products.

Cecum

The cecum is a blind-end sac (Fig. 38–7) into which the ileum empties its contents. The vermiform appendix is attached to the base of the cecum. The appendix has no known use and must be surgically removed if it becomes infected to prevent peritonitis.

Colon

Immediately above the cecum is the ascending colon, which passes upward to become the transverse colon at the right colic flexure (hepatic flexure). It then crosses the abdomen, now called the transverse colon, and becomes the descending colon at the left colic flexure (splenic flexure). At the iliac crest, the descending colon arches backward to form the sigmoid colon (Fig. 38–7). The sigmoid colon is the portion of the colon that crosses from the left side to the

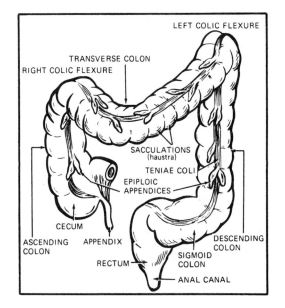

Figure 38–7. Large intestine (anterior view).

midline to become the rectum (Fig. 38–7), which follows the curvature of the lower sacrum and coccyx.

Rectum and Anus

The rectum is about 7 inches long. The distal 1–2 inches are the anal canal (Fig. 38–8). Mucous membrane lines the rectum and is arranged in vertical rows called rectal columns. Each rectal column contains an artery and a vein. These veins frequently enlarge to form hemorrhoids. Two sphincters control the anus (the exterior opening of the rectum). The internal sphincter is composed of involuntary smooth muscle. The external sphincter is voluntary striated muscle.

Layers of the Colon Wall

Epithelial cells form the mucosa of the colon, which is actively involved with absorption of water and some electrolytes. The muscle layers are different from those in the small intestine. The circular layer becomes somewhat spherical (Fig. 38–7), and the longitudinal layer fibers are evenly dispersed in three strips (called teniae coli) around the colon. This results in sacculation, and the resulting pouches are the haustra.

Colonic Motility

The colon moves its contents slowly through the colon system to allow for fluid absorption so that 800–900 ml of chyme liquid is absorbed along with nutrients. Thus, of the 1000 ml of chyme entering the colon, only 150–250 ml of fluid will be evacuated in the stool per day.

Mixing Movements in the Colon

Segmentation of chyme in the large intestine is caused by contraction of the inner muscle layer. There is a slow progress analward with segmentation in the colon. Mixing movements may also be called haustrations. As the circular segmenting contraction occurs, the teniae coli also contract. This provides for more surface contact of the contents to the lumen wall for absorption.

Propulsive Movements in the Colon

These are the result of the haustral contractions but are insufficient to provide for the necessary expulsion of waste products. A mass movement occurs in response to an irritation or distension, usually in the transverse colon. These contractions, as a unit, force the entire mass of fecal material forward. A series of mass movements usually occur for up to 30 min and may then occur again in one-half to one full day.

Mass movements can cause increased colonic motility as a result of intense stimulation of the parasympathetic nervous system, irritation secondary to conditions such as ulcerative colitis, osmotic overload, or simply distension, use of drugs such as morphine sulfate or magnesium sulfate, an increase in bile salts, bacterial endotoxins, and high-residual diets. Hypermotility results in diarrhea and may cause severe fluid loss and electrolyte imbalance.

Mass movements are inhibited by all of the anti-cholinergic drugs and by diets deficient in bulk. This may result in constipation, since the extra length of time in the large intestine allows more fluid absorption.

Colonic Absorption

The colon may increase its absorption rate by three-fold if threatened with large amounts of fluid. Most of the absorption in the colon occurs in its proximal half (the ascending and transverse colon). The distal colon functions principally for storage.

The mucosa of the large intestine has a very high capacity for active absorption of sodium, and the electrical potential created by the absorption of the sodium causes passive chloride absorption. The mucosa of the colon actively secretes bicarbonate and potassium as well.

Bacteria

Bacterial action in the colon causes the formation of gases, which provide bulk and help to propel the feces. Bacteria are capable of digesting small amounts of cellulose, in this way providing a few calories of nutrition to the body each day. These organisms also synthesize some important nutritional factors such as vitamin K, thiamin, riboflavin, vitamin B_{12}, folic acid, biotin, and nicotinic acid. The main anaerobic bacterium in the colon is *Bacteroides fragilis.* The main aerobic bacterium is *Escherichia coli.*

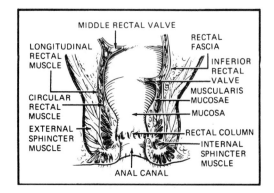

Figure 38–8. Section of the rectum.

Defecation

The stimulus to defecate is the distension of the rectal wall resulting in the stimulation of the myenteric plexus. These nerves cause peristaltic waves in the rectum; the internal anal sphincter relaxes (receptive relaxation), and then the external anal sphincter relaxes so that defecation will occur.

Approximately 150 g of feces are eliminated daily. Feces are three-fourths water and one-fourth solid matter. The organic constituents include undigested food residues, digestive secretions and enzymes, dead cells, bile pigments, and mucus. Thirty percent of the mass consists of bacteria, and another 30% is fat. The nature of the diet does not change the contents of the stool except for the amount of cellulose present. Stereobilinogen gives feces its brown color.

CHEMICAL MESSENGERS OF THE GASTROINTESTINAL SYSTEM

The gastrointestinal chemical messengers can act in one of three ways: under an endocrine stimulus, as a neurotransmitter, or as a neuroendocrine messenger.

An endocrine stimulus is a chemical substance formed in part of the body and carried to another part of the body to alter the functional activity or structure of that part. Examples are gastrin, secretion, gastric inhibitory hormone, insulin, and glucagon.

A neurotransmitter is any specific chemical agent released by a presynaptic cell, upon excitation, that crosses the synapse to stimulate or inhibit the post-synaptic cell. Examples are vasoactive intestinal peptide, acetylcholine, norepinephrine, and serotonin.

A neuroendocrine messenger consists of cells that release a hormone into the circulating blood in response to a neural stimulus. An example is cholecystokinin.

BLOOD SUPPLY OF THE GASTROINTESTINAL TRACT

Arterial Vascularization

The celiac artery, the superior mesenteric arteries, and the inferior mesenteric arteries all branch from the abdominal aorta. Figure 38–9 shows the arterial vascularization of the gastrointestinal tract.

Venous Blood Return

The venous circulation of the gastrointestinal system is unique in that the venous blood enters the portal vein system (Fig. 38–10). All blood from the gas-

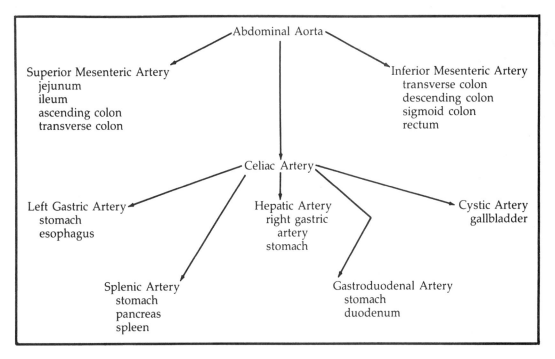

Figure 38–9. Arterial vascularization of the gastrointestinal tract.

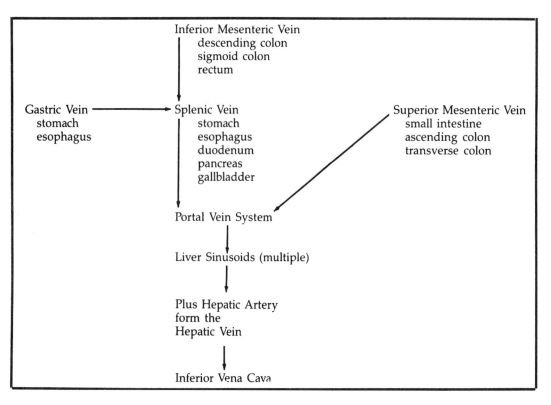

Figure 38–10. Venous return of the gastrointestinal tract.

trointestinal tract enters the portal vein system, which empties into the liver sinusoids. This makes the portal system extremely important for filtering microorganisms and for synthesizing many enzymes and clotting factors needed by the body. The liver also removes various absorbed nutrients, especially glucose and proteins, from the blood and stores them for later use by the body. Generally, the vein corresponding by name to the artery drains the same areas supplied by the artery.

The portal vein drains into the liver sinusoids. These sinusoids join branches of the hepatic artery to form the hepatic vein. In turn, the hepatic veins drain blood from the portal vein and hepatic artery into the inferior vena cava.

INNERVATION OF THE GASTROINTESTINAL SYSTEM

Compared with the other body systems, the gastrointestinal tract is unique in that it has its own separate intrinsic nervous system. The gastrointestinal tract can be influenced by the autonomic nervous system.

The intrinsic nervous system has two layers of neurons connected by specific fibers. The outer layer of neurons is called the myenteric plexus or

Auerbach's plexus. It is located between the longitudinal and circular muscle layers. The inner layer of neurons, called the submucosal plexus or Meissner's plexus, is located in the submucosa.

Generally, the myenteric plexus controls movement of the gastrointestinal tract and the submucosal plexus (Meissner's plexus) controls the secretions of the gastrointestinal tract and sensory function through impulses received by stretch receptors in both the gastrointestinal wall and gastrointestinal epithelium.

Stimulation of the myenteric plexus results in increasing motor tone of the gastrointestinal wall and increasing intensity, rate, and speed of peristaltic waves. Increase in Meissner's plexus activity results in increasing secretions.

The extrinsic nerves of the autonomic nervous system can alter the effects of the gastrointestinal system at specific points or from the mouth to the stomach and then from the distal end of the colon to the anus. Parasympathetic supply for the gut is from the tenth cranial (vagus) and sacral nerves. Acetylcholine is the neurotransmitter from the postganglionic fiber. A few cranial parasympathetic fibers innervate the mouth and pharynx. Extensive parasympathetic innervation exists in the esophagus, stomach, pancreas, and first half of the large intestine. The sacral parasympathetic fibers innervate the distal half of the large intestine, especially the sigmoidal, rectal, and anal portions.

The sympathetic nervous system fibers flow along blood vessels of the entire gut. The sympathetic fibers to the gastrointestinal tract originate in the spinal cord between segments T-8 and L-3. Its neurotransmitter, norepinephrine, inhibits gastrointestinal tract activity. This causes effects opposite those of the parasympathetic neurotransmitter, acetylcholine. If the effects are strong enough, the sympathetic system can virtually halt activity of the gastrointestinal tract.

ACCESSORY ORGANS OF DIGESTION

The accessory organs involved in making chyme suitable for nutrient absorption are the salivary glands, the pancreas, and the biliary system (liver and gallbladder).

Salivary Glands

There are three salivary glands: the parotid, the submandibular, and the sublingual (Fig. 38–11). All of the salivary glands are paired.

Hormones have no influence on the salivary glands. Salivary secretion is controlled by the superior and inferior salivatory nuclei located in the brain stem. Nervous stimuli of the glands occur from the thought, sight, and smell of food.

Pancreas

The pancreas is a soft, fish-shaped lobulated gland lying behind the stomach (Fig. 38–12). The gland is composed of three segments: the head, the body, and the tail.

The pancreas is both an endocrine and exocrine organ. The endocrine portion includes the secretion of insulin from the beta cells and the secretion of glucagon from the alpha cells (see above, "Chemical Messengers of the Gastrointestinal System"). The exocrine portion is related to the gastrointestinal system and produces three enzymes whose release is controlled by two hormones produced in the small intestine.

The main pancreatic duct is the duct of Wirsung, which runs the whole length of the pancreas from left to right and joins the common bile duct on the right.

The exocrine function of the pancreas is composed of acinar glands, which are little sacs called alveoli. These cells are arranged around a small central lumen into which the cells drain the exocrine enzymes that they have synthesized. The central lumens drain into multiple ducts, which eventually drain into the main pancreatic duct. The ampulla of Vater (Fig. 38–13) is the short segment just before the common bile duct enters the duodenum.

The secretions of the acinar glands are digestive enzymes, water, and salts (sodium bicarbonate, sodium, and potassium). These colorless secretions total up to 1200 ml each day and are emptied into the upper portion of the small intestine 4 cm beyond the pylorus. They have a pH of 8.0 to 8.5. The pancreatic (acinar) fluid is composed of three major types of enzymes: amylytic, lipolytic, and proteolytic.

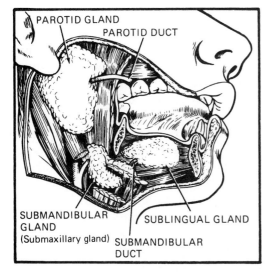

Figure 38–11. Salivary glands.

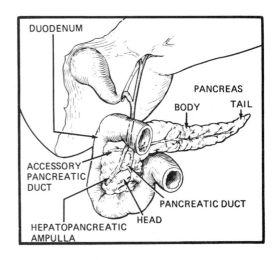

Figure 38–12. Pancreas.

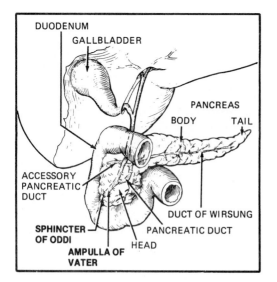

Figure 38–13. Ampulla of Vater and sphincter of Oddi.

At least 10% of the pancreatic enzymes must be present to prevent malabsorption states. During illness or injury the volume of pancreatic fluid usually decreases, and the composition may change.

The amylytic enzyme is predominantly alpha-amylase, first encountered in the saliva. The alpha-amylase is responsible for hydrolysis of carbohydrates. The end products of hydrolysis of carbohydrates are glucose and maltose (a disaccharide of two glucose molecules). The difference between salivary and pancreatic amylase is that the latter is able to digest raw starches as well as cooked starches. Amylase also contains calcium and is excreted in the urine.

The lipolytic enzymes are pancreatic lipase and phospholipase A, which are important in early stages of the digestion of fats. Lipase breaks down triglycerides to free fatty acids, glycerol, and monoglycerides. Bile salts are essential for this function. Phospholipase A hydrolyzes lecithin (a complex lipid) to lysolecithin.

Proteolytic enzymes are actually proenzymes; that is, they must be altered to become biochemically active. The three most important proteolytic proenzymes are trypsinogen, chymotrypsinogen, and procarboxy-peptidase.

Trypsin is involved in the activation of all three proenzymes to enzymes. The proteases are secreted in an inactive form; otherwise, they would act on pancreatic tissue and cause destruction. Once in the intestine, intestinal enterokinase acts on trypsinogen, converting it to trypsin. Trypsin then acts on the other proteases to convert them to active enzymes. These enzymes break amino acid bonds of protein chains, forming small polypeptides and single amino acids.

In addition to the digestive enzymes, pancreatic secretions contain large amounts of sodium bicarbonate, which reacts with the hydrochloric acid emptied into the duodenum in the chyme from the stomach to form sodium chloride and carbonic acid. The carbonic acid is absorbed into the blood and eliminated through the lungs as carbon dioxide. The net result is an increase in the quantity of sodium chloride, a neutral salt, in the intestine. Thus, pancreatic secretions neutralize the acidity of the chyme coming from the stomach. This is one of the most important functions of pancreatic secretion.

Two other important pancreatic enzymes are nuclease and deoxyribonuclease. These enzymes degrade nucleotides within DNA and RNA molecules into free mononucleotides.

Regulation of Pancreatic Secretions

The cells lining the acinar glands contain large amounts of carbonic anhydrase. The alkaline secretions (HCO_3^-) of the duct cells (cells lining the acinar glands) mix with the amylytic, lipolytic, and proteolytic enzymes prior to reaching the major pancreatic duct, the duct of Wirsung.

Secretions of the pancreas are controlled by hormonal and neural factors. There are three phases of secretion: cephalic, gastric, and intestinal. The cephalic phase is activated by the same factors as in the cephalic state of the stomach and is mainly controlled by the vagus nerve (parasympathetic impulses). Stimulation of the vagus nerve (by thought, smell, taste, chewing, and swallowing of food) causes the secretory cells of the pancreas to secrete highly concentrated enzymes with minimal amounts of HCO_3^-. The quantity of fluid secreted, however, is usually so small that the enzymes remain in the ducts of the pancreas and later are floated into the intestinal tract by the copious secretion of fluid that follows secretin stimulation.

The gastric and intestinal phases are interrelated and controlled by two hormones, secretin and cholecystokinin. When the chyme is predominantly undigested proteins and fats, the pancreatic juice will be enzyme rich. When the chyme is mainly acidic (low pH), the pancreatic juice will be HCO_3^- rich. The secretion of cholecystokinin stimulates the enzyme-rich secretion of pancreatic juices; secretin stimulates the release of HCO_3^- and water-rich pancreatic juice. The pancreatic juices enter the duodenum along with the biliary system secretions at the sphincter of Oddi.

Biliary System

The biliary system is composed of the liver and gall-bladder.

Liver

The liver is the single largest organ in the body, weighing 3–4 pounds. It is located in the right upper quadrant of the abdomen, lying up against the right inferior diaphragm.

Gross Structure. The liver is divided into a right and a left lobe by the falciform ligament (Fig. 38–14). The falciform ligament also attaches the liver to the abdominal wall and to the diaphragm. On the inferior liver surface is the quadrate lobe, and on the posterior liver surface is the caudate lobe. Both the quadrate and caudate lobes are small. Most of the liver is covered by peritoneum.

Functional Unit. Each of the hepatic lobes is further divided into numerous lobules. The hepatic lobule is the functioning unit of the liver (Fig. 38–15). Each lobule has a hepatic artery, a portal vein, and a

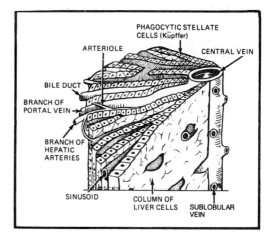

Figure 38–15. Liver lobule.

bile duct known collectively as the portal triad. Between columns of epithelial cells are intralobular cavities called sinusoids. Each sinusoid is lined with Kupffer cells, which are phagocytic cells.

Blood Supply. Each sinusoid receives oxygenated blood from the hepatic arterioles and blood rich in metabolic precursors from the hepatic vein. The blood is filtered by the phagocytic Kupffer cells. Products removed from the blood include amino acids, nutrients, sugars, and bacterial debris. Blood leaves the sinusoid by entering the central lobule vein. It then enters the hepatic veins and follows the normal venous circuit. Approximately 1500 ml of blood enters the liver each minute, making the liver one of the most vascular organs in the body.

Function. The role of the liver in digestion is to synthesize and transport bile pigments and bile salts for fat digestion. The liver cell, the hepatocyte, synthesizes bile (approximately 600 ml/day), which aids in the metabolism of carbohydrates, fats, and proteins. The bile is secreted into bile canaliculi (ducts), which branch and combine, eventually forming the right and left hepatic ducts. Immediately after leaving the liver, the right and left hepatic ducts merge to form the common hepatic duct. The hepatic ducts drain bile salts and the products of hemoglobin and drug metabolism.

The cystic duct of the gallbladder joins the common hepatic duct to form the common bile duct. The common bile duct joins the major pancreatic duct to form the ampulla of Vater just prior to entering the duodenum at the sphincter of Oddi.

The Kupffer cells of the liver sinusoids are typical reticuloendothelial cells. The Kupffer cells are tissue macrophages that are capable of removing and

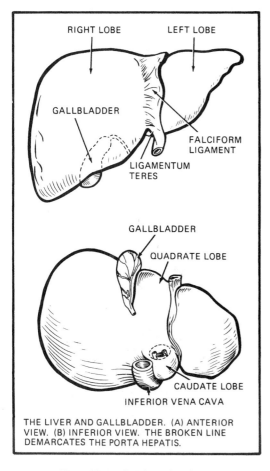

Figure 38–14. Divisions of the liver.

phagocytizing old and defective blood cells, bacteria, and other foreign material from the portal blood as it flows through the sinusoid. This phagocytic action removes the colon bacilli and detoxifies harmful substances that filter into the blood from the intestine.

The liver eliminates bilirubin (by-product of the breakdown of hemoglobin) from the blood through urine and feces. Failure to eliminate bilirubin causes jaundice.

The liver is involved in the metabolism of many hormones by virtue of its role in hormone biotransformation, activation, and excretion. It is particularly involved in the metabolism of steroid hormones such as the estrogens and progesterone, testosterone, glucocorticoids, and aldosterone. Steroid hormones are taken up from the circulation by the liver and then metabolized by hepatic enzymes. The steroid hormones directly influence many of the liver's biochemical and physiologic functions.

A major biochemical function of the liver is the detoxification and metabolism of drugs, vitamins, and hormones. Some compounds are metabolically converted to relatively inactive forms (steroid hormones), whereas others become more biologically active (vitamin D). Of prime importance in maintaining homeostasis and protecting the body against ingested toxins is the ability of the liver to metabolize and detoxify a wide variety of absorbed substances that reach it directly in the portal blood.

The liver is essential in the regulation of carbohydrate metabolism, since it directly receives from the portal circulation most of the ingested carbohydrates and then, by hormonal regulation, controls the concentration of blood glucose in the fed and fasting states. The liver stores glycogen through glycogenesis (glucose to glycogen) and breaks it down in a process called glycogenolysis (glycogen to glucose) as needed. It also synthesizes glucose from amino acids (gluconeogenesis), lactic acid, and glycerol.

The liver is involved in many aspects of lipid synthesis and metabolism. It is a major site of triglyceride, cholesterol, and phospholipid synthesis. It is involved in the formation of lipoproteins, the conversion of carbohydrates and proteins to fats, and the formation of ketones from fatty acids.

The liver's role in protein metabolism includes the deamination of proteins for glucose availability, the formation of urea from ammonia so it may be eliminated from the blood, and the synthesis of plasma proteins such as albumin, haptoglobin, transferrin, and alpha and beta globulins.

The liver is the site of synthesis of the blood-clotting proteins fibrinogen (factor I), prothrombin (factor II), and factors V, VII, and X. It also stores the fat-soluble vitamins (A, D, and K), vitamin B_{12}, iron, and copper.

Gallbladder

The gallbladder (Fig. 38–16) is a saclike storage structure for bile.

Function. Bile is manufactured by the parenchymal cells (hepatocytes) of the liver and secreted by them into the bile canaliculi. The bile then travels to the hepatic duct, to the cystic duct, and then to the gallbladder for concentration (by as much as 12-fold) and storage. Upon stimulation, the gallbladder forces bile into the cystic duct, to the common bile duct, and into the duodenum. The adult gallbladder stores from 30 to 50 ml of bile. The major components of bile are bile acids, bile salts (sodium cholate and chenodenoxycholate), and pigments. The major pigment is mainly bilirubin. Other components include cholesterol, phospholipids (lecithin), alkaline phosphatase, electrolytes, and water.

Bile is responsible for the emulsification of fats and micelle formation. Inside the gallbladder, bile salts react with water, leaving a fat-soluble end to mix with cholesterol and/or lecithin. These formed particles are called micelles. Gallstones may form when the micelles become supersaturated with cholesterol. If bile salts are absent or diminished in the small intestine, normal fat digestion and absorption cannot occur. This results in fat malabsorption and steatorrhea (fatty stools). Most of the bile salts (approximately 80%) are reutilized by reabsorption in the ileum and enter the vascular system to be carried to the liver. The rest are excreted in the feces.

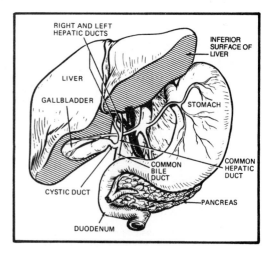

Figure 38–16. Location of the gallbladder.

Bile pigments result from the degradation of hemoglobin. These pigments give the feces its brown color. Absence of bile pigments, as with obstructive jaundice, produces a whitish-gray feces.

Normally bile pigments do not form stones. However, in some diseases, there is an overconcentration of bile pigments, resulting in precipitation of bilirubinate stones. Most of gallstones (approximately 90%) are composed essentially of cholesterol.

Bilirubin is the main bile pigment. Once red blood cells have completed their 120-day sojourn through the circulatory system, they become fragile and rupture, releasing hemoglobin. The hemoglobin is phagocytized by cells of the reticuloendothelial system and thus split into heme and globin. It is from the heme ring that bile pigments are made. Bilirubin is the first pigment to be formed; however, it is soon reduced to free bilirubin and released into the plasma. Once in the plasma, free bilirubin combines quickly with plasma albumin and becomes protein-bound free (fat-soluble) bilirubin. It is now known as unconjugated or indirect bilirubin. Free bilirubin becomes conjugated (or direct) once it is absorbed into the hepatic ducts and combines with other substances. Conjugated bilirubin is now water soluble. Approximately 80% of protein becomes conjugated with glucuronide acid to form bilirubin glucuronide. Another 10% conjugates with sulfate to form bilirubin sulfate, and the remaining 10% conjugates with still other substances. In these three forms, bilirubin is excreted into the bile and passes through the bile ducts. From this point on, bilirubin is found in the plasma, intestinal contents, and urine.

A small amount of conjugated bilirubin formed by the hepatic cells escapes back into the plasma, creating a small portion of plasma bilirubin as conjugated rather than free. Most of the bilirubin passes into the intestines, where bacterial action produces urobilinogen. Some urobilinogen is reabsorbed by the portal blood and returned to the liver, which in turn reexcretes most of this urobilinogen back into the intestines. About 5% of this urobilinogen passes into the urine and is excreted as urobilin (oxidized urobilinogen). Urobilinogen oxidized in the feces becomes stereobilinogen.

Normally the total plasma concentration of both the free and conjugated forms of bilirubin is approximately 0.5 mg per 100 ml of plasma. In normal subjects, almost all of the bilirubin in the plasma appears to be in the unconjugated form. The concentration of bilirubin in the plasma represents a balance between the rate of entry of the pigment into the plasma and the hepatic clearance of bilirubin.

With jaundice, plasma levels of both unconjugated (indirect) and conjugated (direct) bilirubin are measured. If there is either a marked increase in the rate of formation of bilirubin or a defect in any of the processes underlying the hepatic clearance of unconjugated bilirubin (e.g., liver cell dysfunction), then conjugated bilirubin will accumulate in the plasma. In contrast, impairment to biliary flow either at a canalicular or bile ductular level (e.g., biliary tract obstruction) will cause reflux of conjugated bilirubin into the plasma.

Stimulation of the Gallbladder. The sphincter of Oddi opens upon vagal and hormonal stimulation. Vagal stimulation increases bile secretions through the sphincter of Oddi. The sphincter of Oddi in a normal state remains slightly opened, providing for a constant but minuscule amount of bile to enter the small intestine.

During normal digestion, the gallbladder contracts in response to the hormone cholecystokinin, pushing increased amounts of bile through the sphincter of Oddi into the duodenum. The gallbladder does not contract when there is no stimulation by cholecystokinin (e.g., between meals or during starvation diets).

GUIDE TO GASTROINTESTINAL ELEMENTS AND DIAGNOSTIC TESTS

Table 38–1 provides a quick reference to key chemical elements in the gastrointestinal system. Tables 38–2 to 38–5 provide quick references to common gastrointestinal diagnostic tests presented in the next several chapters.

NUTRITION

EDITORS' NOTE

Under normal circumstances, human nutrition relies on a few key concepts. These concepts include minimal caloric needs (about 25 kcal/kg), minimal levels of substrate and vitamin ingestion, and ability of the gastrointestinal system to process the food. The CCRN exam traditionally has not focused heavily on nutritional concepts. This section is designed to provide enough information to cover the major current concepts of caloric need and substrate ingestion (gastrointestinal processing of food has been covered) in order to provide sufficient material for the exam. This sec-

TABLE 38-1. CHEMICAL ELEMENTS IN THE GASTROINTESTINAL TRACT

Chemical Messenger	Origin	Stimulus	Inhibitors	Action
Gastrin (endocrine)	G cells of gastric antrum; duodenal mucosa	Distention of stomach from food Presence of products from protein digestion; vagal stimulation; elevated blood levels of calcium and epinephrine	Acid in stomach	Stimulates secretion of HCl and pepsin; growth of gastric mucosa; relaxes ileocecal sphincter Promotes antral activity Stimulates parietal cells and chief cells
Secretin (endocrine)	Duodenal mucosa	Acid gastric contents entering the duodenum	Lack of acid gastric contents	Stimulates secretion of watery alkaline pancreatic fluid; stimulates pancreatic and hepatic HCO_3^-; augments action of cholecystokinin; decreases gastric acid secretion; stimulates secretion of pancreatic digestive enzymes; may inhibit gastric-emptying time
Cholecystokinin (neuroendocrine)	Duodenal mucosa	Products of protein and fat digestion entering the duodenum	Lack of stimulus	Stimulation of pancreatic enzyme secretion; stimulates gallbladder contraction caused by fat in the intestine; relaxation of the sphincter of Oddi; stimulation of pancreatic growth; inhibits gastric emptying; enhances insulin release; stimulates pepsin secretion; may weakly and selectively stimulate gastric acid secretion; stimulates motility of small bowel; augments secretion in stimulating secretion of alkaline pancreatic juice
Vasoactive intestinal peptide (neurotransmittor or neuropeptide)	Granules located in nerve terminals in the intestinal mucosa	Esophageal distention; intestinal distension; electrical vagal stimulation; intraduodenal fat or acid; serotonin; oxytocin; by intestinal ischemia	None known	Relaxation of smooth muscle; vasodilation, and stimulation of pancreatic and intestinal secretion Stimulates insulin release; intestinal secretion of electrolytes and water; inhibits gastric acid secretion; dilates peripheral blood vessels and lowers blood pressure Mediator of lower esophageal sphincter relaxation and of internal and sphincter relaxation
Gastric inhibitory hormone (endocrine)	Duodenal and jejunal mucosa	Presence of glucose and fat in the duodenum; not affected by acid Released in response to bombesin and to beta-adrenergic stimulation	Lack of stimulus	Enhances insulin release; may inhibit gastric secretion
Insulin (endocrine)	Beta cells of the islets of Langerhans in the pancreas	Presence of glucose in the gut and blood	Low glucose levels	Controls glucose metabolism in the body by controlling the entry of glucose into the fat and muscle cells; increases the quantities of amino acids available in the cells for synthesizing proteins; stimulates the formation of proteins by ribosomes; stimulates the formation of RNA in cells; presence of insulin causes the body to use carbohydrates as fat; in the absence of insulin, fatty acids are mobilized and used in place of carbohydrates
Glucagon (endocrine)	Alpha cells of the islets of Langerhans in the pancreas	Low glucose concentrations (as low as 60 mg/100 ml of blood); severe exercise and/or starvation	Normal-to-high glucose concentrations (greater than 60 mg/100 ml of blood)	Regulates blood glucose level; mobilizes glucose from the liver by glycogenolysis (break-down of the glycogen to glucose); increases gluconeogenesis (conversion of proteins to glucose) by the liver—does this by mobilizing proteins from the tissues of the body and then promotes the uptake of amino acids into the liver as well as conversion of the amino acids into glucose

462

TABLE 38–2. LIVER TESTS BASED ON DETOXIFICATION AND EXCRETORY FUNCTIONS

Type of Test	Associated Pathologies
Serum bilirubin (direct and indirect)	Increased indirect → hemolytic disorders Increased direct → liver or biliary tree disease; multiple blood transfusions; sepsis
Urine bilirubin	Indicates increased direct serum bilirubin and implies liver disease
Sodium sulfobromophthalein dye test	Indicates liver clearance function
Indocyanine green	Measures liver blood flow
Blood ammonia	Increased levels indicate hepatocellular disease and portal hypertension; detects hepatic encephalopathy
Serum bile acids	Sensitive to overall liver function

tion is not a comprehensive review of nutritional concepts. Controversial practices not supported by research (e.g., reducing diarrhea from tube feedings) are not addressed.

Caloric Needs

At rest, humans consume about 25 kcal/kg per day. A 70-kg man, for example, would consume 1750 kcal if he was on bedrest. During normal active states, the energy expended would increase to about 35 kcal/kg per day. Most critically ill patients are near the rest phase of about 25 kcal/kg/day. Temperature elevations are the most common cause of increasing energy expenditure (and caloric needs). Temperature elevations will increase energy needs by about 10% for each degree centigrade elevation.

Each patient should receive at least 25 kcal/kg per day for minimal nutritional support. There are many formulas to calculate (e.g., Harris–Benedict equation) or measure energy expenditure and caloric needs (indirect calorimetry), but for the purpose of the CCRN text, remember only the basic information on approximate caloric needs of the critically ill.

Substrates and nutrients are required in different degrees, depending on the condition of the person. For example, proteins are typically given in levels of about 1 g/kg per day. Some patients may require more than this amount, and nitrogen balance studies should be performed to better determine specific protein needs. Protein deficits, such as albumin levels and total lymphocytes, are often used to assess the severity of malnutrition. Albumin levels less than 2.5 g/dl lymphocytes below 1000 mm^3 indicate potential malnutrition. The CCRN exam, however, currently does not require in-depth knowledge regarding substrate,

TABLE 38–3. TESTS THAT MEASURE BIOSYNTHETIC FUNCTION OF THE LIVER—SERUM

Type of Test	Associated Pathologies
Albumin	Decreased levels may indicate chronic hepatocellular disorders, malnutrition, protein-losing enteropathy, inflammatory bowel disease, and nephrotic syndrome.
Serum globulins (serum protein electrophoresis)	Increased levels indicate chronic liver disease.
Coagulation factors Prothrombin time Partial thromboplastin time Fibrinogen	Elevated in hepatitis, cirrhosis, vitamin K deficiencies, malabsorption, obstructive jaundice, and treatments with broad-spectrum antibiotics
Ceruloplasmin	Elevated values are seen with inflammatory diseases such as cholestatic disorders
Ferritin	Low in iron deficiency; elevated in iron storage diseases such as hemochromatosis
Alpha-1-fetoprotein	Elevated in hepatocellular carcinoma
Serum Enzymes	
Aminotransferases SGPT SGOT	Elevated levels indicate acute hepatocellular disease.
Alkaline phosphatase 5′-Nucleotidase Gamma-glutamyltranspeptidase	Elevated in inflammation of the biliary tree

TABLE 38–4. TESTS USEFUL IN THE DIAGNOSIS OF MALABSORPTION

Type of Test	Associated Pathologies
Stool fat	Steatorrhea
Xylose absorption	Disorders affecting the mucosa of the proximal small intestine
Small intestine biopsy	Value of the differential diagnosis of malabsorption
Schilling's test for vitamin B_{12} absorption	Abnormal in disorders affecting the ileum such as regional enteritis and lymphomas
Secretin test	Used in a diagnosis of pancreatic insufficiency
Serum calcium, albumin, cholesterol, magnesium, and iron	Low level may be indicative of malabsorption.
Serum carotenes, vitamin A, and prothrombin time	May indicate malabsorption of the fat-soluble vitamins
Breath tests (hydrogen and bile acid)	Abnormal hydrogen breath test indicates lactase deficiency. Abnormal bile acid breath test indicates bacterial overgrowth syndromes.
Pancreatic Function Tests	
Amylase	Increased levels are associated with pancreatitis.

TABLE 38–5. GASTROINTESTINAL AND RADIOLOGIC STUDIES

Upper gastrointestinal series	Barium and/or gas is taken orally to show structural or functional problems of the esophagus and stomach. Barium is usually followed through the small bowel with roentgenograms to determine its rate of passage and to look for structural abnormalities.
Lower gastrointestinal series (barium enema)	The large colon is studied with barium and/or gas given per rectum. Sufficient barium and/or gas is given to distend the bowel and show any abnormalities in structure or a tumor.
Cholangiography	Oral cholangiography is based on the ability of the liver to extract from the blood a radiopaque dye that has been absorbed from the intestinal tract and then secrete it into bile. Indicates gallbladder disease. Intravenous cholangiography is based on the slow intravenous injection of a radiopaque dye, its extraction from blood by the liver, and then its rapid excretion into bile. Indicates cystic duct obstruction, most likely from gallstones.
Endoscopy (upper gastrointestinal endoscopy, colonoscopy, proctosigmoidoscopy, and fiberoptic sigmoidoscopy)	Endoscopy is the visualization of the inside of the body cavity by means of a lighted tube. Useful in diagnosing mass lesions, ulcers, strictures, dyspepsia, heartburn, bleeding, or cancers. Also used for biopsies and removal of foreign objects. Widely being used therapeutically for sclerosing, polyp removal, heater probe therapy, and removal of gallstones from the common bile duct.
Percutaneous transhepatic cholangiography	Performed by inserting a long needle into the liver percutaneously, and injecting radiopaque dye into the bile duct. Useful in diagnosing obstructive jaundice.
Endoscopic retrograde cholangiopancreatography	The ampulla of Vater is cannulated through a side-viewing endoscope. A radiopaque dye is injected, and both the pancreatic and bile ducts can be visualized. Allows for diagnosing obstruction, malignancy, and inflammation. Endoscopic sphincterotomy and extraction of gallstones may also be performed.
Percutaneous liver biopsy	Puncture of the liver to diagnose hepatocellular disease, prolonged hepatitis, hepatomegaly, hepatic filling defects, fever, and staging of lymphoma
Angiography	The femoral artery is entered with a large needle that is then exchanged with a catheter that is passed into the celiac artery or one of its branches (superior mesenteric or hepatic). The contrast medium is injected, and films are taken. This procedure allows visualization of the visceral vessels to identify abnormalities of vascular structure and function, to visualize masses, and to note sites of bleeding.
Computed tomography scan	Noninvasive procedure used in identifying masses. Provides a three-dimensional image.
Ultrasound	Noninvasive procedure using sound waves to outline the pancreas, liver, gallbladder, and spleen. It will distinguish fluid from solid structures and will show an abscess or the volume of fluid present in ascites.
Esophageal manometry	Contractions generated by the esophageal wall are measured as luminal pressures. Useful in the evaluation of achalasia, diffuse spasm, scleroderma, and other motility disorders.
Hepatobiliary Imaging	Noninvasive nuclear medicine scan allowing visualization of extra hepatic biliary system and hepatic takeup and excretion of isotope.
Tagged RBC scan	Noninvasive nuclear medicine scan used to assess isotope "tagged" RBCs leakage in acute gastrointestinal hemorrhage.

trace elements, or electrolyte concentrations as they relate to nutrition.

For the purpose of the test, information regarding basic nutritional support methods may be required. Enteral feedings, with the exception of solutions such as Pulmocare and Magnacal, usually have about 1 kcal/ml. Common formulas such as Osmolite, Ensure, and Jevity all have about 1 kcal/ml. Proper nutrition for a 70-kg man would require 1750 ml of full-strength enteral feeding (based on 25 kcal/kg and 1750 cc of enteral feeding = 1750 kcal).

Some enteral preparations have increased caloric values. Pulmocare and Magnacal, for example, have about 2 kcal/ml. In addition, some formulas, such as Pulmocare, have a potential advantage in the higher lipid concentration and subsequent reduced production of carbon dioxide. The reduced carbon dioxide production in theory reduces the stimulation to breathe. Patients with difficulty weaning from mechanical ventilation may do better with a diet high in lipids as a consequence of a lessening of the drive to breathe.

Parenteral solutions have the ability to give higher levels of calories and substrates. Fifty percent dextrose (D_{50}) can give ten times the calories provided by D_5W. One liter of D_{50} can give about 1700 kcal, providing almost all caloric needs of the patient; 500 ml of a 20% lipid solution can give about 900 kcal (based on 9 kcal per gram of lipid and 20 g/dl in the 500 ml of lipids).

Enteral solutions are preferred and should be started as soon as possible after entry into the unit. If the gastrointestinal system is unable to process food, parenteral solutions could be employed as a supplement or replacement for enteral feedings. Complications of enteral feedings, such as diarrhea, may require reduction in enteral volume with supplementation of parenteral solutions. Because of their high osmolality, parenteral solutions must usually be administered in a central vein. Some parenteral preparations, such as $D_{20}W$ or lipids, can be given peripherally. A common practice recently developed is the mixing of all parenteral solutions in a single intravenous bag.

Gastrointestinal Hemorrhage and Esophageal Varices

The content of this chapter addresses the CCRN exam items of acute gastrointestinal hemorrhage and to some extent portal hypertension. Expect two to four questions on the exam regarding this content area.

Hematemesis is gross vomiting of blood. The blood may be fresh, indicated by a bright red color, or may be old, having the appearance of coffee grounds, with a black color. If the blood is excreted in the stool, fresh blood will be maroon and may have clots. Old blood turns feces black (called melena). Hematochezia is the passage of bright red blood through the rectum. Bleeding from the stomach or small intestine usually manifests as melena or maroon stools; bleeding from the colon manifests as maroon or bright red stools.

GASTROINTESTINAL HEMORRHAGE

Upper gastrointestinal hemorrhage is considered to be a bleed from the stomach or small intestine. Peptic disease, the most common cause of upper gastrointestinal bleeding, refers to bleeding either from ulcers or from shallow erosions in the stomach, esophagus, or first part of the small intestine. Lower gastrointestinal hemorrhage is from the colon.

Pathophysiology

Gastrointestinal bleeding occurs when a break in the lining of the gastrointestinal tract erodes arteries, arterioles, or veins. The more serious bleeding usually occurs when arteries are eroded; however, some venous bleeding, such as bleeding from esophageal varices associated with cirrhosis, can be just as catastrophic.

Etiology

Upper gastrointestinal bleeding usually results from ulcers, erosions, acute mucosal tears, or esophageal varices. Ulcers are areas of breakdown in the wall of the gastrointestinal tract that have significant depth. Erosions (e.g., gastritis, duodenitis, or esophagitis), which also represent areas of breakdown in the wall, are much more superficial than ulcers. Approximately 80% of the ulcers are in the duodenum, with duodenal ulcers often causing bleeding.

There are multiple causes of ulcers or erosions, including excessive acid production. Medications that work by decreasing acid production through H_2 inhibition, such as cimetidine (Tagamet) and ranitidine (Zantac), are effective in healing ulcers.

Other causes, such as side effects of medicines (e.g., arthritis medicines, aspirin, and prednisone), stress ulcers associated with surgery, severe burns, head trauma, sepsis, cardiac or respiratory failure, and alcohol use, also have been shown to cause ulcers and erosions. Stress ulcers are usually thought to be from ischemia, since acid production is usually not increased. Another type of ulcer may be due to infection caused by the bacterium *Helicobacter pylori.*

Lower gastrointestinal bleeding usually results from colon tumors (e.g., cancer), diverticuli (which are outpouchings of the colon wall), or abnormal jumbles of arteries and veins (arteriovenous malformations [AVMs]).

Clinical Presentation

The great majority of ulcers and erosions do not cause bleeding. Usually the patient will present with recurring abdominal pain. The pain is usually burning or gnawing in character and is localized either below the xiphoid process, just inferior to the xiphoid in the epigastrium, or in the right upper quadrant of the abdomen. The pain is usually relieved by drinking milk or taking antacids and is usually worse between 30 min and 2 hr after eating. Alcohol, aspirin, caffeine, and spicy foods often worsen the pain.

When gastrointestinal bleeding does occur, it usually manifests either as vomiting of fresh blood or old blood that has been acted on by gastric juices ("coffee grounds") or as bloody bowel movements. A patient who has had a blood loss of less than 1 unit of blood, or 10% of the blood volume, usually will not have dizziness or orthostasis. A loss of more than 1 unit but less than 2 (10–20% of the blood volume) is associated with dizziness and orthostasis. Bleeding of more than 2 units (20% of blood volume) is often associated with shock (hypotension, cold, clammy skin, oliguria). Epigastric pain may or may not be present in gastrointestinal bleeding. A slow bleed may produce only weakness, fatigue, and pallor.

Diagnosis

Diagnosis of the probable site of a bleed can usually be made from the history and physical examination. If "coffee grounds" or blood is vomited, the site of bleeding is the esophagus, stomach, or duodenum. Maroon or red blood with or without clots passed from the rectum is usually indicative of a bleed from the colon, but a severe upper gastrointestinal bleed can sometimes manifest as passage of red blood through the rectum without vomiting of blood. Previous ulcer disease, alcohol, aspirin use, or liver disease can help determine the site of the bleed.

Passage of a nasogastric tube can sometimes be useful in assessing the site and severity of the bleed. Obtaining bright red blood indicates a more recent and usually a more severe bleed than the return of

coffee grounds. However, for a variety of reasons, the nasogastric aspirate is far from perfect for assessing either the source or severity of the bleed.

Upper endoscopy is the best test for diagnosing and possibly treating an upper gastrointestinal bleed. If done within 24 hr, it can detect the site of bleeding in a great majority of patients. Endoscopy involves passage of a long, flexible tube into the esophagus, stomach, and duodenum through which the physician can see the inside lining of the gastrointestinal tract. Sometimes, however, bleeding is massive and a good examination with an endoscope is not possible. In such a case, a radiologic study called angiography is often used.

Bleeding from the colon is often diagnosed by a combination of colonoscopy and different radiologic studies, such as the tagged red blood cell or bleeding scan.

Complications

The major complications of gastrointestinal bleeding are from the hemodynamic effects. Hypotension can cause serious organ damage, including cerebral infarction or myocardial infarction, renal failure, and intestinal infarction. All of these can be prevented if the patient has fluid and/or blood resuscitation given early enough after the onset of the bleed. Therefore, hemodynamic parameters need to be carefully monitored.

Also, aspiration of blood can cause severe respiratory difficulties, especially in unconscious or semiconscious patients. Gastrointestinal content aspiration predisposes patients to adult respiratory distress syndrome. Perforation and peritonitis occur very rarely.

Treatment

The most important aspect of treatment is the maintenance of blood pressure and circulating blood volume. This is accomplished by meticulous attention to pulse, blood pressure, and signs and symptoms of organ perfusion, such as urine output (at least 20–30 ml/hr) and mental status. Serial hemoglobin and hematocrit determinations are made to decide whether and when transfusion of blood is indicated. Large-bore intravenous access should be attained for possible blood product transfusions and also for intravenous fluids. The proper fluids to give to restore blood volume are isotonic solutions, such as normal saline or lactated Ringer's solution, or red blood cells, either as whole blood or as packed red blood cells. After multiple red cell transfusions, fresh frozen plasma or platelet transfusions may also be needed.

Iced saline lavage is controversial in the management of gastrointestinal bleeds, and its use cannot be routinely recommended. Endoscopic therapy has become an important therapeutic modality. Laser, thermal, or electrical coagulation of the bleeding ulcer or erosion has become popular in the treatment of acutely bleeding upper gastrointestinal tract lesions. Radiologic therapy, usually by angiography and infusion of vasopressin or clotting agents, and surgery are sometimes needed to manage gastrointestinal bleeding.

Medical therapy with agents such as cimetidine (Tagamet), ranitidine (Zantac), famotidine (Pepcid), sucralfate (Carafate), and antacids has become the treatment of choice for ulcers and erosions. Although no studies have shown that these agents stop bleeding, they are very effective at healing such lesions. These agents decrease acid production and raise intragastric pH. Antibiotic treatment is used on an increasingly common basis to combat infections by *H. pylori*.

Fortunately, between 80 and 90% of gastrointestinal hemorrhages cease spontaneously, with no more than medications such as cimetidine and ranitidine being used. Patients whose bleeding ceases spontaneously usually do very well, while those who need aggressive therapy are more prone to complications and risk of death.

Classic guidelines for considering surgery are transfusion requirement of greater than 4 units of blood in the first 24 hr, shock, or rebleeding. With the introduction of newer endoscopic therapies, these recommendations may change. Types of surgery may include vagotomy, pyloroplasty, and oversewing or resection of the ulcer. For stress ulcers, total gastrectomy may be needed.

Nursing Intervention

Fluid and electrolyte balance and adequate nutrition are key objectives of nursing treatment. Nursing interventions for hypovolemic shock should also be implemented.

Blood studies should include a complete blood count, type, and cross-match; electrolytes; blood urea nitrogen; and coagulation screen. One to two large-bore (14- to 16-gauge) intravenous lines should be started for rapid fluid and blood replacement.

Anticholinergic medications used to inhibit gastrointestinal action may have side effects such as dizziness, rash, mild diarrhea, leukopenia, blurred vision, headache, and urinary retention. These medications, in addition to the action of antacids, work to increase gastric pH. They will not stop bleeding.

The most important role for the nurse is to monitor the patient's hemodynamic status and observe for signs of continued bleeding. Careful attention to vital signs will guide fluid and blood replacement. Assessment of cardiac and pulmonary status will detect signs of possible fluid overload from too vigorous fluid and blood replacement, as pulmonary edema may develop.

If intra-arterial infusion of vasopressin is used, the patient must be monitored closely for bradycardia, hypotension, water intoxication, and postvasopressin diuresis. Renal status is measured by urinary output, which should be measured at least hourly and should be greater than 30 ml/hr. Tachydysrhythmias are a constant potential complication requiring monitoring and intervention as indicated.

The patency of the nasogastric tube should be maintained to monitor a recurrence of the bleed. Repeated blood from the rectum, return of red blood from a nasogastric tube, or recurrent hematemesis is an indication of continuing or recurrent hemorrhage.

Emotional support of the patient and family will help reduce stress and facilitate cooperation. As the bleeding is brought under control, reassurance will decrease the patient's fear.

ESOPHAGEAL VARICES

Esophageal varices are dilated, engorged, tortuous veins usually seen in the mid to distal esophagus. Varices are usually seen in patients with cirrhosis of the liver. Varices result from increased pressure in the portal veins (the veins that drain the stomach and the small and large intestines). With severe cirrhosis, the blood can no longer pass through the fibrotic liver and finds alternate pathways, through the veins in the distal esophagus. Being engorged, these veins are fragile and have a tendency to bleed, usually massively. Often they bleed within 12 months after they are discovered. Other causes of esophageal varices are splenic, portal, or hepatic vein thrombosis.

Clinical Presentation

Most patients with bleeding esophageal varices have signs of cirrhosis. Jaundice is often present. They usually have ascites, an abundance of intra-abdominal fluid causing abdominal distension. They often have elevated liver function tests, such as bilirubin, lactic dehydrogenase, transaminases (SGOT, SGPT), alkaline phosphatase, and prothrombin time.

Patients usually bleed massively and painlessly, with signs of shock present. They often become disoriented or lapse into coma as a complication of the bleeding and underlying cirrhosis.

Diagnosis

Diagnosis usually requires endoscopy since patients with cirrhosis often will not be bleeding from varices but rather from ulcerations in the esophagus, stomach, or duodenum. The history, physical examination, and laboratory blood studies are suggestive of cirrhosis.

Treatment

Treatment of esophageal varices is frustrating, as the bleeding is difficult to control and often recurs days to months later if initial control is achieved. Initially treatment includes control of shock and maintaining the patient's cardiopulmonary status. Endotracheal intubation may be necessary. Further treatment can be divided into five categories: medical, endoscopic, surgical, radiologic, and balloon tamponade.

Medical Therapy

Medical therapy of a continuous intravenous infusion of vasopressin (Pitressin) is often effective. Vasopressin often is the drug used first. Vasopressin works by reducing portal venous pressure. The dosage is 0.2 to 0.4 unit/min. Vasopressin can cause serious cardiac ischemia and should be used with caution in patients with coronary artery disease. For patients who are receiving intra-arterial vasopressin, cardiac monitoring and frequent neurological assessments are performed because this drug is a very potent vasoconstrictor. Amyl nitrate, an antagonist vasodilator, should be at the bedside so that it is readily accessible if indications of angina pectoris, myocardial infarction, or encephalopathy occur. Patients with known coronary artery disease may be placed on nitroglycerin prophylactically.

Endoscopic Therapy

Endoscopic therapy consists of injecting a sclerosing, fibrosing agent, such as sodium tetradecyl sulfate, into the bleeding vein through the endoscope by a 23-gauge needle. Often effective, sclerotherapy requires considerable expertise in the actively bleeding patient.

Interventional Radiology (Transjugular Intrahepatic Portosystemic Shunt)

The transjugular intrahepatic portosystemic shunt (TIPS) is an interventional radiological procedure that uses the normal vascular anatomy of the liver to create a shunt between the portal and systemic venous systems within the liver (Fig. 39–1). The procedure involves jugular vein access, hepatic vein sheath placement, and portal vein identification. A tract is made through the liver parenchyma between the hepatic and portal veins. The tract is enlarged via balloon dilatation and a metallic stent is deployed, allowing blood to flow from the portal vein to the hepatic vein. Portal hypertension is reduced, minimizing the incidence of variceal bleeding, and has resulted in reduction in mortality rate compared to surgical shunt procedures.

Surgical Therapy

Portosystemic shunt surgery, aimed at bypassing the liver to lower pressure in the varices, is usually effective in stopping bleeding but can carry a 50% higher mortality in acutely bleeding patients.

Radiologic Therapy

Radiologic procedures, though available, are seldom used nowadays in the management of acute variceal hemorrhage.

Balloon Therapy

Balloon tamponade, using versions of the Sengstaken–Blakemore (SB) (Fig. 39–2) or Linton tube, is often effective in stopping acute bleeding. Unfortunately, there is a high incidence of rebleeding once these tubes are removed. These tubes are placed through the nose or mouth into the stomach. They utilize balloons in the early part of the stomach and/or esophagus to place pressure on the bleeding veins. These tubes, however, are fraught with dangers. Aspiration of blood, occlusion of the airway, esophageal necrosis, and esophageal rupture are all potential complications. Balloon pressures must be monitored carefully to prevent or recognize these complications early.

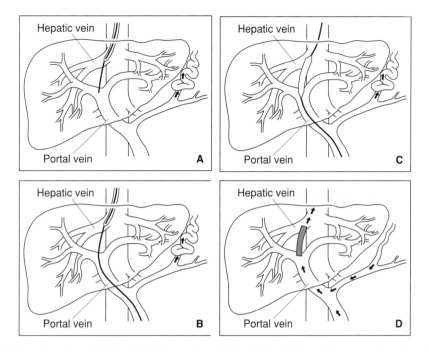

Figure 39–1. Transjugular intrahepatic portosystemic shunt (TIPS) procedure. **(A)** Needle directed through liver parenchyma to portal vein. **(B)** Guidewire passage. **(C)** Balloon dilatation. **(D)** Placement of stent. (Reprinted from the American Medical Association (1991). *JAMA, 266*, 391).

Nursing Intervention

A primary objective of nursing intervention is to control the bleeding to prevent or reverse hypovolemic shock. Attention to the patient's hemodynamic status is crucial. Monitoring electrolyte balance, fluid balance, and nutritional needs will enable early intervention if a problem appears imminent.

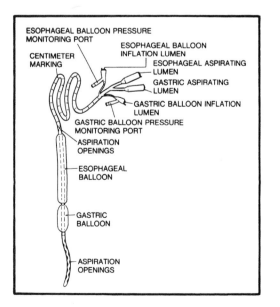

Figure 39–2. Sengstaken–Blakemore tube.

A patient with an SB or Linton tube to provide tamponade is continually observed for signs of asphyxiation or aspiration. These tubes can migrate and occlude the airway, or the patient may aspirate either blood or secretions into the lungs. Suctioning of pharyngeal secretion is required often. If suctioning does not improve the patient's respiratory status, check for breath sounds in the lungs. If no sounds are heard, most often the tube has slipped and is occluding the trachea. The nurse must immediately cut across all three tubes and remove the SB or Linton tube. For this emergency, scissors are often taped to the head of the bed. Many patients with an SB or Linton tube will be prophylactically intubated to prevent airway occlusion. The mortality rate is high for this disease, approaching 33% for all patients with variceal bleeding, despite optimal medical and nursing therapy.

LOWER GASTROINTESTINAL BLEEDING

Etiology

The three major causes of lower gastrointestinal bleeding are diverticulosis, AVMs, and colonic polyps or tumors.

Diverticulosis

Colonic diverticulosis is the presence of outpouchings, usually multiple and most often in the left side of the colon. Diverticulosis is thought partially to result from a relative deficiency of fiber in the American diet. It is very common in the United States, with approximately one-third of the population over the age of 60 affected. It usually is asymptomatic, but the diverticuli can become infected or bleed. The bleeding is usually painless and can be massive. The blood almost always appears red exiting the rectum. Therapy again consists of supporting hemodynamic status via fluids and often blood products, and most often bleeding ceases spontaneously. Diagnosis is usually made by colonoscopy or barium enema examination. Radiologic therapy by angiography and intra-arterial infusion of vasopressin to decrease blood flow to the affected bowel is often effective but rarely needed. Surgery in the form of partial colonic resection is also sometimes necessary to control diverticular hemorrhage. Presently, there is no effective endoscopic therapy.

Arteriovenous Malformations

AVMs, also called angiodysplasia, are closely packed tangles of arteries and veins that have a tendency to bleed. They are usually located on the right side of the colon but can be present anywhere in the colon, small intestine, or stomach. They are a very common cause of lower gastrointestinal bleeding. Diagnosis is usually by colonoscopy, with bright red areas seen on the normally pink colon wall. They can also be noted by angiography, but not by barium enema examination. Therapy is possible with endoscopic laser, thermal, or electric coagulation using a small tube introduced through the colonoscope. Angiographic therapy with intra-arterial vasopressin infusion and surgical resection of the affected portion of the colon are also sometimes necessary. As with diverticulosis, bleeding usually ceases spontaneously. Initial therapy is aimed at stabilizing the patient's hemodynamic status.

Colon Polyps or Tumors

Colon tumors, such as cancer, or polyps, which are thought to be a premalignant growth, are usually asymptomatic. They often bleed, but usually very slowly. These lesions are slightly more likely than diverticuli or AVMs to produce pain with bleeding. Diagnosis is usually by colonoscopy or barium enema. Therapy is with either colonoscopic or surgical removal. As with any gastrointestinal hemorrhage, initial therapy is aimed at stabilizing the patient hemodynamically.

NURSING INTERVENTION

Nursing management of patients with lower gastrointestinal bleeding is aimed at assessment of hemodynamic status. Careful assessment of vital signs, signs of hypovolemic shock, blood cell counts, coagulation studies, and electrolytes should be done frequently. Fluid and electrolyte losses should be replaced. Patients receiving intra-arterial vasopressin should be monitored for cardiac and neurological abnormalities.

Hepatitis, Cirrhosis, Hepatic Failure, and Acute Pancreatitis

EDITORS' NOTE

The content of this chapter addresses the CCRN exam test area including hepatic failure, hepatitis, cirrhosis, and pancreatitis. Expect one to three questions regarding this content area.

HEPATITIS

Viral hepatitis is hepatic inflammation caused by a variety of different viruses with a propensity to infect the liver. The major viruses have specific characteristics that help to differentiate the diseases that they cause. The four major groups of viruses causing viral hepatitis are hepatitis A, hepatitis B, hepatitis D (delta hepatitis), and hepatitis C viruses.

Hepatitis A

Hepatitis A virus (HAV) is an RNA picornavirus that is excreted through the feces of infected individuals. It is spread through fecal–oral contact and is common in developing countries with poor sanitation. Ingestion of clams or oysters has been associated with occasional epidemics. It is a very common infection, with most infections in developing countries occurring early in life. Hepatitis A is often misdiagnosed as a gastroenteritis. Immunity after infection is lifelong. In adults with no prior immunization, the illness is more severe and usually icteric.

The incubation period is between 15 and 50 days. There are two phases of symptoms. The prodromal phase, occurring 2–7 days before the icteric phase, consists of symptoms such as fatigue, nausea, vomiting, and low-grade fever. The icteric phase, usually lasting between 1 and 4 weeks, follows. The icteric phase symptoms consist of darkened urine, light stools, and jaundice. Pruritis is not usually marked. Associated symptoms include anorexia, nausea, vomiting, fever, and relatively mild abdominal pain. A diffuse rash may be present.

The most profound changes are in the liver function tests. Transaminases (SGOT, SGPT) rise dramatically, often into the thousands. Alkaline phosphatase also rises, but usually not to a similar degree. Bilirubin levels can range from normal to markedly elevated. Bilirubinuria is often present. Leukopenia is often seen, as is a mild anemia. Stools can be light colored, and steatorrhea may be present.

Patients are usually fully recovered within anywhere from 6 weeks to 3 months, but may have vague symptoms for up to a year. Rarely, fulminant hepatic failure and death occur. Mortality rates in large epidemics are approximately 19%. Hepatitis A has no progression to chronicity. The virus is excreted in the feces for up to 2 weeks before the icteric period and usually disappears prior to the resolution of the clinical hepatitis. Patients with acute hepatitis A should be placed on enteric precautions.

The antibody response to HAV is the key to diagnosis. The virus elicits both an IgM and an IgG antibody response. HAV-IgM appears in the acute infection and persists for 2–6 months. Detection of HAV-IgM is therefore indicative of infection within the last 6 months. IgG also appears in acute infection but persists for years. Therefore, the presence of IgG indicates a recent or past infection and probably ensures lifelong immunity.

Immune serum globulin is recommended for close personal contacts of an infected patient and in all those exposed to the food and water in an identified epidemic. This treatment has been shown to reduce the rate of infection in exposed subjects.

Hepatitis B

Hepatitis B virus (HBV) is a DNA virus. It consists of a protein coat (known as the surface antigen [HbsAg]), and a core, which contains the double-stranded circular DNA, the e antigen (HbeAg), the core antigen (HbcAg), and the DNA polymerase. Each of these can be detected either in the liver itself or the circulating blood, and various antigens and antibodies have clinical relevance. HBsAg in the blood indicates either an acute or a chronic continuing infection. Surface antibody (HBsAb), however, indicates a resolved infection. HBeAg is associated with a high risk of infectivity and correlates with ongoing viral synthesis. It usually appears transiently during an acute attack. E antibody (HBeAb) is a marker of low infectivity and persists for a few months after the acute infection resolves. HBcAg is not currently detectable, but core antibody (HBcAb) is. IgM HBcAb indicates either acute or chronic infection, and IgG HBcAb is usually a marker for a past, nonactive infection.

Hepatitis B is usually transmitted through blood, but it can also be transmitted through saliva and sperm. It used to be a common cause of transfusion-associated hepatitis, but with present serologic screening of donors, hepatitis B is only rarely transmitted through blood transfusions. Major risk groups for hepatitis B are homosexuals, intravenous drug users, institutionalized persons, and health care professionals.

The incubation period for HBV infection is generally 6–9 weeks. The patient usually is infectious both 1–2 weeks before and during the icteric phase. A serum sickness prodrome may occur, with symptoms such as rash and arthralgias. The clinical course can vary between mild and severe or can be asymptomatic. Fulminant hepatic failure and death can result. Symptoms and laboratory findings are similar to those for hepatitis A. The major difference between hepatitis A and hepatitis B is the 10% rate of chronicity in hepatitis B. While usually asympto-

matic, this condition can lead to cirrhosis or hepatocellular carcinoma.

Therapy for acute hepatitis B is supportive once the infection is established. Prevention is the main focus, as no effective therapy to eradicate the infection exists. Presently there is a very effective vaccine to prevent hepatitis B infection that is composed of the surface antigen. Response to the vaccine and protection against infection are usually excellent. The vaccine is recommended for persons in the previously mentioned high-risk groups.

Persons exposed to hepatitis B, as in accidental needle sticks, should have hepatitis serologies checked. If they are HBsAg and HBsAb negative, then they should be given hepatitis B immune globulin (HBIG). In addition, the hepatitis B vaccine should be given. HBIG needs to be given only once, but the vaccine should be given again in 1 and 6 months. If the HBsAb is positive, the person exposed is already immune, and neither HBIG nor the vaccine need be given. If the HBsAg is positive, the individual is already infected and should be evaluated for acute or chronic hepatitis. Blood and body fluid precautions should be followed when dealing with infected individuals.

Health care workers in high-risk fields, such as intensive care unit nurses and physicians, dialysis staff, and laboratory workers, should be given the hepatitis B vaccine even if no known exposure has occurred. No transmission of infections such as acquired immunodeficiency syndrome has been documented to occur from vaccination.

Hepatitis D

Hepatitis D virus, also called delta hepatitis virus, is a viral particle. It is an RNA virus that infects only patients with coexistent hepatitis B infection. Therefore, a patient may have both hepatitis D and hepatitis B but cannot have hepatitis D alone. It can superinfect patients with either acute or chronic hepatitis B.

Delta hepatitis is uncommon. When present with acute hepatitis B, it usually causes a much more severe clinical hepatitis. Delta hepatitis infection of patients with chronic hepatitis B usually results in an acute exacerbation or worsening of symptoms, in addition to increases in liver function tests.

Because delta hepatitis requires infection with hepatitis B, the way to prevent infection is through immunization of groups at high risk of contracting hepatitis B. At present, there is no vaccine solely for hepatitis D and no satisfactory therapy.

Hepatitis C

Hepatitis C virus, an RNA virus, is the major cause of transfusion-associated hepatitis today. The incubation period varies but is usually about 7 weeks. Many of the infections are asymptomatic; when they are symptomatic, the disease is usually mild. Often the infection is diagnosed by screening liver function tests in an otherwise asymptomatic patient who has received a recent blood transfusion. The clinical manifestations are the same as for a mild case of hepatitis A or B.

Although usually spread through the blood by such means as blood transfusions, clotting factor transfusions, and sharing of needles by drug abusers, some cases have no such risk factors. Sexual transmission is also possible. Rare epidemics from food or water sources have also been described.

Although the initial clinical disease is usually mild, there is a high propensity for the infection to become chronic. It is estimated that up to 50% of acute infections, many of which are asymptomatic, lead to chronic hepatitis and sometimes to cirrhosis.

Hepatitis C antibody can detect chronic, but not acute, cases. Interferon therapy has been shown to be effective in some chronic hepatitis C infections.

Nursing Interventions

Nursing priorities are aimed at reducing demands on the liver while promoting patient well-being, minimizing disturbance in self-concept due to communicability of disease, relieving symptoms and increasing patient comfort, promoting patient understanding of the disease process and rationale of treatment, and being aware of potential complications such as hemorrhage, hepatic coma, and permanent liver damage.

Placing the patient on bedrest with good skin care, providing a quiet environment by possibly limiting visitors, pacing activities, and increasing activity as tolerated can be interventions to prevent decreased mobility from decreased energy metabolism by the liver, activity restrictions, pain, and depression.

Nutritional monitoring is important because of anorexia, nausea, and vomiting from visceral reflexes that may reduce peristalsis. Bile stasis as well as altered absorption and metabolism of ingested foods may also produce these symptoms. Diet is ordered according to the patient's need and tolerance. A low-fat, high-carbohydrate diet is most palatable to the anorexic patient. Protein should be given in low quantities. Counsel the patient to avoid alcoholic beverages. Accurate intake and outputs may be necessary because of severe continuing vomiting and diarrhea. Adequate hydration with intravenous fluids may be necessary. Serum electrolytes must also be monitored.

Particular attention must be paid to the patient's self-concept. Isolation measures are necessary to prevent cross-contamination. Annoying symptoms, confinement, isolation, and length of illness may lead to feelings of depression. Universal precautions should be used by healthcare workers with any patient contact. In addition, members of the healthcare team should have knowledge of patients with acute hepatitis. Patients with acute hepatitis A must be on enteric precautions. Allow times with the patient for listening. Offer diversional activities based on energy levels.

Assess the patient's level of understanding of the disease process and provide specific information regarding prevention and transmission of the disease. Contacts may receive gamma globulin; personal items should not be shared; strict handwashing and sanitizing of clothes, dishes, and toilet facilities are necessary. While liver enzymes are elevated, avoid mucous membrane contact; blood donations should be discouraged. Discuss the side effects of and dangers of taking over-the-counter drugs and prescribed medications. Emphasis should be placed on the importance of follow-up physical examination and laboratory evaluation.

CIRRHOSIS

Cirrhosis is the end stage of many types of liver disease. Basically, cirrhosis is defined as the abnormal fibrous regeneration of the liver, usually in response to chronic damage.

Types and Etiology

There are two major categories of cirrhosis, micronodular and macronodular. The distinction between the two is the size of the regenerating nodules. There are distinct causes under each category, but there can be overlap, with different diseases potentially causing either type. Cirrhosis usually results in increased resistance to blood flow through the liver and failure of the hepatic cells to function properly.

Micronodular cirrhosis is the most common type, and alcoholism is the most common cause of this type of cirrhosis in the United States. However, for unexplained reasons, only a minority of alcoholics develop cirrhosis. Cirrhosis is very unusual with less than 5 years of alcohol abuse, demonstrating that chronic injury is usually necessary for cirrhosis to develop. Alcohol itself directly injures liver cells, but other factors influence the development of cirrhosis.

Macronodular cirrhosis results from any of a variety of causes. Viral hepatitis B is the most common cause of this type of cirrhosis worldwide. Other causes include other types of infection, biliary cirrhosis, iron or copper overload, autoimmune diseases, and idiopathic or cryptogenic cirrhosis. Viral hepatitis A does not progress to cirrhosis.

All types of cirrhosis generally produce a firm, shrunken liver, although at times the liver can be enlarged. Fibrosis, or scarring, is prominent. Splenomegaly can also be present. The scarring provides resistance to normal blood flow through the liver. Loss of hepatocytes can result in hepatic failure.

Clinical Presentation

Usually patients present with gastrointestinal bleeding (often massive), ascites, jaundice, or abnormalities detected on routine blood testing. The patients may have weight loss, poor nutrition, and a history of alcohol abuse. Some patients may have no obvious signs of cirrhosis.

Ascites is usually present in moderate to advanced cirrhosis. The patient notes increased abdominal girth, a discomfort in the abdomen, and often pedal or ankle edema. Numerous factors are involved in ascites formation, including (1) low albumin level (the cirrhotic liver is often unable to make adequate albumin); (2) portal hypertension, resulting in leakage of fluid into the peritoneal cavity and poor fluid resorption; and (3) abnormal renal responses in cirrhosis, which lead to more fluid retention.

Endocrine changes can also be seen. Gynecomastia and testicular atrophy resulting from reduced testosterone levels are often seen in males, and menstrual irregularities are often seen in females. Aldosterone and antidiuretic hormone levels are increased, causing peripheral edema and contributing to ascites formation.

Jaundice is also usually present in advanced cirrhosis. The eyes and skin generally assume a light to bright yellow discoloration as a consequence of elevated levels of bilirubin in the blood.

Other findings include a decreased or abnormal mentation, termed hepatic encephalopathy. This is often seen with an increased serum ammonia level and is caused by toxins usually filtered by the liver. Asterixis (an abnormal flapping of the hands), a hyperkinetic circulation, cyanosis, fetor hepaticus, renal failure, easy bruising, and low platelet and red and white blood cell counts may be seen. Abnormal red clusters of blood vessels on the surface of the skin, termed spider angiomata, can also occur (Fig. 40–1).

Abnormalities in the serum concentrations of the hepatic transaminases and other enzymes (SGOT, SGPT, lactate dehydrogenase, alkaline phosphatase) are usually present. Abnormal coagulation tests (prothrombin and partial thromboplastin times) are often present, since the diseased liver frequently does not make sufficient clotting factors. Acidosis can occur either from shock or from the inability of the liver to clear lactate from the blood.

Diagnosis

Abnormalities in the patient's physical examination and laboratory data (Table 40–1) suggest the diag-

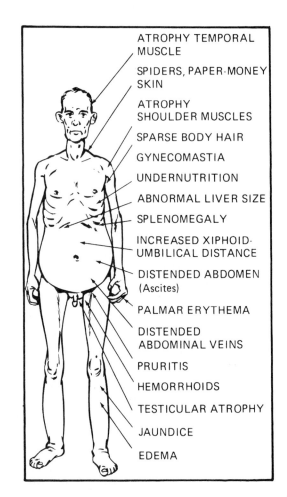

Figure 40–1. Advanced signs of cirrhosis.

TABLE 40–1. LABORATORY TESTS FOR CIRRHOSIS

Decreased Levels	Increased Levels
WBC	Globulin
Hemoglobin	Total bilirubin
Hematocrit	Alkaline phosphatase
Albumin	Transaminase
Serum sodium	Lactate dehydrogenase
Serum potassium	Urine bilirubin
Serum chloride	Fecal urobilinogen
Serum magnesium	Urine urobilinogen
Folic acid	

nosis. A liver biopsy is necessary to confirm the presence of cirrhosis and often determine the cause of the disease.

Treatment

At present, there is no satisfactory treatment to reverse cirrhosis. Treatment is aimed at decreasing any further damage, such as through the cessation of alcohol use. Different therapies, such as prednisone and interferon, are being studied. Protein restriction, fluid and salt restriction, diuretics, and vitamin K therapy are often necessary. Prevention of hepatitis B by immunizing high-risk populations is probably the most important way to decrease the prevalence of cirrhosis worldwide.

Liver transplantation, although costly and necessarily involving lifelong intense medical care, is an option for highly selected patients with cirrhosis.

Nursing Intervention

Monitor the neurological status for behavior changes, increasing lethargy, and neuromuscular dysfunction such as asterixis. Provide a safe environment (siderails up, bed in low position, restraints as needed) for patients who are not completely lucid. Avoid pharmacological sedation despite restlessness and irritable states because of decreased drug clearance. Use verbal reassurance and family involvement.

Monitor serum ammonia levels. Administer neomycin, a poorly absorbed antibiotic, which destroys the normal flora of the large intestine and decreases the formation of ammonia. Also, lactulose, a poorly absorbed sugar, which decreases the bowel pH and increases ammonia excretion through the stool, may be ordered.

Nutritional intervention is mandatory since poor nutrition is influential in the development and progression of cirrhosis. Tube feedings or total parenteral nutrition (TPN) may be necessary. Increase

protein (if there is no impending liver failure) to help regenerate liver tissue if the disease is not too far advanced. Carbohydrates should be increased (up to 2000–3000 kcal/day) to sustain weight and spare use of protein for healing. Vitamin supplements may be necessary.

Check the skin, gums, emesis, and stools often for bleeding and apply pressure at intramuscular sites. Notify the physician of the development of bleeding dyscrasias or an increase in bleeding. Assist patient to minimize trauma by avoiding the use of harsh toothbrushes, forceful nose blowing, and bodily injury.

Monitor fluid retention by weighing the patient daily. Check for dependent edema and maintain accurate intake and output records. Fluid and sodium restrictions may be necessary. Administer diuretics as required. Aldactone an aldosterone antagonist is most frequently used. Recommended diuresis is 1L/day to prevent cardiovascular compromise and hypovolemic shock.

Paracentesis may be indicated in the patient with marked ascites. Paracentesis is generally not the initial treatment of ascites. If paracentesis is performed, note the amount of fluid removed and closely monitor the patient for signs of shock.

Monitor respiratory status for signs of ineffective breathing patterns. General debilitated states place patients at risk for acquired infections. Pressure on the diaphragm due to ascites causes reduced lung volumes, and hypoxemia may occur. Semi-Fowler's or high-Fowler's positions may be necessary. Auscultate lung sounds and turn, position, deep breathe, and position change every 2 hr. Additional laboratory tests to monitor include arterial blood gases (ABGs) and white blood cells (WBCs).

Skin breakdown, which is not uncommon, is due to edema and pruritus. Bathe the patient with moisturizing lotion, not soap. Turn the patient regularly (at least every 2 hr) and ensure rest to prevent an energy drain.

Educate the patient and family on the importance of proper diet, avoidance of alcohol, moderate exercise, and avoidance of any drugs (including over-the-counter medications), especially aspirin, unless the physician approves their use.

HEPATIC FAILURE

Hepatic failure is the result of a very severe acute hepatitis, an advanced cirrhosis, or fatty liver. Causes of fatty liver include alcohol ingestion, starvation, obesity, diabetes mellitus, TPN, and third trimester of pregnancy. Hepatic failure indicates failure of the liver to perform adequately either part or all of its functions.

Pathophysiology

Hepatocytes perform a variety of functions. The liver has a great deal of reserve, and it is estimated that 75–90% of normal liver cell function needs to be lost before liver failure results.

With hepatic failure, the liver is unable to adequately synthesize the plasma proteins. The most commonly deficient proteins are albumin and the coagulation factors. Inadequate albumin can lead to ascites and pedal edema. Deficient coagulation factors can lead to problems of easy bleeding or bruising.

Inability to metabolize substances that the liver normally breaks down leads to increased levels of potentially toxic chemicals in the blood. One of these potentially toxic agents is ammonia (NH_3). Increased levels are seen with mental status changes, i.e., hepatic encephalopathy. Hepatic encephalopathy may be mild or may lead to full coma.

Etiology

Hepatic failure occurs either with severe acute hepatitis or in the face of a chronic cirrhosis. Toxins such as acetaminophen may also cause hepatic failure.

Various factors precipitate hepatic failure in patients with cirrhosis. These include gastrointestinal bleeding, sedatives, chemical imbalances, dehydration, infections (especially spontaneous bacterial peritonitis), alcohol intake, and different anesthetics or surgeries, especially portacaval shunts.

Clinical Presentation

Patients usually present with gastrointestinal bleeding or mental status changes. Mental status changes can be subtle, such as a mild loss in short-term memory or mild confusion, or severe, resulting in coma. In mild changes, writing usually deteriorates (patient writes above and below the line), and the ability to concentrate diminishes. An abnormal flapping of the hands (asterixis) is usually present.

Hepatic encephalopathy can be divided into five stages. Stages 1 and 2 are the early stages, with slurred speech and mild confusion. Stage 3 has marked confusion, and the patient is in a precoma stage. Stage 4 is frank coma. Stage 5 is very deep coma without response to any stimuli.

Diagnosis

Diagnosis is made by recognizing the presence of underlying liver disease and noting the changes in mental status or laboratory values stated previously. Specifically, liver function tests such as SGOT, bilirubin, alkaline phosphatase, albumin, prothrombin time, and partial thromboplastin time are abnormal. Hepatitis A, B, and C studies should be checked to exclude these three infections. The hemoglobin should be checked for signs of gastrointestinal hemorrhage, and the WBC count should be checked as a clue to the presence of infection or sepsis.

Treatment

Hepatic encephalopathy is often amenable to therapy. The most important part of therapy is to reverse any precipitating factors. Treatment consists of changing the bacterial flora of the colon, thus decreasing the production of potentially toxic agents that are absorbed into the bloodstream. Lactulose and neomycin are the two most useful agents.

Correcting electrolyte disturbances such as hypokalemia, protein restriction, and therapy of gastrointestinal hemorrhage are also important factors of therapy. Intravascular volume should be maintained.

Nursing Intervention

Frequent assessment of the patient's neurological status is an index of the response to therapy. Administer medications as ordered, avoiding sedatives and hepatotoxic drugs (e.g., acetaminophen, amino acids). If the patient is comatose, initiate eye care to prevent corneal abrasions.

Monitor intake and output, fluid status, and electrolyte status. Signs of anemia, infection, alkalosis (increasing serum HCO_3^-), melena, or hematemesis should be reported to the physician to provide an opportunity to prevent complications.

Replace dietary protein with calories from glucose. During recovery, introduce protein in very small increments (approximately 20 g at a time). Administer nutrients through tube feedings or TPN.

Monitor respiratory status closely, especially during times of decreasing mental status. Maintain a patent airway and administer oxygen as needed.

Stop all nitrogen-containing drugs and administer neomycin and lactulose. Monitor all side effects of medications and decrease dosages as needed.

Emotional support of the patient (if alert) and the family with realistic responses to the patient's condition is appropriate and essential, since the expected outcome is poor.

ACUTE PANCREATITIS

Acute pancreatitis is an inflammatory disease of the pancreas resulting in enzymatic autodigestion of the pancreas.

Pathophysiology

Acute pancreatitis is thought to result from activation of pancreatic enzymes inside the pancreas itself. Normally, the enzymes are released from the pancreas in an inactive state and are then activated by fluids present in the duodenum. These enzymes normally digest food products, breaking down nutrients into substituents that can be absorbed by the intestinal cells.

In acute pancreatitis, the enzymes are activated before they leave the pancreatic duct and enter the duodenum. It is postulated that an obstruction, usually temporary, leads to activation of these enzymes. Once activated, they act on the pancreatic tissue, causing potentially severe damage to the pancreas. The enzyme trypsin is important mainly in the activation of other pancreatic enzymes. The enzymes phospholipase A_2 and elastase are probably the most important causes of pancreatic damage. Elastase damages blood vessel walls, and phospholipase A_2 acts on acinar cell and fat cell membranes.

Severe edema, necrosis, and hemorrhage can result in the pancreas and can spread to adjacent organs. Fat and pancreatic necrosis leads to an exudative phlegmon, or inflammatory mass, that induces hypoalbuminemia, and calcium sequestration can lead to a loss of ionized calcium.

Etiology

The two most common causes of pancreatitis are gallstones and alcohol, with alcohol the most common cause. Most alcohol-related pancreatitis occurs in heavy drinkers. Alcohol has been shown experimentally to increase the protein content of pancreatic juice, and intraductal protein plugs have been noted to form. This intraductal obstruction has been postulated to lead to activation of pancreatic enzymes. Likewise, gallstones in the distal common bile duct may block off the pancreatic duct, causing an obstruction that can lead to pancreatitis.

There are many other, less common causes of pancreatitis. Some examples are surgical or blunt trauma to the abdomen, hyperlipidemia (especially types I, IV, and V), hypercalcemia, certain drugs such as hydrochlorothiazide, ulcers in the stomach or duodenum, and certain infections. A considerable percentage of cases of acute pancreatitis do not have an identifiable cause and are known as idiopathic.

Clinical Presentation

Pain is the universal symptom. Usually the pain is in the epigastrium and radiates through to the back. The pain can be severe and is eased by sitting forward. Although intense abdominal tenderness may be present, guarding and rebound tenderness are usually not found. The abdomen may also be distended, and bowel sounds may be decreased or absent, as in an ileus pattern. Vomiting is often present, sometimes accompanied by fever, tachycardia, and hypotension. Pleural effusions, usually small, or atelectasis may be present.

Four specific physical findings deserve mention. Grey–Turner's sign (ecchymoses in the flanks) and Cullen's sign (ecchymoses around the umbilicus) are due to hemorrhage and induration. Chvostek's sign (facial muscle twitching when the cheek is tapped) and Trousseau's sign (spasm of the hand with inflation of a blood pressure cuff over systolic blood pressure for greater than 3 min) are manifestations of hypocalcemia.

Diagnosis

Diagnosis is made by the clinical presentation discussed above and an elevated level of amylase or lipase, both pancreatic enzymes, on a serum sample (Table 40–2). Urinary amylase or a urinary amylase/creatinine ratio may also be elevated, but these

---

TABLE 40–2. LABORATORY TESTS TO DIAGNOSE PANCREATITIS

Markedly elevated serum amylase levels, often over 500 units.

Characteristically, amylase levels return to normal 48 hours after onset of pancreatitis.

Supportive laboratory values include:
1. Increased serum lipase levels
2. Low serum calcium (hypocalcemia)
3. WBC counts ranging from 8,000 to 20,000/mm³, with increased polymorphonuclear cells
4. Elevated glucose levels as high as 500–900 mg/100 ml

---

measurements are rarely necessary. Liver function tests are often elevated, usually to a minor degree. Severe cases often have hypocalcemia, anemia, leukocytosis, hypoxemia, hypoalbuminemia, and hyperglycemia.

Other diseases that can be confused with pancreatitis include cholecystitis, ulcers, and myocardial infarction. Amylase measurement usually leads to the correct diagnosis.

Complications

Pancreatitis is a serious disease, and death can result in severe cases. Complications that can lead to major morbidity or mortality include hyperglycemia, hypocalcemia, renal failure, adult respiratory distress syndrome, infection, hypotension, blood coagulation disorders, abscess formation, fistula formation, and pancreatic pseudocyst formation.

Treatment

Treatment involves maintaining the cardiorespiratory status, placing the pancreas at rest, and careful observation and early treatment of any complications that may develop. Monitoring in an intensive care unit may be needed for more serious cases, as well as pulmonary artery (Swan–Ganz) catheter insertion to maintain optimal intravascular blood volume.

The pancreas is placed at rest by strict adherence to an NPO (nil per os, nothing by mouth) regime and often by nasogastric (NG) suction. Pain is treated by meperidine (Demerol) because morphine theoretically may worsen pancreatitis by raising the pressure in the pancreatic duct. Diazepam (Valium) or chlordiazepoxide (Librium) is often needed in alcoholics to prevent delirium tremens. Somatostatin, which inhibits release of pancreatic polypeptides, is often used.

Surgery is infrequently needed, and only acutely in severe pancreatitis. Different techniques used are surgical drainage of abscesses, pancreatic lavage, and subtotal or total pancreatectomy. These procedures carry high morbidity and mortality.

Nursing Intervention

In acute cases, pancreatitis is life threatening and requires both vigorous treatment and nursing care. All vital signs are checked at least hourly. Intake and output should be documented carefully. Insensible losses should be taken into account. Monitor laboratory values such as hematocrit and hemoglobin, blood urea nitrogen, serum protein, creatinine, and electrolytes. Urine should be tested for glucose and acetone. If urine tests positive for glucose, serum glucose should be checked for hyperglycemia. Insulin should be used judiciously.

Observe for muscular twitching, jerking, or irritability. Frequent vomiting and/or gastric suctioning may cause loss of electrolytes, with the possible development of tetany. Calcium is lost because it binds to the fatty acids and is lost in the stool.

Respiratory status is monitored by arterial oxygen saturation levels and arterial blood gases, and hourly auscultation of lungs for crackles, wheezing, and diminished breath sounds. Cardiac monitoring is essential to detect dysrhythmias, which are frequent with shock and/or electrolyte imbalances.

A NG tube is sometimes inserted and connected to suction to prevent a buildup of acid secretions in the stomach. Observe and record color, amount, and nature of NG drainage as well as pH and if blood is present. Mouth and nose care should be given hourly, especially if anticholinergic drugs are administered.

Nutritional support is very important. TPN should be administered in severe cases so as to not stimulate the gastrointestinal tract. Small amounts of clear liquids are allowed when the patient can tolerate the NG tube clamped. Eventually a bland high-protein, high-carbohydrate, low-fat diet with frequent small meals is recommended. Antacids and replacement enzymes should be given.

Medicate the patient to alleviate pain. Give meperidine rather than opiates because opiates produce spasms of the biliary and pancreatic ducts. Observe for side effects of all medications, especially antibiotics.

Emotional support is very important because the pain is severe, the NG tube is uncomfortable, and the monitoring equipment increases apprehension.

Intestinal Infarction, Obstruction, Perforation, and Trauma

EDITORS' NOTE

This chapter addresses the areas of the CCRN exam on bowel infarction, obstruction, perforation, and trauma. Expect one to three questions on the exam in this content area.

INTESTINAL INFARCTION

The intestinal tract receives a rich blood supply. Three major vascular trunks from the aorta supply the intestinal tract: the celiac axis and the superior and inferior mesenteric arteries. Since there is much collateral flow, gradual occlusion of even two of these three major trunks usually does not cause clinical difficulties. Up to 20% of cardiac output after meals is delivered to the intestinal tract.

Because of this rich collateral circulation, mesenteric or intestinal infarction is unusual. Many patients have extensive atherosclerosis of the aorta and intestinal branches, but few have ischemia or infarction.

Pathophysiology and Etiology

Mesenteric ischemia usually results from one of two processes. In the first process, termed occlusive, cardiac output is usually adequate, but an embolus can dislodge from either the heart or aorta and flow into the superior mesenteric artery, lodging a short distance from the aorta and totally occluding blood flow in this area. Another cause could be an acute thrombosis in a vessel with atherosclerosis, much as one sees with coronary occlusion. The result from this sudden occlusion is infarction of part or all of the small intestine and possibly some of the colon. With this sudden occlusion, the collateral circulation is unable to compensate by increasing blood flow to the ischemic bowel.

The second major type, termed nonocclusive, is related to atherosclerosis of the intestinal vasculature. Already there is narrowing of the blood vessels, but in the normal state these narrowings are not clinically significant. When cardiac output or blood pressure is compromised, such as in dehydration, myocardial infarction, atrial fibrillation, or shock from any cause, overall blood supply to the intestines may diminish below a critical level, at which point intestinal infarction can occur. In this type of infarction, the intestinal ischemia is secondary to an overall reduction in cardiac output.

Consequences of either type of ischemia in the intestines are similar. In milder cases, only the mucosa is affected, with sloughing of the mucosa, bleeding, and abdominal pain. With severe ischemia, the submucosal and muscular layers of the intestine can be involved. If the injury is severe, transmural bowel necrosis and perforation can occur. With transmural necrosis, peritonitis will result, and intestinal bacteria enter the bloodstream, causing sepsis. In these circumstances, the disease is usually fatal.

Clinical Presentation

Occlusive mesenteric ischemia usually presents dramatically. The patient often experiences the sudden onset of severe abdominal pain, usually located in the periumbilical area or the epigastrium. There is usually diaphoresis, and the patient prefers to sit up, being more uncomfortable when forced to lie still. The abdomen, in contrast to the impressive appearance of the patient, usually has little tenderness. Guarding, rigidity, and rebound tenderness are usually absent. If diagnosis and treatment are delayed, peritonitis and intestinal perforation result.

Nonocclusive mesenteric infarction, in contrast, does not present dramatically. Often the patient is hospitalized for other diseases. Intestinal infarction is usually preceded by a vague abdominal discomfort with few physical findings. Routine diagnostic studies undertaken for other causes of abdominal pain, such as ultrasound, upper gastrointestinal series, and computed tomography (CT) scans, are usually negative in the course of the disease. With continuing ischemia, infarction and death usually result.

A milder form of nonocclusive ischemia can affect the colon without affecting the small bowel. In these patients, the clinical presentation is similar, but they experience bloody diarrhea and mild crampy pain. These patients usually do not go on to full-thickness infarction, perforation, and death, unlike those whose ischemia involves the small intestine as well.

Diagnosis

In occlusive disease, when the diagnosis is considered, and other causes such as perforated ulcer are excluded, the diagnosis can usually be confirmed at surgery or preoperatively by angiography. Angiography will reveal either an embolus or a thrombosis of the superior mesenteric artery, and surgery will reveal either ischemia or an infarcted small and possibly large intestine.

Nonocclusive disease is usually more difficult to diagnose. Symptoms are not as dramatic, and usually an acute surgical abdomen is not present. Blood analysis often reveals a leukocytosis, increased amylase and lactate dehydrogenase, and decreased pH and bicarbonate, all of which are nonspecific abnormalities. A CT scan may reveal air in the bowel wall or mesenteric vasculature but often is normal. Plain abdominal radiographs are usually of little help. Unfortunately, diagnosis is usually made at autopsy, at which time bowel infarction can readily be appreciated. Diagnosis can also be made during exploratory laparotomy, but at this point, chances of survival are slim.

Treatment

The treatment of occlusive disease has classically been surgical. Embolectomy or thrombectomy with or without bypass is usually performed. Surgical therapy also gives the opportunity to resect any questionable areas of intestine and to evaluate the extent of injury. There have been reports of angiographic management with infusion of thrombolytic (clot-dissolving) agents in patients considered to be poor surgical risks.

Therapy of nonocclusive disease is often also surgical. However, the underlying circulatory abnormality of poor cardiac output or hypotension should first be corrected. Early laparotomy and resection of infarcted intestine are necessary in patients whose pain does not rapidly resolve with correction of the low-flow state.

Delay in diagnosis of either type is almost always associated with a fatal outcome. Even with the diagnosis made and surgical therapy performed in a timely manner, the mortality rate is high.

Nursing Intervention

Careful and astute assessment of patients with unexplained abdominal pain is the key to recognizing intestinal infarction. Monitor the type of pain and relieving factors.

Supportive management of patients with intestinal infarction includes nasogastric suction, appropriate fluid and electrolyte replacement, and administration of antibiotics after cultures have been obtained. Treatment of shock and metabolic acidosis should be managed with fluid therapy, since alpha-stimulating amines such as dopamine can have an adverse effect on intestinal perfusion, precipitating renal failure by reducing blood flow to the kidneys. Dopamine may be used in low doses if a pressor agent is necessary.

The primary objective of initial management should be to prepare the patient for possible surgery before these complications arise. Since most patients with intestinal infarction require surgery, once intestinal stabilization is present and the patient has gone to surgery, the nurse must redirect interventions to postoperative surgical care. Postoperative gastrointestinal surgery interventions will be covered later in this chapter.

INTESTINAL OBSTRUCTION

Intestinal obstruction is one of the most common indications for abdominal surgery. Obstruction is a common problem in the adult population; the patient usually presents with crampy abdominal pain, vomiting, and decreased passage of stool or flatus from the rectum. Intestinal obstruction is divided into gastroduodenal, proximal or distal small intestinal, and colonic.

Pathophysiology

Bowel obstruction often results in problems with fluid balance. Alteration in fluid balance is due to fluid trapped in the intestine and the reduced capacity to ingest and absorb fluids. Often patients have profound dehydration from decreased intake, vomiting, and fluid trapped in the intestinal loops. Serum chemical imbalances can occur specifically with sodium, potassium, chloride, and bicarbonate.

Etiology

In adults, the most common cause of intestinal obstruction is adhesions from previous surgery. When the peritoneal cavity is explored, as in a cholecystectomy or gastric surgery, fibrous bands often form between loops of intestine. Usually these fibrous bands, otherwise known as adhesions, are asymptomatic, but often they can obstruct different segments of the small intestine.

The other major causes of intestinal obstruction in adults are hernias, tumors, and ulcers. A loop of intestine can become incarcerated in a hernia, causing an obstruction. Tumors, usually of the colon, can grow so that they completely block off the lumen of the colon and thus produce obstruction. Ulcers, usually in the distal stomach or duodenum, can also cause a blockage from scarring and fibrosis.

Other, less common causes of obstruction include infections such as diverticulitis, abscesses, inflammation, ischemia, gallstones, or some congenital anomalies.

Clinical Presentation

The presentation depends on the location and etiology of the bowel obstruction. In patients with a gastroduodenal or proximal small intestinal obstruction, vomiting and crampy epigastric pain are the major symptoms. The symptoms will occur early after the obstruction, usually within a few hours. However, if the obstruction is in the distal small intestine or colon, vague, crampy, periumbilical or diffuse abdominal pain is the initial symptom. Patients have vomiting usually hours to days after the start of the pain and may actually present for medical care before

they have any vomiting at all. Commonly, tachycardia and dizziness due to dehydration are present. Later symptoms include decreased bowel movements and gas passage.

Examination often reveals a distended abdomen with hyperresonance or tympany on percussion, sounding like a kettle drum. Bowel sounds are usually increased and high pitched (tinkling), and the abdomen may be diffusely, though usually not severe, tender. There usually is no guarding or rebound tenderness. The fluid vomited may be yellow or green in proximal small bowel obstructions, or darker and feculent-smelling in distal small bowel or colonic obstructions.

Diagnosis

Diagnosis is made on the basis of history, a careful physical examination, and routine abdominal radiographs. The radiographs will usually show dilated small bowel loops with air–fluid levels, or a horizontal line on the radiograph above which air is seen. Surgery usually allows the diagnosis of the cause of the obstruction. Barium contrast, radiographic studies, either of the upper gastrointestinal tract or via a barium enema, are sometimes used for diagnosis prior to surgical therapy.

Treatment

Treatment consists of correcting fluid and electrolyte imbalances. Intravenous fluids are given while carefully monitoring serum electrolyte concentrations, vital signs, and urine output. Passage of a nasogastric tube and applying suction to remove air and fluid can often reverse a small bowel obstruction from adhesions and should be used in virtually all cases of either proximal or distal bowel obstruction. Surgery is often necessary to break the bands of adhesions in obstructions and is almost always necessary in obstructions from tumors. If a hernia can be manually reduced, surgery may not be necessary. If bowel infarction or gangrene has occurred, intestinal resection and antibiotics are needed.

Nursing Intervention

Nursing interventions again are aimed at ensuring hemodynamic stability. Careful observation of fluid and electrolyte balances is of primary importance. Strict records of intake and output, daily weights, vital signs, and serum electrolyte concentrations are maintained.

Careful assessment of the patient's nutritional status must be done on a daily basis to prevent a catabolic state. Since the patient must have nothing by mouth, nutrition will need to be maintained by total parenteral nutrition if surgery is delayed or the obstruction does not resolve within a reasonable length of time.

Since nasogastric suction is very important in relieving a bowel obstruction, patency must always be maintained. Note consistency, type, color, amount, and pH of drainage.

As in intestinal infarction, the primary objective of initial management should be to prepare the patient for possible surgery to relieve the obstruction. Refer to gastrointestinal surgery nursing interventions for postoperative care of patients with bowel obstruction.

GASTROINTESTINAL PERFORATION

Perforation is usually a catastrophic event. The patient usually will have the sudden onset of abdominal pain and will appear very ill. Perforations occur in the stomach, duodenum, appendix, or colon. However, other areas of the gastrointestinal tract can perforate at rare times.

Pathophysiology

Perforation of the intestinal tract results in leakage of intestinal contents into the peritoneal cavity. If the stomach or duodenum perforates, ingested foodstuffs, acids, and enzymes leak into the peritoneal cavity. If the appendix or colon perforates, feces, which contain large amounts of bacteria, are released into the peritoneal cavity. Any of these substances are irritating to the peritoneum and invoke an intense inflammatory reaction, with leakage of fluid and pus into the peritoneal cavity. Fever and leukocytosis result, and severe pain is usually present when the peritoneum becomes inflamed.

Etiology

The most common cause of intestinal perforation in the United States is appendicitis. If diagnosed early, appendicitis usually will not cause perforation. If diagnosis is delayed, the inflamed appendix may rupture, causing either a diffuse or localized peritonitis. Other major causes of colonic perforations are colonic diverticulitis, which represents infection of outpouchings from the colon, or colonic tumors, which can perforate through the bowel wall. The most common cause of gastric or duodenal perforations is ulcers. Small intestinal perforations rarely occur and are usually caused by tumors, congenital malformations, penetrating trauma, or ischemia.

Clinical Presentation

Patients usually present with the acute onset of abdominal pain. The pain is likely to begin in the periumbilical area and spread throughout the abdomen. The patient prefers to lie still, flat on the back, as movement usually accentuates the pain. Fever is often present, respirations are shallow, and a tachycardia may be present. Hypovolemia may be present and manifested as hypotension. Hypovolemia is secondary to fluid exudation into the peritoneal cavity and sequestration in the intestines from an ileus. The patient is often diaphoretic and looks moderately ill. Abdominal exam often reveals a boardlike abdomen with absent bowel sounds. Diffuse tenderness with muscle rigidity and rebound tenderness may be present. In the case of a local perforation that walls off, as occasionally occurs with a perforated appendix or gastric ulcer, the physical findings may be isolated to a certain area of the abdomen.

Diagnosis

Diagnosis usually is made by the history and physical examination. A leukocytosis with a left shift is usually present, and the hemoglobin may be falsely raised from intravascular volume depletion. Serum electrolytes may be abnormal. Plain radiographs of the abdomen often reveal free air underneath the diaphragm on an upright abdominal or chest film. An ileus pattern is often present. Diagnosis of the specific cause is usually made by exploratory laparotomy. In certain cases, either an upper gastrointestinal series or colonic enema with a water-soluble contrast agent, such as diatrizoate will show extravasation of the contrast agent, demonstrating an intestinal perforation.

Treatment

Therapy consists of surgical repair in the vast majority of cases. In some walled-off perforations in poor-risk patients, conservative management may be attempted, with nasogastric suction, intravenous fluids, and parenteral broad-spectrum antibiotics. Prior to surgical therapy, the hemodynamic status may need to be stabilized with intravenous fluids. Antibiotics should be given to treat the peritonitis. The overall prognosis depends on the time from the perforation to definitive therapy, underlying medical disorders, and any complications resulting after the surgery. With prompt diagnosis and treatment, most patients will do well.

Nursing Intervention

Refer to the next section for intestinal infarction and intestinal obstruction nursing interventions.

GASTROINTESTINAL SURGERY

Esophagus

The most common surgical procedures related to the esophagus are those for the treatment of esophageal carcinoma. This disease usually occurs in males over the age of 60. Cigarette smoking and alcohol intake are the two major risk factors. The carcinoma is usually located in the mid-esophagus and is usually epidermoid. Patients usually have dysphagia as the main symptom and a recent unexplained weight loss. At the time of diagnosis, the great majority of tumors have spread beyond the esophagus to the mediastinum, lymph nodes, liver, or pulmonary system. Esophageal tumors frequently are not curable by either surgery, radiation therapy, or chemotherapy.

Surgery is undertaken to either cure the disease or palliate symptoms. Unfortunately, surgery is not always possible. The usual surgical procedure is esophagogastrectomy with primary esophageal-gastric anastomosis. The mortality rate associated with this procedure is anywhere from 2.8 to 17%. Another surgical procedure that was done more frequently in the past is primary esophagectomy with colonic interposition between the cervical esophagus and stomach. Radiation therapy is usually an effective palliative procedure for those who are not operable or have had a recurrence of their tumor. Current studies of chemotherapy do not show much benefit, but further studies of both chemotherapy and radiation therapy are in progress and have shown some success.

Stomach

Gastric surgery is generally performed for three diseases: ulcer disease, gastroesophageal reflux disease, and neoplastic disease.

Many different operations are performed for ulcer disease. One surgery is a vagotomy and pyloroplasty. The vagotomy (severing of the vagus nerve) results in decreased acid production because of the loss of vagally mediated gastric secretion. Pyloroplasty, or widening of the pyloric channel, is necessary to prevent gastric stasis. This surgery generally has a low rate of ulcer recurrence, but a combination of vagotomy and antrectomy has an even lower recurrence rate. In this more complicated surgery, the distal half of the stomach is removed to decrease gastrin production, another stimulus to acid production. Another surgical treatment for ulcers is the highly selective vagotomy, also called the parietal cell or proximal gastric vagotomy. In this operation, the vagal branches to the proximal stomach, the fundus, and body are severed. As this is where acid secretion occurs, this surgery decreases acid production without affecting the motor activity of the distal stomach. This surgery, however, is technically more difficult to perform than the other two.

Gastroesophageal reflux of acid results in problems with esophagitis and esophageal strictures. Usually these conditions can be treated medically, but some cases are refractory to conservative therapy. In such cases, surgery is necessary. One of the operations most commonly performed is the Nissen fundoplication. Fundoplication involves wrapping the fundus of the stomach around the lower esophagus and anchoring the distal esophagus in the abdominal cavity. This greatly reduces reflux of gastric juices into the esophagus, allowing the esophagitis to heal. Another procedure, done less commonly, involves the placement of a plastic ring around the distal esophagus to reduce reflux. This ring is called the Angelchick prosthesis.

Surgery for gastric neoplasms often takes many forms. Adenocarcinoma is the most common malignancy of the stomach. Symptoms often appear late, after spread has already occurred. In lesions that have not spread, the usual procedure is a subtotal gastrectomy, with removal of over half of the stomach. Some tumors are large enough to require a total gastrectomy. In patients with tumors that have already metastasized, gastric bypass in the form of gastrojejunostomy is often needed for palliation.

Small and Large Intestines

Surgery of the small intestine is usually performed for removal of tumors, treatment of hemorrhage, correction of intestinal herniation, or treatment of inflammatory bowel disease. Tumors of the small intestine are rare, and therapy is usually with simple resection of the tumor itself plus a limited margin of normal intestine on either end. Hemorrhage is also uncommon and usually results from arteriovenous malformations, which in most cases form in the colon and not the small intestine. Small intestinal herniation can be either internal or external. Internal herniation is associated with trapping of intestinal loops by adhesive bands that form as a result of previous abdominal surgery. The herniation is referred to as internal because it is within the peritoneal cavity. External herniation involves trapping of an intestinal loop outside the peritoneal cavity, such as in inguinal, femoral, or ventral hernias. Surgical therapy of either type involves freeing the trapped loop of intestine and attempting to prevent its recurrence.

Surgery of the large intestine is usually for appendicitis, colonic carcinoma, diverticulitis, or lower gastrointestinal bleeding.

Appendicitis

Appendicitis is probably the major cause of an acute abdomen in Western civilization. The appendix arises from the cecum and varies in length. The appendix can become inflamed, distend, and perforate. Appendicitis is thought to arise from an obstruction in the more proximal part of the appendix, with stasis and bacterial proliferation distally. The visceral peritoneum initially gets inflamed, with resultant exudation of fluid and proteins. At this stage, pain is localized to the periumbilical area or right lower quadrant. As a response to the infection and inflammation, catecholamine is released, resulting in tachycardia and sweating. With further distension of the appendix and visceral peritoneal inflammation, inflammation of the adjacent parietal peritoneum results. This leads to the findings of localized involuntary abdominal musculature contractions, termed guarding. Rebound tenderness is often present in the right lower quadrant. With continuing obstruction and infection, the pus-filled appendix will perforate. Perforation results in release of pus and bacteria into the peritoneal cavity. An intense inflammation of the peritoneum results, with increased abdominal tenderness. If the infection is still isolated by loops of intestine to the right lower quadrant, the physical findings will be primarily in that site. If, however, the infected fluid spreads throughout the abdominal cavity, then diffuse direct tenderness, rigidity, and rebound tenderness of the abdomen result. At this stage, the

intravascular blood volume will be low, the patient may be hypotensive, and urine output will fall. The patient prefers to lie quietly in bed without moving, and respirations are shallow. The temperature is usually elevated, the white blood cell (WBC) count is elevated with a shift to more immature forms of neutrophils, and the hemoglobin may be raised from hemoconcentration.

Therapy of appendicitis is surgical after fluid and electrolyte resuscitation is initiated. If there has been no perforation, an appendectomy is performed and recovery is usually rapid. If free perforation has occurred, copious irrigation of the peritoneal cavity with an antibiotic solution is required in addition to the appendectomy. Usually the surgical wound must be left open to protect against wound infection. Time to recovery and length of hospitalization are usually greater than in patients without perforation.

Colonic Carcinoma

Colonic carcinoma is presently the second leading cause of cancer death in the United States. Unfortunately, symptoms often appear late in the disease, after spread beyond the colon has occurred, or are ignored by the patient and attributed to other causes. One example of the latter is rectal bleeding, which is often perceived by patients as resulting from hemorrhoids. However, rectal bleeding can also be from a polyp or tumor in the rectum or sigmoid; it should be evaluated by sigmoidoscopy and possibly by barium enema examination. Other possible symptoms of colon cancer include constipation, diarrhea, and colonic obstruction. All of these are results of either a partial or complete mechanical colonic obstruction. Colon cancer may not produce early symptoms, but one early sign can often be found. Presence of microscopic amounts of blood (occult blood) not visible to the naked eye can be noted in many cases of colon cancer. Occult blood can be discovered by card tests, such as Hemoccult. Tests are recommended annually in all people over age 50 in the United States. If colon cancer is detected at an early stage, the likelihood of cure with surgical excision is excellent. However, if the tumor has spread, the chance of surgical cure is poor. Surgical excision involves removal of the tumor with wide margins of uninvolved intestine on either side, with resection of the areas of regional lymphatic drainage. Usually a permanent colostomy is not required, except in carcinoma of the distal rectum.

Diverticulitis

Diverticulitis is a common cause of abdominal pain in patients over the age of 50. It involves infection of one of the outpouchings of the colon prevalent in the older population. Patients may have anywhere from mild abdominal pain and tenderness to diffuse peritonitis from colonic perforation. Therapy is usually with antibiotics and bowel rest, but free perforation or abscess formation may mandate surgical exploration with performance of a temporary diverting colostomy.

Pancreas

Carcinoma of the pancreas is the fourth leading cause of cancer death in men and the fifth most common in women. It usually arises insidiously and is almost always incurable at the time of diagnosis. Risk factors for pancreatic cancer include cigarette smoking, certain dietary and environmental factors, and juvenile-onset diabetes mellitus.

Most patients with pancreatic cancer complain of a vague, dull epigastric discomfort that may radiate through to the back. Insidious weight loss and anorexia are also present. Approximately one-fourth of patients have a palpable abdominal mass. The tumor can spread to the duodenum, liver, lymph nodes, and lungs and can impinge on the stomach. Other symptoms vary with the sites of metastases. If the tumor is compressing on the stomach, gastric outlet obstruction and vomiting are common. If the bile duct is obstructed, jaundice, pruritis, and acholic stools can result. Diagnosis of pancreatic cancer is usually made by CT scan of the abdomen, followed by either percutaneous needle biopsy or surgical exploration.

Most cases of pancreatic cancer are not surgically curable. Those that are resectable require extensive, complicated surgery for attempted cure. The two major procedures undertaken are pancreaticoduodenectomy (Whipple's procedure) and total pancreatectomy. Whipple's procedure involves resection of the head of the pancreas along with contiguous structures. The gastric antrum, duodenal C loop, gallbladder, and lymph nodes are removed. A loop of jejunum is anastomosed to the tail of the pancreas, the stomach, and the common bile duct. The procedure is difficult, and surgical mortality (death within 30 days of surgery) is 5%. Major complications of the procedure have been leakage or hemorrhage at the site of pancreaticojejunostomy. Five-year survival of one large series of patients treated by Whipple's procedure for pancreatic cancer was 20%.

Total pancreatectomy is another option in pancreatic cancer. In this procedure, the same organs are removed as for Whipple's procedure, but a pancreaticojejunostomy is not necessary since the whole pancreas is removed. This procedure is technically simpler to perform than Whipple's procedure. Metabolic management, however, is much more difficult.

Most surgical procedures for pancreatic cancer are palliative rather than curative. The aim is to treat or prevent common bile duct and gastric outlet obstruction. Therefore, anastomosis of the jejunum to either the gallbladder or common bile duct as well as gastrojejunostomy are most often done.

Nursing Intervention

Nursing priorities for patients undergoing gastrointestinal surgery should include promoting optimal physical conditions preoperatively, alleviating psychosocial concerns, meeting nutritional needs, promoting proper gastrointestinal functioning postoperatively, and preventing complications.

Preoperatively, the patient must ideally be hemodynamically stable, have fluid and electrolyte balances in normal limits, be in a reasonable nutritional state (not catabolic), and be emotionally prepared for the impending surgery.

Postoperatively, the first goal of therapy is to ensure hemodynamic and respiratory stability. Maintain an airway by ventilation or oxygen therapy and assess the pulmonary effects of anesthesia. If the patient is not intubated, make sure the patient coughs and deep breathes every 2 hr (make sure you instruct on splinting the incision). Suction the endotracheal tube as needed and note the color, amount, and odor of the secretions. Monitor arterial blood gases or oximetry values if needed.

Assess vital signs at least every 30–60 min initially after surgery. Note urine output and maintain at least 30 ml/hr. If the patient has hemodynamic monitoring, note hemodynamic measurements every hour. Assess intake and output every hour, and monitor serum electrolytes as available. Assess the type and amount of drainage from the nasogastric tube and from incision and drainage tubes. Note any foul odor from any drainage. Assess for possible abdominal fluid accumulation or postoperative hemorrhage.

Maintain nutritional status by TPN if the patient will not tolerate oral or enteral intake within the first several days after surgery. The alimental route for nutrition is restricted because of cessation of peristalsis from intraoperative handling of intestines, anesthesia, and/or potassium loss with resultant decreased smooth muscle contractility. If the patient is not able to eat, maintain the patency of the nasogastric tube and record the characteristics of any drainage. Once bowel sounds are present, liquids, progressing to clear liquids and then to diets low in residue and high in protein, carbohydrates, and calories, may be initiated.

Maintain the integrity of the skin by monitoring for signs and symptoms of infection. Assess vital signs frequently, noting increased pulse, tachypnea, and apprehension. Check dressing and wound frequently during the first 24 hr for signs of bright blood or excessive incisional swelling. Note temperature elevations and elevated WBCs. Monitor for signs of peritonitis (rigidity, guarding, rebound tenderness, and the absence of bowel sounds).

Patients who have had pancreatic resections must have their blood glucose closely monitored.

Emotional support of the postoperative patient is important to both the patient and the family. This is extremely important for patients who have had ostomies placed. Maintain a reassuring, accepting environment and allow the patient time to vocalize fears and altered self-concept.

GASTROINTESTINAL TRAUMA

Blunt or Penetrating Abdominal Trauma

Since violence marks our present civilization, stab wounds and blunt injuries to the abdomen are increasingly seen in emergency rooms, operating rooms, and intensive care units. Injury to the abdomen may occur from a blow to the abdomen in an automobile accident, altercation, or fall. These injuries may occur even though the abdominal wall is still intact. Other penetrating injuries, such as those from a stab wound, may appear superficial and unimportant, but they often are deep and may have lacerated several internal organs. Trauma of any kind is apt to cause bleeding or contusions and may open the bowel lumen to cause peritonitis. In closed abdominal wounds, the spleen, the kidneys, the duodenum (especially the third and fourth portions, which may be squeezed between the steering wheel and the spine), and the liver are injured in approximately that order of frequency; in stab wounds, the liver, stomach, and colon receive most of the injury because of their anterior location.

Diagnosis

Abdominal trauma may cause injury to the liver, spleen, pancreas, gastrointestinal tract, spine, retroperitoneum, kidneys, and pelvic organs. Injuries to the spleen, liver, pancreas, and gastrointestinal tract are the most difficult to diagnose by conventional radiologic methods. A CT scan has been shown to be beneficial for the early diagnosis and accurate evaluation of the extent of internal injuries following abdominal trauma. A CT scan is capable of detecting lacerations, subcapsular hematomas, and ruptures of all abdominal organs and therefore has advantages over organ-specific procedures. In addition, CT scans directly image even small amounts of intra-abdominal hemorrhage, which cannot be identified by other conventional imaging techniques.

At some institutions, a diagnostic peritoneal lavage is done as an emergency procedure for the evaluation of patients who have suffered trauma to the abdomen. By this procedure, it can be determined which patients need laparotomy because of perforated viscera or lacerations of the liver or spleen.

Clinical Manifestations

If the injury is severe (especially with a significant blood loss), the patient may exhibit signs of hypovolemic shock (shallow respirations, weak rapid pulse, and decreased urine output). The patient may have pain, depending on the site and extent of injury. A physical insult to the abdomen is apt to cause cessation of bowel motility. If there is colonic injury, there may be blood in the stool and possible signs of intestinal perforation or obstruction.

In blunt trauma, the pancreas is particularly susceptible to rupture where it passes over the spine, and is often associated with duodenal rupture. With trauma to the pancreas, pancreatitis often follows but is usually asymptomatic. Elevation of serum amylase is not a dependable sign. Traumatic pancreatitis is often recognized only during exploratory laparotomy for gunshot or stab wounds. However, in the nonpenetrating, blunt abdominal trauma, traumatic pancreatitis often goes unnoticed because of the protected retroperitoneal location of the pancreas. This unnoticed pancreatitis may lead to the development of a pseudocyst, a subdiaphragmatic abscess, or massive gastrointestinal hemorrhage. The disease, regardless of whether it is diagnosed during a laparotomy, carries a 14% mortality rate.

Symptoms of liver rupture are similar to those of splenic rupture, but they occur on the right side. There may be pain in the right upper quadrant, some tenderness, and if blood loss is great enough, signs of shock.

Treatment

Initial treatment is aimed at maintenance of the patient's hemodynamic status and prevention of shock. Rapid intravenous fluid and blood replacement may be necessary. Antibiotics may be necessary to prevent peritonitis, especially for open, penetrating wounds.

Surgical intervention must readily be instituted for those who are hemodynamically unstable. Most of these patients will undergo exploratory laparotomy to repair or remove injured organs and surrounding tissue. Vigorous rinsing of the abdominal cavity with an antimicrobial solution is necessary if bowel perforation has occurred. Patients with closed injuries require astute observation for organ failure or hemorrhage necessitating surgical intervention.

Nursing Intervention

Patients with abdominal injury must be carefully observed for coexisting cardiothoracic injury. Signs of pneumothorax, cardiac tamponade, cardiac rupture, and aortic or pulmonary vasculature injuries must be assessed.

Astute assessment of the patient's hemodynamic and respiratory status must be carried out continuously. Fluid and electrolyte replacements are given to counteract third spacing and hypovolemic shock. Anaerobic and aerobic coverage with antibiotics is immediately initiated. Ventilatory and oxygen support may be necessary.

A careful abdominal assessment is performed to evaluate injuries. The nurse must assess for rebound tenderness, muscle rigidity, anorexia, nausea, vomiting, abdominal distension, presence of bowel sounds, and pain. A nasogastric tube should be placed, and changes in drainage should be noticed.

Emotional support is important for the patient and family, since gastrointestinal trauma is usually quite unexpected and coping mechanisms are not readily available.

Other Trauma to the Gastrointestinal Tract

Caustic injury is usually produced by strong alkaline or acidic agents. The ingestion of caustic agents can initiate a progressive and devastating injury to the esophagus and stomach. Most caustic injuries are seen in patients who are very young, psychotic, alcoholic, or suicidal.

Acidic solutions usually cause immediate pain, and unless they are ingested intentionally, they are rapidly expelled. The alkali liquid solutions are often tasteless and odorless and thus are swallowed before protective reflexes can be invoked. Alkali solutions penetrate tissue more rapidly than acid solutions do and are more difficult to treat. Caustic injuries to the gastrointestinal mucosa are classified pathologically in the same manner as skin burns.

Symptoms may be present, especially early after the ingestion. Edema, ulceration, or a white membrane may be present over the palate, uvula, and pharynx. Hoarseness, stridor, dysphagia, epigastric pain, emesis of tissue or blood, tachypnea, and shock may be present. Late symptoms include perforation of the stomach or esophagus, mediastinitis, and peritonitis.

Early treatment includes neutralization of the caustic agent. Acid injuries should be neutralized with large volumes of water or milk. Alkali injuries occur so rapidly that even immediate attempts to neutralize them are probably unsuccessful and should not be undertaken because of the exothermic properties of dilution and neutralization.

Resuscitation should immediately be instituted. Establishment of an airway, fluid and blood resuscitation, and gastrointestinal rest (nothing by mouth) should be first priorities.

Endoscopic evaluation should be performed once the patient is stable to evaluate the extent of the damage. If there is perforation, a thoracotomy or laparotomy may be done to repair injured organs.

The mortality rate after caustic ingestion is 1–3%. However, if the patient survives the acute effects of caustic ingestion, the reparative response can result in esophageal and gastric stenosis and an increased incidence of esophageal cancer.

Esophageal Perforation

The most common causes of esophageal perforation are medical tubes and instruments, forceful vomiting, and foreign bodies. Less frequent are perforations caused by gunshot wounds, necrotizing infections or tumors, and caustic agents.

Perforations are recognized by symptoms of respiratory distress, chest, neck, abdominal, and upper neck pain, and odynophagia. Subcutaneous crepitation, fever, shock, mediastinal crunching sound with the heartbeat, leukocytosis, and radiographic abnormalities may also occur.

The most important determinants of survival are the size and location of the perforation and whether gross contamination outside the esophagus has occurred. Most causes of esophageal perforation are surgically managed to repair the perforation.

42

Management of the Patient with a Gastrointestinal Disturbance

EDITORS' NOTE

This chapter provides an overview of general nursing interventions for patients with any type of gastrointestinal disturbance, including the conditions previously discussed in Chapters 39 through 41. Priority interventions include measures to maintain fluid and electrolyte balance, ensure adequate nutritional intake, maintain bowel elimination, maintain comfort, and prevent infection. The chapter concludes with a brief summary of physical assessment steps when assessing the gastrointestinal system.

INTERVENTIONS TO MAINTAIN FLUID AND ELECTROLYTE BALANCE

1. Maintenance of accurate intake and output. Include number, character, amount, and site of gastrointestinal fluid loss.
2. Monitoring of serum electrolytes per laboratory data. Gastrointestinal fluid losses through tube suction, ostomy drainage, diarrhea, and vomiting can cause losses of essential electrolytes, especially H^-, Cl^-, and K^+, and may produce alkalosis.
3. Correct use of gastrointestinal tubes for decompression and diagnosis. Two types of tubes:
   a. Short tubes. These are used for the stomach and duodenum. Example: nasogastric tubes.

1. Levin (single lumen)
2. Rehfuss (single lumen with metal tube)
3. Salem sump (double lumen)

   The salem sump is most widely used because the second lumen, which is open to air, prevents the development of excessive negative pressure by bringing air into the cavity continuously. Low, intermittent levels of suction are used. The second port of the salem sump (pigtail) must be placed above the patient's midline to prevent reflux into the pigtail. Commercially made anti-reflux valves are available.

   b. Long tubes. These tubes are intended to extend the length of the small bowel. They can be 6 and 10 feet long.
   1. Miller-Abbott
   2. Cantor
   3. Harris

   The tube is threaded from the nose into the stomach and then through the pylorus, where peristaltic activity of the bowel carries it to the desired area. If peristalsis does not carry the tube to the appropriate place, gravity or guidance under fluoroscopy may be used. Once it is in the correct location, the tube is taped securely in place to prevent further migration.

   With all of the gastrointestinal tubes, the material aspirated should be noted for color, odor, and quantity.

4. Maintenance of blood volume during gastrointestinal hemorrhage.

a. Blood volume replacement as needed.
b. Monitor hematocrit/hemoglobin every day and as needed during instability.
c. Monitor amount, color, and area of bleeding.
d. Oxygen therapy as needed.
e. Monitor hemodynamic status.

5. Relief of nausea and vomiting.
a. Monitor for distension; may place nasogastric tube to decompress stomach.
b. Monitor emesis for amount, color, frequency, and presence of blood.
c. Administer antiemetics.
d. Place patient on side to prevent aspiration of vomitus.

INTERVENTIONS TO MAINTAIN NUTRITIONAL STATUS

Patients in the intensive care unit who are unable to eat must be fed enterally or parenterally. Normally, patients at rest require 25 kcal/kg/day. The nurse should assess the calories given versus what is needed.

1. Evaluation of the patient's nutritional status.
   a. History taking
      1. Medical history: illness, surgery, gastrointestinal disease, alcoholism, etc.
      2. Social history: food storage and preparation facilities, money, and education.
      3. Drug history: antibiotics, chemotherapy, anticonvulsants, etc.
      4. Diet history: 24-hr recall.
   b. Anthropometric measures. Physical measurements that reflect growth and development compared with standards specific for sex and age. Compares body fat and skeletal muscle obtained through triceps skinfold, midarm circumference, and midarm muscle circumference measurements.
   c. Types of proteins and biochemical tests
      1. Somatic protein (skeletal). Somatic protein is the protein of voluntary muscles. Indicators of somatic protein losses are low ideal body weight or usual body weight percentages, low fatfold thickness, negative nitrogen balance from nitrogen balance studies, and increased 24-hour urinary creatinine.
      2. Visceral protein. Visceral protein is the protein of the internal organs. Indicators of visceral protein losses are low total lymphocyte count (less than 1000), serum albumin (less than 3.5), and serum transferrin (less than 200 mg/dl).
   d. Measurements of immune function
      Various forms of protein malnutrition have been associated with depression of the immune system.
      1. Lymphocytes: white blood cells that defend against infection. Decrease in number as protein depletion occurs. Decrease for many other reasons also, so they are not nutrition specific.
      2. Antigen skin testing: a test of the immune system's competence, in which an antigen is injected just under the skin. A reaction means that the immune system is working normally.

2. Enteral feeding administration
   A person who has a functioning gastrointestinal tract but is unable to eat enough food may be a candidate for a tube feeding.
   a. Types of tubes: silicone (Silastic) or polyurethane.
   b. Placement of tubes: esophagostomy, gastrostomy, jejunostomy, transnasal, nasogastric, and nasoenteric (nasoduodenal or nasojejunal).
   c. Tube feeding formulas: selected after the client's needs have been identified.
      1. Intact formulas. These contain protein, carbohydrates, and fats of higher molecular weights. A person must be able to digest and absorb nutrients without difficulty to use this type of formula.
      2. Hydrolyzed formulas. These contain smaller molecules of protein, fat, and carbohydrates. They are "predigested" and are recommended for those who lack digestive capabilities or who have a smaller than normal area for absorbing nutrients.
   d. Administration guidelines: Bolus feedings via gravity drip or continuous feedings via pump are used. It is controversial as to which method is preferred. Generally bolus feeds are given into the stomach and continuous feeds into the small intestine. Initial feedings:
      1. Check tube placement before feeding.
      2. Check residual amount in stomach. If greater than 100–150 ml, hold feeding.
      3. Diluting the feeding is controversial. Some institutions may prefer gradual

progression to full-strength external feedings.

4. Check drip rate every 1–2 hr.
5. Feeding should be at or slightly below body temperature. Cold starts vasoconstriction, which reduces the flow of gastric digestive juices.
6. Monitor intake and output.
7. Changing feeding bag and tubing every day.
8. Monitor laboratory data, especially serum electrolytes, two to three times weekly.
9. Flush tube with 50–100 ml of water before and after each feeding to maintain patency.

e. Complications
1. Diarrhea: from bacterial contamination, lactose intolerance, hypertonic formulas, low serum albumin, or drug therapy.
2. Dehydration: from excessive diarrhea, inadequate fluid intake, carbohydrate intolerance, or excessive protein intake.
3. Aspiration pneumonia: from regurgitation of formula that is subsequently inhaled into the lungs or from displacement of feeding tube.
4. Vomiting: from obstruction or delayed gastric emptying.
5. Nausea, cramps, distension: from obstruction, delayed gastric emptying, or intolerance to concentration or volume of formula.
6. Increased glucose levels: from excess glucose loads.

3. Total parental alimentation (hyperalimentation)

If gastrointestinal absorption and delivery of nutrients are inadequate, impossible for prolonged periods of time, or contraindicated, nourishment should be provided parenterally.

Total parental nutrition (TPN) is done with a hypertonic mixture of dextrose, amino acids, electrolytes, vitamins, and trace minerals. It may be given peripherally or through central veins.

a. Nutrient solutions

The concentration and quantity of the solution are gradually increased until a desired state is reached.

A typical TPN solution contains 25–75% dextrose and 3.5–8% amino acids. One liter of a D_{50} solution provides about 1700 kcal daily. Electrolytes, vitamins, and trace minerals are added. The fluid may be concentrated if it is infused through a central line.

b. Lipid emulsions

Lipids supply 9 kcal/g, more than twice the energy supplied by a gram of glucose. They are isotonic. They prevent essential fatty acid deficiency.

c. Administration guidelines
1. Monitor serum electrolytes, albumin levels, and nitrogen balance studies. Increase TPN concentrations as nutritional status warrants.
2. Monitor daily weight and daily intake and output.
3. Monitor serum glucose and urine glucose every four to six hours. May need to administer insulin.
4. Monitor infusion rate every one to two hours. If rate falls behind, monitor for hypoglycemia and spread whatever deficit has incurred over the next 24 hr.

d. Complications
1. Infection or sepsis: Stringent aseptic technique during catheter insertion and dressing changes.
2. Thrombosis of great veins or embolism from the catheter. Remove catheter and start anticoagulation therapy if not contraindicated.
3. Hyperosmolar nonketotic hyperglycemia: Discontinue TPN; give insulin, saline, and D_5W to replace free water.
4. Hyperglycemia: Insulin therapy, slow rate.
5. Hypoglycemia: Check to make sure TPN has not been interrupted or the wrong concentration given.
6. Electrolyte disturbances: Maintain appropriate concentrations.

INTERVENTIONS TO MAINTAIN BOWEL ELIMINATION STATUS

1. Diarrhea
   a. Identify caustic factors.
   b. Record color, amount, and frequency of stools.

   c. Maintain intake and output to prevent dehydration.

   d. Monitor serum electrolytes.

   e. Check for blood in stools.

   f. Administer antidiarrheal medications to decrease intestinal motility if not contraindicated.

   g. Begin nutritional supplement.

2. Constipation
   a. Increase fluid intake if not contraindicated.
   b. Monitor time and consistency of stools.
   c. Administer laxative or enema if not contraindicated. Needed after barium studies.

INTERVENTIONS TO MAINTAIN COMFORT STATUS

1. Pain
   a. Observe for signs and location of pain; determine type and severity.
   b. Administer analgesics or sedatives; morphine sulfate is contraindicated in pancreatitis because it causes spasm of the sphincter of Oddi.

INTERVENTIONS TO PREVENT INFECTION

1. Monitor temperature and white blood cell counts.
2. Use strict aseptic technique when placing lines or changing dressings.
3. Use isolation techniques for specific diseases (e.g., hepatitis).
4. Assess sources of contamination. Culture infected drainage and blood.
5. Use good handwashing techniques to prevent cross-contamination.

PHYSICAL ASSESSMENT

Physical assessment of the gastrointestinal system can be briefly summarized by following the steps listed below:

1. Begin the assessment with inspection of the abdomen. Do not begin palpation, particularly deep palpation, until the last phase of assessment. This will avoid any stimulation of the gastrointestinal system and avoid any initiation of painful stimuli.
2. Auscultation in the second phase of assessment. Bowel sounds are usually heard in all four abdominal quadrants. Observe for a change in sounds or bowel sound intensity and character. Bowel sounds are not always a reliable assessment tool due to the transmission of sound throughout the abdomen.
3. Percussion is the third step in assessment. Usually, the gastrointestinal tract has air present and will result in hearing a resonant or hyperresonant sound. Tympanic sounds can be heard in the stomach, although elsewhere this sound may indicate an obstruction.
4. Palpation, both superficial and deep, are the last phase of assessment. The goal is to detect abnormal organ size, such as liver or spleen enlargement, and to identify if pain is present in the abdomen.

GASTROENTEROLOGY BIBLIOGRAPHY

Achkar, E., Farmer, R.G., Fleshler, B. (1992). *Clinical gastroenterology.* Philadelphia: Lea & Febiger.

Adams, L., & Soulen, M.C. (1993). TIPS: A new alternative for the variceal bleeder. *American Journal of Critical Care, 2,* 3: 196–201.

Bouley, G., et al. (1996). Transjugular intrahepatic portosystemic shunt: an alternative. *Critical Care Nurse, 16,* 1: 23–29.

Halm, M.A. (1996). Acute gastrointestinal complications after cardiac surgery. *American Journal of Critical Care, 5,* 2: 109–118.

Nuone, J. (1995). Acute pancreatitis: an orem approach to nursing assessment and care. *Critical Care Nurse, 15,* 4: 27–35.

Reishtein, J. (1993). Liver failure: Case study of a complex problem. *Critical Care Nurse, 13,* 5: 36–44.

Sugawa, C., Schuman, B.M., Lucas, C.E. (1992). *Gastrointestinal bleeding.* New York: Igaku Shaim.

Winawer, S.J. (1992). *Management of gastrointestinal diseases.* New York: Gower Medical Pub.

PART VI

Gastroenterology Practice Exam

1. Secretion from the salivary glands is primarily regulated by which of the following?
   (A) central nervous system
   (B) autonomic nervous system
   (C) pituitary gland
   (D) hypothalamus

2. Atropine, a parasympathetic inhibitor, would cause which of the following physical symptoms due to parasympathetic action?
   (A) decreased salivary flow
   (B) increased level of consciousness
   (C) increased heart rate
   (D) decreased respiratory rate

3. Achalasia refers to which of the following?
   (A) decreased production of trypsin
   (B) increased backflow of gastric acid into the duodenum
   (C) loss of peristaltic waves in the small intestine
   (D) failure of the gastroesophageal sphincter

4. In which part of the gastrointestinal tract are no enzymes secreted?
   (A) mouth
   (B) esophagus
   (C) stomach
   (D) small intestine

Questions 5 and 6 refer to the following scenario.

A 26-year-old male is admitted to your unit complaining of chest pain unrelated to exercise. The pain is not relieved by rest. No ECG (electrocardiographic) changes are evident. The abdomen is soft and free from pain on palpation. Diet has been normal and no change in stool patterns has been reported. No problems with swallowing have been noted.

5. Based on the preceding information, what is the likely origin of the problem?

   (A) malfunction of the cardiac sphincter
   (B) duodenal ulcer
   (C) pyloric sphincter reflux
   (D) myocardial ischemia

6. What treatment would most likely be instituted in this situation?
   (A) esophageal resection via the thoracic approach
   (B) antrectomy
   (C) vagotomy
   (D) diet change

7. Total gastrectomy would cause the patient to lose which function?
   (A) ability to secrete glucagon
   (B) bile production
   (C) vitamin B_{12} synthesis
   (D) acid-base regulation of chloride and bicarbonate

8. A 44-year-old male has a gastrostomy tube (G tube) placed for nutritional support following diagnosis of a malabsorptive syndrome. He is discharged with the G tube in place. Several weeks later, he is admitted to your unit with complaints of disorientation. The family states that they have been irrigating and aspirating the G tube following tube feedings. This irrigation of the G tube would most likely cause which disturbance?
   (A) metabolic acidosis
   (B) metabolic alkalosis
   (C) respiratory alkalosis
   (D) respiratory acidosis

9. Which substance will increase the production of hydrochloric acid?
   (A) histamine
   (B) atropine
   (C) bicarbonate
   (D) potassium salts

10. Cimetidine or ranitidine acts to reduce stress ulcers by inhibiting the production of which substance?
    (A) histamine
    (B) gastrin
    (C) acetylcholine
    (D) calcium

11. What is the purpose of the intrinsic factor, produced by parietal cells in the stomach?
    (A) promotes absorption of vitamin K
    (B) promotes absorption of vitamin B_{12}
    (C) increases utilization of vitamin C
    (D) synthesizes vitamin D with calcium

12. The normal pH of the stomach falls within which of the following ranges?
    (A) 1 to 3
    (B) 4 to 6
    (C) 6 to 8
    (D) >8

13. In which part of the gastrointestinal system is pepsinogen initially produced?
    (A) mouth
    (B) esophagus
    (C) stomach
    (D) small intestine

14. Which of the following is the most accurate definition of chyme?
    (A) a lipoprotein secreted in the stomach that aids in fat digestion
    (B) gastric cells responsible for negating excessive hydrochloric acid secretion
    (C) a hormone necessary for reducing the desire to eat
    (D) a semiliquid mass of food

15. Gastrin secretion causes which of the following effects?
    (A) increased desire to eat
    (B) inhibited desire to eat
    (C) production of vitamin B_{12}
    (D) increased production of hydrochloric acid

16. Which of the following is a function of cholecystokinin?
    (A) breaks down protein
    (B) inhibits gastric emptying
    (C) stimulates duodenal catabolism of carbohydrates
    (D) inhibits gallbladder activity

17. A vagotomy, through the removal of parasympathetic stimulation, can reduce hydrochloric acid secretion by which of the following mechanisms?

(A) elimination of the cephalic phase of gastric secretion
(B) elimination of the gastric phase of gastric secretion
(C) elimination of the intestinal phase of gastric secretion
(D) altering the ability of the stomach to sense the presence of food

18. Which of the following substrates is most readily processed by the gastrointestinal system?
    (A) fats
    (B) proteins
    (C) carbohydrates
    (D) lipoproteins

19. Approximately how many calories are in a gram of glucose?
    (A) 2 kcal
    (B) 4 kcal
    (C) 6 kcal
    (D) 9 kcal

20. Approximately how many calories are in a gram of fat?
    (A) 2 kcal
    (B) 4 kcal
    (C) 6 kcal
    (D) 9 kcal

21. Approximately how many calories are in a gram of protein?
    (A) 2 kcal
    (B) 4 kcal
    (C) 6 kcal
    (D) 9 kcal

22. D_5W has 5 g of glucose per 100 ml of solution. Approximately how many calories are in 1 L of D_5W?
    (A) 20 kcal
    (B) 200 kcal
    (C) 500 kcal
    (D) 2000 kcal

23. Which of the following enzymes is active in the digestion of proteins?
    (A) amylase
    (B) maltose
    (C) lipase
    (D) trypsin

24. Which of the following enzymes is active in the digestion of fats?
    (A) amylase
    (B) maltose
    (C) lipase
    (D) trypsin

25. Which of the following enzymes is active in the digestion of carbohydrates?
    (A) amylase
    (B) pepsin
    (C) lipase
    (D) trypsin

26. Emulsification (dispersion into small droplets) of fat occurs because of which substance?
    (A) chyme
    (B) lipase
    (C) bile
    (D) cholecystokinin

27. Following a gunshot wound to the abdomen, a 27-year-old male has a complete colectomy with creation of an ileostomy. What nursing measures will be necessary considering the fact that the function of the large intestine has been eliminated?
    (A) administration of proteolytic enzymes via tube feedings
    (B) observation of intake and output since reabsorption of water will be diminished
    (C) administration of proteolytic enzymes via tube feedings and administration of emulsifying agents
    (D) observation of intake and output and administration of emulsifying agents

28. What is the primary function of the small intestine?
    (A) absorption of nutrients
    (B) reabsorption of water
    (C) reabsorption of carbon dioxide
    (D) acting as a reservoir for food

29. Increased colonic motility is produced by which of the following?
    (A) parasympathetic stimulation
    (B) sympathetic stimulation
    (C) central nervous system stimulation
    (D) increased fat content in the diet

30. Which drug would potentially decrease colonic motility?
    (A) nifedipine
    (B) atropine
    (C) digitalis
    (D) gentamicin

31. All venous blood from the intestines eventually drains into which vein?
    (A) gastric
    (B) superior mesenteric
    (C) portal
    (D) celiac

32. The portal vein empties into which structure?
    (A) inferior vena cava
    (B) liver
    (C) large intestine
    (D) bile duct

33. Parasympathetic regulation of the gastrointestinal system is provided by which nerve?
    (A) portal
    (B) phrenic
    (C) hepatic
    (D) vagus

34. The sympathetic neurotransmitter norepinephrine is opposed by which parasympathetic neurotransmitter when regulating gastrointestinal activity?
    (A) epinephrine
    (B) dopamine
    (C) serotonin
    (D) acetylcholine

35. Which of the following is NOT a function of the pancreas?
    (A) secretion of glucagon
    (B) secretion of insulin
    (C) secretion of potassium salts
    (D) secretion of digestive enzymes

36. Which of the following enzymes is NOT secreted by the pancreas?
    (A) pepsinogen
    (B) trypsin
    (C) lipase
    (D) amylase

37. A duodenal feeding tube was placed by the RN on a prior shift. You want to check the placement of the tube in order to confirm that it is in the duodenum rather than the stomach. To check its position, you utilize a pH reading from aspirated tube contents. Which pH range would suggest a duodenal rather than a gastric location?
    (A) 1 to 3
    (B) 4 to 6
    (C) 6 to 8
    (D) >8

38. What is the function of hepatic Kupffer cells?
    (A) phagocytosis
    (B) production of pancreatic lipase
    (C) production of bile
    (D) stimulation of the microenzyme oxidizing system

39. Which of the following are major functions of the liver?
    (A) production of bile and synthesis of amino acids
    (B) production of bile and gluconeogenesis
    (C) synthesis of amino acids and gluconeogenesis
    (D) production of bile, synthesis of amino acids, and gluconeogenesis

40. Which substance causes contraction of the gall-bladder?
    (A) secretin
    (B) cholecystokinin
    (C) bilirubin
    (D) bile salts

41. What is one of the main components of bile?
    (A) bilirubin
    (B) degenerated hepatic cells
    (C) cholecystokinin
    (D) pancreatic lipase

42. A 39-year-old female complains of right lower quadrant pain. Prior to performing an abdominal assessment, in what order should you consider performing the following assessment techniques?
    (A) inspection, palpation, and auscultation
    (B) palpation, auscultation, and inspection
    (C) inspection, auscultation, and palpation
    (D) auscultation, palpation, and inspection

43. Depression of overall protein stores is commonly monitored during a nutritional assessment. Which of the following are measured as part of the routine protein assessment during an analysis of nutritional status?
    (A) total lymphocytes and albumin
    (B) total lymphocytes and lactate
    (C) albumin and lactate
    (D) total lymphocytes, albumin, and lactate

44. A 76-year-old male is receiving tube feeding supplements consisting of Osmolite at 75 ml/h. Approximately how many calories are being administered every 24 hr based on this feeding rate?
    (A) 1200 kcal
    (B) 1800 kcal
    (C) 2400 kcal
    (D) 3000 kcal

45. Vomiting of blood from the gastrointestinal system is denoted by which of the following terms?
    (A) hemoptysis
    (B) hematemesis
    (C) hematopol
    (D) hematochezia

46. At which anatomical location do most ulcers occur?
    (A) stomach
    (B) duodenem
    (C) esophagus
    (D) jejunum

47. Which of the following is thought to be the most common cause of stress ulcers?
    (A) ischemia
    (B) excessive acid production
    (C) mechanical injury
    (D) infections

48. Hydrogen ion blocking agents, such as cimetidine (Tagamet) and ranitidine (Zantac), work by which of the following mechanisms?
    (A) decreasing gastric acid production
    (B) supplying a protective membrane against hydrochloric acid
    (C) increasing bicarbonate production
    (D) blocking the release of catabolic hydrogen enzymes

49. Which of the following treatments is NOT routinely indicated in the treatment of upper gastrointestinal bleeding?
    (A) endoscopy with coagulation of bleeding site
    (B) fluid replacement with crystalloids
    (C) blood transfusions
    (D) iced lavage of the stomach

50. Esophageal varices are the result of increases in which of the following vascular parameters?
    (A) hepatic arterial pressure
    (B) hepatic venous pressure
    (C) portal venous pressure
    (D) superior iliac arterial pressure

51. Portacaval shunts work to decrease bleeding from esophageal varices by which mechanism?
    (A) decreasing portal venous pressure
    (B) improving vena caval blood flow
    (C) improving production of clotting factors
    (D) decreasing blood return to the liver

Questions 52 and 53 refer to the following scenario.

A 61-year-old male is admitted to your unit with the diagnosis of upper gastrointestinal bleeding. He has a history of alcohol abuse and prior gastrointestinal bleeding. His abdomen is distended and his liver is enlarged. He has no complaints of pain. The vomitus is bright red.

52. Based on the preceding information, which condition is most likely to be present?
    (A) diverticuli
    (B) esophageal varices
    (C) duodenal ulcers
    (D) colonic varices

53. The physician elects to place an esophageal balloon (Sengstaken–Blakemore) to aid bleeding control. Which of the following is NOT a potential complication of the esophageal balloon treatment?
    (A) tracheal occlusion
    (B) esophageal necrosis
    (C) esophageal rupture
    (D) reversal of portal blood flow

54. Which of the following is NOT a common cause of lower gastrointestinal bleeding?
    (A) diverticulosis
    (B) colon tumors
    (C) arteriovenous malformations
    (D) hepatic failure

55. Which of the following is NOT a treatment for an upper gastrointestinal tract bleeding?
    (A) vasopressin
    (B) endoscopy
    (C) colon resection
    (D) balloon tamponade

56. A 57-year-old male with the diagnosis of hepatitis A is admitted to your unit. He is also recovering from vascular surgery and has an open wound on his left lower leg. Which type of isolation is likely to be requested for this patient?
    (A) enteric
    (B) respiratory
    (C) wound
    (D) reverse

57. A 69-year-old male has been in your unit for 31 days following an episode of acute respiratory failure. He is receiving nutritional supplementation consisting of 50 ml/h of Pulmocare. His current laboratory information is as follows:

    | albumin | 2.4 g/dl |
    | white blood cell count | 4500 mm^3 |
    | lymphocytes | 20% |
    | Na$^+$ | 130 mEq/l |

    Based on the preceding information, how many calories is he receiving?
    (A) 200 kcal
    (B) 900 kcal

    (C) 2400 kcal
    (D) 2800 kcal

Questions 58 and 59 refer to the following scenario.

A 23-year-old female is admitted to your unit after being found unresponsive by paramedics. She has no overt signs of injury or physical abuse. After starting an intravenous drip, you accidentally stick yourself with the same needle used for the venipuncture.

58. Based on the preceding information, to what type of hepatitis would you most likely be exposed?
    (A) hepatitis A
    (B) hepatitis B
    (C) non-A, non-B hepatitis
    (D) hepatitis D

59. Initial treatment for you, assuming no prior exposure to hepatitis exists, would include administration of which of the following (after appropriate serologic studies of you and the patient had been performed)?
    (A) hepatitis B immune globulin (HBIG) and vaccine
    (B) hepatitis A immune globulin (HAIG)
    (C) non-A, non-B hepatitis immune globulin
    (D) hepatitis A vaccine

60. For which type of hepatitis does an effective vaccine exist?
    (A) hepatitis A
    (B) hepatitis B
    (C) non-A, non-B hepatitis
    (D) hepatitis D

Questions 61 and 62 refer to the following scenario.

A 67-year-old male is admitted to your unit with the complaints of generalized fatigue and weakness. His abdomen is distended with ascites present, producing shortness of breath. The liver is hard but not enlarged. Spider angiomas are noted on his chest and he has atrophied skeletal muscles. Sclerae have an icteric appearance. Vital signs are blood pressure 96/60, pulse 110, and respiratory rate 28.

61. Based on the preceding information, which condition is likely to be responsible for the symptoms?
    (A) acute hepatitis
    (B) cirrhosis
    (C) esophageal varices
    (D) hepatorenal syndrome

62. Which initial treatment would be indicated to help relieve the respiratory distress from the ascites?
    (A) placing the patient in a supine position
    (B) endoscopy

(Answers cont'd.)

(C) protein restriction in the diet

(D) administration of diuretics and sodium restriction

63. All of the following are nursing measures for the patient with acute hepatitis except one. Which one is NOT indicated in the patient with hepatitis?
(A) low-protein, high-carbohydrate diet
(B) monitoring liver enzyme tests
(C) maximizing periods of rest
(D) avoiding periods of rest, initiating active exercise regimes

64. Asterixis is regarded as a sign of the development of which condition?
(A) left ventricular failure
(B) acute calcium disturbance
(C) hepatic encephalopathy
(D) seizures

Questions 65 and 66 refer to the following scenario.

A 53-year-old male is admitted to the unit with the diagnosis of cirrhosis. He currently is confused and disoriented. He has a "flapping" movement of both hands and has jaundiced skin. Laboratory values are as follows:

SGOT	100
SGPT	88
lactate dehydrogenase	250
alkaline phosphatase	165

65. Based on the preceding information, which condition is likely to be developing and causing the behavioral changes?
(A) acute renal failure
(B) loss of cerebral perfusion pressure
(C) loss of cerebral glucose from hepatic failure
(D) hepatic encephalopathy

66. Which treatment would be utilized in the treatment of this patient?
(A) lactulose
(B) high-protein diet
(C) glucose bolus
(D) vitamin D and B administration

67. Pancreatitis is partially monitored by means of which parameters?
(A) pepsinogen levels
(B) amylase values
(C) glucagon values
(D) trypsin levels

68. What is the most common cause of pancreatitis?
(A) liver failure
(B) diabetes

(C) alcohol abuse

(D) intravenous drug abuse

Questions 69 and 70 refer to the following scenario.

A 46-year-old male, with a history of alcohol abuse, is admitted to your unit with the development of severe abdominal pain, with radiation of the pain to his back. The abdomen is tender although rebound tenderness is not present. He is nauseated and has vomited once. Bowel sounds are diminished. Vital signs are blood pressure 98/58, pulse 116, and respiratory rate 34. Laboratory data are as follows:

Na^+	142
K^+	3.8
Cl^-	106
HCO_3^-	22
Ca^{2+}	7.5
Amylase	600

69. Based on the preceding information, which condition is likely to be developing?
(A) superior mesenteric obstruction
(B) cholecystitis
(C) pancreatitis
(D) bowel obstruction

70. Which treatment, aside from pain relief, would be indicated for this patient?
(A) placement on an NPO (*nil per os;* nothing by mouth) regimen with gastrointestinal suction
(B) reduction in the quantity of nitrogen-containing products in the diet
(C) exploratory laparotomy
(D) cholecystectomy

71. Which of the following electrolytes is frequently lost with pancreatitis?
(A) sodium
(B) potassium
(C) bicarbonate
(D) calcium

Questions 72 and 73 refer to the following scenario.

A 69-year-old female is admitted to your unit complaining of excruciating periumbilical pain. Her abdomen is not tender although she does exhibit rebound tenderness. All laboratory values are normal. Vital signs are blood pressure 168/92, pulse 113, and respiratory rate 28.

72. Based on the preceding information, which condition is most likely to be developing?
(A) superior mesenteric arterial obstruction
(B) cholecystitis

(C) pancreatitis

(D) bowel obstruction

73. Which treatment, aside from pain relief, would be indicated for this patient?

(A) placement on an NPO (*nil per os;* nothing by mouth) regime with gastrointestinal suction

(B) endoscopy with cauterization

(C) laparotomy with possible mesenteric embolectomy

(D) cholecystectomy

Questions 74 and 75 refer to the following scenario.

A 76-year-old female is admitted to your unit with vomiting, nausea, and diffuse abdominal pain. The vomitus has a fecal odor. She had a cholecystectomy in the past but has been in good health until the development of abdominal pain 2 days ago. The abdomen has a hyperresonant sound on percussion, with the patient complaining of tenderness to palpation. Laboratory data are normal.

74. Based on the preceding information, which condition is likely to be developing?

(A) bowel obstruction

(B) mesenteric artery occlusion

(C) pyloric stenosis

(D) obstruction of the pancreatic duct

75. Treatment for this condition most likely would include which of the following?

(A) endoscopy for pyloric valve repair

(B) endoscopy with embolectomy of the pancreatic head

(C) laparotomy with possible mesenteric embolectomy

(D) laparotomy for relief of obstruction

76. All of the following can cause intestinal perforation. Which is the most common cause of intestinal perforation?

(A) bowel obstruction

(B) appendicitis

(C) colonic ulcers

(D) gastric ulcers

Questions 77 and 78 refer to the following scenario.

A 29-year-old male is admitted to your unit with complaints of generalized abdominal pain. The pain started yesterday and became worse, but then improved, before worsening again this morning. An abdominal examination reveals diffuse tenderness and "boardlike" rigidity with the patient preferring not to move. An abdominal radiograph reveals free air under the diaphragm. Laboratory data reveal the following:

Na^+	141
K^+	4.2
Cl^-	99
HCO_3^-	25
Amylase	50
WBC	13,000

77. Based on the preceding information, which condition is likely to be present?

(A) pancreatitis

(B) superior mesenteric artery obstruction

(C) intestinal perforation

(D) cholecystitis

78. Which treatment would be indicated for this condition?

(A) A placement on an NPO (*nil per os;* nothing by mouth) regime with gastrointestinal suction

(B) sedation with narcotics while waiting for the pain to subside

(C) upper and lower endoscopy to search for obstructions

(D) exploratory laparotomy

Gastroenterology Practice Exam

1. _____
2. _____
3. _____
4. _____
5. _____
6. _____
7. _____
8. _____
9. _____
10. _____
11. _____
12. _____
13. _____
14. _____
15. _____
16. _____
17. _____
18. _____
19. _____
20. _____

21. _____
22. _____
23. _____
24. _____
25. _____
26. _____
27. _____
28. _____
29. _____
30. _____
31. _____
32. _____
33. _____
34. _____
35. _____
36. _____
37. _____
38. _____
39. _____
40. _____

41. _____
42. _____
43. _____
44. _____
45. _____
46. _____
47. _____
48. _____
49. _____
50. _____
51. _____
52. _____
53. _____
54. _____
55. _____
56. _____
57. _____
58. _____
59. _____

60. _____
61. _____
62. _____
63. _____
64. _____
65. _____
66. _____
67. _____
68. _____
69. _____
70. _____
71. _____
72. _____
73. _____
74. _____
75. _____
76. _____
77. _____
78. _____

PART VI

Answers

1. B p445	21. B p452	41. A p461	60. B p474
2. A p445	22. B p452	42. C p494	61. B p476
3. D p446	23. D p452	43. A p463	62. D p477
4. B p446	24. C p453	44. B p465	63. D p475
5. A p446	25. A p442	45. B p467	64. C p476
6. D p446	26. C p443	46. B p467	65. D p478
7. C p448	27. B p443	47. A p467	66. A p478
8. B p448	28. A p442	48. A p467	67. B p479
9. A p448	29. A p444	49. D p468–469	68. C p479
10. A p448	30. B p444	50. C p469	69. C p483
11. B p448	31. C p445	51. A p470	70. A p483
12. A p449	32. B p446	52. B p470	71. D p479
13. C p448	33. D p446	53. D p470	72. A p482
14. D p448	34. D p446	54. D p471	73. C p482
15. D p449	35. C p447	55. C p468–470	74. A p483
16. B p449–450	36. A p448	56. A p473	75. D p485
17. A p449	37. C p450	57. C p465	76. B p484
18. C p450	38. A p459–460	58. B p474	77. C p484
19. B p450	39. D p459	59. A p474	78. D p484–485
20. D p453	40. A p461		

VII

RENAL

Deborah Klein

43

Anatomy and Physiology of the Renal System

EDITORS' NOTE

Renal patient care problems comprise approximately 5% (10 questions) of the CCRN exam. These 10 questions are spread out over three major areas: life-threatening electrolyte imbalances, acute renal failure, and renal trauma. The following chapters contain information necessary to address each of these areas.

This chapter provides the essential concepts of renal anatomy, information that probably is not directly addressed on the CCRN exam. Understanding the contents of this chapter will, however, prepare you to better appreciate the clinical situations addressed by the CCRN exam. As you review this chapter, do not focus on minute concepts but rather concentrate on general anatomical features relevant to renal concepts that might be addressed in clinical practice.

ANATOMY

Kidney

Location

The kidneys lie in the retroperitoneal space on each side of the vertebrae, with the upper border between T-11 on the right and T-12 on the left. This difference in position results from the natural displacement of the right kidney by the liver. The lower border is at approximately L-3. The posterior surfaces are protected by the last two ribs.

Protective Coverings

The kidneys are protected by coverings that prevent massive blood loss from trauma. The outermost protective covering is pararenal fat that completely surrounds the three coverings of the kidneys. The next layer is the renal fascia, a membrane sheet that surrounds a layer of perirenal fat. This perirenal fat is actually a very dense layer of adipose tissue. It is very compact and surrounds the innermost covering of the kidney, the fibrous renal capsule. The fibrous renal capsule is a thin, resistant membrane that is contiguous with the kidney tissue itself.

Shape and Size

The kidneys are bean-shaped organs with an indentation on their medial surfaces. The indented area is called the hilum. The hilum is the entrance site for the renal artery, lymphatics, and nerves and is also the exit site for the renal vein, ureters, lymphatics, and nerves. The average kidney is 10–12 cm long, 5–6 cm wide, and 3–4 cm thick. Its average weight is about 160–180 g.

Gross Anatomy

The cortex is the outer one-third of kidney tissue (Fig. 43–1). The cortex is composed of the glomeruli of all of the nephrons and the convoluted portions of the distal and proximal tubules. The cortex extends into the medulla between structures called pyramids. These extensions are the renal columns. The cortex itself extends inward from the renal capsule to the base of the pyramids.

The medulla is the inner portion of the kidney. The medulla contains the loops of Henle, the vasa recta, and the collecting ducts. These loops and ducts

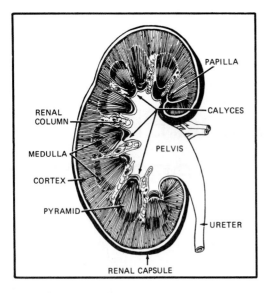

Figure 43–1. Gross anatomy of the kidney.

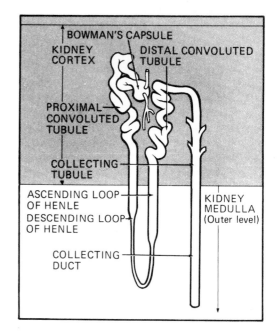

Figure 43–2. Cortical nephron.

are arranged in triangles or pyramids. The tips of the pyramids are called papillae. Groups of papillae merge to form into a single papilla to enter the calyx, which collects urine flow from the collecting ducts. Calyces channel the urine into the renal pelvis. Eventually, the urine flows from the renal pelvis into the ureter.

The number of calyces varies from 8 to 16 per kidney. Therefore, there is no symmetry in renal anatomy.

Nephron

The nephron is the functional unit of the kidney. Each kidney has more than one million nephrons. Up to 75% of the kidney's nephrons can be destroyed before the remaining nephrons are unable to compensate. While compensation is occurring, the functioning nephrons filter a higher solute load. Because of this increased workload, the functioning nephrons hypertrophy. There are two types of nephrons, cortical and juxtamedullary.

Cortical nephrons (Fig. 43–2) have glomeruli that lie close to the cortical surface and have thin, short segments of the loops of Henle. The loops of Henle do enter the medulla but do not go past the outer medulla. Since the loops of Henle in the cortical nephrons are short and do not extend into the inner medulla, they do not participate in the concentration of urine. About 70% of the kidneys' nephrons are cortical nephrons with short or nonexistent loops of Henle.

The juxtamedullary nephrons (Fig. 43–3) are found in the inner one-third of the cortex. They have long loops of Henle that dip deep into the medulla and are surrounded by the peritubular network, the vasa recta. These nephrons have a great capacity to retain sodium and concentrate urine because of the long loops of Henle.

In hypovolemic and hypotensive patients, a large portion of the renal blood flow is shunted from the

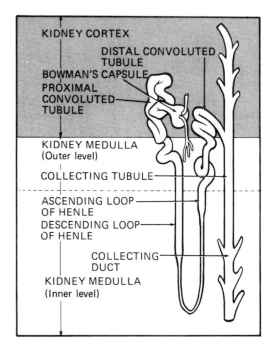

Figure 43–3. Juxtaglomerular nephron.

cortical nephrons to the juxtamedullary nephrons to maintain urine formation.

Structural Anatomy. The nephron, as the functional unit of the kidney, is composed of the glomerulus, the proximal convoluted tubule, the loop of Henle, the distal convoluted tubule, and the collecting ducts.

The glomerulus is a network of capillaries (Fig. 43–4) that are spherical in shape and are formed by the afferent arterioles dividing into between two and eight subdivisions. These subdivisions branch to form as many as 50 capillary loops. The glomerulus is enclosed by an epithelial-lined membrane called Bowman's capsule. The efferent arteriole carries the blood out of the glomerulus.

The proximal convoluted tubule is about 14 mm in length. It receives the contents of the glomerulus. The lumen of the tubule contains tiny threadlike projections that help resorb the glomerular filtrate. The brush border increases the resorptive surface area per unit length of the tubule. The proximal convoluted tubule ends in the medulla of the kidney and becomes the descending limb of the loop of Henle.

The loop of Henle has three distinct portions: a thick descending limb, a thin segment that is the actual loop, and a thick ascending limb. The loops of Henle in the cortical nephron reach just to the inside of the kidney medulla. The loops of Henle in the juxtamedullary nephron reach almost to the tips of the pyramids (the papillae) and then start ascending to become the ascending limb of the loop of Henle. The peritubular capillary network surrounds the loop portion of the juxtamedullary nephron. As the long loop

of Henle dips deep into the medulla, it is surrounded by the vasa recta. Thirty percent of the nephrons in each kidney are juxtamedullary nephrons.

The distal convoluted tubule begins where the ascending limb of the loop of Henle starts twisting. The distal convoluted tubule closely passes its own glomerulus and may even touch it. The distal convoluted tubule continues without convolutions to become the collecting tubule.

The collecting tubule extends to become the collecting duct, which empties into a common collecting duct that in turn empties into the renal pelvis.

Juxtaglomerular Apparatus. All nephrons have a juxtaglomerular apparatus (JGA) that contains three specific components. As the distal convoluted tubule passes between the afferent and efferent arterioles, there are specialized cells (Fig. 43–5) that are tightly packed together. These specialized cells are called the macula densa.

There are also specialized cells on the outside of the afferent and efferent arterioles near their entry point into the glomerulus that are referred to as juxtaglomerular cells. These cells secrete granules of inactive renin.

The area where the distal convoluted tubule passes by or touches the efferent arterioles is the third component of the JGA. The JGA and its actions are covered in a later chapter.

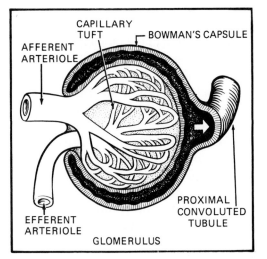

Figure 43–4. Schematic view of the glomerulus.

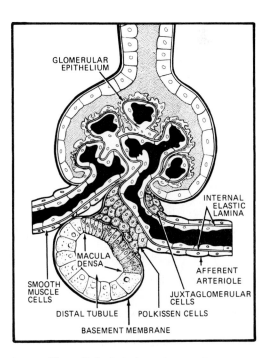

Figure 43–5. Juxtaglomerular apparatus.

Vascular System

One renal artery arises from the aorta to supply both kidneys. (Fig. 43–6). The renal artery enters the kidney at the hilum and bifurcates immediately at the kidney pelvis.

After this first splitting at the kidney pelvis, the renal arteries develop many branches called interlobar arteries. These interlobar arteries, as their name implies, travel between lobes of the renal parenchyma inside the renal columns toward the point where the cortex and medulla meet.

At the interface of the cortex and medulla, the interlobar arteries branch to form the arcuate arteries. These arteries form arcs between the lobes of the parenchyma.

From each arcuate artery, multiple intralobular arteries spread into the cortex. These intralobular arteries form short muscular afferent arterioles that supply the glomeruli. Efferent arterioles drain the blood from the glomerulus and flow through the peritubular capillary network that surrounds the cortical portions of the tubules. The small amount of remaining arterial blood flows into straight capillary loops called vasa recta. These extend down into the medulla to provide arterial blood to the lower parts of the thin segments of the loop of Henle before looping upward to enter the intralobular veins. From the intralobular veins, the blood enters the arcuate veins, the interlobar veins, the renal veins, and the inferior vena cava.

Nerve Supply

The sympathetic nervous system controls constriction of renal arteries. These nerves follow the same course as the arterioles in order to maintain vasoactive tone of the arterioles.

The parasympathetic nervous system innervates the kidney through the vagus nerve fibers arising from the celiac plexus.

Ureter, Urinary Bladder, and Urethra

As the urine leaves the kidney pelvis, it enters the ureter. The ureter, approximately 10 inches in length, moves the urine along by peristaltic action to the urinary bladder, a hollow, muscular organ. It has a normal capacity of 250–500 ml. At the bottom of the bladder is the urethra. It is about 6–8 inches long in males and 1–1.25 inches in females (Fig. 43–7).

PHYSIOLOGY

Physiological processes of the kidney include the formation of urine, the regulation of body water and electrolytes, the excretion of metabolic waste products, the regulation of acid-base balance and blood pressure, and erythropoietin secretion.

Formation of Urine

Three processes are involved in the formation of urine: glomerular filtration, tubular reabsorption, and tubular secretion.

Glomerular Filtration

The kidneys receive 20–25% of the cardiac output. Ninety-five percent of this quantity of blood will go through the glomerulus, where some solutes will be filtered out. An autoregulatory system exists to protect the glomerulus. The afferent and efferent renal arterioles constrict or dilate in response to systemic blood pressure. If systemic blood pressure increases, the afferent arteriole will constrict. This effectively reduces the pressure of the blood entering the glomerulus. In the same way, if systemic blood pressure decreases, the afferent arteriole will dilate to allow more blood to enter the glomerulus.

When the afferent arteriole constricts to reduce the pressure of blood in the glomerulus, the efferent arteriole relaxes (dilates) to allow the blood to leave more rapidly. This helps to control glomerular pressure. Conversely, when systemic pressure drops, the afferent arteriole dilates to let more blood into the glomerulus and the efferent arteriole constricts to help maintain the glomerular pressure. Below a mean arterial blood pressure of about 60 mm Hg, this autoregulatory system fails and the glomerulus suffers the effects of hypotension.

Glomerular filtration is influenced by two factors, filtration pressure and glomerular permeability.

Filtration pressure is determined in part by the anatomical blood flow through the nephron. Each nephron is actually perfused by two capillary beds

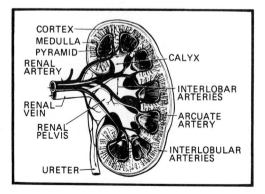

Figure 43–6. Vascular system of the kidney.

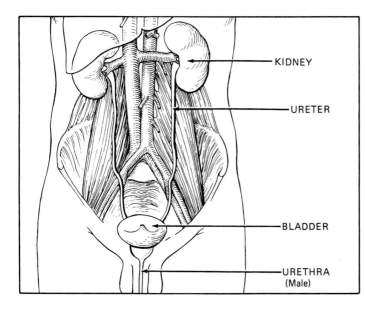

Figure 43–7. Ureter, urinary bladder, and urethra.

(Fig. 43–8). The glomerular capillary bed is perfused by the afferent arteriole with an average hydrostatic pressure of about 60 mm Hg. The peritubular capillary bed is perfused by the efferent arteriole, which resists blood flow. Because of this, the glomerular capillary bed has a high pressure (which may be termed glomerular hydrostatic pressure). The peritubular capillary bed has a low pressure of about 13 mm Hg.

The high pressure in the glomerulus tends to filter fluid out of the glomerulus and into Bowman's capsule. At the same time and following the same principles, the low pressure in the peritubular capillary bed tends to draw fluid from the interstitial spaces into the peritubular capillaries. The high pressures in the glomerulus cause a rapid filtration of fluid. The low pressure of the capillary bed of the peritubular system facilitates rapid uptake of the excreted tubular fluids by the peritubular capillaries. This diminishes backleak and increases net reabsorption.

Blood is brought into the glomerulus by the afferent arteriole. The pressure is close to 60 mm Hg, so fluid is forced from the glomerular capillaries into Bowman's capsule. This fluid is now called the glomerular ultrafiltrate. The fluid is called an ultrafiltrate because protein-size (and larger) molecules cannot filter out of the glomerular capillaries. Those proteins remain in the blood entering the peritubular capillaries from the efferent arteriole. The retained protein molecules cause an increase in the plasma osmotic pressure. The increased plasma osmotic pressure causes the rapid reabsorption of fluid from the peritubular interstitial spaces.

Glomerular permeability is the second influence on glomerular filtration. The glomerular membrane is different from other capillary membranes in the body. The glomerular membrane has three layers: the endothelial layer of the capillary, a basement membrane, and a layer of epithelial cells on the other surface of the capillary (Fig. 43–9). In spite of three layers, the glomerular membrane is 100–1000 times more permeable than the usual capillary. The endothelial cells lining the glomerular capillary are full of thousands of tiny holes called fenestrae. Outside the capillary endothelium is a basement membrane similar to a mesh of fibers. The epithelial cells of the outer layer do not touch each other. The space between the cells is called a slit pore. Any particle greater than 7 nm cannot penetrate the slit pore.

Composition of Glomerular Ultrafiltrate
Normally, the ultrafiltrate is free of protein and red blood cells since they are too large to pass through the slit pores. The semipermeable membrane of the glomerular capillary allows water, nutrients, electrolytes, and wastes to filter into Bowman's capsule.

Glomerular Filtration Rate
In the healthy kidney, the average glomerular filtration rate (GFR) is 125 ml/min. The total quantity of glomerular filtrate per day is about 180 L. More than 99% of this filtrate is reabsorbed in the tubules. The equation for calculating the GFR is the urine concentration of a substance times the urine flow rate divided by the plasma concentration of the same sub-

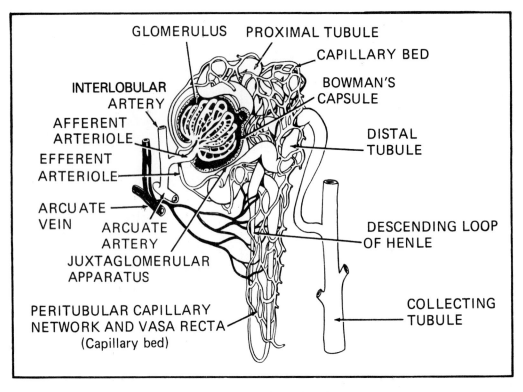

Figure 43-8. Capillary beds of a nephron.

stance. The substance must be freely filtered and not affected by the tubules (Fig. 43–10). The normal adult urine volume is 1–2 L/day.

Factors Affecting the Glomerular Filtration Rate

Any change in the glomerular hydrostatic pressure will alter the GFR. The most common cause of change in the hydrostatic pressure is a change in the systemic blood pressure. A change in systemic blood pressure changes the actual flow of blood into the glomerulus. Alterations in the afferent and efferent arteriole tone (constriction–dilatation) will also affect the glomerular pressure and hence the GFR.

Any alteration in the composition of the plasma, such as an increase in oncotic pressure (the osmotic pressure due to the presence of colloids in a solution), will alter the GFR. Such conditions as hyperproteinemia, hypoproteinemia, hypovolemia, or hypervolemia will also alter the composition of plasma because of alterations in the extracellular fluid (ECF) and intracellular fluid. Thus, these states will alter the GFR.

The GFR will automatically be altered by any abnormality of structure, presence of disease, or ingestion of nephrotoxic substances.

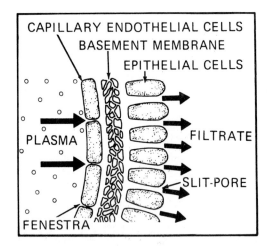

Figure 43–9. Three layers of the glomerular membrane.

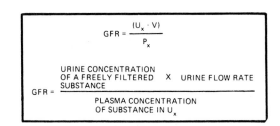

$$GFR = \frac{(U_x \cdot V)}{P_x}$$

$$GFR = \frac{\text{URINE CONCENTRATION OF A FREELY FILTERED SUBSTANCE} \times \text{URINE FLOW RATE}}{\text{PLASMA CONCENTRATION OF SUBSTANCE IN } U_x}$$

Figure 43–10. Equation for calculating the glomerular filtration rate.

Tubular Absorption and Secretion

The glomeruli filter a total of 180 L/day; normal urine output is 1–2 L/day. The tubular function of the nephron is responsible (in part) for determining urinary output.

The nephron uses two processes, absorption and secretion, to convert this 180 L of ultrafiltrate to 1–2 L of urine. These processes may be active or passive and are influenced by hormones, electrochemical gradients, and Starling's law. The following definitions are useful in understanding renal function.

1. Diffusion is the movement of solutes from an area of high concentration to an area of low concentration.
2. Osmosis is the movement of water from an area of high water concentration to an area of low water concentration.
3. Absorption, as discussed here, is the movement of solutes and water from the tubule into the peritubular network (i.e., from the filtrate back into the bloodstream).
4. Secretion, as discussed here, is the movement of solutes and water from the peritubular network into the tubule (i.e., from the bloodstream back into the filtrate).
5. Passive transport is the movement of solutes by diffusion following concentration gradients and electrical gradients.
6. Active transport is the movement of any substance against an electrical or concentration gradient. Active transport requires energy, usually supplied by ATP.

A mnemonic may help unravel the maze of the movement of solutes in the various tubules. Cations are carried by active transport (CAT—carried active transport); anions are passively transported (ANI—a negative ion). Na^+, K^+, and H^+ are the most common cations in the body; Cl^- and HCO_3^- are the most common anions.

As with most rules, there is always an exception. In the collecting duct, chloride (anion) is actively absorbed and the cations are passively absorbed. Table 43–1 traces the formation of urine, starting with the ultrafiltrate and ending with urine after passage through both convoluted tubules, the loop of Henle, and the collecting ducts.

The major function of the loop of Henle is to concentrate or dilute urine as necessary. This is accomplished by the countercurrent mechanism that maintains the hyperosmolar concentration in the renal medulla.

Body Water Regulation

Throughout the discussion of body regulation, the terms osmolarity and osmolality will be used interchangeably. Osmolarity is the concentration of particles in solution. Osmolality is the amount of solvent in relation to the particles.

The volume and concentration of body water content are maintained by the thirst–neurohypophyseal-renal axis. Approximately 60% of ideal body weight is water in males; in females, the proportion is 50–55%. Figure 43–11 shows the distribution of water throughout the body. There are three mechanisms that help regulate body fluid: thirst, antidiuretic hormone (ADH), and the countercurrent mechanism of the kidney.

Thirst. Thirst is the major force in our awareness of a need for water. The thirst center is located in the hypothalamus. Intracellular dehydration causes the sensation of thirst. The most common cause of intracellular dehydration is an increase in osmolar concentration of the ECF. Increased sodium concentration of the ECF causes osmosis of fluid from the neuronal cells of the thirst center. Other important and frequent causes of thirst are excessive angiotensin II in the blood, hemorrhage, and low cardiac output.

The role of the thirst center is to maintain a conscious desire to drink the exact amount of fluid needed to maintain a normal body hydrated state or return a dehydrated state to the normal state of hydration.

Antidiuretic Hormone. ADH works closely with the thirst mechanism. The plasma protein and ECF sodium concentrations determine the osmolality of the ECF. Normal serum osmolality is 280–320 mosm/L. Acid-base control mechanisms of the kidney adjust the negative ion in relation to the extracellular concentration (osmolality) to equal the positive ions in the body. ADH is synthesized in the supraoptic nuclei of the hypothalamus and then drips down the supraoptical–hypophyseal tracts to the posterior pituitary (neurohypophysis), where it is stored. The supraoptic area of the hypothalamus is so close to the

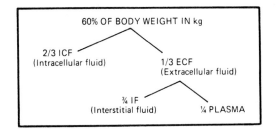

Figure 43–11. Distribution of water throughout the body.

TABLE 43–1. URINE FORMATION

Start	Proximal Convoluted Tubule	Loop of Henle (3 parts)	Distal Convoluted Tubule	Collecting Duct	Finish
Ultrafiltrate	60–80% of ultra-filtrate absorbed **Absorbed** Na+ Cl− Glucose Amino acids All K+ HCO3− H2O passively absorbed **Secreted** H+ Urea Drugs Organic acids HCO3− and H+ (regulates acid-base balance) Ultrafiltrate isotonic to plasma	**I. Descending Limb** H2O absorbed (highly permeable to H2O) Ultrafiltrate fluid becomes increasingly hypertonic **II. Thin segment loop** Permeable to H2O **III. Ascending limb** Cl− absorbed actively; Na+ absorbed Impermeable to H2O Ultrafiltrate is hypotonic	**Absorbed** HCO3− H2O if ADH is present Na+ actively if aldosterone is present **Secreted** K+ H+	**Absorbed** Na+ H2O if ADH is present **Secreted** H+ K+ NH3	Urine flows into renal pelvis, ureters, bladder

Notes:
1. Sulfates, nitrates, and phosphates are absorbed only in amounts sufficient to maintain the ECF concentration.
2. All K+ from the filtrate is absorbed in the proximal tubule.
3. The K+ secreted in the distal convoluted tubule equals about 12% of the K+ in the original filtrate. Under certain circumstances, secretion may exceed the original filtered load.

thirst center that there is an integration of the thirst mechanism, osmolality detection, and ADH release.

The osmosodium receptors respond to changes in osmolality (sodium concentration) in the ECF. An increase in osmolality excites the osmoreceptors. They signal the neurohypophyseal tract that ADH is needed. The posterior pituitary (neurohypophysis) releases the ADH that it has stored. In the presence of ADH, the distal convoluted tubules and the collecting ducts reabsorb water. The reabsorption of the water leaves a hypertonic urine. This cycle will continue until the concentration of the ECF compartment and fluid homeostasis are returned to normal.

If osmolality of the ECF decreases, ADH release is inhibited because the osmoreceptors are not stimulated. Without ADH, the distal tubules and collecting ducts are impermeable to water. Urine will be very dilute because the water cannot be reabsorbed. The urine will continue to be diluted until the loss of water has raised the concentration of the ECF solutes to normal.

Countercurrent Mechanism. The countercurrent mechanism is used to concentrate urine and excrete excessive solutes. Excreting dilute urine is not a problem for the kidney unless there is a neurological dysfunction, an endocrine dysfunction, or traumatic injuries. These conditions may result in an inappropriate release and affect normal kidney function of ADH, aldosterone, and/or cortisol. Concentrating urine to excrete waste solutes is a complex interaction between the long loops of Henle, the peritubular capillaries, and the vasa recta.

The countercurrent multiplier mechanism functions constantly in a loop cycle, with fresh filtrate continuously entering the loop of Henle. At the entry to the loop, the filtrate has a concentration of 300 mosm/L. The medulla increases this concentration so that at the tips of the papillae in the pelvic tip of the medulla, the concentration of the filtrate is 1200–1400 mosm/L.

It is essential for the medullary interstitium to be hyperosmolar. There are four steps in concentrating the solutes to produce this hyperosmolality (Fig. 43–12).

In step 1, chloride ions are actively transported from the thick portion of the ascending limb of the

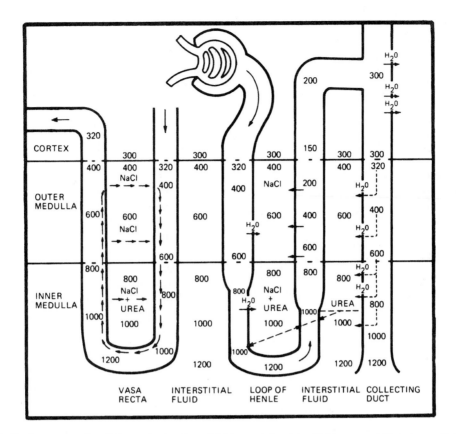

Figure 43–12. Countercurrent multiplier mechanism for maintaining medullary interstitial hyperosmolality and concentrating urine.

loop of Henle into the upper medullary interstitial fluid. The active transport of chloride pulls sodium and some potassium, magnesium, and calcium also.

In step 2, the collecting ducts actively transport sodium into the medullary interstitial fluid. Chloride follows along passively. Steps 1 and 2 increase medullary interstitial fluid hyperosmolality by about 500 mosm.

In step 3, the collecting duct yields urea to the lower medullary interstitial fluid if ADH is present. The hormone makes the collecting duct mildly permeable to urea and very permeable to water. Water leaves the collecting duct to enter the medullary interstitium, resulting in a high concentration of urea in the collecting duct. Urea, following concentration gradients, then diffuses out into the medullary interstitial fluid. This increases the medullary osmolarity by about another 200–400 mosm.

In step 4, water osmosis occurs from the thin (descending) segment of the loop of Henle because of the high urea concentration in the lower medullary interstitial fluid. As the water moves from the loop of Henle, sodium ion concentration in the thin limb increases. Because of the high concentration, sodium and chloride diffuse passively out of the

collecting duct into the lower medullary interstitium. This increases the osmolarity of the medullary interstitial fluid to between 1000 and 1200 mosm.

Excess solutes concentrated in the medullary interstitium must not be allowed to reenter the bloodstream via the peritubular capillary network. This is prevented by sluggish blood flow in these capillaries and a very small amount of blood being present (less than 2% of the total renal blood supply), keeping ion movement to a minimum. Throughout the countercurrent multiplier activity, ion movement from the loop of Henle into the medullary interstitium has been by ionic secretion (ions moving from the tubule lumen) either actively or passively and by diffusion or osmosis.

The ion solutes present in the medullary interstitial fluid must move into the ascending limb of the loop of Henle so that they can be excreted with the urine. This is accomplished by the countercurrent exchange mechanism. The vasa recta are essentially straight tubes forming a long, slender U-shaped blood vessel. Because both sides of the U are highly permeable, fluids and solutes readily exchange places in the high-concentration gradients of the lower medullary interstitium.

As the blood in the vasa recta flows back up the ascending loop of Henle, excess sodium and urea diffuse out of the blood in exchange for water diffusing into the blood. The blood leaves the medulla with almost the same osmolarity as when it entered the descending loop.

The fluid in the loop of Henle becomes more concentrated in the presence of ADH, since water has diffused out. In the ascending thick limb of the loop of Henle and the diluting segment of the distal convoluted tubule, the osmolarity of the filtrate drops. In the distal convoluted tubules and the collecting ducts, the osmolarity depends upon the presence of ADH and aldosterone. If these hormones are present, sodium and water will be absorbed and the tubule fluid will remain concentrated as it passes through the collecting ducts to the renal pelvis to enter the ureter. If the hormones are not present, water will be secreted and a more dilute urine will enter the ureter. Only juxtamedullary nephrons have long loops of Henle; they are responsible for concentrating and diluting the filtrate as urine is formed.

Many diuretics influence the reabsorption of sodium, potassium chloride, and water in the nephron. Table 43–2 presents categories of diuretics.

Excretion of Metabolic Waste Products

The metabolic waste products handled by the kidneys are estimated to be in excess of 200 different substances. These waste products are classified as threshold substances, nonthreshold substances, electrolytes, water, and other substances that may be reabsorbed or excreted by the kidneys according to individual fluctuating needs.

Threshold substances are those that are entirely reabsorbed by the kidneys unless the substances are present in excessive concentration in the blood. Glucose is the most common threshold substance. Amino acids are also threshold substances.

Nonthreshold substances are not reabsorbed by the kidney tubules. Creatinine is the most abundant nonthreshold substance. Urea is included in this category even though urea passively diffuses back into the kidney bloodstream. Proteins and acids of disease processes (lactic acid, ketones) are nonthreshold substances. Water and most electrolytes will be absorbed or secreted according to individual needs.

There are two commonly used tests to determine efficiency of kidney function in handling waste products, blood urea nitrogen (BUN) and creatinine.

The BUN measures the level of urea, a nitrogen waste product of protein metabolism. The BUN is an unreliable test of renal function because the BUN level is affected by many factors. In the presence of liver disease, the BUN will remain low because the liver cannot synthesize urea at a normal rate. Conversely, with normal kidney function, dehydration, gastrointestinal bleeding, sepsis, trauma, drugs, diet, and changes in catabolism may elevate the BUN markedly, to as much as 50 mg/100 ml. Food in the digestive tract may also falsely elevate the BUN.

Serum creatinine is a more reliable index of kidney function. Creatinine is a waste product of muscle

TABLE 43–2. CATEGORIES OF DIURETICS

Category of Diuretic	Drug	Mechanism of Action	Side Effects
Loop diuretics	Furosemide (Lasix) Bumetanide (Bumex) Ethacrynic acid (Edecrin)	Inhibits sodium chloride reabsorption in thick ascending limb of loop of Henle	Hypovolemia, thrombocytopenia, hypokalemia, hyperglycemia, hypochloremic alkalosis, transient deafness
Osmotic diuretics	Metolazone (Diulo, Zaroxolyn) Mannitol (Osmitrol)	Inhibits sodium and water reabsorption by increasing the osmolality of the tubular fluid	Blurred vision, rhinitis, rebound hypervolemia, thirst, urinary retention, electrolyte imbalances
Thiazide diuretics	Hydrochlorothiazide (HydroDiuril, Esidrix)	Inhibits sodium reabsorption in proximal and distal tubules	Rash, leukopenia, acute pancreatitis, thrombocytopenia
Potassium-sparing diuretics	Spironolactone (Aldactone) Triamterene (Dyazide, Dyrenium, Maxzide)	Inhibits aldosterone Promotes sodium excretion and potassium reabsorption in distal tubule causing a mild diuresis	Hyperkalemia, headache, hyponatremia, nausea, diarrhea, urticaria, menstrual disturbances
Carbonic anhydrase inhibitors	Acetazolamide (Diamox)	Inhibits the enzyme carbonic anhydrase in the proximal tubule preventing bicarbonate and sodium reabsorption	Hyperchloremic, acidosis, renal calculi, rash, nausea, vomiting, anorexia

metabolism and is freely filtered. The nephron tubules neither reabsorb nor secrete creatinine. The normally functioning kidney filters creatinine from the blood at a rate equal to the GFR. Since the amount of creatinine produced each day is constant and is proportional to the body's muscle mass, serial serum creatinines are valuable indices of kidney function except in septic patients and patients with muscle-wasting diseases.

Normally, a BUN-to-creatinine ratio of 10:1 is present in serum. A ratio of 20:1 or more is indicative of prerenal insufficiency (water and salt depletion), a high protein catabolism, or low renal perfusion pressures.

An elevation of both BUN and creatinine above the normal ratio indicates renal disease. In these patients, a creatinine clearance is usually performed. Creatinine clearance is probably the most reliable index of kidney function available. Normal creatinine clearance is 125 ml/min. Urine is collected for 12 or 24 hr or for a specified period of time, and a blood serum sample is drawn halfway through the urine collection. If the BUN, creatinine, and creatinine clearance tests are normal, the kidneys are functioning adequately in excreting metabolic waste products from the body.

Regulation of Acid-Base Balance

The body acid-base balance is maintained by the lungs, blood buffers, and the kidneys. The kidneys regulate acid-base balance by controlling the bicarbonate ion (HCO_3^-) and, in much lesser quantity, the hydrogen ion (H^+).

A normal diet contains some acids (phosphates and sulfates) that must be excreted. In addition, protein catabolism is markedly increased in the critically ill. Protein catabolism adds to the acid load of the body. Products of protein catabolism are eliminated by the kidneys.

Four mechanisms provide for the excretion of acid and regulation of acid-base balance by the kidneys.

The first mechanism is direct excretion of hydrogen ions. Hydrogen ion is excreted in a very minute amount (less than 1 mEq of hydrogen ion per day) and has only a minor role in acid-base control. A passive secretion of hydrogen ion occurs in the proximal tubules. An active secretion of hydrogen ion occurs in the distal tubules.

The second mechanism is excretion of hydrogen with urine buffers. Nonvolatile acids are excreted in this process. The glomerulus filters these acids and bicarbonate. The phosphate acids filtered are an example of the process for excreting hydrogen ion with a urine buffer.

$$H_2CO_3 + Na_2HPO_4 \rightarrow NaHCO_3 + NaH_2PO_4$$

| carbonic acid | bisodium phosphate | sodium bicarbonate | sodium biphosphate |

The carbonic acid combines with bisodium phosphate and yields sodium bicarbonate and sodium biphosphate. The sodium bicarbonate breaks down into sodium and bicarbonate and is reabsorbed as needed. The sodium biphosphate adds a hydrogen ion to become a molecule and is excreted in urine. The net result of the phosphate and sulfate wastes filtered by the glomerulus is the addition of a hydrogen ion per molecule excreted. Up to 20 mEq per day may be excreted with these buffers.

The third mechanism of acid-base control by the kidneys is excretion of acids by using ammonia (NH_3). Chemically, ammonia is produced in renal tubular cells and diffuses into tubular fluid, where carbonic acid combines with ammonia and actually produces two factors that benefit acid-base control.

$$NH_3 + H_2CO_3 \rightarrow NH_4 + HCO_3$$

| ammonia | carbonic acid | ammonium ion | bicarbonate ion |

Ammonium (ammonia with one additional hydrogen ion) combines with anions.

$$2NH_4HCO_3 + Na_2SO_4 \leftrightarrow 2NaHCO_3 + (NH_4)_2SO_4$$

| ammonium bicarbonate | sodium sulfate | sodium bicarbonate | ammonium sulfate |

The ammonium sulfate, which now has two hydrogen ions, is excreted in the urine. The sodium bicarbonate is available to buffer in the body as needed. Up to 50 mEq of acid per day may be excreted by using ammonia.

In the fourth mechanism, production and reabsorption of bicarbonate, new bicarbonate ion is manufactured in the distal convoluted tubule as needed. The formula is:

$$H_2O + CO_2 \overset{CA}{\leftrightarrow} H_2CO_3 \overset{CA}{\leftrightarrow} H^+ + HCO_3^-$$

| water | carbon dioxide | carbonic acid | hydrogen ion | bicarbonate ion |

The process of forming a new bicarbonate can start in the distal tubule. Carbon dioxide results from dissolved carbon dioxide in the renal venous blood. The carbon dioxide combines with water present in the distal tubule to form carbonic acid. This is termed the hydration of carbon dioxide with the catalyst carbonic anhydrase (CA).

Carbonic anhydrase speeds up the chemical reaction without actually entering into the chemical reaction. The brush border of the proximal convoluted tubule contains a great deal of carbonic anhydrase; the distal convoluted tubule does not. The formation of carbonic acid is very rapid in the proximal tubule. The carbonic acid produced ionizes more slowly in the distal tubule.

The carbonic acid ionizes into hydrogen ion and bicarbonate ion to buffer as needed. If the body is acidotic, the hydrogen ion is excreted in the urine. The bicarbonate is absorbed into the ECF along with sodium. If the body is in acid-base balance, the carbonic acid dissociates into water and carbon dioxide. The water joins the urine, and the carbon dioxide rapidly diffuses into the ECF.

In acidotic states, there is an increase in hydrogen ion secretion in the distal tubule that accompanies an increased excretion of acid buffers, phosphates, and sulfates. Ammonium formation is the predominant control mechanism. Because more acid is being excreted in the urine, urine pH may be as low as 4.4.

In alkalotic states, there is a decrease in hydrogen ion secretion in the distal tubules. This is accompanied by an excess bicarbonate excretion in the urine, resulting in urine that is alkaline (pH greater than 7.0).

Regulation of Blood Pressure

The kidneys participate in regulation of blood pressure through four different mechanisms: by maintaining ECF volume and composition, by regulating aldosterone, through the renin-angiotensin mechanism, and by regulating prostaglandin synthesis.

Maintaining Extracellular Fluid Volume and Composition

The autoregulatory system of the afferent and efferent arterioles responds to change in blood pressure to maintain consistent perfusion of the glomerulus. When this system fails, plasma flow may increase by two mechanisms. Vasoconstriction will maintain or elevate the blood pressure for a short period of time. If no more defense mechanisms exist, then only intravenous fluids (crystalloids or colloids) will alter the volume flow or composition of the plasma and the ECF. As the flow of plasma decreases, the patient becomes hypotensive, hypoxic, and hypoperfused. As the plasma flow deficit and the extracellular deficits are corrected, the patient becomes more closely normotensive.

Aldosterone Effect on Blood Pressure

The main effect of aldosterone is to maintain normal sodium concentration in the ECF. As sodium is the most abundant cation in the ECF, all other cations and anions will be present in varying ratios to the sodium. Aldosterone promotes reabsorption of sodium in both the distal convoluted tubule and the collecting ducts of the kidneys. Sodium will "drag along" water, bicarbonate, chloride, and other ions as it is reabsorbed. This mechanism helps to restore extracellular and intracellular fluid volumes, alter the composition of the compartments as needed, and subsequently, in a normal healthy kidney, maintain the blood pressure.

Renin-Angiotensin Mechanism

Any factor that decreases the glomerular filtration rate will activate the renin-angiotensin system. The most potent effect is upon systemic blood pressure.

Once activated, the juxtaglomerular apparatus (JGA), located adjacent to the glomeruli, releases inactive renin. Factors triggering the release of inactive renin (e.g., decreased blood pressure and decreased sodium content in the distal tubule) reflect a diminished GFR. Once released, the inactive renin acts on angiotensinogen to split away the vasoactive peptide, angiotensin I. Angiotensin I is split to angiotensin II in the presence of a converting enzyme found primarily in the lung and liver but also located in the kidney and all blood vessels.

Angiotensin II is a potent vasoconstricting agent. Angiotensin II in the circulatory system causes a severe constriction of peripheral arterioles and a milder constriction in the venous system. It also causes a constriction of renal arterioles. This results in the kidneys reabsorbing sodium and water and expanding the ECF volume.

Angiotensin II also stimulates the release of aldosterone to enhance sodium and water reabsorption, thus supporting an increase in circulating volume. This increase in sodium stimulates the thirst mechanism in an effort to reestablish circulating blood volume.

On rare occasions, some factors initiate the release of renin and the release is never turned off. The continuous presence of renin may maintain an active system known as malignant hypertension. The key to treating malignant hypertension is to cut off the release of renin.

Prostaglandins

It was once thought that prostaglandins were originally located in the seminal vesicles and produced by the prostate gland (thus their name). Prostaglandins are unsaturated fatty acids found in most cells but highly concentrated in the kidneys, brain, and gonads. Prostaglandins or their precursors are synthesized in the medullary interstitial cells and the collecting tubules of the kidneys. Prostaglandins promote a vasodilation of the renal medulla to maintain renal perfusion during severe or prolonged systemic hypoperfusion.

Red Blood Cell Synthesis and Maturation

Renal erythropoietic factor is an enzyme that is released by a hypoxic kidney as a result of decreased oxygen supply. After being released into the bloodstream, the erythropoietic factor reacts with a glycoprotein to break away as erythropoietin. Erythropoietin circulates in the blood for about 24 hr. During this time, it stimulates red blood cell production by the bone marrow. After five or more days, a

TABLE 43–3. BLOOD AND URINARY DIAGNOSTIC STUDIES FOR EVALUATION OF THE RENAL FUNCTION

Study	Significance
Blood	
Hematocrit/hemoglobin	Reflects bleeding or lack of erythropoietin
Creatinine	Reflects renal disease
Blood urea nitrogen (BUN)	Normal BUN to creatinine ratio is 10:1
	Ratio in excess of 20:1, suspect dehydration, catabolic state
	Elevation in both BUN and creatinine results from decreased GFR
Electrolytes	
Arterial blood gases	
Clotting profile	
Osmolality	
Protein, albumin, glucose, cholesterol	
Urine	
Specific gravity (normal 1.003–1.030)	Less than 1.010, suspect DI, overhydration, or CHF
	Greater than 1.030, suspect proteinuria, glycosuria, x-ray contrast media, or severe dehydration
Creatinine clearance (24 hr urine collection)	Estimates percentage of functioning nephrons
Culture and sensitivity	Presence or absence of infection
pH (normal 4–8)	Alkaline urine seen with infection
Glucose	Present when renal threshold for glucose exceeded
Acetone	Present during starvation and DKA
Protein	Present in nephrotic syndrome and renal failure caused by myeloma proteins
Spot electrolytes (sodium, potassium, and chloride)	Assesses ability of renal tubules to conserve sodium and concentrate urine
Urinary sediment	
Casts	Protein that takes on the shape of the tubule in which it is formed
Hyaline casts	Present in large amounts in proteinuria
Erythrocyte casts	Diagnostic for active glomerulonephritis
Leukocyte casts	Diagnostic for infection
Granular casts	Result from degenerating erythrocyte or leukocyte casts
Fatty casts	Present in large amounts in lipoid nephrosis and nephrotic syndrome
Renal tubular casts	Present in acute renal failure
Renal epithelial cells	Present in large amounts during ATN and nephrotic injury
Erythrocytes	Present in large amounts in active glomerulonephritis, interstitial nephritis, infections
Bacteria	Presence determined by Gram stain
Leukocytes	Present in infection and interstitial nephritis
Crystals	Present in diseases of stone formation or following ethylene glycol intoxication
Eosinophils	Present during an allergic reaction in kidney

DI, diabetes insipidus; CHF, congestive heart failure; DKA, diabetic ketoacidosis; ATN, acute tubular necrosis.

TABLE 43–4. RADIOLOGIC STUDIES USED IN EVALUATING RENAL FUNCTION

Study	Significance
Abdominal radiograph	Determines position, shape, and size of kidney
Intravenous pyelogram (IVP)	Visualizes urinary tract to diagnose partial obstruction, renovascular hypertension, tumor, cysts, and congenital abnormalities
Renal scan	Determines renal perfusion, function, and presence of obstruction and masses
Retrograde pyelography	Determines presence of obstruction in upper region of urinary collecting system
Retrograde urethrography	Evaluates urethra
Cystoscopy	Detects bladder or urethral pathologic processes
Renal arteriography	Identifies tumors and status of renovascular disease
Ultrasonography	Identifies hydronephrosis and fluid collections
Computed tomography (CT)	Identifies tumors and other pathologic conditions that create variations in body density
Magnetic resonance imaging (MRI)	Provides direct imaging in several planes conducive to detecting renal cystic disease, inflammatory processes, and renal cell carcinoma
Kidney biopsy	Determines cause and extent of lesions

maximum rate of red blood cell production is achieved. The life of the red blood cell is approximately 120 days.

Either the kidney itself or some other factor that is the precursor of erythropoietin synthesizes the erythropoietic factor by releasing an enzyme called renal erythropoietin factor. Bone marrow by itself does not respond to hypoxia by producing new red blood cells.

Patients with chronic renal failure have hemoglobins of 5 and 6 g. The diseased kidneys are unable to respond to hypoxia and cannot produce erythropoietin factor. It is believed that possibly 10% of erythropoietin is formed in some place other than the kidney.

Diagnostic studies used in evaluating renal function are presented in Tables 43–3 and 43–4.

44

Renal Regulation of Electrolytes

EDITORS' NOTE

This chapter contains information from the CCRN section on life-threatening electrolyte imbalances. You will find more detail in this chapter than the test requires. However, understanding this detail is helpful in answering the questions presented on the exam. Expect two to four questions from this chapter on the exam.

One of the major functions of the kidney is to maintain electrolyte homeostasis. Within 1 hr of cessation of kidney function, physiological deterioration of the body begins because of a lack of electrolyte regulation. Electrolytes are in a precarious balance in the critically ill patient. Continuous monitoring is essential to recognize imbalances early, to prevent generalized deterioration, and to assist the kidneys in reestablishing homeostasis.

The electrolytes of major concern are sodium, potassium, calcium, phosphate, magnesium, and chloride. Electrolyte imbalances are a result of (1) excessive ingestion or reabsorption of an electrolyte or (2) the lack of ingestion or excessive excretion of an electrolyte. Most body fluid imbalances are caused by a dysfunction in the regulation of electrolytes and water by the kidney.

SODIUM

Sodium Regulation

Sodium (Na^+) is the most prevalent cation in the body's extracellular fluid compartment. Na^+ directly influences the fluid (water) load of the body and exists in the body in combination with an anion, usually chloride. Sodium is important in maintaining extracellular fluid osmotic pressure, serum osmolarity, and acid-base balance. Intracellularly, it plays a major role in chemical pathways. Sodium also controls muscle contraction. The normal serum sodium level ranges between 135 and 145 mEq/L. To maintain this level, sodium is reabsorbed from four parts of the kidney. The majority of filtered sodium is reabsorbed in the proximal convoluted tubules; lesser amounts are reabsorbed in the loop of Henle, in the distal convoluted tubule, and in the collecting ducts. Reabsorption of sodium increases with a decreased glomerular filtration rate (GFR) as seen with hypoperfusion states (shock, myocardial infarction).

Aldosterone has the greatest influence on sodium excretion. Aldosterone is a mineralocorticoid secreted by the adrenal cortex. It is the most potent natural inhibitor of sodium excretion. Aldosterone production and release is stimulated by high potassium levels, steroids (ACTH), and angiotensin II. Aldosterone acts on the distal convoluted tubule and the collecting duct to promote reabsorption of sodium and excretion of potassium. Without aldosterone present, the distal tubule and the collecting ducts cannot closely regulate the amount of sodium reabsorbed. The increased reabsorption of sodium in the presence of aldosterone also results in reabsorption of water.

Diuretic therapy is usually thought of in relation to potassium. However, the loop diuretics (furosemide [Lasix], ethnacrynic acid [Edecrin], and bumetanide [Bumex]) block the chloride pump in the thick portion of the ascending limb of the loop of Henle. When chloride reabsorption is blocked, sodium cannot diffuse out of the ascending limb. Other factors that can increase the excretion of sodium include an increased GFR, decreased aldosterone secretion, and increased antidiuretic hormone (ADH) levels.

Hypernatremia

A serum sodium level above 145 mEq/L is termed hypernatremia. Most cases of hypernatremia are due not to Na^+ disturbances but to fluid disturbances. Hypernatremia may be seen with dehydration. Treatment is centered on giving fluid, not removing sodium. If there is a pure water loss or decreased intake causing the hypernatremia, the hematocrit will be elevated, serum chloride will be above 106 mEq/L, urine specific gravity will be greater than 1.025, and urine sodium levels will be low. Hypernatremia may also be associated with fluid volume excess with a gain of both sodium and water, but a relatively greater gain of sodium. Hypernatremia is a significant electrolyte disturbance because of the neurological and endocrine disturbances that result. Hypernatremia may cause some depression of cardiac function.

Etiology

With the exception of disturbances in vascular fluid levels, any condition leading to polyuria with conservation of sodium results in hypernatremic dehydration. The most common cause is the lack of or insufficient ADH secretion (e.g., diabetes insipidus). Increased insensible water loss (e.g., from severe burn injuries) and hypertonic enteral feedings may lead to hypernatremia. Potassium depletion (from vomiting, diarrhea, or nasogastric suction) and uncontrolled diabetes mellitus with osmotic diuresis secondary to hyperglycemia may also create a hypernatremia.

The comatose patient is a high-risk patient for hypernatremia, since the thirst mechanism cannot be recognized or expressed. Excessive administration of osmotic diuretics and sodium bicarbonate (in treating lactic acidosis) may also cause an iatrogenic hypernatremia. Overuse of high sodium-containing laxatives and antacids may also precipitate a hypernatremia. Hypernatremia may also be seen with renal dysfunction. If the kidneys are too damaged to filter and excrete sodium, sodium and fluid retention may result.

Clinical Presentation

Hypernatremia generally occurs with dehydration. Signs include dry, sticky mucous membranes, thirst, oliguria, fever, tachycardia, and agitation. The patient may demonstrate behavior changes, hypotension, decreased cardiac output, convulsion, or coma; death may result. As long as renal function is intact, hypernatremia rarely produces increased mortality. Patients with hypernatremia associated with sodium and fluid volume excess present with edema, increased blood pressure, dyspnea, and weight gain.

Treatment

Fluid administration with free water (nonelectrolyte solutions like D_5W) in a dehydrated patient is the key to diluting the sodium and halting the progression toward hypovolemic shock. Identifying and treating the underlying cause is the key to successful treatment of hypernatremia with fluid retention. The challenge is to stabilize the patient's hypertension, prevent pulmonary edema, and maintain neurological stability. Diuretics and limitation of fluid intake are indicated.

Hyponatremia

Hyponatremia is present when the serum sodium level is less than 130 mEq/L. Usually, the plasma chloride will be less than 98 mEq/L. Hematocrit may be decreased due to water excess.

Etiology

Hyponatremia is due to either (1) an excessive amount of water or (2) sodium depletion. Excessive amounts of water can occur in many situations. The postgastric or postintestinal surgery patient who has nasogastric suction in use and who is receiving intravenous D_5W may become hyponatremic in only 2 or 3 days. Repeated tap water enemas may result in hyponatremia. Occasionally, patients drink too much plain water.

The syndrome of inappropriate ADH (SIADH) release may precipitate a hyponatremia. In this instance, the stimulus that activated ADH release is never turned off. The presence of ADH results in the kidneys reabsorbing water continuously and diluting the body's sodium levels. Water retention diluting serum sodium levels may also occur with congestive heart failure, cirrhosis of the liver, or nephrotic syndrome. A low cardiac output precipitates water retention by the kidneys.

Hypovolemic hyponatremia due to sodium depletion or loss is commonly caused by the overuse of the thiazide diuretics, furosemide (Lasix), and monnitol (Osmitrol). Diarrhea, Addison's disease, gastric suction, hyperglycemia (with a glucose-induced diuresis), vomiting, and extreme diaphoresis without intravenous replacement of sodium may also cause hypovolemic hyponatremia.

Clinical Presentation

The clinical presentation of hyponatremia depends on the magnitude, rapidity of onset, and cause. In general, the faster the serum sodium drops and the lower the serum sodium level, the more likely that symptoms will be severe.

Hyponatremia with Water Retention

In hyponatremia with water excess, signs of water intoxication are usually present. They include apathy, coma, confusion, headache, generalized weakness, hyporeflexia, convulsions, and death. Increased blood pressure and edema are usually present.

Hyponatremia with Dehydration

If the hyponatremia is associated with decreased extracellular fluid, the symptoms are essentially the same as for heat prostration. Apprehension and anxiety are followed by a feeling of impending doom. The patient is weak, confused or stuporous, and may have abdominal cramps and nausea. Mucous membranes are dry. Azotemia develops and progresses to oliguria. In severe cases, vasomotor collapse occurs with hypotension, tachycardia, and shock.

An interesting clinical presentation exists in cases of hyponatremia associated with dehydration. As dehydration progresses, fluid moves from the extracellular to the intracellular compartment. A finger pressed over the sternum will result in a fingerprint. This "fingerprinting of the sternum" indicates that much extracellular fluid has been excreted and plasma fluid has moved into the intracellular spaces from the vascular system. Without appropriate intervention, the patient may die very quickly. In less severe cases, symptoms may include lassitude, apathy, headache, anorexia, nausea, vomiting, diarrhea, muscle spasms, and cramps.

Treatment

The goal of treatment is to reestablish normal serum sodium levels slowly in order to avoid cerebral injury. Fluid restriction or low-dose diuretic therapy is the treatment of choice if the hyponatremia is due to excess vascular fluid. Diuretics, if used, are given cautiously to avoid cerebral injury. Cerebral injury could occur from too rapid expansion of brain cells from the water removal. In instances other than SIADH, replacement of sodium with normal or hypertonic saline may also be indicated. Close monitoring of all body systems, along with monitoring of serial serum sodium levels, is essential during this period.

In SIADH, the treatment is to restrict water intake while attempting to aid the kidneys in excreting water normally. In susceptible SIADH patients, hypertonic saline administration may induce congestive heart failure.

POTASSIUM

Potassium Regulation

Potassium (K^+) is the most prevalent intracellular cation in the body. The normal serum potassium level is 3.5–5.0 mEq/L. Potassium maintains osmolarity and electrical neutrality inside the cell and helps maintain acid-base balance. Intracellular homeostasis is needed for converting carbohydrates into energy and for reassembling amino acids into proteins. Transmission of nerve impulses is dependent on potassium. The muscles of the heart, lungs, intestines, and skeletal muscles cannot function normally without potassium.

All of the potassium filtered by the glomeruli is reabsorbed in the proximal convoluted tubule. Potassium that is excreted is secreted from the interstitial medullary space into the distal convoluted tubules. It amounts to about 10–12% of the original potassium volume of the ultrafiltrate in the proximal convoluted tubules. The amount of potassium excreted depends largely on the volume of urine. About 85% of the potassium is excreted in the urine, and about 15% is excreted in the intestines. Even in hypokalemia (decreased potassium), a large urine volume will contain potassium, further compounding problems. Sodium and potassium will compete with each other for reabsorption. The normal ratio of potassium to sodium ion reabsorption is 1:35.

Sodium and potassium are intimately related, and factors that affect sodium reabsorption and excretion also affect the potassium level. Potassium levels are commonly raised by intravenous fluids containing potassium chloride. Although the kidneys act readily to conserve sodium, potassium is poorly conserved, especially in patients who are critically ill.

Factors that enhance excretion of potassium include an elevated intracellular potassium level, which may be caused by an acute metabolic or respiratory alkalosis that forces potassium into the cells and hydrogen out of the cells. Diuretics and other factors resulting in high-volume flow rates in the distal convoluted tubule result in increased excretion of potassium. Aldosterone functions as a feedback mechanism on the distal convoluted tubule and collecting ducts to reabsorb sodium and excrete potassium when the extracellular fluid potassium level is increased. The enhancement of sodium reabsorption may force potassium excretion.

Potassium maintains an extracellular-to-intracellular fluid gradient. This gradient is affected by the adrenal steroids, hyponatremia, glycogen formation, testosterone, and pH changes. The most significant of these influences is the pH. Serum potassium moves inversely to the pH. If the pH falls, potassium concentration increases. If the pH rises, potassium concentration decreases in part because of the ionic charge of potassium and hydrogen. Serum potassium must be evaluated with the arterial blood gases to avoid compounding problems of potassium therapy.

Hyperkalemia

Hyperkalemia is a potassium level greater than 5.5 mEq/L. It is due to an inability of the kidney tubules to excrete potassium ions. Tubular damage or increased potassium load that exceeds the kidney's ability to handle the quantity of potassium results in hyperkalemia.

Etiology

Hyperkalemia may be due to acute and chronic renal disease, low cardiac output states, acidosis, sodium depletion, or large muscle mass injury. Any factor that destroys cells (e.g., burns, trauma, or crush injuries) will release the intracellular potassium, causing hyperkalemia. Excessive ingestion of potassium chloride (found in antacids and salt substitutes), adrenal cortical insufficiency, and the hemolysis of banked blood may also cause hyperkalemia.

Clinical Presentation

Hyperkalemia causes a dilated and flaccid heart accompanied by a bradycardia. Generalized muscle irritability or flaccidity, which may be severe enough to be a flaccid paralysis, and numbness of extremities are present. There may be abdominal cramping, nausea, and diarrhea. Generally, the patient is apathetic and may be confused.

Electrocardiogram (ECG) tracings show a tall, peaked or tent-shaped T wave with potassium levels of 5.5–7.5 mEq/L. In marked hyperkalemia (potassium of 7.5–9 mEq/L), there is a flattening and widening of the P wave, a prolonged PR interval, and usually depression of the ST segment. In severely advanced hyperkalemia (potassium of 8–9 mEq/L and often more than 10 mEq/L), the P

waves disappear and intraventricular conduction disturbances occur, producing intraventricular and supraventricular dysrhythmias progressing to ventricular tachycardia, ventricular standstill, or fibrillation and death.

Treatment

A serum potassium level above 5.5 mEq/L requires immediate intervention. Treatment is initiated to prevent increasing bradycardia and cardiac arrest. The objective of treatment is to reduce the serum potassium to a safe level as rapidly as possible. Cardiac monitoring is essential.

Intravenous 10% glucose with regular insulin will temporarily drive potassium into the cell. Intravenous sodium bicarbonate will buffer cellular hydrogen and allow potassium to move intracellularly. Calcium chloride will oppose the cardiotoxic effects of hyperkalemia. However, calcium therapy is contraindicated in patients on digoxin. Kayexalate is given orally or as an enema to rid the body of potassium. Kayexalate forces a one-for-one exchange of sodium for potassium in the intestinal cell wall; however, the patient must be monitored for sodium retention. Sorbitol is used to induce an osmotic diarrhea through semiliquid stools.

These measures are all emergency procedures to provide time to ascertain the cause of the hyperkalemia. If the cause is physiological or if the hyperkalemia is refractory, dialysis is indicated. If the cause is overingestion, the emergency measures may be sufficient and the patient may need only additional conservative treatment, close monitoring, and instruction on how to prevent recurrences.

Hypokalemia

Hypokalemia is a serum potassium level of less than 3.5 mEq/L. Hypokalemia occurs when potassium loss is greater than potassium intake.

Etiology

Hypokalemia may be due to alkalosis, which stimulates hydrogen ion retention and potassium ion secretion in the distal convoluted tubules of the kidney. Diuretic therapy, without potassium replacement, endocrine dysfunction (increased ACTH, thyroid storm) and renal dysfunction (tubular acidosis) may all cause hypokalemia.

High potassium losses, gastric and intestinal surgery, nasogastric suctioning, diarrhea, prolonged vomiting, and intestinal diseases predispose the patient to hypokalemia unless replacement therapy is maintained.

Clinical Presentation

Hypokalemia has many of the same signs as hyperkalemia. There is a general malaise and muscle weakness which may progress to a flaccid paralysis. Anorexia, nausea, and vomiting may accompany a paralytic ileus. Mental status may range from drowsiness to coma. Hypotension may be present and may lead to cardiac arrest. If the patient is on digitalis, signs of digitalis toxicity may be present because hypokalemia potentiates the effect of digitalis.

Cardiac dysrhythmias are most commonly atrial unless the hypokalemia is profound, in which case premature ventricular beats are found. Other ventricular dysrhythmias are rare unless digitalis toxicity is present. ECG tracings most commonly show a prominent U wave. Depression or flattening of the ST segment or inversion of the T wave may be apparent. An inverted T wave may fuse with the U wave, giving the appearance of a prolonged QT interval. There is a generalized irritability of the heart in hypokalemic states.

Weakness of the muscles results in shallow respiration that may progress to apnea. In hypokalemia, death may be due to respiratory arrest.

Treatment

Emergency treatment of severe hypokalemia is the slow intravenous administration of potassium chloride (approximately 10–20 mEq/h) while monitoring the patient's ECG patterns for dysrhythmias due to hyperkalemia. Monitoring of symptoms, serum potassium levels, and arterial blood gases is imperative to prevent an iatrogenic hyperkalemia.

Nonemergency treatment is to replace potassium with intravenous fluids containing potassium chloride or with oral potassium supplements. Oral supplements should be diluted to prevent gastrointestinal irritation and to facilitate absorption. The patient is monitored for adequate intake and output, cardiac status, potassium levels, and signs of alkalosis or impending digitalis toxicity.

CALCIUM

Calcium Regulation

The normal serum calcium (Ca^{2+}) concentration is 8.5 to 10.5 mg/dl. Calcium, with phosphorus, makes bones and teeth rigid and strong. Calcium is integral to determining the strength and thickness of cell membranes. Calcium exerts a quieting action on nerve cells, thus maintaining normal transmission of nerve impulses. Calcium also activates specific enzymes of the blood-clotting process and those involved in the contraction of the myocardium.

Ninety-eight percent of calcium filtered by the kidneys is reabsorbed along the same pathways as sodium. There are four major factors influencing calcium reabsorption: parathyroid hormone (PTH), vitamin D, corticosteroids, and diuretics.

Parathyroid Hormone

If the serum PTH level is increased, there is increased reabsorption of ionized calcium from renal tubules. Reciprocally, the PTH increases phosphate excretion and increases calcium absorption from the gastrointestinal tract. PTH will mobilize calcium from the bones when the kidneys cannot or do not reabsorb sufficient calcium.

Vitamin D

Vitamin D must be present in an activated form to promote absorption of calcium from the small intestines. Vitamin D is ingested in food, especially milk. The vitamin must then be activated by ultraviolet (sun) light changing a chemical in the skin. This vitamin is additionally changed in the liver. Finally, the kidneys convert the vitamin to 1,25-dihydroxycholecalciferol, also known as activated vitamin D. The activated vitamin D promotes absorption of calcium from the small intestines. PTH stimulates this activation process, since a low serum level of calcium precludes an increase of calcium absorption in the kidney without PTH.

Corticosteroids

Corticosteroids are suspected of interfering with the activation of vitamin D, possibly in the liver, and decreasing the amount of calcium absorbed from the small intestines.

Diuretics

Diuretics can cause increased excretion of calcium and the other electrolytes. If a fluid volume loss results in a decreased total body fluid volume, there will be a decreased GFR, resulting in reduced calcium excretion.

Hypercalcemia

Etiology

Hypercalcemia exists when the serum calcium level is above 10.5 mg/dl. Increased renal reabsorption of calcium may cause hypercalcemia. It may also be the result of increased intestinal absorption of calcium due to excessive dietary calcium intake or excessive vitamin D ingestion.

Hyperparathyroidism caused by parathyroid adenoma will cause hypercalcemia by increasing bone release of calcium and by continuously stimulating the kidneys to reabsorb calcium. This also occurs in carcinoma of the parathyroid glands. Milk-alkali syndrome can occur in peptic ulcer patients treated for a prolonged period with milk and alkaline antacids, particularly calcium carbonate.

Multiple myelomas and metastatic carcinoma of the bone cause hypercalcemia secondary to the release of calcium from the bone into the serum. Prolonged bedrest or immobilization potentiates the movement of calcium from the bones, teeth, and intestines. This process is more conspicuous in patients with Paget's disease. Frequently, the calcium is deposited in joints, in muscle tissue close to joints, and in the kidneys as calcium stones.

Drugs, especially thiazide diuretics, inhibit calcium excretion leading to hypercalcemia in susceptible patients. Renal tubular acidosis, thyrotoxicosis, and hypophosphatemia may all cause hypercalcemia in susceptible patients.

Clinical Presentation

Neurological changes include subtle personality changes in early and mild hypercalcemia progressing to lethargy, confusion, and coma as the severity of the hypercalcemia increases. Neuromuscular changes progress from weakness and hypotonicity to flaccidness.

The renal system may be affected by the formation of calcium calculi with varying amounts of urine output, depending on the location of the calculi, which may cause thigh or flank pain. Polyuria and polydipsia are often present because the increased calcium inhibits the action of ADH on the distal tubules and the collecting ducts.

Gastrointestinal symptoms include anorexia, nausea, vomiting, and constipation. Hypercalcemia stimulates gastric acid secretion and may lead to peptic ulcers. The hypotonicity caused by hypercalcemia results in decreased intestinal motility and constipation.

Cardiac changes are less common in hypercalcemia than in hyperkalemia. The earliest ECG change is a shortening of the QT interval due to shortening of the ST segment. Digitalis and calcium are synergistic. Sudden death in hypercalcemia is often attributed to ventricular fibrillation due to this synergism.

An ocular abnormality known as band keratopathy may occur as a result of deposition of calcium crystals in the cornea. Calcium is deposited at the lateral borders of the cornea in the shape of parentheses. If the calcification is extensive, calcium will be deposited in semilunar bands across the cornea connecting the parentheses. This band keratopathy may be seen by the naked eye.

Treatment

The objective of treatment is to reduce the serum calcium level. Normal saline intravenous solutions and diuretics will increase the GFR and thus excretion of calcium, provided there are no obstructive calculi. These treatments require accurate intake and output monitoring.

Drug therapy includes corticosteroids (which antagonize vitamin D and decrease gastrointestinal absorption of calcium), mithramycin (which actually depresses mobilization of calcium from the bones), and phosphates (which will bind to calcium in the intestines and precipitate calcium when administered intravenously).

Neurological and cardiac monitoring are essential in assessing the efficacy of treatment. Some underlying causes (such as multiple myeloma) will tend to make hypercalcemia refractory to treatment. In such cases, the goal of therapy becomes keeping the calcium level as low as possible.

Hypocalcemia

Etiology

Hypocalcemia is a clinical condition in which the serum calcium level is less than 8.5 mg/dl. Hypocalcemia usually develops from an excessive loss of calcium as a result of, for example, diarrhea, use of diuretics, malabsorption syndromes, or hypoparathyroidism. Chronic renal failure is probably the most common cause of hypocalcemia. If calcium is lost in peritoneal dialysis or hemodialysis, hyperphosphatemia may occur. This enhances a peripheral deposition of calcium. Calcium deposits keep calcium from being available to raise serum levels. There is also an inability of the patient with chronic renal failure to absorb calcium from the intestines secondary to a lack of activated vitamin D. Alkalosis can cause hypocalcemia because the calcium becomes bound to albumin and thus remains inactive in the serum.

Chronic malabsorption syndromes may cause hypocalcemia. These syndromes are found following gastrectomies, in small bowel diseases, in patients with a high fat diet (fat impairs calcium absorption), and in patients with a magnesium deficiency (magnesium inhibits PTH).

Malignancies may also cause hypocalcemia. These include osteoblastic metastases (whereby calcium is used for abnormal bone synthesis) and medullary carcinoma of the thyroid (causing an increased secretion of thyrocalcitonin, which in turn stimulates osteoblasts and prevents calcium from entering the serum).

Hypoparathyroidism of any cause results in hypocalcemia, since there is a decreased secretion of PTH. The most common causes are surgical removal of the parathyroid glands, adenoma of the parathyroid glands, depleted magnesium levels (inhibits PTH), and idiopathic hypoparathyroidism.

A vitamin D-deficient state (or nonactivated vitamin D) is often seen in chronic renal failure, liver failure, and rickets. Without activated vitamin D, calcium is not absorbed from the intestines. Acute pancreatitis causes a precipitation of calcium in the inflamed pancreas and in intra-abdominal lipids.

In hyperphosphatemia, phosphates and calcium bind together and precipitate in tissues. This is commonly found in chronic renal failure as a result of decreased excretion of phosphates. Increased oral intake of phosphates rarely causes hyperphosphatemia if renal function is normal.

Clinical Presentation

Neuromuscular irritability is the overwhelming symptom present and the most dangerous. Muscle tremors and cramps are present in mild hypocalcemia. As the calcium level drops, tetany and generalized tonic–clonic seizures occur. Neuromuscular irritability causes labored, shallow respirations. Wheezing will be present if bronchospasms have occurred. Bronchospasms may lead to laryngospasm and tetany of the respiratory muscles, resulting in respiratory arrest. Monitoring of the neurological status by testing Chvostek's and Trousseau's signs is important.

To test for Chvostek's sign, tap your finger over the supramandibular portion of the parotid gland, which is located in the subcutaneous tissue of the cheek. If the upper lip twitches on the side of stimulation, the test is positive. To test Trousseau's sign, apply a blood pressure cuff to the arm and inflate it until a carpopedal spasm occurs. If no spasm appears in 3 min, the test is negative. To test this result, remove the blood pressure cuff and have the patient hyperventilate (more than 30 breaths/minute). The respiratory alkalosis that develops may produce the carpopedal spasm. This indicates a positive test.

The neuromuscular irritability frequently causes a decreased cardiac contractility leading to a cardiac arrest. The earliest ECG change is a lengthening of the QT interval due to a lengthening of the ST segment. Significant dysrhythmias due to hypocalcemia are extremely rare. The neuromuscular irritability may also cause biliary colic and paralytic ileus.

An alteration in blood clotting may be seen in hypocalcemia. Since calcium is necessary for normal blood clotting, hypocalcemia is often accompanied by bleeding dyscrasias.

Treatment

The aim of treatment is to raise the calcium level to normal as rapidly as possible to halt or prevent tetany.

In cases of tetany or impending tetany, intravenous 10% calcium gluconate or calcium chloride is administered. The patient must be on a cardiac monitor because a rapid infusion may enhance digitalis toxicity and because hypocalcemic patients are often also hyperkalemic. Vitamin D supplements are administered if a deficiency is present.

Monitoring serum calcium, phosphate, and potassium levels along with ECG monitoring and neurologic monitoring (using Chvostek's and Trousseau's signs) will evaluate the efficacy of patient treatment.

PHOSPHATE

The normal serum level of phosphate (PO_4) is 3.0–4.5 mg/dl. The phosphate ion is found in bones and is a major factor in intracellular production of ATP (energy). Phosphate combines with proteins and lipids to form important intracellular molecules. Intracellular phosphate ions may react with DNA and RNA molecules. Phosphate acts as a buffering agent for urine, is responsible for bone growth, promotes white blood cell phagocytic action, and is important in platelet structure and function.

Phosphate Regulation

Phosphate levels are influenced by two major factors, PTH secretion (increases renal excretion of phosphate ions) and calcium concentration. Calcium and phosphate have a reciprocal relationship. If calcium levels increase, phosphate levels decrease; conversely, if calcium levels decrease, phosphate levels increase.

Reabsorption of phosphates occurs actively in the proximal convoluted tubule in the presence of sodium. Without sodium, phosphates will not be reabsorbed.

Excretion of phosphates is regulated by PTH and the GFR. PTH inhibits reabsorption of phosphates in the proximal tubule, so phosphates will be excreted. With a decrease in the GFR, phosphate excretion will decrease; with an increase in the GFR, phosphates excretion will increase.

Hyperphosphatemia

Etiology

A serum phosphate level above 4.5 mg/dl constitutes hyperphosphatemia. Inability to excrete phosphates or excessive ingestion of phosphates are the two pathologic processes of hyperphosphatemia. The inability to excrete phosphates may be due to a decreased GFR or to renal failure.

Excessive ingestion of phosphates may be due to routine use (or abuse) of phosphate-containing laxatives and enemas or use of cytotoxic agents for the treatment of leukemias and lymphomas. Hypoparathyroidism causes hyperphosphatemia secondary to the effects of PTH on the kidney. Occasionally, over-administration of intravenous or oral phosphates will induce a hyperphosphatemia.

Clinical Presentation

Clinical presentation of hyperphosphatemia is the same as for hypocalcemia. Elevated phosphate levels enhance the movement of calcium into bone. If seizures occur, they are due to hypocalcemia caused by hyperphosphatemia. Remember that calcium and phosphate have a reciprocal relationship.

Metastatic calcification occurs when calcium and phosphates chemically combine to form calcium phosphate, which then precipitates in arteries, soft tissue, and joints.

Treatment

The objective of therapy is to decrease the serum phosphate level. This is accomplished by giving aluminum hydroxide gels or calcium antacids that combine with phosphate, limiting the amount of phosphate available for absorption in the intestines.

Hypophosphatemia

Etiology

Hypophosphatemia is a serum phosphate level of less than 3.0 mg/dl. Any factor that increases the cellular uptake to form sugar phosphates will decrease serum levels of phosphate. For example, prolonged intense hyperventilation can depress serum phosphate by inducing respiratory alkalosis. Sepsis and diabetic ketoacidosis, also contribute to hypophosphatemia. A decreased phosphate absorption from the intestines (malabsorption syndromes), severe diarrhea, loss of proximal convoluted tubular function with renal phosphate wasting as seen in Fanconi's syndrome, and rickets that are vitamin D resistant may also cause hypophosphatemia.

Chronic alcoholism results in a dietary deficiency of phosphates and may interfere with the absorption of any phosphates present. Abuse (including overuse) of phosphate-binding gels such as Amphojel and hyperparathyroidism (causing renal phosphaturia) cause hypophosphatemia.

Long-term hyperalimentation may contribute to hypophosphatemia if phosphates are not included in the solution in adequate amounts. Use of the high glucose content in hyperalimentation solutions requires phosphates. This is no longer a common etiology.

Clinical Presentation

Complaints of general malaise, anorexia, and vague muscle weakness may be of chronic or acute onset. With chronic onset, muscle wasting is apparent. With acute onset, rhabdomyolysis (a diffuse muscle-wasting necrosis) is due to a depletion of intracellular ATP and a concurrent decrease in all ATP-mediated processes. Hypercalcemia and hypercalciuria, with associated symptoms, are indicators of acute phosphate depletion due to hyperparathyroidism (PTH increases serum calcium by removing it from bone and decreases serum phosphate by excretion in the urine).

Hypoxia occurs because of a deficit in red blood cell phosphate content necessary for the formation of 2,3-DPG. With a decrease in 2,3-DPG, a decrease in the dissociation of oxygen from hemoglobin is seen and tissue hypoxia results.

Complicating hypophosphatemia may be osteomalacia, severe metabolic acidosis, and insulin resistance resulting in hyperglycemia. This syndrome is rare and usually seen in chronic alcoholism. It is a severe intravascular hemolysis caused by a phosphate depletion that results in a decrease of 2,3-DPG in red blood cells.

Treatment

The objective of therapy is to replace the phosphates, first by intravenous administration and then orally. Use of phosphate-binding gels is discontinued, and then treatment of the underlying cause of hypophosphatemia is started.

MAGNESIUM

The normal serum level of magnesium (Mg^{2+}) is 1.5–2.5 mEq/L. The magnesium ion is the second major intracellular cation. Magnesium acts as a coenzyme in the metabolism of carbohydrates and proteins. It regulates neuromuscular excitability and phosphate levels. It is stored in bone, muscle, and soft tissue.

Magnesium Regulation

Renal reabsorption of magnesium is essentially the same as for calcium. The presence of sodium directly affects the reabsorption in the proximal tubules. Without sodium, there is no reabsorption of magnesium. PTH appears to have a minimal effect on reabsorption. Reabsorption processes of calcium and magnesium are mutually suppressive.

Hypermagnesemia

Etiology
Hypermagnesemia is a serum magnesium level above 2.5 mEq/L. This is extremely rare. Reabsorption is similar to the calcium process. Absorption of excessive sodium (due to any cause) in the renal tubules may "drag" an excessive amount of magnesium back into the blood.

Chronic renal disease and untreated diabetic acidosis are the usual causes. Addison's disease, hyperparathyroidism, excessive magnesium administration, and overuse of magnesium-containing antacids are other causes of hypermagnesemia.

Clinical Presentation
Lethargy, coma, depressed respirations, hyporeflexia, and hypotension are the usual symptoms. All of the symptoms of hyperkalemia may be present. ECG changes consist first of prolonged PR intervals, followed by widening of the QRS complex as the magnesium concentration rises. Death usually occurs with a concentration of 6 mEq/L or more.

Treatment
Attempts to lower magnesium levels by hemodialysis with a hypomagnesium dialysate have been successful.

Hypomagnesemia

Etiology
A magnesium level of less than 1.5 mEq/L is a state of hypomagnesemia. Any inhibition of absorption of magnesium from the gastrointestinal tract or of reabsorption from the renal system may account for hypomagnesium. Severe malabsorption syndromes, acute pancreatitis, chronic alcoholism, primary aldosteronism, diabetic ketoacidosis, diuretic therapy, and renal disease are the usual causes.

Clinical Presentation
Neuromuscular and central nervous system hyperirritability characterize hypomagnesemia. Muscle tremors, delirium, convulsion, and coma are seen. Positive Chvostek's and Trousseau's signs, tachycardia, increased blood pressure, depressed ST segments, and prolonged QT intervals are also seen. Hypomagnesemia may result in digitalis-induced dysrhythmias.

Treatment
The objective of treatment is simply to provide sufficient magnesium to raise the serum level. Low magnesium levels have been implicated in the development of ventricular dysrhythmias and have been treated more aggressively in recent years. Usually 1–2 g of magnesium can be given by intravenous administration.

CHLORIDE

Cloride Regulation

Normal serum chloride (Cl), level is 98–106 mg/dl. Chloride is reabsorbed by the kidney at all of the sites for sodium reabsorption. Chloride moves freely with the gastric and intestinal fluids and is reabsorbed accordingly.

Anion Gap

Excretion of chloride is influenced by the acid-base balance. In acidosis, chloride is excreted while bicarbonate is reabsorbed. In alkalosis, chloride is reabsorbed while bicarbonate is excreted. Chloride can be used in combination with bicarbonate and sodium to obtain an estimated "anion gap." While an anion gap never really exists, since cations and anions must balance to maintain electrochemical neutrality, an anion gap appears to be present if only sodium, bicarbonate, and chloride are measured. A normal anion gap is less than 15 mEq and is obtained by subtracting bicarbonate and chloride from sodium. For example, a patient with a sodium of 140, bicarbonate of 25, and chloride of 100 would have a anion gap of 15 (140 − [(100 + 25)∧] = 15.

The value in computing an anion gap is simple. If an anion gap exceeds 15, a specific type of metabolic acidosis exists. If the anion gap exceeds 15, either a lactic, keto, or chronic renal failure acidosis exists. The reason the anion gap appears to increase is due to the loss of bicarbonate to buffer the acidosis without the simultaneous increase in chloride. In lactic, keto-, and chronic renal failure acidosis, anions other than chloride increase to offset the loss of bicarbonate.

Hyperchloremia

Etiology
Hyperchloremia is a serum chloride level above 106 mg/dl. An excessive ingestion of chloride or an excessive kidney reabsorption of chloride ions are the pathophysiological changes in hyperchloremia.

Clinical Presentation
The symptoms are the same (or very similar) to those of hypernatremia.

Treatment
The objectives of treatment are to reduce the chloride level, which is most often achieved by the treatment for metabolic acidosis.

Hypochloremia

Etiology
Hypochloremia is a serum chloride level of less than 98 mg/dl. Chloride ions are lost through excessive vomiting or gastric suction without replacement of electrolytes. This results in a physiological metabolic alkalosis. The bicarbonate ion and chloride ion normally balance each other in kidney function.

Clinical Presentation
Symptoms of hypochloremia include changes in sensorium, possible neuromuscular irritability, and usually slow, shallow respirations.

Treatment
The objective of treatment is to replace the lost chloride ions either orally or intravenously and to treat the metabolic alkalosis to reestablish acid-base balance.

45

Diagnosis and Treatment of Acute Renal Failure

EDITORS' NOTE

The content of this chapter is designed to address CCRN exam questions on acute renal failure (e.g., acute tubular necrosis). Expect about two to four questions on the exam regarding material covered in this chapter.

Acute renal failure (ARF) refers to a sudden loss of renal function that may or may not produce oliguria or anuria with a concurrent increase in plasma creatinine and blood urea nitrogen (BUN). Oliguria is present if less than 400 ml of urine is produced per day. This is an obligatory water loss, i.e., the minimum amount of urine needed to rid the body of its daily wastes. The mortality rate for ARF ranges from 40 to 70%.

PATHOPHYSIOLOGY

Acute renal failure can be classified as prerenal, intrarenal, or postrenal.

Prerenal ARF is defined as a decreased renal perfusion secondary to decreased cardiac output. Decreased renal perfusion causes a decrease in renal artery pressure leading to a reduced afferent arteriole pressure. Afferent arteriole pressures of less than 100 mm Hg may decrease the glomerular filtration rate (GFR), resulting in oliguria and/or anuria.

Hypovolemia is the most common cause of acute renal failure in the critically ill patient.

Intrarenal ARF is caused by disease or injuries of the nephron from the glomerulus to the collecting duct. The most common cause of intrarenal failure is acute tubular necrosis (ATN). Subsequently, these intrarenal conditions can be cortical or medullary in nature.

Cortical conditions involve swelling of the renal capillaries and cellular proliferation. Infectious, vascular, and/or immunologic processes cause edema and some resultant cellular debris that obstructs the glomeruli, resulting in a fall in urine output.

Medullary involvement specifically affects the tubular portions of the nephron, causing necrosis. The extent of medullary damage differs depending on the cause of the necrosis: nephrotoxic injury or ischemic injury. Nephrotoxic injury affects the epithelial cells, which can regenerate after the nephrotoxic injury is resolved. Ischemic injury extends to the tubular basement membrane and may involve peritubular capillaries and other parts of the nephron. Ischemic injury is more serious, since the tubular basement membrane cannot regenerate. Ischemic injury occurs when the mean arterial pressure falls below 60 mm Hg for over 40 min secondary to massive hemorrhage or shock.

Postrenal ARF usually indicates an obstruction at or below the level of the collecting ducts. The obstruction may be partial or complete. If the obstruction is complete, the blockage and subsequent backup of urine flow involve both kidneys. Eventually, urine output is decreased as a result of decreased glomerular filtration.

ETIOLOGY

Prerenal failure has many causes. One major cause is hemorrhage resulting in hypovolemia with fluid and electrolyte imbalance. Other causes include excessive use of diuretics and decreased glomerular perfusion after an acute myocardial infarction or congestive heart failure. Occasionally, following anesthesia and surgery, increased renal vascular resistance and/or the hepatorenal syndrome occurs. Sepsis progressing to septic shock results in vasodilation and a resultant hypovolemia. Embolism or thrombosis may cause a bilateral renal vascular obstruction, resulting in decreased or no perfusion to the kidneys.

The causes of intrarenal failure can be fairly well categorized as either cortical or medullary. Table 45–1 summarizes the multiple causes of cortical and medullary intrarenal failure.

Causes of postrenal ARF are obstructive in nature and include prostatic hypertrophy; bladder, pelvic, or retroperitoneal tumors; renal calculi; ureteral blockage (after surgery or instrumentation); urethral obstruction; bladder infections; or a neurogenic bladder.

PHASES

There are four phases in the cycle of ARF: onset, oliguric, diuretic, and recovery.

TABLE 45–1. CAUSES OF INTRARENAL FAILURE

Cortical Nephron Failure	Medullary Nephron Failure
Infections	Nephrotoxic causes
Poststreptoccal	Heavy metals
glomerulonephritis	Pesticides
Acute pyelonephritis	Fungicides
Goodpasture's syndrome	Hemoglobinuria
Systemic lupus erythematosus	Myoglobinuria
Malignant hypertension	Hypercalcemia
	Antibiotics
	Aminoglycosides
	Cephalosporins
	Tetracyclines
	Penicillins
	Amphotericin
	Ischemic causes
	Crush injuries
	Burns
	Sepsis
	Cardiogenic shock
	Postsurgical hypotension
	Hemorrhage with multiple trauma

Onset or Initial Phase

The onset or initial phase precedes the actual necrotic injury and is associated with decreased cardiac output, renal blood flow, and GFR. If mean arterial blood pressure falls below 60 mm Hg for over 40 min, the risk of development of ARF is high. A consistent increase in cardiac output will produce a consistent increase in renal blood flow and protect the patient from ARF.

Oliguric Phase

The oliguric phase reflects the obstruction of tubules from edema, tubular casts, and cellular debris. Damage to the tubules makes absorption and secretion of solutes variable. If the obstruction and damage are severe enough, a backleak of filtrate through the epithelium may occur, returning the filtrate into the circulation.

During the oliguric phase, laboratory reports will indicate rising levels of urea, creatinine, and potassium. Serum and urine osmolality are increased. Hypervolemia and electrolyte imbalances caused by retention of the metabolic waste products are the greatest dangers to the patient. This phase lasts 8–14 days.

Diuretic Phase

The diuretic phase indicates the beginning of the return of tubular function. The diuretic phase lasts about 10 days. The greatest danger to the patient in this phase is excessive loss of water and electrolytes. Extreme diuresis is due to the osmotic diuretic effect produced by the elevated BUN and the inability of the tubules to conserve sodium and water, resulting in an output of 3000 ml or more of urine per 24 hr. Hypokalemia is usually present.

Recovery Phase

The recovery phase begins when the diuresis is no longer excessive. There is a gradual improvement in kidney function. This improvement may continue for 3–12 months. The end result may be a permanent reduction in the GFR, which may or may not be sufficient to maintain adequate renal function without dialysis. ARF may progress to chronic renal failure, but this is uncommon unless the patient has an underlying kidney disease or is advanced in age.

CLINICAL PRESENTATION

Oliguria may or may not be present in ARF. Fifty percent of ARF patients and many ATN patients are anuric. Therefore, urine volume alone is not an adequate guide to renal function. Progressive azotemia (an excess of urea or other nitrogenous bodies in the blood) occurs as a result of decreased GFR in spite of apparently adequate urine output. ARF should be diagnosed before uremic signs are present. Table 45–2 summarizes the clinical presentation of uremia.

DIAGNOSIS

Diagnosing ARF or ATN may be difficult, especially in the nonoliguric patient. Factors that must be considered in a diagnosis include urinary volume, urinary sediment, BUN levels, serial serum creatinines, creatinine clearance, arterial blood gases, trauma, and postsurgical status.

Urinary Volume

Normal urinary output is about 0.5 ml/kg/h. In prerenal failure urine volume is decreased. In ATN, daily urine output may be constant or may gradually increase or decrease. Complete anuria suggests obstruction or cortical necrosis. It may occur in acute glomerulonephritis and complete postrenal obstruction but is very rare otherwise. Different degrees of obstruction are suggested by large and irregular daily urine volumes. Partial obstruction can cause progressive azotemia, even though there may be normal or increased urine volume.

Laboratory Data

In prerenal failure, urinary sodium (Na^+) is less than 20 mEq/L as the kidneys attempt to conserve sodium and water. Urinary osmolality, which reflects the concentrating ability of the kidney, is elevated. Urinary osmolality is usually greater than 500 mosm (normal level is 300–900 mosm). Specific gravity, a less sensitive indicator of concentrating power than osmolality, is also elevated. Specific gravity is greater than 1.020. There is minimal or no proteinuria. There is normal urinary sediment. The BUN increase is greater than the creatinine increase (20:1; normal ratio is 10:1). Normal serum creatinine is about .8–1.8 mg/dl and normal BUN is about 10–20 mg/dl. The fractional excretion of sodium (FeNa) is less than 1% in prerenal failure.

$$FeNa = \frac{\dfrac{Urine}{Na} \Big/ \dfrac{Plasma}{Na}}{\dfrac{Urine}{Creatinine} \Big/ \dfrac{Plasma}{Creatinine}} \times 100$$

In cortical intrarenal failure, urinary sodium is less than 10 mEq/L. Specific gravity will vary with moderate to heavy proteinuria. Serum BUN and creatinine will be elevated (10–15:1). Hematuria is present with erythrocyte casts and leukocytes. In medullary intrarenal failure or ATN, urinary sodium is greater than 20 mEq/L, an abnormal sign when urine output is low. Normally the kidneys conserve sodium in an attempt to maintain extravascular water. In ATN, when urine output is low, the expected conservation of sodium fails to occur, resulting in a normal urinary sodium level (40–220 mEq/L). Urinary osmolality decreases (below 500 mosm), reflecting the inability of the kidneys to concentrate the urine. Simultaneously, the specific gravity also decreases, usually between 1.008 and 1.012. Minimal to moderate proteinuria is present with an elevated serum BUN and creatinine. The FeNa is above 1% in ATN. Urinary sediment consists of numerous renal tubular epithelial cells, tubular casts, and a rare erythrocyte.

In postrenal failure there are scanty sediment, rare white cells, red cells, hyaline casts, and fine gran-

TABLE 45–2. UREMIC SIGNS OF ACUTE RENAL FAILURE

Respiratory	**Metabolic**
Deep or rapid respiratory rate (metabolic acidosis)	Electrolyte imbalance
Bilateral rales	
Pulmonary edema	
Cardiovascular	**Integument**
Tachycardia	Dry skin
Dysrhythmias	Uremic frost (excretion of urea)
Pericarditis	Pruritus
Friction rub	Increased susceptibility to infection
	Edema
Neurological	**Hematological**
Decreased level of consciousness	Anemias
Confusion	Uremic coagulopathies
Lethargy	Bruising
Stupor	
Gastrointestinal	
Nausea	
Vomiting	
Anorexia	
Constipation or diarrhea	
Abdominal distension	

ular (>40 mEq/L) casts. Urinary sodium is elevated, specific gravity varies, and BUN and creatinine are elevated (10–15:1).

MANAGEMENT OF PATIENT CARE PROBLEMS

There are four major problems of patient care in renal failure: an increase in the products of catabolism, severe electrolyte imbalance with associated acidosis, fluid overload, and infection.

Increase in the Products of Catabolism

Protein catabolism increases in the critically ill and stressed patient. A decrease in proteins available for catabolism will retard the rate of azotemia, decrease the incidence and severity of acidosis, and decrease the occurrence and levels of hyperkalemia in the serum. Caloric requirements of the patient must be met mainly through an adequate carbohydrate diet intake.

Serum Electrolyte Imbalance and Acidosis

Sodium intake is restricted unless there is a serum sodium deficit. No salt substitutes are used because of their potassium content. Careful management of fluids and sodium intake will prevent overhydration, congestive heart failure, hyponatremia, and water intoxication.

Hyperkalemia is a significant imbalance seen in ARF. Hyperkalemia is further compounded as a result of catabolism associated with fever. It also occurs as a result of decreased potassium excretion caused by volume depletion or drugs. Metabolic acidosis can also cause hyperkalemia. The fall of the pH forces hydrogen ions into the cells and potassium into the extracellular fluid.

Fluid Overload

It is essential to determine the patient's state of hydration and to continually monitor this state. Indicators of overhydration include weight gain, edema, anasarca, ascites, increased blood pressure, jugular vein distension (JVD), and dyspnea. Indicators for dehydration include weight loss, decreased blood pressure, poor skin turgor, no evidence of JVD, and decreased central venous pressure.

Fluids are restricted to amounts equal to urine output plus 400 ml for insensible fluid loss. It is important that accurate daily weights be taken using the same scales. It is also important to remember that 1000 ml of fluid weighs about 2.2 lb or 1.0 kg.

Infection

Since proper kidney function affects all body systems, the chance of infection is greatly increased in renal failure patients. The body defense systems do not function properly, and the patient is predisposed to urinary tract infections, septicemia, pneumonia, and wound or skin infections (due to the severe pruritus that some patients experience). Good nutritional intake by the patient and proper hygiene will help prevent infections. If fever develops, culture and sensitivities of blood, urine, sputum, or any wound should be performed to identify the invading organism. Once the organism is identified, appropriate antibiotic therapy is started with antibiotic doses adjusted to renal function.

DIALYSIS

As the patient develops systemic symptoms of renal failure, the need for dialysis is assessed. The purposes of dialysis are to (1) remove the by-products of protein metabolism, including urea, creatinine, and uric acid, (2) remove excess water, (3) maintain or restore the body's buffer system, and (4) maintain or restore the body's concentration of electrolytes. Dialysis is defined as the diffusion of dissolved particles from one fluid compartment to another across a semipermeable membrane. Three principles are utilized in dialysis: osmosis, diffusion, and filtration and are achieved through peritoneal dialysis, hemodialysis, and continuous renal replacement therapies (CRRT).

Osmosis is the movement of fluid across a semipermeable membrane from a less concentrated solution to a more concentrated solution. Diffusion is the movement of particles (or solutes) across a semipermeable membrane from a more concentrated solution to a less concentrated solution. Filtration is the movement of particles or solutes across a semipermeable membrane through the utilization of hydrostatic pressure.

Peritoneal Dialysis

In peritoneal dialysis, the peritoneum is the semipermeable membrane. The peritoneum is a strong, smooth, colorless, serous membrane that lines the abdominal cavity with a parietal layer and wraps the abdominal organs with a visceral layer (Fig. 45–1).

The dialysate is instilled into the abdominal cavity between these two layers of peritoneum through a catheter. The visceral peritoneum is contiguous with the intestinal wall and the capillary beds of the intestines. The dialysate is instilled into the peritoneal space, bathing the intestines. Osmosis, diffusion, and filtration occur readily after "dwelling" in the abdomen.

Indications

There are many instances in which peritoneal dialysis may be used. In acute renal failure, peritoneal dialysis may be used to treat the renal failure or to prevent uremia while ascertaining an underlying cause or while stabilizing a patient for surgery.

Chronic renal failure patients who have had a recent infection may undergo peritoneal dialysis to prevent localization of the infection at the fistula site. Patients in whom there is no vascular access route for hemodialysis may undergo peritoneal dialysis until an access route is available.

Circulatory overload from renal impairment with congestive heart failure is amenable to peritoneal dialysis. Refractory hyperkalemia and metabolic acidosis and intoxication from dialyzable drugs and poisons are also indicators for peritoneal dialysis.

In chronic renal failure, peritoneal dialysis may postpone the need for chronic hemodialysis. In patients with diabetes, chronic hemodialysis may cause blindness associated with diabetic retinopathy. Patients awaiting renal transplantation may utilize peritoneal dialysis because it is less expensive than

hemodialysis. Some patients undergo peritoneal dialysis instead of hemodialysis because of religious beliefs and the desire to avoid blood transfusions associated with hemodialysis emergencies.

The use of peritoneal dialysis in peritonitis is a controversial topic. Some nephrologists believe in adding antibiotics to the dialysate in addition to using oral or intravenous antibiotics. The rationale is to bathe the infected area itself with antibiotics. Other nephrologists believe that peritonitis is justification for stopping peritoneal dialysis. The rationale here is to treat the patient with intravenous antibiotics to prevent septic shock from developing or to prevent weakening (to the actual point of rupture) of an inflamed, infected visceral peritoneum and the contiguous intestinal wall.

Contraindications

Any patient with blood-clotting dyscrasias should not undergo peritoneal dialysis until the blood-clotting problems have been resolved. Patients with fresh post-operative vascular prostheses, such as a fresh femoral–popliteal bypass, are not candidates for peritoneal dialysis. The procedure may result in graft failure at the site of anastomosis, resulting in exsanguination.

Patients who have had recent peritoneal surgery or those with postoperative abdominal drains are not candidates for peritoneal dialysis. The peritoneum may not be strong enough to hold the dialysate without rupture or tearing of the peritoneum, and abdominal drains preclude any dwell time since the dialysate would flow out of the drains.

Abdominal adhesions or any other condition where a danger of puncturing viscera exists is a contraindication to peritoneal dialysis. Pregnant women should not undergo peritoneal dialysis because of the increased risk for fetal distress.

Advantages

Peritoneal dialysis can be performed at the bedside. The expensive, elaborate equipment and highly skilled personnel utilized for hemodialysis are not needed in peritoneal dialysis. Because it requires more time to effectively remove metabolic wastes and restore electrolyte and fluid balance, it is less stressful for pediatric and elderly patients and can be initiated quickly. There is no need for systemic anticoagulation.

Disadvantages

Peritoneal dialysis is slower to rid the body of waste products than hemodialysis. Exchanges of 2000 ml

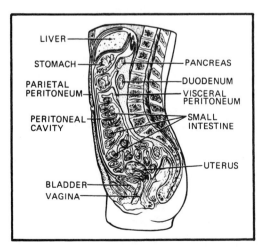

Figure 45–1. The peritoneal space (female).

performed every 3 hr achieve approximately the same solute clearance as a 4-hr hemodialysis treatment performed every other day. Prolonged peritoneal dialysis results in a protein depletion and may result in ascites, poor wound healing, and decreased resistance to infection. Peritonitis, usually resulting from Staphylococci or gram-negative organisms, may develop with repeated treatments. With peritonitis, some physicians will stop the peritoneal dialysis and others will continue with the addition of an antibiotic to the dialysate.

Dialysate

The dialysate solution concentration is selected by the physician. The more concentrated the solute concentration, the greater the osmotic forces exerted to remove fluid and waste products. Osmotic forces are determined by the concentration of glucose in the dialysate, usually ranging from 1.5 to 4.25%. During the administration of 4.25% dialysate, the serum glucose must be monitored because glucose can diffuse into the serum.

The temperature of the dialysate influences the effectiveness of peritoneal dialysis; urea clearance is 35% greater at body temperature (98.6°F) than at room temperature (75°F). Body temperature dialysate will also enhance patient comfort.

The volume of the dialysate influences effectiveness. An exchange volume of 3 L of dialysate in 1 hr almost doubles the urea clearance achieved with 1 L per hour. Most adults are comfortable with 2 L per exchange, and a few can tolerate 3 L.

The physician will order the amount of heparin to be added to the dialysate to prevent fibrin or blood from clotting the catheter. The amount of potassium chloride added depends on the patient's serum potassium level, state of digitalization, and arterial blood gases.

Some physicians add lidocaine, usually 50 mg/2 L of dialysate, for generalized abdominal discomfort. Some physicians also add antibiotics if peritonitis is present or suspected.

Procedure and Nursing Care

To help obtain the patient's cooperation, the nurse should explain the procedure, making the patient aware of the discomforts of, limited mobility during, and duration of the procedure. The patient is weighed before the procedure and either daily or after the last exchange.

The patient should void or be catheterized immediately before the physician inserts the catheter. Using strict sterile technique at the bedside, the physician inserts the catheter midline of the abdomen between the umbilicus and the symphysis pubis. Once the catheter is in place, 2 L of warmed dialysate is unfused and drained as soon as it is instilled to ensure patency of the catheter. Outflow should drain in a steady stream.

When catheter patency is confirmed, the warmed dialysate is infused, allowed to dwell in the abdomen, usually for 20–45 min, and then allowed to drain via gravity as completely as possible. One exchange usually takes about an hour. Turning the patient side to side may enhance the drainage of dialysate.

At the end of the dwell time, the dialysate is assessed for color. Normally, it is clear, pale yellow. If the drainage is cloudy, suspect infection or peritonitis. If it is brownish, suspect bowel perforation. Blood-tinged dialysate during the first four exchanges is normal. However, if after four exchanges the dialysate is still bloody, discontinue and notify the physician. The patient may have abdominal bleeding or a uremic coagulopathy.

Periodic cultures of the dialysate drainage are obtained to assess for infection, and the tip of the catheter is cultured when it is removed.

Monitoring vital signs every 15 min during the first hour and then every 1–2 hr is the usual procedure if the vital signs are stable. The outflow period is the most likely time for abnormal or changing vital signs. Signs of impending shock, fluid overload, and pulmonary edema will be most apparent in this outflow period.

One of the most important aspects of peritoneal dialysis is the intake–output record maintained by the nurse. Hospital policies vary in the format for recording peritoneal dialysis intake and output. Information needed is the time the exchange was started, the number of the exchange, the amount of fluid infused, the dwell time, the amount of fluid drained, and the fluid balance.

Fluid balance is crucial. If 2000 ml is instilled and only 1750 ml drains out, the patient fluid balance is +250 ml. If the next exchange instills 2000 ml and drains 1900 ml, the patient fluid balance for the exchange is +100 ml. The present balance is now +350 ml. Assume that the third exchange is with a 4.5% dialysate (hypertonic solution). The amount instilled was 2000 ml, and the output drainage was 2275 ml. The patient balance for this exchange is –275 ml. The patient gave back more fluid than was instilled in this exchange. However, in the continuous fluid balance columns, the patient is still at a fluid balance of +75 ml. Intake–output records are maintained for each exchange and overall for total exchanges.

Complications

Infection is one of the most common complications of peritoneal dialysis. Insertion of the catheter under sterile technique and closed sterile instillation and drainage of dialysate will help reduce infection. Daily sterile changes of the dressing over the tube insertion site helps decrease the chance of infection. Perhaps the most effective way to prevent infection is to keep the procedure time to 36 hr or less.

Volume depletion occurs if the dialysis is too effective and removes several hundred milliliters of fluid per exchange. This will result in hypotension. Water removal may cause hypernatremia if the 4.25% glucose dialysate is used. Nursing intervention includes monitoring for signs of increasing sodium retention.

Volume overload may occur during peritoneal dialysis. When the patient is severely hyponatremic, sodium and water move into the third space. As third spacing resolves by sodium and water returning to the intravascular bed, cardiovascular overload may occur. Shortening the dwell time and repositioning the patient may help. If not, the patient may need hemodialysis.

Hyperglycemia may be severe if hypertonic fluid is used in the diabetic patient. Hyperosmolar coma and death have occurred. If hyperglycemia develops, the dialysis is discontinued until the blood sugar is controlled. Suspect hyperglycemia if the patient complains of thirst or if there is a deterioration in the patient's level of consciousness.

Metabolic alkalosis may occur if dialysis is continued for a long time. Dialysate fluid contains sodium lactate or acetate (45 mEq/L), which is converted to sodium bicarbonate in the body.

Digitalis intoxication is a serious complication. It is a result of lowering the serum potassium and at the same time correcting hypocalcemia, hyponatremia, and acidosis. The dose of the digitalis is usually reduced in uremic patients. Serum levels of cardiac glycosides are not affected by routine dialysis. Disequilibrium syndrome occurs more often in hemodialysis and will be covered in the discussion of hemodialysis.

Respiratory insufficiency may occur as the 2 L of dialysate are infused into the abdomen and push the abdominal viscera against the diaphragm, resulting in decreased depth of respirations. There is also an increased risk for atelectasis and pneumonia.

Severe pain at the end of inflow or outflow must be assessed. The pain may be caused by the temperature of the dialysate, incomplete draining of the previous exchange, early development of peritonitis, or instillation of too much dialysate.

Hemodialysis

Hemodialysis is a process of removing metabolic waste products of the body by use of extracorporeal circulation. The patient's blood is transferred by tubing from the patient to a machine that functions like a kidney to filter out waste products and then return the filtered blood to the patient by another tube. Hemodialysis uses the same principles of osmosis, diffusion, and filtration that are used in peritoneal dialysis.

Indications

Hemodialysis has the same indications as peritoneal dialysis. Other reasons for performing hemodialysis include acute renal failure due to trauma or infection, chronic renal failure no longer controlled by medication and diet, when rapid removal of toxins, poisons, and drugs is essential, and when peritoneal dialysis is contraindicated.

Contraindications

Labile cardiovascular states that would deteriorate with rapid changes in extravascular fluid volume are the major contraindications to hemodialysis.

In the past, patients who could not tolerate systemic heparinization could not be hemodialyzed. Today, however, the heparin is infused into the dialysis machine to keep blood anticoagulated within the machine. Before the blood is returned to the patient, protamine is infused to neutralize the heparin as the blood is returned to the patient. This process is called regional heparinization (Fig. 45–2).

For the patient without a condition that would be worsened by heparin, intermittent heparinization is used. In these cases, 2000–5000 units of heparin are infused at the start of hemodialysis, and 1000–2000 units of heparin are added for each hour that the patient is on the machine. These patients must be monitored closely for signs of bleeding.

There are three ways to access a patient's blood for hemodialysis: an arteriovenous (AV) shunt, single- or double-lumen catheters, and an AV fistula. The AV shunt (Fig. 45–3) consists of two Silastic catheters; one is inserted in an artery, and the other is inserted into a nearby vein. Blood is channeled from the artery to the dialysis machine and back to the vein. Part of the shunt lies subcutaneously, and part lies outside the skin.

When the patient is not undergoing hemodialysis, blood flows directly from the artery through the shunt and into the vein. Shunts are inserted under local anesthesia. The favored sites are the arm, wrist,

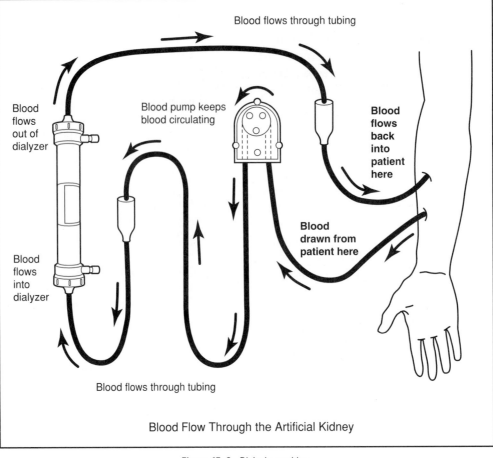

Figure 45–2. Dialysis machine.

legs, and ankles. In the upper extremity, the preferred vessels are from the radial artery to the cephalic vein. In the lower extremity, the preferred vessels are from the posterior tibial artery to the great saphenous vein.

Dialysis catheters (Fig. 45–4) are short-term shunts. They can be placed in the femoral vein or subclavian vein. With femoral access, one or two cannulas may be placed in the femoral vein. During dialysis, one catheter is used to channel blood to the dialysis machine and the other catheter is used to channel blood from the dialysis machine back to the patient. One bifurcated catheter can also be used. Peripheral pulses must be frequently assessed in the cannulized extremity. The patient must be maintained on bedrest. Assessment for signs of bleeding or hematoma formation is done frequently. If the catheter(s) is to remain after dialysis, low-dose heparin is utilized to maintain catheter potency.

Subclavian access also provides immediate short-term or long-term access. One bifurcated catheter is utilized with heparin irrigations to main-

tain catheter potency between dialysis treatments. Patient activity is not restricted with subclavian access. However, the patient must be monitored for signs of a pneumothorax.

Fistulas have a longer life span than do AV shunts and tend to preserve the blood vessels in which they are placed. Fistulas are less restrictive than other forms of vascular access and therefore offer greater freedom to the patient. The fistula can be formed by the patient's vessels or by a graft (Fig. 45–5). Examples of graft materials are bovine carotid, woven Dacron, and umbilical vein. If grafts are used, they are tunneled under the skin in a U shape (Fig. 45–6). The surgical procedure involves anastomosis of the artery directly to the vein, utilizing most frequently a side-to-side technique. Fistulas need to mature over a 10–14-day period. During this time, the vein adapts to the high pressure of the arterial blood by dilatation and thickening of the venous wall. When the fistula matures, the vein will be able to withstand the insertion of large-bore needles (14–16 gauge). The insertion of needles in the arterial and venous

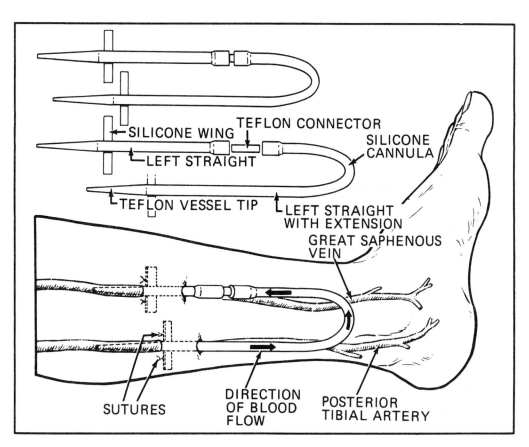

Figure 45–3. Arteriovenous shunt.

arms of the fistula permits attachments to the dialysis machine.

Complications associated with the AV fistula are infection, clotting, venous hypertension, and steal syndrome. Infection at the fistula site has direct access to systemic circulation and can precipitate septicemia. Localized infections present as reddened, tender, warm areas over the fistula, particularly at the anastomosis or needle puncture sites. Clotting sometimes causes severe pain and numbness in the affected arm; it can be confirmed by the absence of the bruit and thrill at the fistula site.

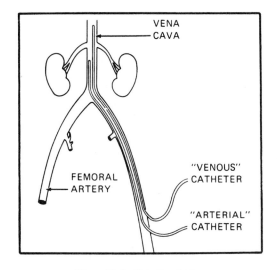

Figure 45–4. Dialysis catheters.

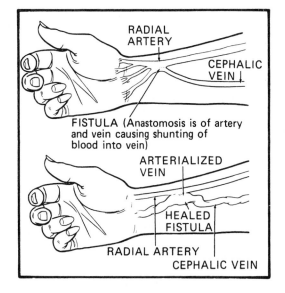

Figure 45–5. Anastomosis to form an arteriovenous fistula.

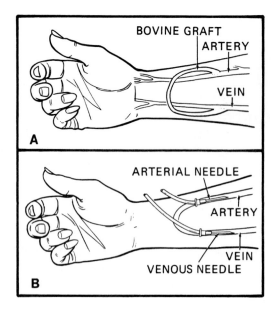

Figure 45–6. A graft in place **(A)** and placement of needles in a graft for hemodialysis **(B)**.

In venous hypertension, there is too much blood in the extremity distal to the fistula. This may cause ulcerations and may necessitate a fistula revision. In the steal syndrome, there is insufficient blood to the extremity because of excessive diversion of arterial blood to the vein at the anastomosis. Symptoms include coldness and poor function of the extremity. In severe cases, gangrene with necrosis of the extremity tips may develop. The steal syndrome is corrected by revising the fistula.

Once an access site is available, an evaluation of the patient's most recent electrolytes is made to determine what adjustments in the dialysate bath are to be made. An accurate predialysis weight of the patient is determined daily. By weighing the patient postdialysis, it is possible to calculate exactly how much fluid was removed or added.

Nursing Care

Infection is prevented by cleaning the shunt site daily using sterile technique and also by cleaning the fistula site until the incision is healed. If the shunt or fistula becomes infected, culture and sensitivity tests are done to identify the infecting organism. Once the organism is identified, intravenous antibiotics are started. If the shunt or fistula remains infected, it is removed and a new shunt or fistula is created.

The prevention of thrombosis is always a challenge. Anything that decreases blood flow increases the chance of thrombosis. Some examples are hypotension, hypovolemia, tourniquets, blood pres-

sure cuffs, tight clothing and jewelry, heavy handbags and packages, and dehydration.

If the shunt is patent, one can see bright red blood flowing freely through it and it feels warm to touch. There should not be any layering of the blood components (cells at the bottom, clear serum at the top). Proximal to the insertion site, one should feel a thrill (the turbulence of the arterial blood). With a stethoscope, one should hear a bruit (arterial blood turbulence). If either the thrill or bruit is absent, notify the physician immediately.

If the shunt becomes clotted, the physician may insert a catheter to remove the clot. After patency has been established, routine use of heparin will maintain patency.

To prevent hemorrhage due to shunt disconnection, clamps are attached to the dressing to ensure immediate availability. If the catheter becomes unconnected, the arterial cannula is clamped first to control excessive blood loss from the arterial system and then the venous cannula is clamped.

The precautions taken for shunts are also taken for fistulas. A thrill and bruit should be present. The arm with a fistula is not used for intravenous fluids, blood pressure monitoring, venipuncture, or injections. The fistula is cleansed daily using sterile technique. Bleeding, skin discoloration, or drainage is reported to the physician.

Complications

Problems associated with hemodialysis occur most often during the initial stages or during a procedure lasting more than 4 hr. Hypotension is caused by dehydration, sepsis, or blood loss. The patient may already be hypotensive or may rapidly become hypotensive when dialysis is initiated. This is treated by reducing the blood flow, discontinuing ultrafiltration (fluid removal), and giving fluids. If the patient does not respond to this method of treatment, dialysis is discontinued.

Cardiac dysrhythmias may be caused by potassium intoxication, but usually no specific electrolyte derangement can be identified. In some instances, dysrhythmias may be related to the development of transient myocardial ischemia as evidenced by premature ventricular contractions. Treatment consists of decreasing the blood flow and using appropriate medication as indicated. The dialysis procedure must be stopped if the dysrhythmia is severe or does not respond to treatment. Congestive heart failure in most instances is secondary to fluid overload, which can be reversed by ultrafiltration.

Disequilibrium syndrome may occur in reaction to the slowed clearance of urea from the cerebrospinal fluid during dialysis. Fluid shifts that occur to restore equilibrium result in cerebral swelling. Symptoms include headache, nausea, vomiting, restlessness progressing to disorientation, twitching, and seizures. Treatment focuses on prevention.

Air embolism may occur through an arterial or venous site as a result of a leak in the dialysis tubing, a loose connection, or the disconnection of dialysis tubing. With arterial air embolism, air travels the arterial system to a point distal to the entry site. In the head, the emboli enter the small vessels of the brain. Seizures may occur followed by rapid brain cell damage. Death will occur if critical areas of the brain are destroyed.

Venous emboli migrate back to the lungs and may cause pulmonary emboli. In the sitting patient with dialysis access in the lower extremities, air enters the venous system of the leg and travels to the inferior vena cava, then up through the right atrium to the superior vena cava, and then finally to the head. In this case, the symptoms are the same as for arterial emboli in the brain.

If the patient is lying flat when air is introduced, the air enters the right atrium and moves into the right ventricle. Essentially, the air is trapped in the right ventricle and cannot be propelled from the heart. Blood cannot enter the pulmonary system. The lack of pulmonary blood return to the left atrium quickly stops the pumping of blood into the systemic circulation.

Symptoms of air embolism include deep respirations, coughing, cyanosis, unconsciousness, and then cessation of breathing. Auscultation over the heart reveals a "mill wheel" sound during both phases of contraction. This is the sound of air turbulence in the heart.

Once air embolism has occurred, rapid corrective action is imperative. There are several important differences in the resuscitation of a patient with an air embolism as compared with the usual cardiopulmonary resuscitation. The patient must be placed in Trendelenburg position and turned on the left side. Once resuscitated, the patient must be kept in the Trendelenburg left side position until the air is absorbed. This will prevent movement of the air into the cerebral tissues and heart and promote movement toward the feet (air will be higher than fluid). The absorption time will vary, but it usually takes from days to weeks; the mortality rate is extremely high.

Continuous Renal Replacement Therapy

Continuous renal replacement therapy (CRRT) is designed to relieve fluid overload in critically ill patients. The process uses the patient's arterial blood pressure, without the use of an external pump, to deliver blood to a low-resistance hemodialyzer for fluid and low-molecular-weight substance removal. CRRT is an inexpensive and efficient method of treating fluid and electrolyte problems in the intensive care unit (ICU) setting.

Indications
The principal indication for CRRT is the treatment of patients with acute oliguric renal failure. Because fluid volume alteration and electrolyte removal is a slow process, CRRT is especially beneficial in treating acute volume overload in patients with unstable cardiovascular systems unresponsive to diuretic therapy, as occurs in acute pulmonary edema, congestive heart failure, postcardiac surgery, and recent myocardial infarction.

Continuous renal replacement therapy is also indicated in patients who require large quantities of parenteral fluid such as in hyperalimentation, intravenous antibiotic administration, and the continuous administration of vasopressors. CRRT is also considered when other forms of dialysis are contraindicated. CRRT may also be used to treat hyperkalemia, azotemia, and drug or poison intoxication.

Contraindications
Contraindications to CRRT are an inability to tolerate anticoagulation and a hematocrit greater than 45%. Both of these problems precipitate clotting in the hemofilter. Lack of vascular access is also a contraindication of CRRT.

Advantages
Continuous renal replacement therapy has distinct advantages over hemodialysis. It allows the elimination of large amounts of fluid without the osmolar changes associated with hemodialysis, thus maintaining extracellular fluid status. During hemodialysis rapid water removal causes the extracellular fluid to become hypotonic in relation to the hypertonic environment of the cell. Extracellular fluid is drawn into the cell, creating a depleted or hypovolemic state. The slow consistent process of CRRT maintains osmolality and cardiovascular stability. Another problem occurring with hemodialysis but absent with CRRT is the reduction in the platelet and white

blood cell count as the patient's blood comes into contact with cuprophane, cellulose acetate, or regenerated cellulose membrane. CRRT can be managed by the critical care nurse at the bedside rather than by hemodialysis staff.

Disadvantages

The main disadvantage of CRRT is its limited ability to remove waste products and excess solutes with minimal volume replacement.

Hemofiltration Process

Three modes of CRRT are readily available in the ICU setting: slow continuous ultrafiltration (SCUF), continuous arteriovenous hemofiltration (CAVH), and continuous arteriovenous hemodialysis (CAVHD). All three modes use the same equipment: a highly porous hemofilter, arterial and venous blood lines, and a fluid collection device (Fig. 45–7). CRRT is dependent on the rate of blood flow, which is determined by the mean arterial blood pressure (MAP). A MAP of at least 60 mm Hg is needed to maintain the system.

Cannulation of a large artery and vein is performed by the physician, usually at the femoral site. A hemofilter and blood lines are primed with heparinized saline. Blood flow begins at the arterial site and passes through the blood line to the hemofilter. The hemofilter separates plasma water and certain solutes from the blood and passes the ultrafiltrate to a graduated measuring device. Blood, minus the ultrafiltrate, is then returned through the venous blood line to the venous site.

Slow Continuous Ultrafiltration. Slow continuous ultrafiltration (SCUF), the removal of molecules dissolved in plasma, is based on the principle of convection. Some elements in the plasma water are conveyed across the semipermeable hemofilter as a result of the differences in hydrostatic pressure. Albumin and protein-bound substances are retained in the plasma and returned to the patient. SCUF removes filterable solutes in proportion to plasma water: large amounts of plasma water removed result in large amounts of filterable solutes removed (ultrafiltration). SCUF, therefore, does not alter the concentration of solutes in the blood.

Continuous Arteriovenous Hemofiltration. Continuous arteriovenous hemofiltration (CAVH) uses the principles of convection and replacement. The concentration of the ultrafiltrate is lowered by replacing the ultrafiltrate with a solution free of unwanted solutes (e.g., potassium-free lactated Ringer's solution). The infusion rate of this replacement fluid is determined by the ultrafiltration rate, intake, output, and desired fluid removal. CAVH can filter up to 20 L/24 h. An infusion pump placed on the arterial blood line may be used to increase the rate of ultrafiltration production.

Continuous Arteriovenous Hemodialysis. Continuous arteriovenous hemodialysis (CAVHD) uses the principles of convection and diffusion. It provides more solute (urea, creatinine) clearance; therefore, it is used in uremic patients with high catabolic rates (acidosis, hyperkalemia). Urea clearance is approximately twice that of CAVH. A peritoneal dialysate solution is used to create a diffusion gradient, enhancing the removal of urea and creatinine into the dialysate solution and out of the hemofilter into the ultrafiltrate. The higher the glucose concentration in the dialysate solution (1.5%, 2.5%, 4.25%), the greater the solute and fluid removal.

Nursing Care

Access sites are cleansed and inspected daily for signs of infection. Patency of the system can be assessed by inspection and palpation. Both the arterial and venous blood lines should be warm and a thrill palpable. Signs that the system is no longer patent include a decrease in the production of ultrafiltrate, a darkened or streaked filter, and blood-tinged ultrafiltrate. Laboratory values, daily weights, and hourly records of intake and output are performed.

Complications

The insertion site is inspected frequently for signs of infection, infiltration, and bleeding. If any of these occur, the access will be changed and appropriate antibiotic therapy instituted. The tubing and catheter are kept free of kinks. A kinked catheter will decrease blood flow and greatly increase the risk of clotting as blood stagnates in the hemofilter.

Disconnection of the system from the hemofilter, blood lines, or access catheter may result in exsanguination. The system must be reconnected under sterile conditions. The circuit is clamped off to prevent air from entering the system. If air has entered the system, it is allowed to pass through the filter and must be removed through the blood infusion port (venous) so that it is not delivered to the patient.

The large doses of heparin required for CRRT place the patient at risk for bleeding. The danger can be minimized by monitoring clotting profiles.

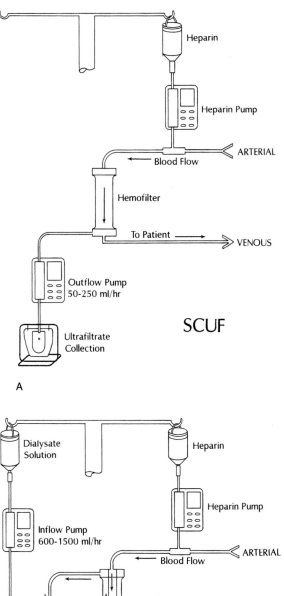

A

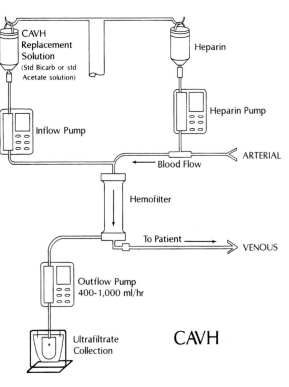

B

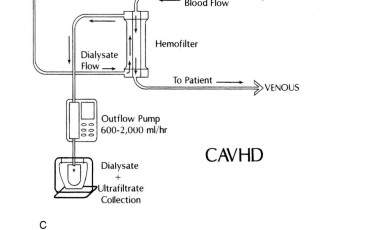

C

Figure 45–7. Modes of continuous renal replacement therapy (CRRT). **(A)** Slow continuous ultrafiltration (SCUF). **(B)** Continuous arteriovenous hemofiltration (CAVH). **(C)** Continuous arteriovenous hemodialysis (CAVHD).

Problems with the ultrafiltration rate may develop from problems with the patient or circuit. If the patient is hypovolemic or hypotensive, the force that pushes the blood through the circuit will be reduced. This will decrease the amount of ultrafiltrate generated. This also contributes to clot forma-tion in the hemofilter, resulting in slower filtration and less ultrafiltrate production. To minimize these complications, the filter is always kept below the level of the patient's heart and the collecting system low enough to the floor that the ultrafiltrate moves with the assistance of gravity.

Renal Trauma

Trauma or injury to the kidney is frequently seen with colon, spleen, liver, and pancreatic injuries. It is most often detected while evaluating the presence of injuries to the abdomen, flank, or lower thorax. Renal trauma occurs most frequently in men between the ages of 20 and 40 years. The mortality rate is approximately 6–12%, with the greatest risk to those who are elderly, who have pre-existing renal disease, or who abuse drugs and alcohol.

ETIOLOGY

Most injuries to the kidney are nonpenetrating (blunt) injuries. The most common mechanism of injury is a motor vehicle accident. Acceleration–deceleration forces occur as the victim makes contact with the steering wheel or dashboard as the vehicle stops and the kidney continues to move forward, tearing blood vessels. Falls, accidents during contact sports, and physical assaults also may cause renal injury.

Penetrating injuries to the kidney are caused by knife or gunshot wounds. They are associated with a high incidence of intraperitoneal visceral injury, hemorrhage, fistulas, and infections.

ASSESSMENT

All trauma victims require a standardized primary and secondary survey followed by a focused assessment of each area that has been injured. In addition, a complete history of the incident must be ascertained from the patient, family, or people who responded to the accident.

Any injury to the flank, lower thorax, or abdomen arouses suspicion of possible renal trauma.

Areas of pain are identified and compared to complaints of pain at the scene of the accident. Patients with renal injury often complain of pain or tenderness in the flank, upper abdomen, or back. It may radiate to the groin or shoulder and may be accompanied by nausea. A history of hypertension is determined, as renal injuries may cause hypertension later.

The lower rib area, flanks, lumbar spine, and abdomen are inspected for ecchymoses, abrasions, contusions, or lacerations. Ecchymosis over the flank and lower back area, Turner's sign, is indicative of retroperitoneal hematoma. Entry and exit sites of any penetrating injuries are noted because they provide clues to potential internal organ injuries.

The external genitalia, perineum, and urethral meatus are inspected for blood or ecchymosis. If blood is found surrounding the urinary meatus, insertion of a urinary catheter is contraindicated until urethral damage is ruled out. If a urinary catheter has been inserted, the urine is inspected for clots or blood. Gross hematuria indicates genitourinary injury and requires further investigation. The presence of gross or microscopic hematuria suggests renal injury, however, there is no correlation between the degree of hematuria and the extent of injury.

Auscultation of the abdomen is performed in all four quadrants. Auscultation is performed before palpation to avoid stimulating any abdominal sounds or inducing pain. The absence of bowel sounds may indicate extravasation of blood. Normally, percussion of the abdomen produces tympany. Dullness on percussion may indicate the accumulation of blood, urine, or other fluid in the abdominal cavity. Dullness over the flank may be related to a retroperitoneal hematoma.

Any abdominal rigidity, pain, or tenderness during palpation indicates inflammation or injury to the abdominal wall. Pain upon rapid withdrawal of the examiner's hands, or rebound tenderness, occurs with intra-abdominal inflammation. Costovertebral angle tenderness is also assessed. With the patient in a sitting or lateral decubitus position, the palm of one hand is placed over each costovertebral angle and struck with the ulnar surface of the opposite fist. Kidney infection or injury is suspected if pain is felt.

DIAGNOSTIC PROCEDURES

A thorough history and physical assessment leads to a high index of suspicion of renal trauma. Table 46–1 presents an overview of common diagnostic studies performed to further evaluate renal trauma.

TABLE 46–1. DIAGNOSTIC PROCEDURES

Type	Comments
Hematological	
Blood urea nitrogen (BUN)/creatinine	Elevation of BUN indicates catabolism and/or hypovolemia
	Elevation of BUN and creatinine indicates poor renal function
Hematocrit/hemoglobin	Decrease indicates hemorrrhage
Leukocytes	Elevated slightly with increased polymorphonuclear leukocytes (neutrophils, eosinophils, basophils) from local renal tissue injury
Electrolytes	Vary
Urological	
Volume	May be decreased in renal trauma or obstruction
	Decreased in hypovolemia
Urinalysis	Blood and protein may be present or absent in renal trauma
Radiological	
Intravenous pyelogram (IVP)	The kidneys are compared by the injection of contrast media
	Abnormal findings: Delayed excretion, extravasation of dye, distortion of the calyces, or incomplete filling
Renal angiography	Provides more information on the integrity of the renal vasculature
Computed tomography (CT)	Determines the extent of injury in three dimensions
Kidneys, ureter, and bladder films (KUB)	Visualizes renal outline and lower rib fractures
Renal scan	Determines status of renal blood flow and presence of parenchymal injury

CLASSIFICATION OF RENAL TRAUMA

Renal trauma is classified according to severity: contusion, laceration, fracture, and vascular injury. Renal contusions account for 60–80% of all renal injuries. They result from blunt trauma and present with hematuria, ecchymosis over the flank or lower thorax, subcapsular hematoma, and costovertebral angle pain with palpation. An intravenous pyelogram (IVP) is indicated to assess the severity of injury. Management for this minor injury includes bedrest, increased fluid intake, monitoring of urinary volume, concentration, urinalysis results, hematology results, and vital signs.

A laceration is a disruption in renal tissue that may involve only the cortical layer or may extend into the renal collecting system (calyces). Patients present with flank trauma, hematuria, and may have other injuries. An IVP is performed to determine the extent of extravasation. Management may be conservative by allowing the laceration to heal on its own, treating it the same as a minor renal injury, and performing renal scans. Uncontrolled bleeding or increased urinary extravasation requires surgical intervention.

A complete renal tear or fracture involves diffuse rupture of both poles and midportion of the kidney. These patients present in hemorrhagic shock due to massive bleeding. Trauma is present in the flank area with an expanding flank mass. Multiple system injuries are usually present. If an IVP shows extravasation, a renal arteriogram is then performed. Surgery is performed immediately to remove all or part of the damaged kidney.

Renal vascular injuries include a tear or laceration in the renal vasculature or a thrombosis of the renal artery. Lacerations of the renal vasculature result from penetrating trauma (gunshot or stab wound) and are considered life-threatening. Since the kidneys receive 20–25% of the cardiac output, massive hemorrhage into the retroperitoneal space may occur. These patients present in hemorrhagic shock and require emergency surgery to repair or remove the kidney as well as fluid resuscitation.

Thrombosis of the renal artery occurs when the intima is torn, forcing blood between the intima and the intact media. A thrombus forms, occluding the blood vessel. It usually results from a deceleration injury. The patient presents with flank pain, with or without hematuria. Auscultation of bruits in the upper abdominal quadrants may be found. Renal artery thrombosis may not be apparent for several days or weeks following injury, when hypertension secondary to excessive release of angiotensin appears. Renal arteriography reveals the vascular defect that is then repaired surgically.

TREATMENT AND NURSING INTERVENTION

Initial management following renal trauma is the same for all types of injuries, including maintaining a patent airway, providing oxygenation, controlling hemorrhage, establishing intravenous access, correcting blood losses, and monitoring vital signs and laboratory results. If the patient is unable to void, a urinary catheter is placed. If a catheter cannot be passed because of resistance, radiological examination of the urinary tract is indicated. Catheters should never be forced, since obstruction is indicative of injury or hematoma.

Minor renal trauma is managed with bedrest, monitoring of hematocrit, hemoglobin, hematuria, urinalysis, urine concentration, and vital signs, providing analgesics, and administering antibiotics. Ambulation begins once gross hematuria clears. Healing takes 4–6 weeks.

Major renal trauma is usually managed surgically. Postoperative care includes maintaining fluid and electrolyte balance, ensuring patency of any drains or tubes, and monitoring for signs of hemorrhage. Urine is monitored for amount, color, clarity, and specific gravity. Hematuria is common except following a nephrectomy. Daily weights and monitoring of intake and output from indwelling catheters and nephrostomy tubes are also performed. All tubes and drains must be kept patent to prevent abscess formation or increased intracalyceal pressure resulting in tissue damage. Signs of hemorrhage include flank pain or mass, increased bloody drainage from tubes, decreased hematocrit and hemoglobin, and clinical signs of shock.

COMPLICATIONS

The most common complication of renal trauma is hypertension. Renal injury causes scarring of the renal parenchyma, which may result in narrowing of the renal vasculature and a decrease in renal blood flow. The renin-angiotensin mechanism is then activated causing increased blood pressure.

Extravasation of urine increases the risk of infection. Signs of extravasation include midline bulging from a distended bladder, abdominal distension, thigh expanding from fluid, abdominal pain, rebound tenderness, and hematuria (not always present).

Other complications include infection, secondary hemorrhage, and acute tubular necrosis (ATN). Hemorrhage/hypovolemia decreases renal blood flow and contributes to oliguria or anuria. Massive muscle breakdown from crush injuries may contribute to rhabdomyolysis, which obstructs the renal tubules and causes ATN.

RENAL BIBLIOGRAPHY

Baer, C.L., & Lancaster, L.E. (1992). Acute renal failure. *Crit Care Nurse Q*, *14*, 4: 1–21.

Calhoun, K.A. (1990). Serum potassium concentration abnormalities. *Crit Care Nurse Q*, *13*, 3: 34–38.

Clochesy, J.M., Breu, C., Cardin, S., Rudy, E.B., Whittaker, A.A. (1993). *Critical Care Nursing*. Philadelphia: W.B. Saunders Co.

Douglas, S. (1992). Acute tubular necrosis: diagnosis, treatment, and nursing implications. *AACN Clin Issues in Crit Care Nurs*, *3*, 3: 688–697.

Graves, L. (1990). Disorders of calcium, phosphorus, and magnesium. *Crit Care Nurse Q*, *13*, 3: 3–13.

Guyton, A. (1991). *Textbook of Medical Physiology*, 8th ed. Philadelphia: W.B. Saunders Co.

Innerarity, S.A. (1990). Electrolyte emergencies in the critically ill renal patient. *Crit Care Clin North Am*, *2*, 1: 89–99.

Isley, W.L. (1990). Serum sodium concentration abnormalities. *Crit Care Nurse Q*, *13*, 3: 82–88.

Metheny, N.M. (1992). *Fluid and Electrolyte Balance: Nursing Considerations*, 2nd ed. Philadelphia: J.B. Lippincott Co.

Price, C.A. (1992). An update on continuous renal replacement therapies. *AACN Clin Issues in Crit Care Nurs*, *3*, 3: 597–604.

Smith, L.J. (1992). Peritoneal dialysis in the critically ill patient. *AACN Clin Issues in Crit Care Nurs*, *3*, 3: 558–568.

Smith, M.F. (1990) Renal trauma: adult and pediatric considerations. *Crit Care Clin of North Am*, *2*, 1: 67–77.

Renal Practice Exam

1. A 51-year-old male is in the unit following a fall from a 15-foot ladder. He landed on his back and complains of pain between T-7 and T-12. Neurological tests, including a head CT (computed tomography) scan, are negative. Abdominal CT shows no fracture or active bleeding. He is alert and oriented and has no difficulty breathing. The following information is available:

Urine and stool	*Blood*
Increased RBCs	Hgb 13
Stool guaiac negative	Hct 39
	WBC 7900
	Amylase 50

   Based on the preceding information, which organ is most likely to have been injured?
   (A) spleen
   (B) kidney
   (C) pancreas
   (D) descending colon

2. Which intervention is most likely to occur?
   (A) oxygen therapy and SpO_2 monitoring
   (B) urinary catheter
   (C) nasogastric tube to suction
   (D) head CT

3. A 64-year-old female is in the ICU with the diagnosis of possible sepsis secondary to a urinary tract infection. Upon admission she was markedly short of breath with an a/A ratio of .14, a FI02 of 80% and a PaO2 of 72. She was intubated due to increased work of breathing. Shortly after admission, she became hypotensive and had a pulmonary artery catheter inserted to aid her management. Over the next two days, she was aggressively treated with normal saline fluid bolus (with a subsequent 10 Kg weight gain), antibiotics and dobutamine. Based on the information below, what effect has taken place in terms of her electrolytes?

Na	121
K	4.9
Cl	94
HCO_3	25

   (A) not enough chloride has been given
   (B) she has received too much fluid
   (C) she has become dehydrated
   (D) she needs more sodium in her IV fluids

4. A 78-year-old male is in the unit with a diagnosis of CHF. He has received increasing amounts of lasix over the past 3 days due to low urine output. Based on the information below, the MD believes a contraction alkalosis has developed. Do the following electrolytes agree with this observation?

Na	144
K	4.3
Cl	90
HCO_3	39

   (A) yes, based on the increased sodium level
   (D) yes, based on the decreased chloride and increased bicarbonate levels
   (C) no, based on the high potassium
   (D) no, since the key electrolyte, magnesium, is not given

5. The right kidney is slightly lower than the left. What is the reason for this difference?
   (A) the right kidney is larger because of the presence of more nephronal structures
   (B) the left kidney is displaced upward by the spleen
   (C) the right kidney is displaced downward by the liver
   (D) the left kidney is drawn upward by the diaphragm

6. The kidneys have the ability to regulate blood flow partially via local regulatory mechanisms. If

the systemic blood pressure falls, how does the kidney maintain perfusion?
(A) decreasing nephronal resistance to glomerular filtrate
(B) afferent arteriole dilation and efferent arteriole constriction
(C) efferent arteriole dilation and afferent arteriole constriction
(D) decreasing glomerular filtration rate and increase active secretion levels

7. Fluid is forced from the glomerulus, forming an ultrafiltrate. Into which compartment is the fluid forced?
(A) Bowman's capsule
(B) proximal tubule
(C) collecting ducts
(D) distal tubule

8. Which of the following elements is NOT filtered during glomerular filtration?
(A) sodium
(B) potassium
(C) proteins
(D) creatinine

9. From a renal perspective, secretion can be defined by which of the following descriptions?
(A) movement of solutes and water from the peritubular network into the tubule
(B) movement of solutes and water from the tubule into the peritubular network
(C) movement of high-molecular-weight particles into the urine
(D) acceleration of electrolyte elimination at the glomerulus

10. Glomerular filtration is affected by all of the following factors. Which has the most significant effect on glomerular filtration rate?
(A) osmotic pressure of the blood
(B) hydrostatic pressure of the blood
(C) dilation of the afferent arteriole
(D) constriction of the efferent arteriole

Questions 11 and 12 refer to the following scenario.

A 37-year-old male is in your unit following a motor vehicle accident. During the initial 24 hr, he was hypotensive and developed acute renal failure. His current laboratory data reveal the following information:

	Serum	Urine
NA$^+$	126 mEq/L	59 mEq/L
K$^+$	3.9 mEq/L	
osmolality	290 mosm	485 mosm
creatinine	3.0 mEq/L	

11. Based on the preceding information, which condition is likely to be present?
(A) dehydration
(B) fluid overload
(C) acute renal failure
(D) glomerulonephritis

12. Which laboratory data are abnormal?
(A) serum creatinine
(B) urinary osmolality
(C) serum osmolality
(D) urinary Na$^+$

13. Which of the following corresponds most closely to normal serum osmolality?
(A) 50 to 100 mosm
(B) 100 to 250 mosm
(C) 280 to 320 mosm
(D) 320 to 410 mosm

14. Which of the following corresponds most closely to the range of normal serum sodium values?
(A) 40 to 60 mEq/L
(B) 60 to 75 mEq/L
(C) 80 to 120 mEq/L
(D) 135 to 145 mEq/L

15. Which of the following corresponds most closely to the range of normal serum potassium values?
(A) 1 to 2 mEq/L
(B) 2.5 to 3.5 mEq/L
(C) 3.5 to 5.0
(D) 5 to 6.5 mEq/L

16. Which of the following corresponds most closely to the range of normal urine sodium values?
(A) 40 to 220 mEq/L
(B) 220 to 320 mEq/L
(C) 335 to 445 mEq/L
(D) 455 to 470 mEq/L

17. Which of the following corresponds most closely to the range of normal serum calcium levels?
(A) 1 to 3 mg/dl
(B) 4.5 to 6.5 mg/dl
(C) 6 to 8 mg/dl
(D) 8.5 to 10.5 mg/dl

18. An 81-year-old male has been in the intensive care unit for 45 days because of surgical complications from a ruptured bowel. The physician suspects that he may have nutritional impairment despite hyperalimentation. Laboratory tests reveal the following serum electrolyte information:

Na$^+$	141 mEq/L
K$^+$	3.9 mEq/L

Cl^-	102 mEq/L
HCO_3^-	25 mEq/L
Ca^{2+}	8.9 mg/dl
Mg^{2+}	4.3 mg/dl

Which of the preceding laboratory values is/are abnormal?

(A) Mg^{2+}
(B) Ca^{2+}
(C) Cl^- and Na^+
(D) K^+ and HCO_3^-

19. Which of the following corresponds most closely to the range of normal phosphate levels?
(A) 3 to 4.5 mg/dl
(B) 4.5 to 6.5 mg/dl
(C) 6 to 8 mg/dl
(D) 8.5 to 10.5 mg/dl

20. Creatinine level is a valuable indicator of glomerular filtration rate for which reason?
(A) Once filtered in the glomerulus, creatinine is not reabsorbed in the tubular system.
(B) Creatinine only enters the glomerulus when glomerular filtration pressures exceed 60 mm Hg.
(C) Creatinine filtration is unaffected by renal disease.
(D) Creatinine is formed in the glomerulus and only decreases in filtration causing creatinine levels to change.

21. What is the effect of ADH (antidiuretic hormone) on renal function?
(A) It inhibits water reabsorption in the distal tubules and collecting ducts.
(B) It increases water reabsorption in the distal tubles and collecting ducts.
(C) It increases fluid excretion from the glomerulus.
(D) It blocks the effect of loop diuretics, such as furosemide (Lasix).

22. Which of the following would stimulate the release of ADH (antidiuretic hormone)?
(A) decreased serum osmolality
(B) increased serum osmolality
(C) increased serum creatinine
(D) decreased urine sodium

23. The countercurrent mechanism in the nephron is designed to accomplish which purpose?
(A) retaining creatinine
(B) eliminating hydrogen ions
(C) concentrating urine
(D) increasing water loss

24. Most water reabsorption occurs in which part of the nephron?
(A) proximal tubules
(B) loop of Henle
(C) distal tubules
(D) collecting ducts

25. A 46-year-old male is in your unit following an episode of ARD (acute respiratory distress) after radiation therapy for large cell lung cancer. His urine output decreases on day 3 of his intensive care unit stay to 20 ml/h. The physician asks you to call him if the patient's BUN (blood urea nitrogen)/creatinine ratio becomes abnormal. The following laboratory data are available:

serum BUN	64
serum creatinine	2
urine Na^+	76

Based on this information, is the BUN/creatinine ratio abnormal and should you contact the physician?
(A) The BUN/creatinine level is normal; do not call the physician.
(B) The BUN/creatinine level is low; call the physician.
(C) The BUN/creatinine level is high; call the physician.
(D) BUN/creatinine ratios cannot be calculated without urinary creatinine and BUN values.

26. Which of the following corresponds most closely to the range of normal serum creatinine levels?
(A) 0.8 to 1.8
(B) 2 to 2.9
(C) 3.2 to 4
(D) 4.5 to 5

27. Which of the following corresponds most closely to the range of normal serum BUN levels?
(A) 10 to 20 mg/dl
(B) 20 to 30 mg/dl
(C) 30 to 40 mg/dl
(D) 40 to 50 mg/dl

28. In the presence of oliguria, a BUN/creatinine ratio greater than normal suggests that which condition has developed?
(A) prerenal failure
(B) renal failure
(C) postrenal failure
(D) acute tubular necrosis

29. Aldosterone exerts an effect on renal function at which anatomical site?

(Answers cont'd.)

(A) proximal tubule
(B) loop of Henle
(C) distal tubule
(D) glomerulus

30. The juxtaglomerular system is responsible for releasing which substance?
(A) erythropoietin
(B) aldosterone
(C) secretin
(D) angiotensin

31. Angiotension II exerts which of the following physiological actions?
(A) vasoconstriction
(B) vasodilation
(C) increases glomerular filtration rate
(D) promotes ADH (antidiuretic hormone) secretion

32. A 34-year-old male with chronic renal failure has a hemoglobin level of 7.4 g/dL and a hematocrit of 23%. His blood pressure is 160/92 and his heart rate is 98. What is the most likely explanation for the hemoglobin and hemotocrit values?
(A) The values are abnormally elevated because of hemoconcentration.
(B) The values are abnormally low because of a reduced cardiac output.
(C) The values are normal.
(D) The values are decreased because of loss of erythropoietin.

33. Which substance has the most significant effect on sodium regulation?
(A) renin level
(B) aldosterone level
(C) glomerular filtration rate
(D) serum pH

34. What is the primary action of aldosterone?
(A) inhibits sodium excretion
(B) promotes sodium excretion
(C) blocks water reabsorption
(D) stimulates vasoconstriction

35 What is the primary cause of hypernatremia?
(A) vascular water deficits
(B) excessive vascular free water
(C) excessive serum sodium levels
(D) loss of serum chloride

36. The lack of ADH (antidiuretic hormone) causes which effect on serum electrolytes?
(A) increase in sodium levels
(B) decrease in sodium levels
(C) decrease in hydrogen ion levels
(D) increase in serum bicarbonate levels

37. Which of the following is NOT a common sign of hypernatremia?
(A) tachycardia
(B) dry mucous membranes
(C) poor skin turgor
(D) distended neck veins

38. Administration of which of the following is a normal initial treatment for hypernatremia?
(A) diuretics and fluid restriction
(B) nonelectrolyte (free water) solutions
(C) normal saline
(D) potassium salts

39. Hyponatremia is most often caused by which of the following?
(A) excessive sodium levels
(B) decreased sodium levels
(C) excessive vascular volume
(D) decreased vascular volume

40. The most dangerous symptoms of hyponatremia center on which organ system?
(A) central nervous system
(B) cardiac system
(C) renal system
(D) respiratory system

41. Excessive secretion of ADH (antidiuretic hormone) could produce which of the following electrolyte changes?
(A) increased serum osmolality
(B) increased serum sodium
(C) decreased serum sodium
(D) decreased hydrogen

42. Treatment of severe hyponatremia (less than 120 mEq/L) consists of administration of which of the following?
(A) diuretics
(B) nonelectrolyte (free water) solutions
(C) normal saline
(D) potassium salts

43. Hypokalemia is associated with which acid-base disturbance?
(A) metabolic acidosis
(B) metabolic alkalosis
(C) respiratory acidosis
(D) systemic acidosis

44. Which of the following ECG (electrocardiographic) changes is NOT associated with hyperkalemia?
(A) peaked T waves
(B) depressed P waves
(C) PVCs (premature ventricular contractions)
(D) widening QRS complex

45. Which of the following is NOT recommended for the treatment of hyperkalemia?
(A) Kayexalate
(B) glucose/insulin infusion
(C) dialysis
(D) ammonium chloride

46. Hypokalemia is associated with which of the following ECG changes?
(A) peaked T waves
(B) depressed P waves
(C) PVCs (premature ventricular contractions)
(D) widening QRS complex

47. The concentration of which electrolyte is inversely related to that of calcium?
(A) sodium
(B) potassium
(C) phosphate
(D) magnesium

48. Which mechanism is calcium NOT involved in regulating?
(A) coagulation
(B) formation of bone
(C) transmission of electrical impulses
(D) absorption of vitamin D

49. A 51-year-old male with a history of alcoholism has marked muscle irritability. The following laboratory data are available:

Na^+	135 mEq/L
K^+	4.8 mEq/L
Ca^{2+}	3.7 mg/dL
Mg^{2+}	1.8 mg/dL

Which of the following electrolytes is most likely to be the source of the muscle hyperirritability?
(A) sodium
(B) calcium
(C) potassium
(D) magnesium

50. Chvostek's sign is tested by which maneuver?
(A) tapping the flexor tendon over the knee
(B) tapping the supramandibular area
(C) stroking the sole of the foot
(D) measuring clotting times after venipuncture

51. Trousseau's sign is a test for which electrolyte deficiency?
(A) hypophosphatemia
(B) hypercalcemia
(C) hypocalcemia
(D) hypokalemia

52. Which organ or organ system is involved in the regulation of phosphate elimination?

(A) liver
(B) respiratory system
(C) renal system
(D) spleen

53. A 75-year-old female is admitted to your unit with pneumonia and malnutrition. Her chief complaint currently is weakness and inability to perform her normal "chores." She has stated that she has not eaten well for the past several months. The following information is available:

Na^+	150 mEq/L
K^+	3.6 mEq/L
Cl^-	110 mEq/L
Mg^{2+}	2.1 mg/dl
Ca^{2+}	9.2 mg/dl
PO_4^{3-}	2.3 mg/dl

Which of the preceding levels is a likely source of her weakness?
(A) low phosphate
(B) high sodium and chloride
(C) low magnesium
(D) high calcium

54. Which of the following does NOT have phosphate as a component?
(A) ATP (adenosine triphosphate)
(B) ADP (adenosine diphosphate)
(C) 2,3-DPG (2,3-diphosphodiglyceride)
(D) PTH (parathyroid hormone)

55. Which electrolyte is directly related to the reabsorption of magnesium?
(A) potassium
(B) calcium
(C) sodium
(D) phosphate

56. Which of the following is a primary treatment to reduce magnesium levels?
(A) normal saline bolus
(B) dialysis
(C) mechanical ventilation
(D) calcium carbonate administration

57. Hypomagnesemia is manifested clinically by which of the following symptoms?
(A) muscle irritability
(B) muscle fatigue
(C) nausea
(D) positive Turner's sign

58. A 61-year-old male admitted with the diagnosis of COPD (chronic obstructive pulmonary disease) has the following set of laboratory data for arterial blood gases and electrolytes:

PO_2	63 mm Hg
PCO_2	71 mm Hg
pH	7.37
HCO_3^-	39 mEq/L
Na^+	146 mEq/L
Cl^-	87 mEq/L

The COPD-induced blood gas changes have altered the electrolytes as well. Based on the preceding information, which electrolyte change occurred because of the PCO_2 elevation?
(A) decrease in pH
(B) chloride increased
(C) sodium increased
(D) increased HCO_3^-

59. Elevated chloride levels are associated with which condition?
(A) alkalosis
(B) acidosis
(C) hyponatremia
(D) hypercalcemia

60. Left ventricular failure will cause which effect on the BUN/creatinine ratio?
(A) It will cause the ratio to rise. (BUN rises faster than creatinine.)
(B) It will cause the ratio to fall. (BUN rises slower than creatinine.)
(C) It will have no effect on the ratio but will elevate creatinine levels.
(D) It will reverse the ratio.

61. A 74-year-old female is admitted to your unit with possible sepsis and renal failure. The following laboratory information is available:

urinary Na^+	13
urinary osmolarity	1000
urine output	15 ml/h

Based on these data, what is likely to be occurring?
(A) prerenal azotemia
(B) acute tubular necrosis
(C) postrenal obstruction
(D) vasomotor nephropathy

62. A 61-year-old female is in your unit after being admitted from a nursing home. At the time of admission, it was noted that she seemed confused, although she is currently alert and oriented. She has had a "cold" for the past several days. Her laboratory data are as follows:

Na^+	155
K^+	3.6
Cl^-	122
HCO_3^-	24

What is the most likely reason for the abnormal sodium level?
(A) excess total sodium
(B) decreased total potassium
(C) dehydration
(D) fluid excess

63. Which of the following patients has an increased anion gap?

	1	2	3	4
Na^+	132	142	121	153
K^+	3.2	4.8	4.1	3.5
Cl^-	93	108	89	113
HCO_3^-	25	17	19	26

(A) patient 1
(B) patient 2
(C) patient 3
(D) patient 4

64. What is the clinical value in establishing whether or not an anion gap exists?
(A) The finding permits determination of a metabolic alkalosis.
(B) The finding permits determination of a metabolic acidosis.
(C) The finding permits identification of respiratory acidosis.
(D) The anion gap acts as a marker of acute renal failure.

Questions 65 and 66 refer to the following scenario.

A 61-year-old male has a two-day history of abdominal pain with nausea and vomiting. He has intermittent chest pain, which is unrelieved by nitrates, changes in position, or rest. He has a history of CHF (congestive heart failure) and underwent a CABG (coronary artery bypass graft) 2 years ago. Currently he has a urine output of 15 ml/h. He has had a urine output of 200 ml over the past 24 hr. Currently he has the following vital signs:

blood pressure	88/56
pulse	114
respiratory rate	32

He has a pulmonary artery catheter in place, from which the following information is available:

cardiac output	3.7
cardiac index	2.4
arterial pressure	20/8
PCWP	6
CVP	2

The following laboratory data are also available:

SMA-6

Na^+	153
K^+	3.6
Cl^-	120
HCO_3^-	19
creatinine	2.2
glucose	154
BUN	35
osmolality	320

He has the following blood gas values:

PaO_2	82
$PaCO_2$	28
pH	7.30
HCO_3^-	20
SvO_2	52%
PvO_2	32

Urinary electrolyte values are as follows:

Na^+	35
osmolality	845
creatinine	48

Other laboratory data include the following:

albumin	3.6
hemoglobin	15.6
lactate	2.2

65. Based on the preceding information, what is the potential problem and the likely reason for the decrease in urine output?
    (A) prerenal azotemia from hypovolemia
    (B) prerenal azotemia from left ventricular failure
    (C) acute tubular necrosis
    (D) ATN from hypovolemia

66. What would be the most effective therapy to improve this patient's renal function?
    (A) fluid bolus
    (B) dobutamine therapy
    (C) diuretics
    (D) renal dose dopamine

67. A 31-year-old female is in the intensive care unit following multiple gunshot wounds to her face and abdomen. She has been in the unit for 4 days and during the fourth day her urine output decreases to 200 ml for the entire day. She is alert and oriented yet cannot communicate because of an endotracheal tube. The following information is available to you:

Na^+	132
K^+	4.1

Cl^-	99
HCO_3^-	20
creatinine	2.5
BUN	43
osmolality	295
urinary creatinine	50
urinary osmolality	343

Based on the preceding information, what is the most likely cause of her decreased urine output?
(A) prerenal azotemia from hypovolemia
(B) prerenal azotemia from rhabdomyolysis
(C) acute tubular necrosis
(D) ureter obstruction

68. As you are orienting a preceptor, she asks you about the treatment your patient is receiving for an infection. She tells you she remembers being taught that aminoglycosides (your patient is receiving gentamicin) can cause renal failure. Yet your patient has a normal urine output (2100 ml/day) and the following laboratory values:

Na^+	142
K^+	4.6
Cl^-	103
HCO_3^-	21
creatinine	3.2
BUN	54
osmolality	278
urinary osmolality	297
urinary Na^+	49

She asks if this patient is at any risk for developing renal failure. Based on the preceding information, what would you answer?
(A) As long as the urine output is greater than 30 ml/h she is not in danger of renal failure.
(B) As long as her creatinine level is no greater than 2.5 mg/dl she is not at risk for acute renal failure.
(C) Based on the information, she already has signs of acute renal failure.
(D) Although she may be at risk for renal failure, a renal ultrasound scan would be required to make a definitive diagnosis.

69. A 65-year-old male is in the intensive care unit for a CVA (cerebrovascular accident) and possible CHF (congestive heart failure) secondary to systemic hypertension. He is currently intubated after developing a respiratory acidosis in the emergency room. During the second day in the unit, he begins to put out over 2000 ml of urine on your shift. The following laboratory information is available:

Na$^+$	158
K$^+$	3.4
Cl$^-$	112
HCO$_3^-$	23
creatinine	1.8
BUN	29
osmolality	341
urinary osmolality	343
urinary Na$^+$	28

Based on the preceding information, what condition is likely to be developing?

(A) prerenal azotemia
(B) acute renal failure
(C) diabetes insipidus
(D) inappropriate secretion of ADH (antidiuretic hormone)

70. Measurement of which of the following is helpful in differentiating acute renal failure from PRA (prerenal azotemia)?

(A) FENa
(B) BUN
(C) urinary osmolality
(D) serum Na$^+$

71. During the care of a patient undergoing peritoneal dialysis, the infusate has not completely drained. Which method would be acceptable to help facilitate drainage?

(A) applying continuous low-pressure suction
(B) turning the patient from side to side
(C) manipulating the peritoneal catheter
(D) applying manual pressure to the abdomen

72. Which of the following is NOT considered an indication for continuous arteriovenous hemofiltration?

(A) treating acute volume overload in congestive heart failure
(B) fluid removal when diuretic therapy has failed

(C) acute hyperkalemia
(D) as a replacement for hemodialysis in the non-university hospital setting

73. Which of the following will continuous arteriovenous hemofiltration NOT remove?

(A) fluid
(B) albumin
(C) sodium
(D) potassium

Questions 74 and 75 refer to the following scenario.

A 72-year-old male is in your unit with chronic CHF (congestive heart failure). He has become increasingly resistant to diuretic therapy. CAVH (continuous arteriovenous hemofiltration) is started to help alleviate his symptoms. After one day on CAVH, the filtrate from the CAVH begins to diminish. The arteriovenous filter is warm to the touch and pulsates with each pulse. You notice that the filter is on an IV pole about 12 inches above the patient's heart level. His blood pressure is 100/62, pulse 98, respiratory rate 24, temperature 37.5°C.

74. Based on the preceding information, which condition is likely to be developing?

(A) inadequacy of pump inflow rates
(B) obstruction of the CAVH filter
(C) obstruction of the arteriovenous catheter
(D) inadequate arterial pressure

75. What measures could you take to correct the situation?

(A) add potassium to the dialysate until the flow problem is corrected
(B) add glucose to the dialysate to develop an osmotic pressure gradient
(C) increase the outflow pump rate
(D) lower the filter to heart level

PART VII

Renal Practice Exam

1. _____	20. _____	39. _____	58. _____
2. _____	21. _____	40. _____	59. _____
3. _____	22. _____	41. _____	60. _____
4. _____	23. _____	42. _____	61. _____
5. _____	24. _____	43. _____	62. _____
6. _____	25. _____	44. _____	63. _____
7. _____	26. _____	45. _____	64. _____
8. _____	27. _____	46. _____	65. _____
9. _____	28. _____	47. _____	66. _____
10. _____	29. _____	48. _____	67. _____
11. _____	30. _____	49. _____	68. _____
12. _____	31. _____	50. _____	69. _____
13. _____	32. _____	51. _____	70. _____
14. _____	33. _____	52. _____	71. _____
15. _____	34. _____	53. _____	72. _____
16. _____	35. _____	54. _____	73. _____
17. _____	36. _____	55. _____	74. _____
18. _____	37. _____	56. _____	75. _____
19. _____	38. _____	57. _____	

PART VII

Answers

1.	B	p548	20.	A	p519	39.	B	p524	58.	D	p520
2.	B	p549	21.	B	p515	40.	B	p525	59.	A	p532
3.	B	p536	22.	B	p515–516	41.	C	p515–516	60.	A	p519, 534–535
4.	B	p532	23.	C	p516	42.	A	p525			
5.	C	p509	24.	B	p517–518	43.	B	p527	61.	A	p535
6.	B	p512	25.	C	p535	44.	C	p526	62.	C	p524
7.	B	p513	26.	A	p535	45.	D	p526	63.	B	p531–532
8.	C	p513	27.	A	p535	46.	D	p528	64.	B	p532
9.	A	p515	28.	A	p534	47.	C	p529	65.	A	p534–536
10.	B	p513	29.	C	p520	48.	D	p529	66.	A	p524
11.	B	p535	30.	D	p520	49.	B	p529	67.	C	p535–536
12.	A	p536	31.	A	p520–521	50.	B	p529	68.	C	p535–536
13.	C	p515	32.	A	p522	51.	C	p529	69.	C	p252
14.	B	p523	33.	B	p523	52.	C	p529–530	70.	A	p535–536
15.	B	p525	34.	A	p520	53.	A	p530	71.	B	p538
16.	A	p535	35.	A	p524	54.	B	p529–530	72.	D	p543
17.	D	p527	36.	A	p515	55.	C	p531	73.	B	p544
18.	A	p531	37.	D	p524	56.	B	p531	74.	B	p546
19.	A	p529	38.	B	p524	57.	A	p531	75.	D	p546

VIII

MULTIORGAN PROBLEMS

Thomas S. Ahrens/Donna Prentice

47

Sepsis and Multiorgan Dysfunction Syndrome

EDITORS' NOTE

Sepsis and multiorgan dysfunction syndrome (MODS) are a new part of the CCRN exam. This section, along with burns and toxic ingestions, makes up 10% of the CCRN exam (20 questions). This chapter addresses the areas of sepsis and MODS, a section that may have anywhere from 5 to 15 questions on the CCRN exam. Due to the relevance of sepsis and MODS to critical care, it is a valuable area to learn. Understanding these two major concepts involves becoming familiar with relatively complex cellular activities.

In this chapter, a brief summary of these complex activities are given in an attempt to maintain a simplified approach that covers essential CCRN content.

It is unlikely the specific detail in this chapter will be heavily addressed on the CCRN exam. Try to understand the major terms and the general sequence of events that occur in sepsis. If you understand the major therapies and symptoms of sepsis, you will probably be adequately prepared for the exam.

Concepts in sepsis and multiorgan dysfunction are changing rapidly. Even definitions and terminology are changing in an attempt to keep pace with the improved understanding of concepts involving conditions such as sepsis. In this chapter, definitions and terminology will be employed which are consistent with a recent joint American College of Chest Physicians–Society of Critical Care Medicine com-

mittee recommendation. These terms and definitions are listed in Table 47–1. The major reason for these new definitions is the better understanding of the body's response to both infections and inflammation. The key new terms are systemic inflammatory response syndrome and multiorgan dysfunction syndrome (MODS). MODS replaces the term multisystem organ failure (MSOF). MODS is proposed as a more accurate term, since dysfunctions of organs exist along a continuum, rather than being healthy or in failure, as MSOF implies. These definitions are in addition to the slightly revised definition of sepsis.

The rationale for adopting these new terms is based on important diagnostic and therapeutic concepts. To effectively treat any of the above conditions, you need to understand their causes. With the current definitions, the appropriate origin is not always clear. For example, conditions that previously were termed "sepsis" were frequently associated with an inflammatory process but without any active infection. Sepsis, by definition, must have an active infectious source. Consequently, patients were being diagnosed as having sepsis when they did not meet the definition. In this type of patient, the use of antibiotic therapy or even more advanced therapies, such as monoclonal antibodies, may not be effective, since no active infection is present.

Over the next several pages, sepsis and MODS will be briefly explained. From this explanation, an understanding of the appropriate nursing, diagnostic, and therapeutic actions will be possible. This information should prepare you for the CCRN exam in the area of sepsis and MODS.

TABLE 47–1. DEFINITIONS USED IN SEPSIS

Infection Microbial phenomenon characterized by an inflammatory response to the presence of microorganisms or the invasion of normally sterile host tissue by those organisms.

Bacteremia The presence of viable bacteria in the blood.

Systemic inflammatory response syndrome The systemic inflammatory response to a variety of severe clinical insults. The response is manifested by two or more of the following conditions:
    Temperature >38°C or <36°C
    Heart rate >90 beats/min
    Respiratory rate >20 breaths/min or $Paco_2$ <32 mm Hg
    WBC >12,000 cells/mm^3 or <4000 cells/mm^3, or >10% immature (band) forms

Sepsis The systemic response to infection. This systemic response is manifested by two or more of the following conditions as a result of infection:
    Temperature >38°C or <36°C
    Heart rate >90 beats/min
    Respiratory rate >20 breaths/min or $Paco_2$ <32 mm Hg
    WBC >12,000 cells/mm^3 or <4000 cells/mm^3, or >10% immature (band) forms

Multiorgan dysfunction syndrome Presence of altered organ function in an acutely ill patient such that homeostasis cannot be maintained without intervention.

SEPSIS

Sepsis is one of the leading causes of increased morbidity and mortality in critical care. Sepsis is still a confusing entity for clinicians in that it is a difficult condition to identify, it is difficult to predict who is at risk, and it is even more difficult to treat the condition. Sepsis can present in a mild or severe (septic shock) form, with mortalities ranging anywhere from 20% to 80%, depending on the form of sepsis present. Part of the problem with sepsis is identifying when it is present and why it occurs. In this chapter, potential causes of sepsis are presented along with physical symptoms and responses. Current concepts in treating sepsis will be discussed, as well as controversies in management of the septic patient.

Etiology

Sepsis is defined as the systemic response to infection. It not only is the direct result of an infection but also reflects an inflammatory response produced by the immune system. Sepsis can originate from any antigen, bacterial, viral, or fungal, although by far the most common sources are bacterial. The most significant infections seen in critical care are usually gram-negative bacterial infections (e.g., *Pseudomonas aeruginosa*, *Klebsiella*, *Serratia*, and *Escherichia coli*), although some gram-positive infections (e.g., *Staphylococcus aureus*) are also responsible for sepsis.

The antigen eventually causing sepsis must take hold in tissues and start to grow in order to produce an infectious process. For example, an antigen can exist on the skin (colonization), or even in the blood, but will not produce an infection until it resides and grows in normal tissue. Normally, most infections are controlled by the immune system, and further progression does not take place. However, in sepsis, the initial infection progresses to a more advanced state. The urinary and respiratory systems are the most common sites for initial infections.

Septic Cascade

From the initial infection, an extension of the infectious response occurs. The extension involves a series of events, primarily an inflammatory response sequence as well as a direct physiological response to the infection. The extension can be viewed as a cascade of events, which probably becomes self-perpetuating after a certain point. Several events occur that characterize the septic process and subsequent inflammatory response. These events are briefly summarized below. In addition, Table 47–2 shows the primary factors involved in the septic cascade.

The exact sequence of events in sepsis is unclear, although one potential scenario is as follows (Fig. 47–1). The antigen (e.g., bacteria) is attacked by a macrophage (e.g., a segmented neutrophil). The macrophage ingests and destroys most of the antigen. By-products of the damaged antigen, such as endotoxin, are released. The immune system responds to the antigen and the by-products by producing substances designed to control the continued growth of the antigen. For example, the complement system (particularly C3a and C5a) is activated to stimulate neutrophil activity. In addition, platelet activation and aggregation are promoted, perhaps as an attempt to isolate the infection. The neutrophil or other macrophage (e.g., monocytes) will initiate a sequence

TABLE 47–2. MAJOR IMMUNE SYSTEM MEDIATORS

Arachidonic acid   Phospholipid from cell walls that can produce leukotrienes, thromboxane A_2, and prostaglandins.

Complement   There are two major types, C3 and C5, which have similar actions. Causes mast cells to release vasodilatation mediators, stimulation of arachidonic acid, increased neutrophil and monocyte activity, increased capillary permeability, stimulation of TNF release, and decreased systemic vascular resistance.

Interferons   Increase TNF and interleukin release, activate B-cell activity for antibody formation, and increase neutrophil and monocyte activity.

Leukotrienes   Several different types exist, although the primary actions are to increase platelet aggregation, cause vasoconstriction (reducing capillary blood flow), and increase pulmonary vascular resistance. Stimulate prostacyclin, probably as a feedback control mechanism.

Prostaglandin E_2   Inhibits interleukin-1, causes vasodilation, and can inhibit TNF production.

Prostaglandin I_2   Inhibits platelet aggregation and thrombus formation. Causes vasodilatation and decreased capillary permeability.

Thromboxane A_2   Increases platelet aggregation, leading to capillary obstruction. Increases capillary permeability, vasoconstriction, and bronchoconstriction.

Tumor necrosis factor (TNF)   Stimulated from endotoxin or similar substance. Primary action is to increase production

---

of events also designed to control the antigen. The major immunologic responses are listed below.

Arachidonic Acid Sequence

In response to the infection, macrophage (neutrophil and monocyte) activity (polymorphonuclear leukocytes [PMNs]) in the area increase. PMNs attempt to control the infection through a variety of processes, including release of highly destructive molecules such as oxygen free radicals. Another method used by the PMNs is through the breakdown of arachidonic acid. As arachidonic acid is generated, it is further degraded. The degradation of arachidonic acid takes place by one of two pathways, the cyclo-oxygenase or lipo-oxygenase pathway (Fig. 47–2). From the cyclo-oxygenase pathway, two important by-products, thromboxane A_2 and prostacyclin (a prostaglandin), are generated. From the lipo-oxygenase pathway, various leukotrienes (e.g., leukotrienes B_4, C_4, D_4, and E_4) are released.

Both leukotrienes and thromboxane A_2 generate a series of reactions, including an increased tendency for platelet aggregation, increased capillary permeability, and vasoconstriction. Prostacyclin (the precursor to specific prostaglandins) produces essentially the opposite responses, i.e., a decreased tendency for platelet aggregation, decreased capillary permeability, and vasodilatation.

Down-Regulation of the Immune/Inflammatory Response

An important aspect of the immune/inflammatory response is the body's ability to neutralize toxic products produced by the immune system. The ability of components of the immune system to control infections is based on the generation of substances that destroy virtually any substance which with they

come into contact, including normal cells. For example, oxygen radicals, once released, will damage or destroy any cell with which they come in contact. The body will attempt to produce neutralizing substances, such as peroxidases for oxygen radicals, to avoid injury to normal tissues. One theory of sepsis holds that the down-regulation of the immune system malfunctions and allows normal tissue to be damaged by the immune responses.

T-Cell Response

The macrophage also stimulates T-cell activity by alerting the T cell to the presence of an ingested antigen through markers on the macrophage cell surface. The T cell senses these markers and promotes the formation of interleukin-2 (IL-2). From IL-2, specific interferons as well as granulocyte-macrophage colony-stimulating factor are released. IL-2 is an active cardiovascular modifier. With release of IL-2, the systemic vascular resistance (SVR) decreases and cardiac output increases.

Tumor Necrosis Factor

Tumor necrosis factor (TNF) is thought to be produced in response to a substance such as endotoxin. TNF produces platelet aggregation, increased capillary permeability, neutrophil activation, and stimulation of the release of IL-1, IL-6, and IL-8. It is thought that TNF may mediate the central response to sepsis, although the exact mechanism for this is unclear. It is also a pyrogenic (fever-producing) substance.

In addition to these responses, the body generates increased quantities of endorphins (endogenous opiate release). The opiate release produces vasodilation (a reduction in SVR) and changes in capillary permeability.

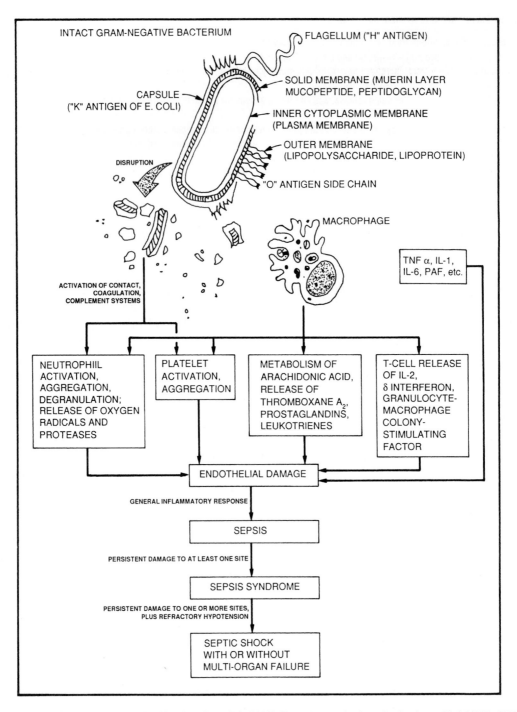

Figure 47–1. The septic cascade. (Modified from Bone, R.C. (1991). The pathogenesis of sepsis. *Ann Intern Med*, 115(6), 460.)

Effect of Immune Response on Endothelial Cells

All of the above activities are designed to help control the growth of antigens. If properly released, the immune/inflammatory response does not injure normal tissue. However, if the response is not controlled, normal cells can be injured. The most likely cells to be at risk of injury in the immune response are the endothelial cells of the blood vessels. If the endothelial layer of blood vessels is damaged, every organ is threatened, since control of vascular fluid and oxygen and nutrient supply may be disrupted.

The immune response is initially a local response. Under normal circumstances, the above responses control antigen growth. Keep in mind, however, that

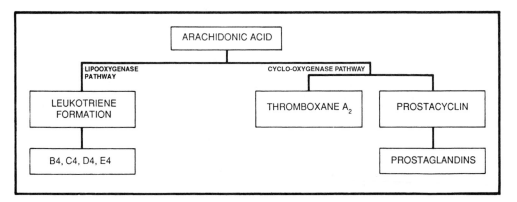

Figure 47–2. Arachidonic acid sequence.

all of these processes, which are designed to control antigen growth, can also damage endothelial cells.

If the immune response spreads beyond a local level, either because the infection is too great to be controlled or because down-regulation fails to occur, the immune response may spread systematically. It is the systemic spread that is probably the first major indicator of a septic process.

Extensions of Sepsis

As the septic process manifests, at least one organ will be affected. If the inflammatory response spreads to more than one organ, MODS is likely to occur. In addition, if the systemic spread produces hypotension (see definition in Table 47–1), septic shock is likely to occur. Survival from septic shock is dependent on many factors, with a reduced survival associated with patients who are over 65 years old, immunosuppressed or malnourished.

Clinical Presentations

The physical presentation is a combined result of the factors causing sepsis. For example, by-products of arachidonic acid produce systemic vasodilatation, pulmonary hypertension, increased pericapillary shunting, and leakage of fluid from the capillaries (producing third-spacing of fluid and edema). The actual physical symptoms produced by these events vary, making clear identification of when the septic process starts difficult.

Several substances, such as TNF, are direct pyrogenic substances. Temperature elevation is common in sepsis, although hypothermia can exist. Temperature elevation is not so much an indicator of sepsis as it is a reflection of the responses of the immune system to the initial infection and the subsequent inflammatory responses.

The patient generally is tachycardiac as a result of an increased cardiac output. The cardiac output increases secondary to a decrease in SVR. The increase in cardiac output is somewhat contradictory, since sepsis has been demonstrated to produce myocardial depressant factors. The increase in cardiac output is probably a consequence of an increased end diastolic volume, since ejection fraction is usually reduced.

The patient may have pulmonary symptoms reflective of increased extravascular lung water secondary to increased capillary permeability (such as seen in the adult respiratory distress syndrome). If pulmonary symptoms are present, they may result in refractory hypoxemia (PaO_2 unresponsive to oxygen therapy), generalized crackles heard upon auscultation, shortness of breath, and increased secretion production.

As the septic process continues, any organ system can be affected. For example, a change in level of consciousness may reflect central nervous system involvement, or acute renal or hepatic failure can result. Physical signs of these organ systems failing are the same as if the organ failed for other reasons. Specific signs of individual organ failure can be found in chapters addressing each organ. If the septic process is severe and involves multiple organs, MODS can result.

Treatment

Treatment of sepsis currently is designed to treat the infectious process, control undesirable immune responses, and provide support to any organ system in failure. No curative therapy for sepsis currently exists because of the inability to address the first two objectives. The potential to cure sepsis exists with new therapies designed to control the original infection or immune response, such as monoclonal anti-bodies. Improved treatment of sepsis is theoretically possible with agents designed to reduce the immune response, such as ibuprofen and naloxone, although research has not verified their role at this time. While great promise exists in eventually controlling sepsis, unfortunately for now most therapy for sepsis is aimed at treating symptoms rather than curing the septic patient.

Therapies that Control the Septic Process

Specific Mediators of the Immune Response Ibuprofen. Ibuprofen is a thromboxane A_2 inhibitor. Theoretically, it should improve capillary blood flow by blocking capillary vasoconstriction and increased clotting tendencies. Ibuprofen has not been as successful as originally believed in the treatment of sepsis.

Naloxone (Narcan). With the release of endogenous opiates, naloxone should improve the symptoms produced by sepsis by blocking the response of the opiates. While theoretically promising, naloxone has not been effective in clinical trials.

Prostaglandins. An area of interest in treating septic symptoms is the use of derivatives of prostacyclin. Prostacyclin derivatives (prostaglandins E_1 and E_2) will possibly reduce pulmonary hypertension, reduce coagulopathies, and improve cardiac performance. Studies have indicated conflicting responses to prostaglandins, although clinical results are promising.

Monoclonal Antibodies. The only way to actually cure sepsis is to eliminate the original infection while simultaneously controlling the septic cascade originating from the sepsis. While no drugs are available at this time, within the next few years several drugs that specifically address the infectious agent are likely to be released. Most of these agents are in the category of monoclonal antibodies. Two such antibodies (HA-1A and E5) are examples of monoclonal antibodies for sepsis. These antibodies are specifically designed to neutralize gram-negative bacteria, the most common cause of sepsis. Although the potential of these agents is exciting, their availability is currently limited.

Antibiotic Support. To treat the underlying infectious process that is causing the septic response, spe-cific antibiotic support is required. Cultures are necessary to identify the infectious antigen. If the infectious agent is unknown, broad antibiotic coverage is given. This treatment frequently employs two or three types of antibiotics, e.g., gram-positive coverage (such as a penicillin or cephalosporin), gram-negative coverage (such as an aminoglycoside like gentamicin), and broad gram-negative and gram-positive coverage (imipenem).

Supportive Therapy for Sepsis

General systemic support is usually provided by addressing specific symptoms. While none of these therapies will correct the septic process, they have the potential to improve patient comfort and "buy time" for the other therapies to help control the original problem.

Temperature Changes. Excessive temperature elevation (over 102°F or 39°C) may be treated if the patient is uncomfortable or has excessive oxygen consumption. Oxygenation should be monitored through mixed venous blood gases (SvO_2, MvO_2) in order to assess the effect of treating temperature elevations.

Fluid Administration. One of the current therapies for sepsis is the administration of potentially large amounts of fluids. Fluid boluses (e.g., normal saline) may be employed in an attempt to maintain capillary blood flow. These therapies may be used even when the cardiac output is normal or elevated, based on the assumption that capillary blood flow is altered and can be maintained only with supranormal blood flow (cardiac outputs).

In sepsis, pulmonary capillary wedge pressures may remain low despite large amounts of fluid administration. This is likely due to the leaking of fluid from the capillaries into the interstitial spaces. Fluid administration may be best controlled by monitoring the critical oxygen delivery point.

Critical Oxygen Delivery Point. In sepsis, particularly septic shock, it has been theorized that a critical oxygen delivery point (DO_2) exists. Research has not directly supported this concept yet. This point is characterized by the development of a dependence of oxygen consumption on oxygen delivery (Fig. 47–3). This dependence is a result of loss of capillary blood flow.

Under normal circumstances, cells use only the required amount of oxygen for metabolic activities.

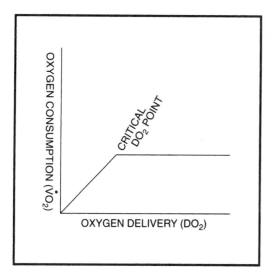

Figure 47–3. The critical oxygen delivery (DO_2) point.

If more oxygen is provided, such as with an increase in cardiac output with dobutamine, the cells will not use more oxygen just because it is available. Normally then, oxygen consumption should be independent of changes in oxygen delivery.

In pathologic states, such as hypoperfusion (from left ventricular failure or hypovolemia) and sepsis, blood flow to cells can be interrupted. The interruption can be due to many factors, such as severely reduced blood flow or microemboli. Whatever the factor, cells will be deprived of oxygen. This point is identified by noting a dependence of oxygen consumption on oxygen delivery. Oxygen consumption dependence on oxygen delivery reflects changes in capillary blood flow. For example, if oxygen delivery falls to abnormally low levels (hypovolemia, left ventricular failure) fewer cells will receive blood flow (and oxygen) with the result of a decrease in oxygen consumption. In sepsis, oxygen delivery is greater than normal secondary to elevated cardiac outputs. However, capillary blood flow is disrupted by local vasoconstriction and microemboli.

If oxygen delivery is increased and oxygen consumption simultaneously increases, it is a reflection of restoration of blood flow to capillary beds. Therapies for patients who have a dependence of oxygen consumption or oxygen delivery is focused on increasing oxygen delivery until oxygen consumption once again becomes independent. As long as VO_2 increases when DO_2 increases, it implies more cells are using oxygen again due to re-established blood flow. When VO_2

does not increase when DO_2 increases, the cellular supplies of oxygen are likely to be adequate.

Therapy to treat sepsis and septic shock, used to increase oxygen delivery until VO_2 is independent of DO_2, has been suggested to improve patient outcome. Studies are still progressing in this area.

To monitor the critical oxygen delivery point, pulmonary artery (Swan-Ganz) catheters are required, preferably fiberoptic catheters to monitor SvO_2 levels at the same time.

Inotropic Support. Normally, when the cardiac output is elevated, as in septic states, one would not expect administration of inotropes. However, some studies have suggested that inotropes (such as dobutamine) be used to help exceed the critical oxygen delivery point. The administration of dobutamine (or other inotropes) is titrated to achieve an optimal balance between oxygen delivery and consumption.

Vasopressors. If the blood pressure falls and is not maintained by fluids and inotropes, vasopressors may be used. The vasopressor generally utilized is either norepinephrine (Levophed), dopamine (Intropin), or phenylephrine (Neosynephrine).

Steroids. Steroid use has been demonstrated to be ineffective in the treatment of sepsis. Despite theoretical advantages, several large studies have indicated that steroids have no major role in the treatment of sepsis.

Nutritional Support. Aggressive support of the septic patient is important to avoid development of malnutrition. Both enteral and parenteral support may be employed to provide adequate calories. Sepsis tends to produce highly catabolic states, requiring adequate protein replacement. Carbohydrates and fats should be administered in adequate levels, with an avoidance of excessive carbohydrates in order to decrease the respiratory work generated by carbohydrate catabolism.

General Supportive Measures. Diuretics may be employed if acute renal failure develops. If acute renal failure is present, the cardiac system will be supported by inotropes rather than by fluid therapy.

If hepatic failure exists, therapies designed to reduce hepatic work will be necessary. For example, low-protein diets and lactalose may help reduce symptoms of hepatic failure.

Sepsis is a difficult clinical entity to understand and treat. Symptoms are inconsistent and not clear enough to differentiate sepsis from other conditions. While our understanding of the events that occur in sepsis is improving, treatments are limited in helping improve outcomes for the patient who develops sepsis. While great promise exists for better therapies over the next several years, current therapy is centered on supportive rather than on curative treatment.

SEPTIC SHOCK

Septic shock is a continuation of the septic process. In this situation, however, hypotension develops and is resistant to most therapies. Aggressive fluid resuscitation, inotropic support, and vasopressor application may be required. In septic shock, the likelihood of success in ameliorating these symptoms is limited. Mortality from septic shock is high because of the lack of definitive treatments for the original septic problem.

Septic shock usually presents with hypotension secondary to a markedly reduced SVR. Clinically the patient presents with a reduced blood pressure (less than 90/60), tachycardia, tachypnea, warm skin (due to peripheral vasodilatation) and reduced urine output. It was originally thought that septic shock may progress to a terminal phase in which the cardiac output falls and the SVR increases, although recent evidence suggests that this stage does not necessarily occur prior to death from septic shock.

MULTIORGAN DYSFUNCTION SYNDROME

This new category is based upon the understanding that organ dysfunction can take place without actual organ failure. It is probably a precursor to multisystem organ failure, although actual organ failure is likely a preterminal event. MODS may be an extension of the septic process. Widespread organ dysfunction occurs secondary to endothelial injury from the septic cascade. While all organs are affected, the three most common in terms of dysfunction are the lungs, liver, and kidneys. The central nervous system is also commonly affected, as evidenced by a decrease in level of consciousness or change in behavior.

Multiorgan dysfunction syndrome can be classified as either primary or secondary. Primary MODS is the result of direct injury or insult to an organ. The organ failure is the result of the injury or insult, such as acute respiratory failure secondary to aspiration of gastrointestinal contents. The subsequent failure of other organs stems from the primary organ injury. Secondary MODS is a result of organ failure from a distant or unknown site. The organs that fail have not received any direct injury or insult.

Treatment for MODS is supportive of the organs failing, in conjunction with use of any of the therapies described above. It is important to remember that support of an organ is not curative. Consequently, supporting a patient on mechanical ventilation for respiratory failure secondary to sepsis may not improve survival. Perhaps all that is gained is a prolongation of life for several days until the systemic response causes other organs to fail.

48

Toxic Emergencies

EDITORS' NOTE

Toxicology is another new area for the CCRN exam and will probably engender only one to four questions. Questions are likely to center on the immediate critical care setting, although a knowledge of emergency room care may be useful. This section provides a brief but intense review in the area of toxicology. The information provided may be more than you will need for the CCRN exam; however, since this area is new to the CCRN exam, it may be best to overprepare. The other option is not to study this area in any depth and take the risk of missing these few questions; the choice is yours. Once again, do not focus on minor details but try to understand the major concepts in assessing and managing the acute-overdose patient.

Toxic emergencies are grouped in four categories: poisonings, overdoses, drug abuse, and alcoholism. Of the more than one million poisonings that are reported in the United States each year, 54.1% involve children under the age of 6. Most are caused by household products and constitute 10% of all emergency room visits.

A poison is defined as any substance which, when introduced into an organism, acts chemically upon the tissue to produce serious injury or death. There are four routes of entry: ingestion, inhalation, injection, and surface absorption. This chapter will focus primarily on ingestion.

Poisonings most commonly involve household products such as petroleum-based agents, cleaning agents, and cosmetics. Medications are the next most frequent source, followed by toxic plants and conta-

minated food. Table 48–1 lists agents that are the leading causes of death by poisoning.

Toxic effects of ingested substances can be delayed or immediate. Delayed effects are dependent on the rate of absorption and metabolism from the gastrointestinal tract. Since most absorption occurs in the small intestine, toxins may remain in the stomach for up to several hours if a large amount of food is present. Medications or other substances that slow gastrointestinal motility may interfere. Some medications or toxins are more rapidly absorbed than others. Immediate effects of a toxin can be seen with the ingestion of corrosive substances such as strong acids or alkalis or with highly toxic and rapidly absorbed toxins such as organophosphates (pesticides) or cyanide.

ASSESSMENT

Patient assessment begins with the taking of a history. This should include the five W's: (1) who (patient age and previous medical history, including allergies and current therapies); (2) what (inquire about the suspected agent[s] or toxin[s] to which the patient has access, then obtain management information from local poison control centers); (3) when (determine the approximate time of ingestion, corroborating with others in contact with the patient); (4) where (it is important to know the surroundings or circumstances in order to prepare for complications, as in the case of an overdose that takes place in a running car in a garage or in a tub full of water); and (5) why (assess the patient's psychiatric stability to account for inaccuracies in history or the intent of the depressed patient to deliberately mislead).

573

TABLE 48–1. AGENTS RESPONSIBLE FOR THE HIGHEST POISONING MORTALITY

Category	No. of Deaths/Year	Percentage of All Exposures in Category
Antidepressants	140	0.559
Analgesics	126	0.078
Stimulants and street drugs	64	0.320
Sedatives/hypnotics	78	0.153
Cardiovascular drugs	70	0.345
Alcohols	53	0.122
Gases and fumes	46	0.225
Asthma therapies	34	0.265
Hydrocarbons	31	0.053
Chemicals	27	0.051
Cleaning substances	25	0.016
Pesticides (including rodenticides)	14	0.023

Adapted from Litovitz, T.L., Schmitz, B.F., Bailey, K.M. (1990). 1989 Annual Report of the American Association of Poison Control Centers, National Collection System. *Am J Emerg Med*, 8, 394–442.

These questions are important tools in assessment because many initial intake histories are incorrect with respect to agent, time, or amount.

Emergency Versus Hospital Admissions

Criteria for an intensive care unit admission may vary, but as a general rule, an emergency admission referral is made based on certain criteria: (1) overdose is substantial or highly toxic chemical is involved; (2) patient exhibits signs of acute poisoning; (3) patient is asymptomatic, but the suspected agent is rapidly absorbed, such as in the case of diphenoxylate (Lomotil; delayed absorption) or tricyclics; (4) patient is suicidal.

Hospital admission is usually required if any of the following criteria are met: (1) patient is symptomatic and has electrocardiographic changes after tricyclic ingestion; (2) patient is unresponsive to verbal stimulation; (3) endotracheal intubation was required; and (4) systolic blood pressure is below 80 mm Hg.

Patient Assessment

The examination should include vital signs with a temperature and respiratory rate. Cardiopulmonary stabilization and anticipation of possible deterioration should also occur during initial assessment. Cardiac monitoring, pulse oximetry, and use of a large-bore intravenous line should be considered.

Respiratory Assessment

Respiratory rate and depth can be affected by a number of agents. Check for airway patency. An increased rate and depth can be attributed to sympathomimetics such as cocaine, amphetamines, or caffeine. Noting the rate and pattern may be your first clue to an acid-base disorder. Tachypnea may result in primary alkalosis from salicylates or as a compensation for a dangerous metabolic acidosis that can occur from ethylene glycol, methanol, or other agents.

Assessment of lung sounds is an important part of serial assessments to note the presence of crackles or wheezes in patients who may have aspirated or are in congestive heart failure. Table 48–2 lists agents associated with tachypnea.

Cardiovascular Assessment

Evidence of cardiac dysrhythmias, hypotension, or hypertension requires advanced cardiac life support as well as intensive care observation. Continuous cardiac monitoring is required, since life-threatening dysrhythmias can occur rapidly with such agents as tricyclics. Certain agents require cardiac monitoring (Table 48–3); others predispose to hypotension (Table 48–4).

Neurological Assessment

A depressed level of consciousness is a major complication in the overdose patient. Describe the patient's response to stimuli, presence or absence and type of reflexes, as well as vital sign disturbance. Other causes of decreased level of consciousness (trauma, diabetes, anoxia, sepsis, and others) should be investigated. The Glasgow Coma Scale is helpful and commonly used in neurological assessment. A summary of common neurological assessments is provided in Table 48–5. When noting pupillary size and response during your examination of the patient, be aware that certain toxins can cause characteristic eye changes (Table 48–6).

TABLE 48–2. AGENTS ASSOCIATED WITH TACHYPNEA

Carbon monoxide	Drug-associated metabolic
Salicylates	acidosis
Pentachlorophenol	Drug-associated hepatic failure
Cyanide	

Tables 48–2 to 48–26 are adapted from Bryson, P.D. (1989). *Comprehensive Review of Toxicology*. Rockville, MD: 2nd ed. Aspen Publications.

TABLE 48–3. COMMON AGENTS ASSOCIATED WITH HYPERTENSION AND TACHYCARDIA

Anticholinergics	Withdrawal Syndromes	Sympathomimetics
Tricyclics	Alcohol	Amphetamines
Antihistamines	Methyldopa	Caffeine
Antipsychotics	Beta blockers	Cocaine
Mushrooms	CNS depressants	Clonidine
Plants	Sedatives/hypnotics	LSD
Over-the-counter medicines		Theophylline
		Phencyclidine
		Monoamine oxidase inhibitors

TABLE 48–5. COMPONENTS OF NEUROLOGICAL EXAMINATION OF THE PATIENT

Focal signs
Gag reflex
Mental status
    Affect
    Behavior and appearance
    Intellectual functioning
    Perceptual disorders
    Thought process and content
Ocular changes
    Nystagmus
    Pupillary size

Seizures

Seizures are best managed by treating the underlying cause (e.g., hypoxia, hypoglycemia, or hyponatremia). Diazepam, phenytoin, and phenobarbital can be effective in controlling seizures from nonspecific causes or until underlying causes can be corrected. Physostigmine may be useful in cases of life-threatening anticholinergic poisonings. Halothane or thiopental can be used for refractory seizures not responsive to the above treatments. The use of general anesthetics is reserved for cardiopulmonary stabilization when conventional methods fail. Although general anesthesia will allow for physiological stabilization, it will not stop the seizures. During generalized seizures, airway protection and maintaining oxygenation are vital. Seizures may be a clue to drug withdrawal; they may be seen after administration of naloxone to a comatose patient who is narcotic dependent, or fumazenil if benzodiazepine, tricyclic antidepressant, or benzodiazipine dependent. Table 48–7 lists factors that may precipitate seizures. Common treatments for patients with altered mental status are listed in Table 48–8.

TABLE 48–4. COMMON AGENTS ASSOCIATED WITH HYPOTENSION

Hypotension and Tachycardia	Hypotension and Bradycardia
Carbon monoxide	Beta blockers
Cyanide	Calcium channel blockers
Narcotics	Clonidine
Nitrites	Digoxin
Phenothiazines	Organophosphates
Sedatives/hypnotics	
Tricyclics	
Iron	
Disulfiram	

Gastrointestinal Assessment

Gastrointestinal disturbances are most frequently associated with the agents listed in Table 48–9. Common symptoms associated with gastrointestinal poisoning center around the loss of gastrointestinal fluids and subsequent hypovolemia. Electrolyte imbalances can occur as well. Blood loss can result from irritation of the gastric mucosa or from a Mallory–Weiss tear of the esophagus during protracted vomiting. Gastrointestinal decontamination is of vital importance in treatment of a toxic ingestion. Radiographic studies can be diagnostic with agents that may be radiopaque (Table 48–10).

Hepatic and Renal Assessment

Laboratory studies are essential to assess potential damage to hepatic and renal systems. Liver func-

TABLE 48–6. SUBSTANCES CAUSING CHARACTERISTIC EYE CHANGES

Mydriasis	Substances Causing Miosis
Anticholinergics	Cholinergics
Glutethimide (Doridan)	Clonidine (Catapres)
Meperidine (Demerol)	Insecticides
Mushrooms (anticholinergics)	Mushrooms (cholinergics)
	Narcotics
Withdrawal of abused substances	Nicotine
	Sympathomimetics
Phenothiazines	Phencyclidine (PCP)

Toxins Causing Nystagmus (Acronym: SALEM TIP)		
S	Sedatives/hypnotics, solvents	T Thiamine depletion, Tegretol (carbamazepine)
A	Alcohol	
L	Lithium	I Isopropanol
E	Ethanol, ethylene glycol	P Phenylcyclidine, phenytoin (Dilantin)
M	Methanol	

TABLE 48–7. COMMON AGENTS CAUSING SEIZURES (ACRONYM: WITH LA COPS)

W	Withdrawal
I	Isoniazid
T	Theophylline
H	Hypoglycemia agents, hypoxia
L	Lead, lithium, local anesthesia
A	Anticholinergics, amphetamines
C	Camphor, carbon monoxide, carbamazepine, cholinergics, cocaine, chlorinated hydrocarbons, cyanide
O	Organophosphates
P	Phencyclidine, phenothiazines, phenytoin, propoxyphene
S	Salicylates, strychnine, sympathomimetics

TABLE 48–9. AGENTS CAUSING GASTROINTESTINAL DISTURBANCES

Salicylates	Mushrooms
Acetaminophen	Mercury
Lithium	Arsenic
Iron	Phosphorus
Contaminated food	Colchicine

tion tests (e.g., SGPT, SGOT, and alkaline phosphatase) are useful in assessing hepatic functioning. Although jaundice is a latent indicator of liver failure, it is seen with the agents listed in Table 48–11.

When assessing the renal system, urine output, the presence of myoglobinuria or hematuria, as well as laboratories studies (blood urea nitrogen, creatinine) are significant in determining renal failure. Table 48–12 lists agents that are potentially renal toxic.

Skin and Mucous Membrane Assessment

Skin and mucous membrane assessment can provide important clues in determining the causative agent. Observe for burns or erosion of oral mucosa as well as cutaneous bullous lesions. Evidence of unaccounted-for puncture wounds and contusions may be indicative of snake bites, drug abuse, or trauma. Table 48–13 lists some of these agents.

The sense of smell can also provide diagnostic clues when one is dealing with an unknown toxin or can help confirm suspicions. Some agents that have a characteristic odor are listed in Table 48–14.

TREATMENT

The goals in treatment of a patient with a known or suspected toxic ingestion are to remove the agent(s), detoxify the patient, and prevent absorption of the suspected agent(s).

Removal of Toxic Agents

Removal can be done with the use of an emetic (ipecac) or through gastric lavage.

Emesis

Syrup of ipecac is the preferred emetic currently used in the United States. It acts locally on the gastric mucosa and centrally on the chemoreceptor trigger zone to stimulate vomiting.

The recommended dose is 30 ml for adults and 15 ml for children 1–12 years of age. This dose may be repeated once if emesis has not occurred in 20–30 min. Although chronic use of ipecac can cause neurological and cardiac complications, ipecac poses little toxicity in the recommended dose.

Ipecac should never be used if a specific oral antidote for the suspected agent is available (*N*-acetylcysteine); if the patient exhibits potential for or history of gastrointestinal bleeding (salicylates), absent gag reflex (sedatives, narcotics), or impending coma or seizures (sedatives, tricyclics); or if the patient has ingested rapidly absorbed or caustic agents (tricyclics, alkalis, acids). Complications of

TABLE 48–8. SUGGESTED THERAPY FOR PATIENTS WITH ALTERED MENTAL STATUS (ACRONYM: DONT)

	Drug	Dosage
D	Dextrose	Adult: 50 ml of $D_{50}W$ Child: 1 ml/kg of same solution diluted 1:1
O	Oxygen	As necessary
N	Naloxone	2 mg IV
T	Thiamine	50 to 100 mg IM or IV

TABLE 48–10. AGENTS THAT MAY BE RADIOPAQUE (ACRONYM: BET A CHIP)

B	Barium
E	Enteric-coated tablets
T	Tricyclic antidepressants
A	Antihistamines
C	Chloral hydrate, cocaine, condoms, calcium
H	Heavy metals
I	Iodides
P	Phenothiazines, potassium

TABLE 48–11. COMMON AGENTS CAUSING HEPATOTOXICITY

Acetaminophen
Arsenic
Carbon tetrachloride
Iron
Toluene (solvent in airplane glue)

TABLE 48–13. AGENTS CAUSING BULLOUS LESIONS

Caustics	Environmental Agents	Sedative/Hypnotic Agents
Acids	Carbon monoxide	Barbiturates
Alkalis	Snake venom	Diphenoxylate (Lomotil)
	Insect venom	Glutethimide (Doriden)
		Meprobamate (Equanil, Equagesic*)
		Methaqualone (Quaalude)

*Equagesic is not a pure meprobamate; it is a compound of meprobamate and aspirin.

ipecac include Mallory–Weiss tear of the esophagus, drowsiness, electrolyte imbalance from protracted vomiting, delay in giving activated charcoal or a specific oral antidote, diarrhea, and aspiration. Table 48–15 lists agents for which induced emesis or gastric lavage is not advised. There are certain hydrocarbons that are exceptions for induced emesis or gastric lavage (Table 48–16). Because of the high toxicity of these substances, the risk of aspiration is justified.

Gastric Lavage

Gastric lavage is another method for removal of toxins.

Equipment needed consists of an orogastric tube, 26–28 Fr for children or 32–40 Fr for adults with large distal and lateral holes. Large-bore orogastric tubes allow pill fragments to be retrieved and decrease the chance of tube occlusion from pills or food particles. Various kits are available for the instillation and retrieval of lavage fluid. In adults, warm tap water can be used because it does not alter serum electrolytes or osmolality. In children, warm saline is recommended. Warm lavage fluid is preferred because it decreases gastric peristalsis and increases the rate of pill dissolution, allowing the stomach contents to pass more easily through the tube. Lavage is performed until the fluid is clear, which usually requires 5–20 L of fluid.

The technique for performing lavage requires that the patient be placed in the Trendelenburg, left lateral decubitus position with knees flexed. This position allows for optimum relaxation of the abdominal wall and can reduce the risk of aspiration should vomiting occur. A local anesthetic may be used in the oropharynx to diminish the gag reflex prior to passage of the lavage tube. Warming the lavage tube and treating it with a water-soluble lubricant can ease its passage. As the tube is gently

advanced, the patient is instructed to swallow. Coughing, inability to speak, cyanosis, or respiratory distress can indicate unintentional endotracheal intubation. Proper placement should be confirmed prior to instillation of the lavage fluid.

Auscultation of the stomach while air is instilled into the passed tube plus retrieval of stomach contents ensures proper localization of the tube. For patients whose gag reflex is absent, exhibit central nervous system depression, or are comatose, airway protection is required prior to gastric lavage. For those patients, endotracheal intubation is usually required. After passage of the tube and confirmation of its placement, the stomach is initially aspirated of contents.

TABLE 48–12. COMMON AGENTS ASSOCIATED WITH RENAL TOXICITY

Amanita phalloides (mushrooms)
Antibiotics
Ethylene glycol

TABLE 48–14. AGENTS WITH CHARACTERISTIC ODORS

Odor	Agent
Acetone	Ethyl alcohol
	Isopropyl alcohol
	Lacquer
Bitter almond	Amygdalin
	Apricot pits
	Cyanide
	Laetrile
Burned rope	Marijuana
Carrot	Cicutoxin
Garlic	Arsenic
	Arsine gas
	Organophosphates
	Selenium
	Thallium
	Dimethyl sulfoxide
Mothballs	Naphthalene
	Paradichlorobenzene
Peanuts	Rodenticides
Pear	Chloral hydrate
	Paraldehyde
Pungent aromatic	Ethchlorvynol
Rotten egg	Hydrogen sulfide
	Mercaptans
	Sewer gas
Shoe polish	Nitrobenzene
Violets	Turpentine
Wintergreen	Methyl salicylate

TABLE 48–15. SUBSTANCES FOR WHICH INDUCED EMESIS OR GASTRIC LAVAGE IS CONTRAINDICATED

Caustic Agents	Petroleum Distillates
Acids, alkalis, ammonia, coffee pot cleaners, drain cleaners, automatic dishwasher detergent, hair bleaches, lye, metal cleaners, mildew removers, oven cleaners, rust removers wart removers, toilet bowl cleaners	Furniture polish, gasoline, kerosene, linseed oil, lighter fluid, mineral spirits, naphtha, oils, paint and lacquer thinners, petroleum solvents, pine oil cleaners, turpentine, wood stains

Larger aliquots (300–500 ml) of lavage fluid for adults tend to open the rugae of the stomach, thus exposing pill fragments or toxins that may be in the rugal folds. Abdominal massage (during gastric lavage) at the left upper quadrant is recommended when concretions or bezoars are possible. A concretion or bezoar occurs when numerous pills clump together into a solid mass in the stomach (Table 48–17).

Since gastric lavage is an invasive procedure, it carries certain risks and complications. The risk versus benefit should be determined before this procedure is performed. Complications of gastric lavage are listed in Table 48–18.

Cathartics

Cathartics are used to decrease the transit time for the nonabsorbed toxin, thereby minimizing absorption in the bowel. Osmotic cathartics are classified as saline or saccharide. They include sorbitol, magnesium sulfate/citrate, sodium sulfate, disodium phosphate, and are preferred to the stimulant types such as cascara, castor oil, senna, or bisacodyl. Although the use of cathartics is based primarily on empirical and anecdotal evidence, most toxicologists agree with their use as a means of decreasing gastrointestinal transit time for toxins. Contraindications for cathartics are noted in Table 48–19.

TABLE 48–16. EXCEPTIONS: HYDROCARBONS THAT NEED TO BE EVACUATED FROM THE BOWEL (ACRONYM: CHAMP)

C	Camphor-based hydrocarbons
H	Halogenated hydrocarbons
A	Aromatics
M	Heavy metals
P	Pesticides

TABLE 48–17. AGENTS CAUSING CONCRETIONS (ACRONYM: BIG MESS)

B	Barbiturates
I	Iron
G	Glutethimide
M	Meprobamate
E	Extended-release theophylline
SS	Salicylates

Detoxification and Prevention of Absorption

Activated Charcoal

Activated charcoal is made from the distillation of various types of organic matter, which is then activated by heating to temperatures in excess of 600°C in the absence of air. This cleans and expands the charcoal, increasing its surface area and resulting in enhanced absorption ability. Activated charcoal appears as an inert, fine black powder. It is tasteless and odorless, and has a gritty consistency. It is available as a powder, as an aqueous slurry, or in a suspension of 20% activated charcoal in 70% sorbitol. It can be given either orally or through a lavage or nasogastric tube. The charcoal slurry tends to be thick and gritty and is not very palatable when administered orally. It can be difficult to pass through a small-bore nasogastric tube because of its thick consistency. Therefore, whenever lavage is required, it is advantageous to instill the activated charcoal prior to removal of the lavage tube.

Charcoal dosing should provide a 10:1 ratio of charcoal to toxin to provide optimal binding. Because of the inaccuracies of ingested doses of toxins, an arbitrary dose of 1–2 g/kg of body weight is recommended. Activated charcoal adsorbs not only toxins but other therapeutic drugs as well.

Activated charcoal is thought to be a safe, inert, nontoxic material. No harmful effects have been shown from exposure to skin; however, aspiration can be harmful. Although activated charcoal is use-

TABLE 48–18. COMPLICATIONS OF LAVAGE

Aspiration

Respiratory distress

Gastric erosion

Epistaxis

Laryngospasm

Esophageal tear

Mediastinitis

Bolusing of toxins from the stomach into the small bowel

TABLE 48–19. CONTRAINDICATIONS FOR USE OF CATHARTICS

Adynamic ileus

Current diarrhea

Intestinal obstruction

No saline cathartics in patient with history of congestive heart failure or salt restrictions

No magnesium sulfate in patient with potential for renal failure

No oil-based cathartics (hazardous if aspirated)

Caution in the very young and very old

In patient with severe fluid and electrolyte imbalance

ful in adsorbing many toxins, there are agents that it does not appear to adsorb (Table 48–20).

Enhanced Elimination

Enhanced elimination of certain drugs may be assisted by making use of certain pharmacokinetic parameters that affect drug excretion. These include forced diuresis (with or without ion trapping), multiple-dose charcoal, dialysis, hemoperfusion, and plasmapheresis.

Forced Diuresis

This method involves enhanced elimination of the agent through urinary excretion. Normally, excretion takes place through glomerular filtration, active tubular secretion, and tubular reabsorption. This method deals with inhibiting tubular reabsorption only by diluting the concentration gradient between the blood and the urine. This will lessen the time of the agent's exposure to the reabsorptive sites in the distal tubules. Sodium must be carefully monitored and replaced when dealing with Lithium toxicity.

Ion-Trapping Methods

Ion-trapping methods cause a solution to become more alkaline or acidic, so that the substance is trapped in the kidney and excretion is enhanced. Weak acids are more ionized in an alkaline solution, and weak bases are more ionized in an acidic solu-

TABLE 48–21. DRUGS RESPONSIVE TO ENHANCED DIURESIS OR ION TRAPPING

Alkaline Diuresis	Acid Diuresis
Phenobarbital	Phencyclidine
Salicylates	Amphetamines
Primidone	

tion. If a difference in pH occurs across a membrane, ion trapping will occur. The toxin will collect in the compartment where ionization is greater because the nonionized form crosses the lipid–cell membrane interface more readily than the ionized form does (Table 48–21).

Alkaline diuresis can be achieved by the administration of sodium bicarbonate in intravenous fluids. Administer fluid amounts to keep urine flow to 3–6 ml/kg/h. Add two to three ampules of sodium bicarbonate to each liter of D_5W. Use enough bicarbonate to achieve a urinary pH of 7.5 or greater. Careful observation of electrolytes is required during diuresis. This is useful for agents that cause metabolic acidosis (Table 48–22).

The risks of acid diuresis currently outweigh the possible benefits. The compounds used to achieve acidification also have the potential to cause acute tubular necrosis secondary to rhabdomyolysis.

TABLE 48–22. AGENTS THAT CAUSE METABOLIC ACIDOSIS (ACRONYM: A MUD PILE CAT)

A	Alcohol
M	Methyl alcohol
U	Uremia
D	Diabetic ketoacidosis
P	Paraldehyde
I	Iron, isoniazid
L	Lactic acidosis
E	Ethylene glycol
C	Carbon monoxide, cyanide
A	Aspirin
T	Toluene

TABLE 48–20. AGENTS NOT ADSORBED BY ACTIVATED CHARCOAL

Alkali	N-Methyl carbamate	Sorbitol
Boric acid		Magnesium sulfate
DDT		
Iron salts	Sodium metasilicate	Tolbutamide
Mineral acids	N-Acetylcysteine (?)	Hydrocarbons
Lithium		
Ethanol		

TABLE 48–23. DRUGS RESPONSIVE TO MULTIPLE-DOSE CHARCOAL

Carbamazepine (Tegretol)	Meprobamate
Cyclic antidepressants	Nadolol (Corgard)
Dapsone	Phenobarbital
Digitoxin	Phenylbutazone
Aspirin	
Theophylline	

TABLE 48–24. IMMEDIATE INDICATIONS FOR HEMODIALYSIS REGARDLESS OF CLINICAL CONDITION

Amanita phalloides (mushroom) ingestion

Ethylene glycol

Methanol

Heavy metals in soluble compounds

TABLE 48–25. DRUG CRITERIA FOR DIALYSIS

Low molecular weight

Water solubility

Small volume of distribution

Small degree of protein binding

Dialyzable active metabolites

TABLE 48–26. AGENTS RESPONSIVE TO DIALYSIS

Alcohols	Calcium	Meprobamate	Ammonia
Potassium	Methanol	Salicylates	Ethylene glycol
Barbiturates	Antibiotics		Quinidine
Lithium			

Multidose Charcoal

Multiple doses of activated charcoal appear to be effective in enhancing elimination of certain drugs that undergo enterohepatic or enterogastric circulation. The usual recommended dose for adults is 20–100 g every 2–8 hr until serum drug levels have been reduced to a subtoxic range (5–10 g every 4–8 hr is recommended for children). To avoid repeated doses of a cathartic, activated charcoal without the added cathartic is essential for this method. Also,

remember that charcoal will enhance the elimination of therapeutic drugs such as digoxin, theophylline, and carbamazepine (Table 48–23). Careful evaluation of these drug levels is warranted, and the drugs may need to be replaced during this procedure.

Extracorporeal Methods of Elimination Hemodialysis

Hemodialysis can be useful in further clearance of certain substances from the body. It is usually reserved for the patient who has not responded to more conservative and conventional methods.

Patient criteria to determine the need for hemodialysis include the following: stage 3 or 4 coma, hypotension not corrected by adjusting circulating volume, impending renal or hepatic failure, severe acid-base disturbance not responding to therapy, marked hyper- or hypothermia, and severe electrolyte imbalance not responsive to therapy. Certain agents are highly toxic, and immediate hemodialysis is needed even if the patient appears stable (Table 48–24).

Various pharmacological properties of the drug(s) or toxin(s) to be eliminated enhance their ability to be dialyzed from the body. These factors are listed in Table 48–25.

Because of their pharmacological properties, the drugs listed in Table 48–26 are responsive to hemodialysis. Keep in mind that although these agents can be dialyzed, hemodialysis and other extracorporeal measures should be used only when conventional and more conservative measures fail. Dialysis is always indicated for serious methanol and ethylene glycol poisoning even if the patient seems fine.

TABLE 48–27. AGENTS AND ANTIDOTES

Drug/Toxin	Antidote/Dose	Comment
Acetaminophen	*N*-Acetylcysteine 140 mg/kg PO (loading) 70 mg/kg PO every 4 hr × 17 doses (maintenance)	No ipecac; charcoal may be given early after ingestion. Most effective within 12 hr.
Anticholinergics	Physostigmine Adult: 0.5–5.0 mg (IV slowly) Child: 0.5 mg or 0.02 mg/kg IV slowly (1–5 mg IV) (absolute last resort)	Observe for seizures or bradycardia.
Beta-adrenergic blockers	Glucagon: 1–5 mg IV	
Benzodiazepines (Valium, Dalmane, Tranxene)	Flumazenil (Romazicon) Initial: 0.2 mg IV over 15 sec Follow-up: 0.2 mg every 60 sec to 3 mg in 1 hr/1 mg in 5 min	Observe for seizures.
Bromide	Sodium chloride	
Carbamate insecticides	Atropine Adult: up to 5 mg IV every 15 min Child: 0.05 mg/kg IV	Physiological; blocks acetylcholine

continued

TABLE 48–27. *(Continued)*

Drug/Toxin	Antidote/Dose	Comment
Carbon monoxide	Oxygen: 100% reduced half-life of carbon monoxide to 1.5 hr	Hyperbaric chamber at 3 atm reduces half-life to 23 min.
Cardiac glycosides	Fragment, antigen-binding antibody therapy, Digibind	Use in severe dysrhythmias, digitoxicity with K$^+$ > 5–6.0 mEq/L. Toxic dose ingestion: Adult: 10 mg Child: 4 mg
Chronic mercury, copper	Penicillamine: 1–4 g	Cuprimine is readily absorbed orally.
Cyanide	Amyl nitrite (pearls) every 2 min	Methemoglobin plus cyanide
	Sodium nitrite Adult: 300 mg IV Child: 10 mg/kg	Causes hypotension. Dose assumes normal Hg.
	Sodium thiosulfate Adult: 12.5 g IV slowly Child: 1.5 mL/kg	Forms harmless sodium thiocyanate.
Ethylene glycol, methanol	Ethyl alcohol (in conjunction with dialysis) 1 ml/kg of 100% ethanol in glucose (loading) 0.1 ml/kg/per hr diluted to maintain level at 100 mg%	Competes for alcohol dehydrogenase; prevents formation of formic acid and oxalates.
Gyromitra mushrooms	Pyridoxine: 25 mg/kg IV slowly	
Heavy metals Lead Mercury Gold Arsenic	Succimer (DMSA) IV BAL (British antilewisite): 5 mg/kg IM ASAP	Effective chelating agents; form stable, nontoxic, excretable cyclic compounds.
Iron	Deferoxamine (Desferal) 40–90 mg/kg IV (initial) not to exceed 1 g 10–15 mg/kg/per hr	Deferoxamine mesylate forms excretable ferrioxamine complex. IV is preferred; secondary possibility of hypovolemia and hypotension.
Isoniazid	Pyridoxine: gram for gram with initial dose; if unknown, 5 g IV	
Narcotics/opiates, including diphenoxylate (Lomotil) and propoxyphene (Darvon)	Naloxone: 0.01 mg/kg IV	Frequent repeated doses may be needed; may precipitate acute withdrawal.
Nitrites	Methylene blue: 1–2 mg of 1% solution IV over 5 min	Exchange transfusion may be needed; blocks acetylcholine.
Organophosphates	Atropine* Adult: up to 5 mg IV every 15 min Child: 0.05 mg/kg IV Pralidoxime (2-PAM): Initial dose: Adult: 1 g IV Child: 25–50 mg/kg IV	Breaks alkyl phosphate-cholinesterase bond
Tricyclic antidepressants	Sodium bicarbonate*	Protein binding of drug occurs at alkalotic pH.
Venoms Black widow Pit vipers	Antivenom One vial in 50 ml saline over 30 min May require large dose due to lower neutralizing antibody titers in antivenom	Indicated for patients <12 or >65 years old or with serious medical history For systemic or severe local envenomations Observe for serum sickness, since antivenoms are of equine origin.†
Warfarin (Coumadin)	Vitamin K Adult: 5–25 mg IM or IV Child: 1–5 mg IM	Promotes hepatic biosynthesis of prothrombin

*Both may need to be given for several days.
†Will not appear in ICU.

Hemoperfusion

Hemoperfusion is another method of clearing toxins from the body by passing blood through charcoal columns or resins. Plasma extraction ratios are significantly higher for hemoperfusion than for hemodialysis. The advantage of hemoperfusion is that it is not as restricted by physical drug characteristics, such as molecular weight, water solubility, and protein binding, that limit hemodialysis.

The use of hemoperfusion is controversial but is indicated for a massive ingestion when the extracellular distribution is significant and the plasma level of the toxin is at its maximum. Hemoperfusion is generally successful with the same agents that respond to hemodialysis and preferred for theophylline toxicity.

Antidotes

Certain drugs and toxins have specific antidotes that counteract their harmful effects. It is best to use an antidote if available, although reversal of certain drugs can precipitate withdrawal symptoms and seizures. Table 48–27 provides a list of drugs and antidotes as well as specific precautions needed.

49

Airway Obstruction

EDITORS' NOTE

The CCRN exam may include one to four questions on airway obstruction. Airway obstruction might also be addressed in the context of other clinical conditions or situations, such as postextubation. This brief chapter should be adequate to prepare you for the questions on the CCRN exam addressing airway obstruction.

UPPER AIRWAY OBSTRUCTION

Upper airway obstruction is one of the highest-priority emergencies a critical care clinician can encounter. The prompt recognition and treatment of a partially or fully obstructed airway can literally mean the difference between life and death for the patient. Multiple conditions may be responsible for acute upper airway (superior to the primary carina) compromise, all of which require prompt diagnosis followed by definitive therapy to re-establish air flow.

Identifying Characteristics

Upper airway obstruction may present either as an obvious life-threatening emergency or in a more subtle fashion, depending on the degree of occlusion as well as its cause. The classic finding in a patient with a partial airway obstruction at or above the larynx is a high-pitched crowing or harsh whistle with inspiration termed stridor. In contrast, an intrathoracic obstruction in the trachea is signaled by expiratory stridor due to the natural narrowing of the airway with expiration. Clinically, the obstructed patient may also present with dyspnea, clutching the throat

("choking sign"), facial swelling, neck vein prominence, pallor or cyanosis, coughing, wheezing, sore throat, altered voice or phonation, dysphagia (difficulty swallowing secretions, which can lead to drooling), or accessory muscle contraction. Foreign-body aspiration is frequently accompanied by paroxysmal coughing. With complete obstruction the patient is unable to breathe, cough, or speak and rapidly degenerates into a state of unconsciousness.

Etiology

The underlying causes of upper airway obstruction are varied. As one might expect, foreign-body aspiration is the leading cause of upper airway obstruction. Infectious processes such as epiglottitis, retropharyngeal abscess, laryngeal diphtheria, Ludwig's angina (a progressive submaxillary cellulitis that involves the neck and floor of the mouth, frequently following dental disease), tonsillitis, pharyngitis, mononucleosis, and otitis can all cause asphyxiation by obstruction. More commonly, the infection may actually erode a blood vessel, causing massive hemorrhage, or a purulent pocket may rupture. Noninfectious laryngeal edema may result from trauma, inhalation of noxious gases, burns, or anaphylactic shock (caused by inhalants, bee stings, drugs, contrast media, blood products), or follow removal of an endotracheal tube. Neck surgery, trauma, diagnostic procedures (carotid angiography), or erosion of a blood vessel by the invasion of cancerous or infectious cells may result in retropharyngeal hemorrhage.

Treatment

In cases of severe upper airway obstruction a mixture of helium and oxygen may be administered to provide temporary support pending a definitive diagnosis and treatment plan. Severe or complete obstruction requires immediate airway control. Following institution of the head tilt and jaw thrust maneuver to minimize the soft tissue contribution to obstruction, the larynx and oropharynx must be inspected and any obstructive material (blood, vomitus, foreign matter) removed via suctioning. If adequate ventilation is not then achieved with a bag-valve-mask device driven by 100% oxygen, an airway must be emergently established with the placement of an endotracheal tube or by a tracheostomy or cricothyrotomy.

NEAR-DROWNING

An estimated 9000 lives are lost from drowning each year. Additionally, there are 75,000 near-drowning victims annually. Near-drowning is defined as a submersion injury after which the patient survives for at least 24 hr. Drowning, on the other hand, is defined as a submersion injury that causes death within 24 hr.

Identifying Characteristics

Although each near-drowning victim presents somewhat differently depending on the previous health state, quantity and type (fresh, salt, chlorinated, polluted) of water aspirated, length of time submersed, and the temperature of the water, there is a predictable sequence of events that occurs during the submersion injury. Initially, the victim begins to cough and gasp as water enters the mouth and nose, which results in a variable amount of water being swallowed. Simultaneously, as water is aspirated into the larynx, laryngospasm develops, which helps to protect the airway from further aspiration of water. Subsequently, the laryngospasm causes asphyxia, which results in the victim losing consciousness. Hypoxemia then leads to the development of metabolic acidosis. If the victim dies during the laryngospasm phase, it may be called a "dry" drowning, or suffocation, because a large quantity of water was not aspirated to this point. However, it is estimated that only 10–15% of drowning cases are "dry" drownings. For the other 85–90% of victims who aspirate at some point during the submersion injury, the loss of consciousness is thought to cause relaxation of the laryngeal muscles, which allows aspiration of water. However, it is also thought that the hypercarbic or hypoxic drives stimulate inhalation or aspiration of water, thus resulting in a "wet" drowning.

Earlier, it was believed that the inhalation of salt water, with its increased concentration of electrolytes and thus the ability to draw fluid into the lungs, resulted in an electrolyte imbalance and pulmonary edema. Fresh water, on the other hand, was thought to produce hemodilution and hemolysis from the hypotonic fluids. It is now believed that most near-drowning victims do not aspirate sufficient quantities of water to produce these changes. It is thought that it is the amount of aspirated water and not the type of water that results in pulmonary changes during the submersion injury. The aspiration of water decreases pulmonary compliance. Whether surfactant is washed out of the alveoli with fresh-water aspiration or is denatured by salt water entering the alveoli, an intrapulmonary shunt develops and hypoxia occurs. Therefore, the focus of attention with submersion injuries should be the management of hypoxia.

The other inherent problem with submersion injuries is hypothermia. A danger of hypothermia is the development of lethal cardiac dysrhythmias that may result in cardiac arrest. However, hypothermia may be beneficial if it occurs before the development of hypoxia. It is thought to be neuroprotective as evidenced by those who have survived ice-water submersions for longer than thirty minutes, especially children.

Treatment

Patient care for the near-drowning victim includes early endotracheal intubation with the administration of 100% oxygen at 5–10 cm PEEP (positive end expiratory pressure). Early intubation may also protect the airway from aspiration of gastric contents, which is likely with submersion injuries. In cold-water submersion injuries cardiac dysrhythmias should be anticipated and aggressively managed. Standard resuscitation protocols should be used in the management of cardiac arrest. Because the metabolic acidosis may be severe, the administration of sodium bicarbonate may be warranted. After resuscitation, monitoring for the development of bronchospasm is necessary and the treatment of bronchospasm, if it develops, must be aggressive. Pulmonary artery catheterization and monitoring may be necessary in management of pulmonary edema.

Burns are among the most devastating injuries that a nurse can encounter. Burns can affect multiple organ systems, beyond what appears to be the area involved. Unfortunately, burns are relatively common and are the third leading cause of accidental death in adults.

Burns can be the result of thermal, chemical, electrical, or inhalation injury. According to the American Burn Association, more than 2.5 million people in the United States experience thermal injury each year. Approximately 100,000 of those are hospitalized, and 12,000 will die. Burn mortality has improved: a 70% body surface area (BSA) burn today has the same 50% mortality that a 30% BSA burn had in 1970. The best rate of survival exists for persons between the ages of 5 and 34. The very young and very old have the worst prognosis. The median age for a burn victim is 22. Because of the loss of body image and self-esteem, burns can leave both physical and emotional scars that prevent a person from returning to or becoming a productive member of society. Burns typically require a prolonged rehabilitation phase. The medical and societal costs of burns are truly great.

The common variable in all burn injuries is skin damage. The skin is one of our largest organ systems. It is composed of two layers, the epidermis and dermis. The epidermis is the outer, thinner layer. The dermis is a deeper, thicker layer that contains the hair follicles, sweat glands, sebaceous glands, and sensory fibers. (Fig. 50–1)

The skin is our first defense against infection and injury. It protects us from the environment, prevents loss of body fluids, regulates body temperature, and provides sensory contact with the environment through pain, touch, pressure, and temperature.

Burns are classified by the extent of BSA affected and the depth of skin damage. The extent of a burn is a product of the temperature generated by the heat source and the exposure time. The center of the burn wound has the most contact with the heat source. The cells have been coagulated and are necrotic. This area is referred to as the zone of coagulation. Lying next to the zone of coagulation is the zone of stasis. This area has cells that have been injured but are not necrotic. If proper resuscitation occurs, these cells will survive; however, they will usually become necrotic within 24–48 hr and extend the severity of the burn. The outermost area of the burn wound is the zone of hyperemia. These cells have suffered the least injury and usually recover in 7–10 days. The rule of nines formula is used to estimate the BSA involved (Fig. 50–2), but this method gives only a gross estimate. More exact BSA involvement can be calculated with the use of more detailed charts (e.g., Lund and Browder); however, the charts must be available for use and are not easily commit-

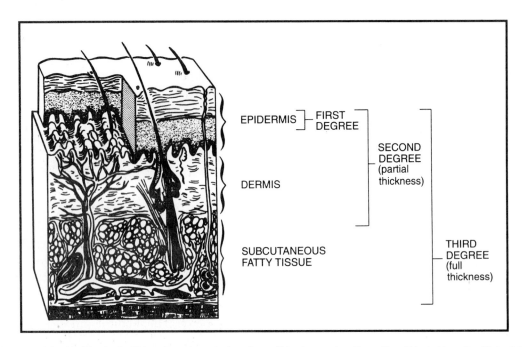

Figure 50–1. Anatomy of the skin. The depth of injury determines whether a burn will heal or require skin grafting. (Adapted from Rue III, L., & Cioffi, W. (1991). Resuscitation of thermally injured patients. *Crit Care Clin North Am, 3*(2), 183.)

ted to memory. BSA can also be estimated with the use of the victim's palm, which is equal to 1% of the BSA. This is a useful method with scattered or irregular patterns of burns. The extent of BSA involved is used to calculate the patient's fluid replacement needs.

CLASSIFICATION

Depth of the burn will determine to what degree or whether any skin grafting is needed. Variable destruction of skin can occur. Formerly burns were classified as first, second, or third degree. More recently, burns have been subdivided into partial- and full-thickness wounds (Table 50–1 and Fig. 50–1). The partial-thickness wounds are further divided into superficial and deep wounds. First-degree burns damage the epidermis or superficial layer of the skin. The wounds appear pink, dry (no blistering), and slightly edematous and are painful. Clinically, first-degree burns are of little importance and are not typically considered in fluid replacement.

Second-degree or partial-thickness burns destroy the epidermis and varying degrees of the dermis. The wounds appear blistered and are painful, and blanching will be detected.

Third-degree or full-thickness burns destroy both the epidermis and dermal layers of the skin. These burns may extend into the subcutaneous tis-

sue to muscle and may even reach bone. The wounds appear dry, hard, and leathery, and no blanching is detected as a result of destruction of the capillary bed. A common misconception is that the wound is painless since the nerve endings are destroyed. However, the patients may experience deep somatic pain from ischemia or inflammation. Wound edges may also be hypersensitive in making the transition from third-degree to less severely burned areas.

INITIAL MANAGEMENT

The initial management of a burn victim is to stop the burning process. This is usually accomplished before the patient receives hospital care, but, depending on the type of burn, irrigation may still be necessary once the patient reaches the hospital. All clothing must be removed, including jewelry, which can retain heat and have a tourniquet-like effect on limbs and cause neurovascular compromise. As with all trauma patients, attention must then be given to airway management, assistance with breathing, and support of circulation as needed. The possibility of other injuries must also be assessed, with management as appropriate. Since major burn victims are often intubated at the scene or in the emergency room, a history must be obtained from either witnesses, rescue personnel and/or family members.

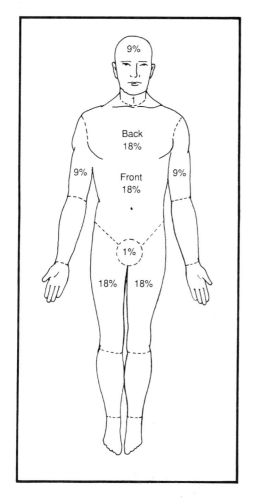

Figure 50–2. The rule of nines. (From Kravitz, M. (1988). Thermal injuries. In *Trauma Nursing*, Ed. Cardona, V.; Hurn, P.; Mason, P.; et al. Philadelphia: W.B. Saunders, 709.)

BURN SHOCK

Burn shock has both a cellular and a hypovolemic component. Burns of less than 20% BSA have primarily a local response, whereas major burns of greater than 20–25% BSA have a systemic response. The greater the percentage of burn, the greater the systemic response.

Initially, burn patients experience a rise in capillary hydrostatic pressure and an increase in capillary permeability. Rapid fluid shifts occur, with fluid moving from the intravascular space to the interstitium, causing edema formation within the wound and a decrease in circulating blood volume. The cardiac output can decrease as much as 50% in the first hour if adequate resuscitation is not initiated. Catecholamine release may further compromise cardiac output by causing the heart to pump against increased systemic vascular resistance. The greatest fluid shifts occur during the first 6–8 hr postburn. Adequate and rapid fluid replacement is required to prevent hypovolemic shock. As a result of decreased cardiac output, the systemic vascular resistance increases in an attempt to preserve some organ perfusion and protect the blood pressure. This increase in systemic vascular resistance, however, further depresses cardiac output. Myocardial depressant factors may also play a role in lowering cardiac output, but attempts to isolate them have been inconclusive.

Fluid requirements are based on the percentage of BSA burned. The clinician must keep in mind that

TABLE 50–1. CLASSIFICATION OF BURN DEPTH

Degree of Burn	Depth of Tissue Penetration	Characteristics
First-degree	Partial-thickness	Injury to the superficial epidermis, usually caused by over-exposure to sunlight or brief heat flashes. Classically, can be described as a sunburn. Wounds are red and dry, blanch, and are painful to touch, although superficial blisters may be present. Wounds will heal within 7 days, shedding the dead skin layers, and will leave no residual scar.
Second-degree	Superficial partial-thickness	Injury is to the epidermis and upper layers of the dermis. Wounds characteristically appear red, wet, or blistered, blanchable, and extremely painful. Will heal within 3 weeks from epidermal regeneration from remaining remnants found in the tracts of hair follicles and sweat and sebaceous glands. Will not scar unless unduly manipulated or infected.
	Deep partial-thickness	Injury is through the epidermis and may affect isolated areas of the deep dermal strata from which cells arise. This wound may appear red and wet or white and dry, depending on the extent of deep dermal damage. It heals without grafting but requires > 3 weeks and closes with suboptimal cosmesis. Excision and split-thickness skin grafting are recommended for optimal and timely wound closure.
Third-degree	Full-thickness	Injury has destroyed both the epidermis and the dermis. The wound appears white, will not blanch, and is anesthetic. Tough, nonelastic and tenacious coagulated protein (eschar) tissue may be present on the surface. This wound will not heal without surgical intervention, unless it is extremely small and healing can occur through contracture. Excision of the nonviable tissue with split-thickness skin grafting is necessary to close the wound optimally and to minimize contracture.

(From Desai, M., & Herdon, D. (1991). Burns. In *Current Therapy of Trauma*. Ed. Trunkey, D., & Lewis F. St. Louis: B.C. Decker, 317.)

this is only an estimate, and the patient's response to therapy must be closely monitored to assist with fluid replacement and adjust fluid rates accordingly. Many formulas exist to calculate fluid replacement (Table 50–2). The most frequently used calculation is the Parkland formula, which is 4 ml/kg per % BSA of lactated Ringer's solution. Most agree that colloids are not to be used during the first 24 hr since the degree of capillary leakage is so severe that the large colloid molecules will also pass through the capillaries. Fifty percent of the calculated fluid requirement is given in the first 8 hr postburn; the remaining 50% is given over the last 16 hr. It may be necessary for the critical care nurse to catch up on fluid requirements that have not been adequately met early in the patient's care. Remember that fluid replacement is based on the first 24 hr after injury, not after hospital admission. The nurse must inquire about prior fluid administration and time of injury as well as obtain an accurate weight. Clinical indicators of adequate fluid resuscitation are maintenance of a stable blood pressure with a urine output of 0.5–1.0 ml/kg/h. Invasive hemodynamic monitoring is usually required only in high-risk patients who have underlying cardiopulmonary disorders or those who are not responding as predicted. Patients who may require higher than expected fluid requirements are those with inhalation injury, underlying dehydration preburn, or electrical burns. The most common reason for low urine

output and low blood pressure is inadequate fluid resuscitation. However, if invasive hemodynamic monitoring indicates that fluid volume is adequate, inotropic agents may be necessary. Because of the large amount of catecholamine released postburn, larger than normal doses of inotropic agents may be necessary since some down-regulation of the receptors may occur.

Capillary integrity returns to normal by 24–36 hr postburn, resulting in decreased loss of fluid and protein into the wounds. If fluid resuscitation has been adequate, cardiac output will return to normal and then proceed to a hyperdynamic level at which cardiac output is above normal. The goal of fluid therapy changes as compared with the first 24 hr and is now meant to maintain organ perfusion. Inadequate fluid resuscitation can lead to acute tubular necrosis, stress ulcers, and conversion of partial-thickness wounds to full-thickness wounds. Colloids may now be given to help replace the plasma volume deficit. Approximately 10% of red blood cell mass is decreased after thermal injury. Most is lost as a result of direct destruction by heat but other reasons may include hemorrhage, wound stasis, and increased fragility of the red blood cells. Because of the large sodium load given in the first 24 hr, patients usually have a whole-body excess of sodium. Fluid management is aimed at helping the patient excrete the large sodium and water load obtained during initial resuscitation. Rapid sodium

TABLE 50–2. FORMULAS FOR FLUID REPLACEMENT/RESUSCITATION

	FIRST 24 HR			SECOND 24 HR		
	Electrolyte	Colloid	Glucose in Water	Electrolyte	Colloid	Glucose in Water
Burn budget of F.D. Moore	1000–4000 ml lactated Ringer's solution and 1200 ml 0.5N saline	7.5% of body weight	1500–5000 ml	1000–4000 ml lactated Ringer's solution and 1200 ml 0.5N saline	2.5% of body weight	1500–5000 ml
Evans	Normal saline, 1 ml/kg/% burn	1.0 ml/kg/% burn	2000 ml	One half of first 24-hr requirement	One half of first 24-hr requirement	2000 ml
Brooke	Lactated Ringer's solution, 1.5 ml/kg/% burn	0.5 ml/kg/% burn	2000 ml	One half to three quarters of first 24-hr requirement	One half to three quarters of first 24-hr requirement	2000 ml
Parkland	Lactated Ringer's solution, 4 ml/kg/% burn				20–60% of calculated plasma volume	
Hypertonic sodium solution	Volume to maintain urine output at 30 ml/hr (fluid contains 250 mEq Na/L)			One third of salt solution orally, up to 3500 ml limit		
Modified Brooke	Lactated Ringer's solution, 2 ml /kg/% burn				0.3–0.5 ml/kg/% burn	Goal: maintain adequate urinary output
Burnett Burn Center	Isotonic or hypertonic alkaline sodium solution/% burn/kg			D$_5$ 1/4 NS maintenance	Colloid 0.5 ml/ % burn/kg	D$_5$W (% burn) (TBSAm^2)

(From Hudak, C., Gallo, B., Berg, J. (1990). *Critical Care Nursing*, 5th ed. Philadelphia: JB Lippincott, 766.)

shifts should be avoided, since cerebral edema may result. The patient's weight and serum sodium level are used to guide fluid replacement.

Overresuscitation should be avoided, since it can have serious consequences such as pulmonary edema or excessive wound edema inhibiting perfusion either locally or distally to the wound. Decreased local wound perfusion can cause conversion of wounds from partial to full thickness. Decreased perfusion distally can lead to neurovascular compromise of extremities.

Current research is looking into alternatives in fluid resuscitation. One possibility is the use of high-osmolar solutions such as hypertonic lactate saline, 7.5% sodium chloride, or 6% dextran 70. In theory, high-osmolar solutions will cause a rapid shift of fluid from the intracellular compartment to the intravascular space, expanding plasma volume. This improvement in cardiovascular performance, however, may be only transient. The potential risks of high-osmolar solutions are cellular dehydration and hypernatremia.

The ability of hypertonic solutions to produce less wound edema may be advantageous, particularly in patients with inhalation injuries, circumferential full-thickness burns of extremities, and intracranial injuries. Serum sodium levels must be monitored closely since serum sodium exceeding 160 mEq/L is associated with oliguria and mental status changes.

FLUID REMOBILIZATION PHASE

Fluid remobilization or diuresis usually begins 48–72 hr postburn and lasts 1–3 days. Fluid shifts from the interstitial space into the intravascular compartment, causing great increase in blood volume. As a result, urine volume will increase. Caution should be used with fluid volume replacement, since giving large amounts during this phase may lead to fluid overload. The nurse must assess the patient for signs of volume overload such as venous distension, crackles, and frothy sputum. Patients with impaired renal or cardiovascular function are at high risk during this time, since they may be less likely to handle the large fluid shifts. Most patients return to preburn weight by postinjury day 10. Remember that loss of skin integrity will increase water loss by evaporation.

OTHER INITIAL MANAGEMENT

Patients with a greater than 15% BSA burn should have a nasogastric tube inserted and hooked to low continuous suction. These patients are prone to paralytic ileus. Gastric prophylaxis should be initiated, since burn patients are prone to stress ulcers.

Pain relief is an essential treatment for burn victims. Typically, narcotics are given intravenously in small doses until pain relief is achieved. Because of the unpredictability of circulation and absorption, intramuscular and subcutaneous routes should not be utilized.

Edema formation related to initial fluid shifts occurs both locally at the wound sites and systemically in burns of greater than 20% BSA. Edema formation may cause neurovascular compromise to the extremities; therefore, frequent assessments are necessary to evaluate pulses, skin color, capillary refill, and sensation. Arterial circulation is at greatest risk on circumferential burns. The Doppler flow probe may be one of the best ways to evaluate compromise. Elevating extremities may help decrease some of the edema formation. An escharotomy may be required to restore arterial circulation, prevent ischemia and necrosis, and allow for further swelling. Eschar, which forms from full-thickness burns, is tight, leathery, and nondistensible and does not have pain fibers. The escharotomy can be performed at the bedside, utilizing a sterile field and scapel (Fig. 50–3). Care should be taken to avoid major nerves, vessels, and tendons. The incision should extend through the length of the eschar, over joints, and down to the subcutaneous fat. The incision is placed laterally or medially on the extremity. If a single incision does not restore circulation, bilateral incisions will be required.

Circumferential burns can also cause problems when they occur on the chest. Adequacy of ventilation must be assessed continually. Ventilatory excursion may be restricted, requiring a chest escharotomy. Bilateral incisions should be made down the anterior axillary line. If burns are extensive, the incision may be extended onto the abdomen. The incisions are then connected by a transverse incision along the costal margin.

WOUND MANAGEMENT

Treatment of other life-threatening conditions takes priority over burn wound management. Initially, the burn wound should be covered with clean sheets. Ice is never used to treat burns because of the susceptibility to hypothermia or frostbite. If transfer to a burn center is anticipated (Table 50–3), it is not necessary to debride or apply topical antimicrobial agents within the first 24 hr.

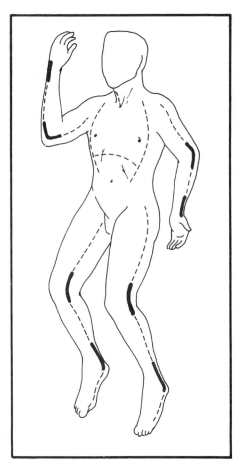

Figure 50–3. Preferred sites of escharotomy incisions. (Redrawn from Rye, L.W., & Cioffi, W.S. (1991). Resuscitation of thermally injured patients. *Crit Care Nurs Clin North Am 3*; 181–189.)

Besides hypovolemia, the major threat to the patient is sepsis of the burn wound. The incidence of infection varies with burn size, patient's age and current health, and type of bacteria. None of the topical antimicrobials sterilizes the wound, but they do control bacterial proliferation and provide the best control over bacterial growth. The most common topical antimicrobial agents are mafenide acetate (Sulfamylon), silversulfadiazine (Silvadene), or 0.5% silver nitrate soaks. The nonviable eschar is an ideal environment for bacterial growth. Systemic antibiotics have little control over this bacterial growth, since they are unable to reach the injured tissue. Systemic antibiotics are reserved for severe wound infections.

Once a patient is hemodynamically stable, wound care begins. All burned areas are cleansed once or twice daily with normal saline or an antimicrobial liquid detergent. Loose and necrotic tissue is gently removed, with care taken not to damage viable tissue or cause excessive bleeding. Large blisters (greater than 2 cm in diameter) are debrided. Once the wounds are cleansed, a topical antimicrobial agent is applied. One of two methods is utilized, depending on the philosophy of the burn center. The open method applies the antimicrobial agent sterilely and leaves the wound open to the air. Advantages of this method are that it allows for constant wound assessment, eliminates painful dressing changes, and may limit bacterial proliferation. The closed method also applies an antimicrobial agent, but then covers the wound with a gauze dressing. Advantages include less heat loss and faster eschar separation.

The common recommendation is that if a burn wound will not heal in 10–14 days, excision should be undertaken to improve functional and cosmetic results, decrease length of hospital stay, and reduce cost of care. Superficial partial-thickness burns, if protected from infection, usually heal in 7–10 days, with a functional and cosmetic result that cannot be improved upon by excision and grafting. Deep partial-thickness burns will require 10–21 days to heal. When healed, hypertrophic scar formation often results. The amount of scar is proportional to the time required for healing. Full-thickness burns have no surviving skin appendages and so require excision and grafting to achieve definitive closure.

Excision of burn tissue is usually done by a tangential technique. Blood loss associated with this procedure can be large, with some estimates at 9% of circulating blood volume per percentage of body surface excised. The end point of excision is the presence of uniformly dense capillary bleeding from the entire burn wound bed. Since approximately 20% of burn wound debridements induce bacteremia, systemic antibiotics are administered prophylactically in the perioperative period. Patients with burns of greater than 50% BSA will require staging of successive operations to achieve complete burn excision and coverage. The use of meshed autografts, or a biologic dressing or a skin substitute followed by autograft, or, more recently, the application of cultured epidermal autografts, permits timely closure of even massive burn wounds that have been excised.

INHALATION INJURY

With any burn situation the clinician must consider the possibility of an inhalation injury since 80% of all fire victims die of smoke inhalation. Death at the scene of a fire is almost always a result of smoke inhalation. The degree of thermal injury, however, is

TABLE 50–3. BURN CLASSIFICATIONS BY THE AMERICAN BURN ASSOCIATION

Injury Severity	Identifying Criteria	Recommended Treatment Facility
Minor burns	Partial thickness of ≤15% TBSA No full thickness No involvement of eyes or ears	Emergency rooms—outpatients
Moderate burns	Partial thickness of 15–25% TBSA Full thickness of <10% TBSA not involving the hands, face, eyes, ears, feet, or genitalia	General hospital or may be outpatients

Major burns	Partial thickness of >25% TBSA
	Full thickness of >10% TBSA
	True electrical injuries
	Injury to hands, face, eyes, ears, feet, or genitalia
	Concomitant injuries, e.g., inhalation injury, fractures,
	    or other trauma
	High–risk patients, e.g., <2 years old, >50 years old,
	    or with pre-existing conditions
		Burn unit or center

TBSA, total body surface area.
(From Desai, M., & Herdon, D. (1991). Burns. In *Current Therapy of Trauma.* Ed. Trunkey, D., & Lewis, F. St. Louis: B.C. Decker, 317.)

not an indication of presence or absence of inhalation injury. Inhalation injury can occur from direct thermal injury or inhalation of carbon monoxide or other toxic gases that result from incomplete combustion.

Patients at risk for smoke inhalation are anyone with the history of being in a closed space where fire was present and/or flame burns of the face, neck, and chest. Early recognition and intervention is critical to the patient's early survival. Suspect smoke inhalation if you observe singed nasal hairs, mucosal burns of the nose, lips, mouth, or throat, carbonaceous or sooty material in sputum, or hoarseness. If inhalation injury is suspected the patient should be intubated immediately. Airway edema can occur rapidly, making it impossible to insert an endotracheal tube.

Direct thermal damage occurs usually just to the upper respiratory tract. Heat is dissipated by the upper respiratory tract in the nasal pharynx and upper airways. Cellular damage occurs, leading to tissue swelling and edema. Airway obstruction can result. Direct thermal injury below the glottis is rare but may occur with steam exposure. Pulmonary edema develops in 5–30% of inhalation injury patients. The lower respiratory tract injury is most often the result of inhalation of noxious gases. Destruction of surfactant can occur, resulting in a high incidence of adult respiratory distress syndrome.

Carbon monoxide is a product of incomplete hydrocarbon combustion. Carbon monoxide has a 200 times greater affinity for hemoglobin than oxygen. As a result, carbon monoxide attaches to hemoglobin, displacing oxygen and making less oxygen

available to the cells. The oxyhemoglobin dissociation curve shifts to the left so the oxygen on the hemoglobin is not readily given up to the cells. Carbon monoxide also attacks the cytochrome oxidase system, which affects mitochondrial activity further decreasing cellular oxygenation. The result can be massive tissue hypoxia. A pulse oximeter (SpO_2) will provide an inaccurate assessment of hemoglobin oxygen saturation. The pulse oximeter sees oxyhemoglobin and carboxyhemoglobin as the same, so the (SpO_2) reading will be falsely elevated. Carboxyhemoglobin levels should be drawn on admission to the emergency department and repeated every 4 hr until the level returns to normal.

Treatment of inhalation injuries includes first the maintenance of a patent airway. Prophylactic intubation carries little risk when compared to the danger of complete airway obstruction. The greatest risk of laryngeal and upper airway edema is 12–36 hr postinjury. Oxygen therapy should be instituted early. Carbon monoxide elimination can be decreased from 4 hr to 45 min with an inspired oxygen concentration of 100%. Hyperbaric oxygen therapy can shorten the time even greater. Ventilatory support with positive end expiratory pressure and continuous positive airway pressure will be required since the patient often experiences decreased lung compliance and atelectasis. Following airway edema and pulmonary edema the third stage of an inhalation injury is bronchopneumonia. Bronchopneumonia occurs 3–10 days postexposure in 15–60% of the patients and carries a mortality rate of 50–80%. A high incidence of sepsis is associated with the development of bronchopneumonia. Antibiotics should be given for documented infections.

ELECTRICAL BURNS

Electrical burns result from electrical energy being converted to heat. Electrical injuries are divided into high-voltage (greater than 1000 volts) or low-voltage injuries. In the United States, alternating current (AC) is the most common, with direct current (DC) found predominately in industry. Alternating current is more dangerous than direct current.

The point of contact will receive the greatest heat. Electricity will travel through the body in the path of least resistance. Nerves offer the least resistance followed by blood vessels, then muscle, with bone offering the most resistance. Electrical burns can be difficult at best to assess. The skin may appear intact except for entrance and exit wounds, while the underlying tissues may be injured to the point of necrosis.

Electrical burns can cause vascular disruption, resulting in hemorrhage and/or thrombus formation. Underlying edema and swelling can cause compartment syndrome. Breakdown of muscle can result in myoglobin being released into the circulation (rhabdomyolysis). Myoglobinuria is suspected if pink to dark red pigment is noted in the urine. If not excreted, myoglobin can precipitate in the renal tubules and cause renal failure. Myoglobinuria is treated by keeping urine output up with crystaloids mannitol, and administration of sodium bicarbonate since myoglobin is excreted better in alkaline urine.

Since estimation of the extent of the burn is difficult, generally fluids are given to maintain urine output of 75–100 ml/h. If urine is clear, fluids can be given to maintain a urine output of 30–50 ml/h. Peripheral pulses, skin color, capillary refill, and sensation are assessed hourly to monitor for compartment syndrome. Fasciotomies may be necessary if vascular compromise occurs.

A 12-lead electrocardiogram (ECG) is obtained on admission, followed by continuous ECG monitoring since dysrhythmias may develop. Wound care is the same as with thermal burns.

CHEMICAL BURNS

Chemical burns result from direct contact with agents such as acids, alkalis, and/or petroleum-based products. The severity of chemical injury is related to the agent, concentration, volume, and duration of contact. Alkaline chemicals cause the most serious burns. Treatment consists of removing saturated clothing, brushing any powder from the skin, and irrigating with large amounts of water or normal saline. Irrigation should be continued until the patient experiences a decrease in pain in the wound. Alkaline substances require longer irrigation than acids. It may be necessary to contact a regional poison control center to determine the best methods to neutralize the chemicals. Personnel caring for patients exposed to chemical agents must always wear protective clothing in the form of a gown, gloves, goggles, and mask to avoid personal contact with the chemical.

Petroleum burns (gasoline or diesel fuel) can often produce full-thickness burns that initially appear to be partial-thickness. Systemic toxicity may appear with evidence of pulmonary, hepatic, or renal failure. Care must be taken not to ignite the gasoline or diesel fuel. Tar or asphalt burns should be cooled with water but will require a petroleum product like mineral oil to dissolve the substance.

Hydrofluoric acid burns can be life-threatening since inhalation of this acid can cause pulmonary edema. The activity of fluoride in soft tissue combines with calcium or magnesium to produce an insoluble salt. Copious irrigation may be followed with a local injection of 5–10% calcium gluconate. Relief of pain following injection is immediate.

MULTISYSTEM ORGAN DYSFUNCTION BIBLIOGRAPHY

Advanced Burn Life Support Provider's Manual. (1990). Nebraska Burn Institute.

Bishop, M.H., Shoemaker, W., Appel, P., et al. (1993). Relationship between supranormal circulatory values, time delays and outcome in severely traumatized patients. *Crit Care Med, 21* (1), 56–63.

Bone, R. (1991). Pathophysiology and treatment of septic shock. *JAMA, 266*(4), 548–554.

Bone, R. (1994). Sepsis and SIRS. *Nephrol Dialysis Transplant, 9* (Suppl. 4), 99–103.

Burgess, M. (1991). Initial management of a patient with extensive burn injury. *Crit Care Clin North Am, 3*(2), 165–179.

Cardona, V., Hurn, P., Mason, P., et al. (1994). *Trauma Nursing from Resuscitation Through Rehabilitation.* Philadelphia: W.B. Saunders.

Carey, P.D., Windsor, C.J., Walsh, C.J., et al. (1994). Multi-agent therapy in the treatment of sepsis-induced microvascular injury. *Br J Surg, 81*, 1752–1756.

Cooney, R., Owens, E., Juraskinski, J., et al. (1994). Interleukin-1 receptor antagonist prevents sepsis-induced inhibition of protein synthesis. *Am J Physiol,* E636–E641.

Duncan, D. & Driscoll, D. (1991). Burn wound management. *Crit Care Clin North Am., 3*(2), 199–220.

Goodwin, C.W. (1995). Fluid management and nutritional support of the burn patient. In *Current Surgical Therapy.* Ed. Cameron, J.L. St. Louis: C.V. Mosby.

Litovitz, T.L., Schmitz, B.F., & Bailey, K.M. (1989). Annual Report of the American Association of Poison Control Centers, National Data Collection System.

Metheny, N. (1992). *Fluid and Electrolyte Balance: Nursing Considerations.* Philadelphia: J.B. Lippincott.

Mira, J., Fabre, J., Baigorri, F., et al. (1994). Lack of oxygen supply dependency in patients with severe sepsis. *Chest, 106*(5), 1524–1531.

Pass, H.I., Mew, D., Pass, H., & Temeck, B. (1995). The macrophage, TNF and other cytokines. *Chest Surg Clin North Am, 5*(1) 73–90.

Pruitt, B.A. (1995). Burn wounds. In *Current Surgical Therapy* Ed. Cameron, J.L. St. Louis: C.V. Mosby.

Rangel-Frausto, M., Pittet, D., Costigan, M., et al. (1995). The natural history of the systemic inflammatory response syndrome. *JAMA, 273*(2), 117–123.

Rue, L., & Cioffi, W. (1991). Resuscitation of thermally injured patients. *Crit Care Clin North Am, 3*(2), 181–189.

Schiller, H., Reilly, P., & Bulkley, G. (1993). Antioxidant therapy. *Crit Care Med, 21*(2), S92–S102.

Sibbald, W., & Vincent, J.L. (1995). Roundtable conference on clinical trials for the treatment of sepsis. *Chest, 107*(2), 522–527.

Trunkey, D., & Lewis, F. (1991). *Current Therapy of Trauma.* Philadelphia: B.C. Decker.

Wang, P., Ba, Z.F., & Chaudry, I. (1994). Nitric oxide. *Arch Surg, 129,* 1137–1143.

Welch, G. (1991). Anesthesia for the patient with thermal injury. *Curr Rev Nurse Anesth, 14*(12), 94–99.

Zainal, G. (1994). Nutrition of critically ill people. *Inten Crit Care Nurs, 10,* 165–170.

PART VIII

Multisystem Organ Dysfunction Practice Exam

Questions 1 and 2 refer to the following scenario.

A 71-year-old male is admitted to the intensive care unit with hypotension of unknown origin. His past medical history includes recent surgery for prostate cancer. Because of an initial lack of response to treatment for the hypotension, he has a fiberoptic pulmonary artery catheter placed. At 0800, he is unresponsive, with a Glasgow Coma Scale score of 4. His skin is warm and dry, and lung sounds reveal generalized crackles. His vital signs and pulmonary artery catheter reveal the following information. The physician requests dobutamine to be added to his treatment. One hour after the dobutamine, a repeat set of hemodynamics reveals the following:

	0800	0900
blood pressure	102/68	104/66
pulse	101	106
cardiac output	8.9	9.4
cardiac index	5.4	5.6
PA	42/22	44/23
PAOP	16	16
CVP	12	13
SvO_2	0.86	.85
PaO_2	67	74
SaO_2	0.92	.93
$PaCO_2$	36	38
FIO_2	0.70	.70
PEEP	+10	+10
pH	7.35	7.34
Hgb	11	11
Lactate	4.5	4.5
DO_2	1207	1289
VO_2	79	110

1. Based on this information, was the addition of dobutamine effective?
   - (A) yes, since an increase in DO_2 occurred
   - (B) yes, since an increase in VO_2 occurred
   - (C) no, since the blood pressure did not increase
   - (D) no, since the SvO_2 and lactate are unchanged

2. If tissue oxygenation improved on this patient, which parameters would you most likely see change?
   - (A) decrease in the SvO_2
   - (B) increase in pH
   - (C) decrease in lactate
   - (D) increase in SaO_2

3. A 74-year-old female is in the intensive care unit with the diagnosis of possible sepsis secondary to pneumonia. Upon admission she was markedly short of breath with an FIO_2 of 80% and a PaO_2 of 72. She was intubated because of increased work of breathing and placed on assisted mandatory ventilation (AMV), with the following settings:

FIO_2	80%
PEEP	+8 cm H_2O
Tidal volume (Vt)	800 ml
Ventilator rate	10 breaths/min
Total rate	32 breaths/min
Peak airway pressure	48 cm H_2O

Shortly after admission, she became hypotensive and had a fiberoptic pulmonary artery catheter inserted to aid in her management. She is placed on dopamine at 7 µg/kg/min to support her blood pressure and normal saline is being administered intravenously at 150 ml/h. Listed below are her first three sets of hemodynamic and other clinical information:

	0610	0705	0820
PaO_2	87	78	92
SpO_2	0.98	0.96	0.98
$PaCO_2$	35	32	33
pH	7.33	7.31	7.30
HCO_3^-	21	20	20
blood pressure	88/52	92/56	90/56
pulse	114	116	112
cardiac output	8.6	8.9	9.3
cardiac index	4.1	4.2	4.7
PA	42/32	46/35	39/29
PCWP	14	15	12
CVP	9	10	10
SvO_2	0.78	0.83	0.85
Lactate		5.6	

Based on the above information, is she improving, deteriorating, or stable?
- (A) improving, based on the stable SpO_2
- (B) stable, based on the blood pressure
- (C) worsening, based on the increasing SvO_2
- (D) improving, based on the improved PaO_2

4. A blood culture report returns for a 73-year-old male who is in the intensive care unit for possible sepsis. The report states that he has *Escherichia coli* (a gram-negative bacterium) in the blood. He currently is receiving gentamicin, imipenem, and cefoxitin. Based on the report, what should be done about the antibiotic coverage?
- (A) discontinue all drugs and start moxalactam
- (B) maintain the current regime
- (C) remove the imipenem and cefoxitin
- (D) remove the gentamicin

Questions 5 and 6 refer to the following scenario.

A 69-year-old female is admitted to your unit with probable septic shock after sustaining a ruptured diverticulum in her large intestine. The following information is available:

blood pressure	80/52
pulse	121
respiratory rate	38
temperature	38°C
cardiac output	8.9
cardiac index	5.6
stroke index	46
PA	24/11
PCWP	8
CVP	2
PaO_2	78
$PaCO_2$	29

pH	7.32
HCO_3^-	16
lactate	5.1
SvO_2	81%
SpO_2	95%

5. Based on this information, which treatment(s) is/are likely to be implemented first?
- (A) normal saline fluid bolus of 300 ml/30 min and dobutamine at 5 µg/kg/min
- (B) dobutamine at 5 µg/kg/min and administration of antipyretics
- (C) normal saline fluid bolus of 300 ml/30 min and administration of antipyretics
- (D) all of the above

6. Treatment with which of the following is most likely to reverse the effects of the sepsis?
- (A) HA-IA antibody
- (B) ibuprofen
- (C) dopamine
- (D) fluid bolus of either crystalloid or colloidal solutions

7. A 64-year-old female is in the intensive care unit with the diagnosis of possible sepsis secondary to a urinary tract infection. Upon admission she was markedly short of breath with an a/A (arterial/alveolar) ratio of 0.14, an FiO_2 of 0.80, and a PaO_2 of 72. She was intubated because of increased work of breathing. Shortly after admission, she became hypotensive and had a pulmonary artery catheter inserted to aid in management. Over the next 2 days, she was aggressively treated with normal saline fluid bolus (with a subsequent 10-kg weight gain), antibiotics, and dobutamine. Based on the following information, has the therapy been successful to this point?

	Day 2	**Day 3**	**Day 4**
PaO_2	87	78	92
$PaCO_2$	35	32	37
pH	7.33	7.31	7.33
HCO_3^-	21	20	22
blood pressure	88/52	92/56	90/56
pulse	114	116	112
cardiac output	8.6	8.9	9.3
cardiac index	5.1	5.2	5.5
PA	42/32	46/35	39/33
PCWP	14	15	17
CVP	9	10	10
SvO_2	0.55	0.53	0.52
lactate	4	4.6	4.6

(A) yes, as illustrated by an increased cardiac index

(B) yes, as illustrated by an increased PaO_2

(C) no, as illustrated by an unimproved SvO_2

(D) no, as illustrated by an increase in PCWP

Questions 8 to 10 refer to the following scenario.

A 64-year-old female is admitted to your unit following a house fire in which she suffered circumferential full-thickness burns of both legs and partial-thickness burns to her front torso. She is confused and cannot describe what happened. The following laboratory data are available:

PaO_2	88
$PaCO_2$	33
pH	7.36
HCO_3^-	21
FIO_2	0.28

8. Based on this information, how much of her body surface area was burned?
   (A) 15%
   (B) 27%
   (C) 39%
   (D) 54%

9. Which of the following would be considered initial therapies for this situation?
   (A) administration of large volumes of lactated Ringer's
   (B) silver sulfadiazine ointment to burn wounds
   (C) IV analgesia
   (D) all of the above

10. Which other initial therapies are important for this patient?
    (A) neurovascular checks of extremities and gastric prophylaxis/
    (B) ice packs to burn wounds
    (C) IV antibiotics
    (D) diuretics

11. Hypertonic solutions in burn resuscitation offer which of the following advantages?
    (A) delayed need for nutritional support
    (B) less wound edema
    (C) lower serum sodium and lower serum osmolality
    (D) less sepsis

12. Which of the following is the most common reason for low urine output associated with burns?
    (A) underresucitation
    (B) myoglobinuria

(C) sepsis
(D) interstitial edema

13. Monoclonal antibodies are of potential benefit in treating which of the following conditions?
    (A) sepsis and acute renal failure
    (B) sepsis and ARDS (adult respiratory distress syndrome)
    (C) acute renal failure and ARDS
    (D) all of the above

Questions 14 and 15 refer to the following scenario.

A 26-year-old male was working in his basement with an acetylene torch when the flame started a fire in some nearby paper and wood. He states that the flame flashed toward his face but he quickly ran to the other side of the basement and got a fire extinguisher. The fire was not initially controlled by the extinguisher, so he ran outside. He is now admitted to your unit with second-degree upper torso and arm burns. In addition to the burns on his chest, his face is red with loss of facial hair. The following laboratory data are available:

pH	7.30
PaO_2	79
$PaCO_2$	29
HCO_3^-	19
FIO_2	0.30
SaO_2	0.83
CoHgb	0.16
MetHgb	0.01

14. Which of the following information would be suggestive of smoke inhalation in this patient?
    (A) MetHgb level of 1% and PaO_2 of 79
    (B) SaO_2 of 83% on FIO_2 of .30
    (C) Singed facial hair and CoHgb level of 16%
    (D) $PaCO_2$ of 29

15. Which treatment would most likely be given at this time?
    (A) increase FIO_2 to 100% and intubation
    (B) paraffin soaks to his facial burns
    (C) following pulse oximeter for oxygenation status
    (D) decrease the amount of fluids given for resuscitation

16. In the patient with smoke inhalation, what is the most likely time period during which pulmonary complications may develop?
    (A) first 4 hr postinhalation
    (B) 4 to 8 hr postinhalation
    (C) 12 to 36 hr postinhalation
    (D) 24 to 48 hr postinhalation

17. A 26-year-old woman with 26% BSA deep partial-thickness burns to her arms and chest is scheduled for split-thickness skin grafting on postinjury day 7. The nurse should anticipate which of the following?
    (A) prophylactic IV antibiotics perioperatively
    (B) administration of blood products following the procedure
    (C) potential for faster wound healing and better cosmetic appearance
    (D) all of the above

18. A 17-year-old male is admitted to your unit following an electric shock injury. His friends state that he was climbing a sign when a pole he was carrying touched a power line. He fell from the sign and was unresponsive. His friends immediately brought him to the emergency room. Based on the preceding description, which conditions could be anticipated to be present during the first 24 hr of intensive care unit admission?
    (A) cardiac dysrhythmias
    (B) lower fluid requirements since open wounds are small
    (C) little to no pain
    (D) elevated COHgb

Questions 19 and 20 refer to the following scenario.

A 23-year-old male is admitted to your unit following a fire at his place of work, a paint factory. He has burns across his chest, arms, and upper legs. He is responsive to verbal stimuli and currently denies any pain. His wounds appear white and no blanching is detected. His vital signs are as follows:

blood pressure	104/62
pulse	134
respiratory rate	32

19. Based on the preceding information, which type of burn is likely to be present?
    (A) first-degree
    (B) superficial partial-thickness
    (C) second-degree with loss of upper layer of dermis
    (D) full-thickness

20. Which of the following would be the most likely initial therapy in this situation?
    (A) administration of topical silver sulfadiazine
    (B) administration of large volumes of intravenous lactated Ringer's
    (C) administration of 100% oxygen
    (D) placement of a Swan-Ganz catheter to assess fluid status

21. Which of the following is considered most useful for stabilizing hemodynamics in the immediate postburn resuscitation period?
    (A) Hespan
    (B) lactated Ringer's
    (C) normal saline
    (D) albumin

Questions 22 and 23 refer to the following scenario.

A 46-year-old male is in your unit following a fire in which the chair in which he was sitting was ignited by a cigarette. He is burned over 40% of his body (mostly back and lower extremities) with partial-thickness and full-thickness burns. It is now 24 hr since he sustained the burns. He complains of pain in both feet, but particularly his right. His right leg is covered with eschar. He has no Doppler pulse in his right foot.

22. Based on the preceding information, which method of pain relief would be the most appropriate?
    (A) escharotomy
    (B) intramuscular Demerol
    (C) ace wraps to lower extremites to decrease swelling
    (D) elevation of legs

23. In this patient, what would be the advantage to performing an escharotomy?
    (A) pain relief and improvement in circulation
    (B) faster healing of burn wound
    (C) reduction in postburn scarring
    (D) decreases need for IV antibiotics

24. Which of the following organs is/are likely to be affected in multisystem organ dysfunction?
    (A) liver and kidney
    (B) liver and lungs
    (C) kidney and lungs
    (D) all of the above

25. The effects of tumor necrosing factor, leukotrienes, and thromboxane A_2 are similar in the systemic responses they initiate. Which of the following are consistent with the actions produced by these substances?
    (A) vasoconstriction and increasing cardiac ejection fraction
    (B) vasoconstriction and promoting platelet aggregation
    (C) increasing cardiac ejection fraction and promoting platelet aggregation
    (D) all of the above

26. A 19-year-old female is admitted to your unit after an argument with her parents. Her parents

state that they found her in her room with an empty bottle of Tylenol on her nightstand. Which of the following is the initial treatment for an overdose of acetaminophen?

(A) ipecac
(B) lavage and N-acetylcystine
(C) dialysis
(D) charcoal only

27. Which of the following are considered symptoms of aspirin poisoning?
(A) initial pH > 7.45 and gastrointestinal bleeding
(B) tachypnea
(C) gastrointestinal bleeding and late pH <7.35
(D) all of the above

28. Tricyclic poisoning can produce lethal consequences from which of the following effects?
(A) quinidine-like effects
(B) neurological injury secondary to seizures
(C) parasympathetic stimulation
(D) noncardiogenic pulmonary edema

29. Which of the following is a useful diagnostic sign when trying to determine the severity of a tricyclic poisoning attempt?
(A) presence of seizures
(B) tricyclic blood levels
(C) QRS complex narrowing
(D) widening pulse pressure

30. A burn involving the entire length of both lower extremities would constitute a burn over what percentage of the entire body?
(A) 9%
(B) 18%
(C) 36%
(D) 52%

31. A 20-year-old male is admitted to your unit following a suicide attempt after breaking up with his girl friend. He ingested an unknown drug or drugs and is currently combative but with a reduced level of consciousness. A large-bore nasogastric tube has been inserted in an attempt to lavage his stomach. Which of the following nursing actions should be initiated at this point?
(A) protection against aspiration
(B) intubation and mechanical ventilation
(C) sedation to reduce the combativeness
(D) all of the above

Questions 32 and 33 refer to the following scenario.

A 47-year-old male is admitted to the hospital following complaints of severe muscle weakness of the lower extremities. Neurological examinations are negative, including MRI (magnetic resonance imaging) of the head and back. While on the medical floor, his level of consciousness changes and he is arousable only by deep stimuli. He requires intubation and mechanical ventilation. The following laboratory and vital sign information is available:

blood pressure	88/54
pulse	126
respiratory rate	24 (on assisted mandatory ventilation)
temperature	39°C
PaO_2	78
FIO_2	0.50
HCO_3^-	18
white blood cells	31,000
BUN	38
SGOT	433
pH	7.33
$PaCO_2$	32
Hgb	13
creatinine	2.6
SGPT	512
alkaline phosphatase	199

32. Based on this information, which condition is likely to be developing?
(A) Guillain-Barré syndrome
(B) ARDS (adult respiratory distress syndrome)
(C) systemic inflammatory response syndrome
(D) amyotrophic lateral sclerosis

33. Treatment for this condition is most likely to include which of the following?
(A) increased intravenous fluids
(B) plasmapheresis
(C) dopamine
(D) beta blockers, such as propranolol or esmolol

34. Which of the following are the most characteristic responses of the cardiovascular system to sepsis?
(A) increased ejection fraction and increased cardiac output
(B) increased ejection fraction and reduced systemic vascular resistance
(C) increased cardiac output and reduced systemic vascular resistance
(D) all of the above

Questions 35 and 36 refer to the following scenario.

A 54-year-old female is in your unit following acute hepatic failure from hepatitis C, to be evaluated for a liver transplant and for management of a persistent fever (temperature >39°C). She becomes hypotensive (84/50) and tachycardic (130). A fiberoptic pulmonary artery catheter is placed and reveals the following:

cardiac output	12.9
cardiac index	7.2
PA	30 12
PCWP	8
CVP	3
SvO_2	0.88

35. Based on the preceding information, which condition would explain her current clinical status?
    (A) portal hypertension
    (B) left ventricular failure
    (C) hypovolemia secondary to loss of plasma proteins
    (D) sepsis

36. Which of the following would explain the SvO_2 value of 0.88?
    (A) increased oxygen consumption and increased oxygen delivery
    (B) increased oxygen consumption and pericapillary shunting
    (C) increased oxygen delivery and pericapillary shunting
    (D) all of the above

37. Since the initial recognition of sepsis as a distinct disorder, particularly in the past 30 years, treatment has frequently been ineffective because of the inability to isolate a central mediating agent. Of the following, which has the most potential to be a central mediating agent in the development of sepsis?
    (A) arachidonic acid
    (B) monoclonal antibodies
    (C) prostaglandins
    (D) tumor necrosing factor

Questions 38 and 39 refer to the following scenario.

A 19-year-old soldier is brought to your hospital from a Middle Eastern country for treatment of an unidentifiable source of inflammation. He is restless and responsive only to deep pain and appears to be uncomfortable. His urine output has been 400 ml for the past 24 hr. The following physical and laboratory information is available:

blood pressure	100/54
pulse	133
respiratory rate	38
temperature	39.5°C
white blood cells	19,300

red blood cells	3,500,300
Hgb	11
Hct	32
Na^+	155
K^+	3.9
Cl^-	111
HCO_3^-	26
urinary Na^+	9
urinary osmolality	878

38. Based on the preceding information, the physician wants to start a fluid bolus with 500 ml of D_5W. Which of the following findings support this decision?
    (A) red blood cell count of 3,500,300 and Na^+ level of 155
    (B) red blood cell count of 3,500,300 and clinical picture of systemic inflammation
    (C) Na^+ level of 155 and clinical picture of systemic inflammation
    (D) all of the above

39. Given an unknown source of inflammation, which of the following therapies would most likely be prescribed?
    (A) aminoglycosides (e.g., gentamicin) and anti-inflammatory agents (e.g., methylprednisolone)
    (B) aminoglycosides and cephalosporins (e.g., cefoxitin)
    (C) antiinflammatory agents and cephalosporins
    (D) all of the above

Questions 40 and 41 refer to the following scenario.

A 38-year-old female is in your unit with a fever of unknown origin. She became acutely short of breath on the step-down floor and was transferred to the unit. She required intubation and mechanical ventilation when her shortness of breath could not be relieved. Her present ventilator settings are AMV (assist/control), rate 12 (total rate 34), tidal volume 700 ml FIO_2 0.70. Her mental status is confused and she is restless and pulling at her tubes, requiring her to be restrained. She currently has the following vital signs and laboratory data:

blood pressure	136/82
pulse	127
respiratory rate	34
temperature	38.8°C
PaO_2	65
$PaCO_2$	34
pH	7.31
HCO_3^-	17

40. One of your fellow nurses states that, in systemic inflammatory responses like the preceding situation, oxygen consumption and energy requirements are increased. Another nurse says that that is not always true, that only in some instances are energy requirements increased. Which of the preceding pieces of information suggests that this patient has increased energy expenditure and oxygen consumption?
    (A) respiratory rate of 34 and PaO_2 of 65
    (B) respiratory rate of 34 and temperature of 38.8°C
    (C) PaO_2 of 65 and temperature of 38.8°C
    (D) all of the above

41. Which of the following therapies would be designed to help reduce the energy expenditure in this patient?
    (A) changing to IMV (intermittent mandatory ventilation) from AMV and administering sedation, such as a benzodiazepine (e.g., 1–2 mg Versed)
    (B) changing to IMV from AMU and administering an antipyretic, such as acetaminophen (Tylenol)
    (C) administering sedation and an antipyretic
    (D) all of the above

Questions 42 and 43 refer to the following scenario.

A 76-year-old male on postoperative day 5 following a colon resection for a bowel obstruction develops a fever of 39°C. He has no overt signs of infection. During the evening he becomes hypotensive and is transferred to your unit. A pulmonary artery catheter is placed and the following information is available:

blood pressure	84/50
pulse	116
respiratory rate	29
temperature	39°C
PaO_2	88
FIO_2	0.50
PA	20/8
PCWP	5
cardiac output	9.1
cardiac index	6.0
SvO_2	0.81
PvO_2	50

Based on this information, the physician states that she believes the symptoms are consistent with the diagnosis of sepsis.

42. Which of the following clinical signs are consistent with the diagnosis of sepsis?
    (A) SvO_2 of 0.81 and a cardiac index of 6.0
    (B) SvO_2 of 0.81 and a PCWP of 5
    (C) cardiac index of 6.0 and a PCWP of 5
    (D) all of the above

43. Which of the following would be indications of an improvement in the septic condition?
    (A) decrease in PCWP
    (B) increase in PaO_2
    (C) decrease in SvO_2
    (D) increase in cardiac index

44. Which of the following are the two most common sources of infection in the critically ill population?
    (A) urinary tract infection and respiratory system infection
    (B) urinary tract infection and central nervous system infection
    (C) respiratory system infection and central nervous system infection
    (D) they are all equal in the incidence of infections

Questions 45 and 46 are based on the following scenario.

A 22-year-old male is admitted following an electrical burn. An entrance wound is found on his left hand and an exit wound is noted on his right foot. He has two 16-gauge IVs in place and is receiving lactated Ringer's solution at 300 ml per hour. During your shift you notice his urine output is 50 ml for the past hour and is becoming red in color. You notify the physician who suspects myoglobinuria.

45. Which of the following treatments would you expect based on this diagnosis?
    (A) increase IV fluids until urine output is 75–100 ml/h
    (B) alkalinization of urine by adding sodium bicarbonate to IV fluids
    (C) administration of mannitol
    (D) all of the above

46. The major complication of myoglobinuria is
    (A) muscle wasting
    (B) renal failure
    (C) low hemoglobin requiring blood transfusion
    (D) increased wound edema

PART VIII

Multisystem Organ Dysfunction Practice Exam

1. _____
2. _____
3. _____
4. _____
5. _____
6. _____
7. _____
8. _____
9. _____
10. _____
11. _____
12. _____

13. _____
14. _____
15. _____
16. _____
17. _____
18. _____
19. _____
20. _____
21. _____
22. _____
23. _____
24. _____

25. _____
26. _____
27. _____
28. _____
29. _____
30. _____
31. _____
32. _____
33. _____
34. _____
35. _____

36. _____
37. _____
38. _____
39. _____
40. _____
41. _____
42. _____
43. _____
44. _____
45. _____
46. _____

1.	D	*p571*	13.	B	*p570*	25.	B	*p567*	36.	C	*p570–571*
2.	A	*p571*	14.	C	*p591*	26.	B	*p580*	37.	D	*p567*
3.	C	*p571*	15.	A	*p591*	27.	D	*p574–576*	38.	C	*p570, 524*
4.	C	*p570*	16.	C	*p591*	28.	A	*p574–575*	39.	B	*p570*
5.	A	*p570*	17.	D	*p590*	29.	B	*p576*	40.	B	*p570–571*
6.	A	*p570*	18.	A	*p592*	30.	C	*p587*	41.	C	*p570*
7.	C	*p571*	19.	D	*p586*	31.	A	*p577*	42.	D	*p569*
8.	D	*p587*	20.	B	*p587*	32.	C	*p568–569*	43.	C	*p571*
9.	D	*p588–589*	21.	B	*p588*	33.	A	*p570*	44.	A	*p572, 566*
10.	A	*p589*	22.	A	*p589*	34.	C	*p571*	45.	D	*p592*
11.	B	*p589*	23.	A	*p589*	35.	D	*p569*	46.	B	*p592*
12.	A	*p588*	24.	D	*p572*						

Comprehensive Practice Exam—1

In this edition, you have two practice exams to utilize in your preparation for the CCRN exam. You may use them in any way you like, however, you might want to take the first exam and review the questions you missed. Then, after further study, you could take the second exam.

The practice of taking exams should help you improve your score on the CCRN exam. Remember, no practice exam will exactly simulate the actual CCRN exam. However, the exams you are seeing here have been prepared by clinicians who have taken the CCRN exam and are familiar with the format and general type of questions asked. Good luck as you take these last two exams. We sincerely hope that they will help you in your preparation for the CCRN exam.

Questions 1 and 2 refer to the following scenario.

A 63-year-old male is admitted to your unit with an anterior wall MI (myocardial infarction). His blood pressure is 92/56 with a heart rate of 102. During your discussion with the physician, the question arises of whether treatment to increase the blood pressure should be started. One drug suggested is dopamine.

1. What would be the effect of adding a vasopressor such as dopamine?
   (A) decrease CVP (central venous pressure) and myocardial oxygen consumption
   (B) increase systemic vascular resistance and myocardial oxygen consumption
   (C) increase PAOP (pulmonary artery opening pressure) and decrease myocardial oxygen consumption
   (D) increase cardiac output and decrease PAOP

2. How would you make a determination of whether the blood pressure is low enough to be of clinical concern?

(A) assess the cardiac output and measure blood gases for a PaO_2 value
(B) assess the cardiac output and assess level of consciousness
(C) measure blood gases for a PaO_2 value and assess level of consciousness
(D) all of the above

Questions 3 and 4 refer to the following scenario.

A 57-year-old male is admitted to your unit with the complaint of epigastric discomfort. He says that he took "a couple of swigs of Maalox" but the discomfort has not gone away. The pain has been present for about the past 4 hr. An admission ECG (electrocardiogram) has been obtained and is shown on page 608.

3. Based on the preceding information, what is likely to be occurring?
   (A) anterior myocardial ischemia
   (B) no ECG abnormality is present
   (C) inferior wall injury pattern
   (D) pericarditis

4. Which therapy is most likely to resolve the cause of this condition?
   (A) thrombolytic therapy
   (B) nitroglycerin
   (C) H_2 blocker
   (D) oxygen therapy

Questions 5 and 6 refer to the following scenario.

A 62-year-old male is admitted to your unit with the symptoms of shortness of breath and orthopnea. He has an S_3 heart sound, bilateral dependent pulmonary crackles, and distended jugular veins. His 12-lead ECG shows no ST-segment changes, although Q waves are present in II, III, and aVF. A pulmonary artery catheter is placed and reveals the following information:

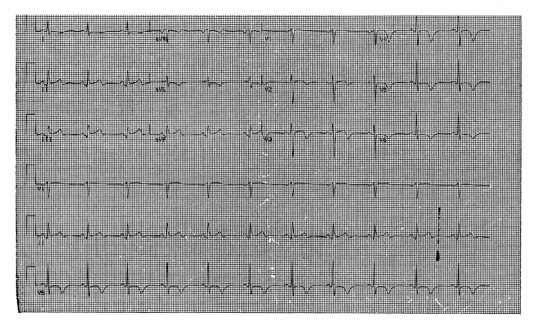

Figure for Questions 3 and 4.

blood pressure	104/68
pulse	110
PA	38/24
PAOP	22
CVP	14
cardiac output	4.1
cardiac index	2.2

5. Based on the preceding information, which condition is likely to be developing?
   (A) cardiogenic shock
   (B) hypovolemic shock
   (C) biventricular (congestive) failure
   (D) pulmonary hypertension secondary to right ventricular failure

6. Which of the following would be an appropriate treatment choice?
   (A) dobutamine
   (B) dopamine
   (C) normal saline fluid bolus
   (D) diltiazem

7. A physician is attempting to insert a central line and states that the internal jugular approach is superior since there is less chance of causing a pneumothorax. If you were to listen to the lung after the insertion attempt to assess for a pneumothorax, where would be the best location to hear the superior border of the lung?
   (A) slightly above the clavicle
   (B) slightly below the mediastinum

   (C) at the second ICS (intercostal space)
   (D) near the fourth ICS

Questions 8 and 9 refer to the following scenario.

A 28-year-old male is in the intensive care unit following a fall from a one-story rooftop 3 days ago. At the time he suffered a fractured left femur and right humerus. No neurological or chest trauma occurred. He has large contusions over his right lower flank. During the last 24 hr, his urine output has fallen to 300 ml. He has had a 1-lb increase in weight since yesterday. Vital signs are as follows:

blood pressure	140/86
pulse	106
respiratory rate	25
temperature	38.3°C

Laboratory studies reveal the following information:

Na^+	136
K^+	4.3
Cl^-	103
HCO_3^-	22
creatinine	2.8
BUN	36
urinary Na^+	72
urinary osmolality	302

8. Based on the preceding information, which condition is likely to be developing?
   (A) hypoperfusion with renal dysfunction (prerenal)

(B) acute tubular necrosis
(C) postrenal failure
(D) hypovolemic induced prerenal failure

9. What would the primary treatment include at this point?
(A) fluid bolus
(B) dialysis
(C) diuretics
(D) CAVHD (continuous arterial/venous hemodialysis)

10. Elevations in intracranial pressure can be caused by which of the following?
(A) hypovolemia
(B) hypercarbia
(C) hyperventilation
(D) hypotension

11. Interpret the following ECG rhythm strip.
(A) atrial tachycardia with block
(B) third-degree block
(C) second-degree block, type I
(D) atrial flutter with block

Questions 12 and 13 refer to the following scenario.

Early in the afternoon, another nurse asks you to examine her patient since she "looks different" than earlier and her blood pressure is lower than that recorded that morning. When you examine the patient, you notice that her right breast is larger than her left. Upon auscultation of her chest, you notice diminished breath sounds on the right and distant heart sounds. The nurse states that no new procedures have been performed, although a central line was inserted earlier in the day. The patient is confused, although this has been noted throughout her admission. She is now more restless, however, with her pulse oximeter displaying a value of 0.94 on 5 L/min of nasal oxygen. Her vital signs are as follows:

blood pressure	98/62
pulse	107
respiratory rate	31
temperature	36.8°C

12. Based on the preceding information, which condition is likely to be developing?
(A) pericardial tamponade
(B) sepsis
(C) pneumomediastinum
(D) right-sided pneumothorax

13. Which therapy should be instituted to treat the condition?
(A) pericardiocentesis
(B) anterior chest tube
(C) mediastinal chest tube
(D) No therapy is necessary; the patient requires only observation at this time.

14. Reverse isolation is frequently initiated when which immunologic finding is noted?
(A) lymphocyte count of 1500–3000/mm^3
(B) temperature elevation of 104°F
(C) left-sided shift in the differential
(D) granulocyte count of less than 500/mm^3

Questions 15 and 16 refer to the following scenario.

A 34-year-old male is in your unit following changes in behavior at home. His wife states that he has been on a liquid diet and has been drinking 5 L of water a day in an attempt to lose weight. He has generally been in good health and has not recently been to a physician. She states that her husband has had to to "go to the bathroom" more often since the diet started. His vital signs and laboratory data are listed below.

blood pressure	148/88
pulse	104
respiratory rate	26

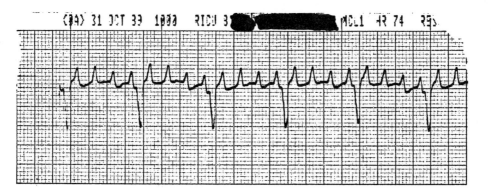

Figure for Question 11.

temperature	37.3
Na^+	108
K^+	3.8
Cl^-	78
HCO_3^-	21
osmolality	264

15. Based on the preceding information, which condition is likely to be developing?
    (A) malnutrition
    (B) acute high-output renal failure
    (C) hypo-osmolality-induced CNS (central nervous system) deterioration
    (D) hyponatremia-induced behavior changes

16. Which therapy should be initiated to treat this condition?
    (A) increased calories
    (B) diuretics
    (C) 1000 ml of 3% NaCl (sodium chloride)
    (D) vasopressin

17. Which of the following is used in clinical settings to estimate preload of the left ventricle?
    (A) CVP (central venous pressure)
    (B) SVR (systemic vascular resistance)
    (C) MAP (mean arterial pressure)
    (D) PAOP (pulmonary artery opening pressure)

Questions 18 and 19 refer to the following scenario.

A 21-year-old male college student is admitted to your unit following a fall from a tree during a prank. He is alert and oriented and complains of shortness of breath and chest pain on the right. He states that he landed on his right chest, a point confirmed by other witnesses. On physical examination, he has no overt trauma to the chest, breath sounds are diminished on the right, and the trachea is deviated to the left. His ECG shows nonspecific ST changes and analysis of his blood gases reveals the following:

pH	7.48
$PaCO_2$	28
PaO_2	69
FIO_2	room air

18. Based on the preceding information, which condition is developing?
    (A) myocardial contusion
    (B) open pneumothorax
    (C) tension pneumothorax
    (D) tracheal rupture

19. Which treatment would be indicated for his condition?
    (A) open thoracotomy
    (B) chest tube insertion
    (C) emergent tracheostomy
    (D) pericardiocentesis

20. A 49-year-old male is in your unit following surgery for colon cancer. During your shift, he develops a fever (39°C) and an increased white blood cell count (15,000). Levels of which of the following will be elevated if this is a new infection?
    (A) lymphocytes
    (B) monocytes
    (C) neutrophils
    (D) antibodies

Questions 21 and 22 refer to the following scenario.

A 24-year-old male is admitted to your unit after developing severe muscle weakness. His condition has been related to excessive ingestion of black licorice. His vital signs and electrolyte report are as follows:

blood pressure	134/72
pulse	106
respiratory rate	24
temperature	37°C
Na^+	147
K^+	1.8
Cl^-	116
HCO_3^-	22

21. Based on the preceding information, which other clinical symptoms may be present in this person?
    (A) tall peaked T waves on the ECG
    (B) PVCs (premature ventricular contractions) on the ECG
    (C) behavioral changes
    (D) decreased level of consciousness

22. Which therapy would be useful in treating this condition?
    (A) diuretics
    (B) sodium bicarbonate ($NaHCO_3$)
    (C) potassium chloride (KCl)
    (D) sodium chloride (NaCl) fluid bolus

23. A 48-year-old male is admitted to your unit following an episode of hematemesis. He states that he has had three such episodes prior to coming to the hospital. Based on this information, he is likely to be in a hypovolemic state and to experience loss of stroke volume.

Which of the following components of cardiac output will compensate for the loss of stroke volume?
(A) heart rate
(B) SVR (systemic vascular resistance)
(C) MAP (mean arterial pressure)
(D) CVP (central venous pressure)

24. A compensated respiratory acidosis would demonstrate which two blood gas findings?
(A) elevated $PaCO_2$ and decreased HCO_3^-
(B) decreased $PaCO_2$ and PaO_2
(C) increased HCO_3^- and decreased $PaCO_2$
(D) increased $PaCO_2$ and HCO_3^-

25. Upon performing an abdominal examination on your patient, you notice tympanic sounds upon percussing the left lower quadrant. Which sounds should be heard in the left lower quadrant under normal circumstances?
(A) tympanic
(B) resonant
(C) dull
(D) flat

26. A 55-year-old male has a history of systemic hypertension. Which of the following ECG changes are characteristic of chronic hypertension with left ventricular hypertrophy?
(A) large Q waves in II, III, and aVF
(B) a reversed R:S ratio in lead V_1
(C) large S waves in V_1 and large R waves in V_5
(D) ST segment elevation in all precordial leads

Questions 27 and 28 are based on the following scenario.

A 61-year-old female is admitted to your unit at 1500 after repair of an abdominal aortic aneurysm. Her admission vital signs and hemodynamics are stable and within normal limits. At 2000, she complains of abdominal discomfort unrelated to incisional pain. Her breath sounds are clear, her skin is cool, and she has no shortness of breath. The following hemodynamic information is available:

blood pressure	100/60
pulse	112
PA	23/10
PAOP	6
CVP	2
cardiac output	3.6
cardiac index	2.0

27. Based on the preceding information, which condition is likely to be developing?

(A) left ventricular failure
(B) hypovolemia
(C) sepsis
(D) cardiogenic shock

28. Which initial treatment would best support her hemodynamic function?
(A) furosemide (Lasix)
(B) dobutamine
(C) normal saline bolus
(D) dopamine

29. The primary effects of sepsis include which of the following?
(A) loss of consciousness
(B) increased pH
(C) increasing PaO_2 levels
(D) altered capillary permeability

Questions 30 and 31 refer to the following scenario.

A 24-year-old male is in your unit following a fight in which he received multiple stab wounds to his chest and abdomen. He is now in his fourth postoperative day and is being considered for transfer to the floor. On your shift, he develops a fever of 38.6°C. He complains of increasing shortness of breath and you note that his pulse oximeter reading has decreased from 0.99 to 0.92 in the last hour. A chest film reveals wide-spread infiltrates in both lungs. He is alert and oriented, although he states that he feels "tired." His heart rate is 122 (up from 84) and his respiratory rate is 33 (up from 18). Blood gas analysis and laboratory data reveal the following:

pH	7.33
$PaCO_2$	30
PaO_2	67
HCO_3^-	18
FIO_2	0.50
white blood cells	15,400
segmented neutrophils	66
lymphocytes	19
monocytes	11
other	4

30. Based on the preceding information, which condition is likely to be developing?
(A) recurrent atelectasis
(B) mucous plugging
(C) sepsis
(D) generalized pneumonia

31. Which therapy is most likely to be effective in improving the clinical situation?

(Answers on pg. 612.)

(A) oxygen therapy
(B) postural drainage and percussion
(C) aerosol therapy
(D) antibiotic administration

Questions 32 and 33 refer to the following scenario.

A 59-year-old male is admitted to your unit with chest pain for the last hour. It is unrelieved by rest or nitroglycerin. He is short of breath and mildly orthopneic. A 12-lead ECG indicates ST segment elevation in V_1 through V_4 with ST segment depression in II, III, and aVF. No Q waves are present.

32. Based on the preceding symptoms and ECG findings, which condition is likely to be developing?
    (A) Prinzmetal's angina
    (B) inferior MI (myocardial infarction)
    (C) CHF (congestive heart failure); no MI can be occurring because of the absence of Q waves
    (D) anterior MI

33. Which of the following treatments is most likely to prevent further myocardial damage?
    (A) tPA (tissue plasminogen activator)
    (B) nitroglycerin (TNG)
    (C) dobutamine
    (D) furosemide (Lasix)

Questions 34 and 35 refer to the following scenario.

A thin, 64-year-old female was admitted to your unit with severe shortness of breath accompanying her diagnosis of COPD (chronic obstructive pulmonary disease). She had complained of gradually increasing shortness of breath over the past 2 days. Her oral tempature is 38°C. Her chest film indicates a consolidation in the left lower lobe. She has the following blood gas values:

pH	7.36
PaO_2	52
$PaCO_2$	33
HCO_3^-	26
FIO_2	0.40

34. Based on the preceding information, which condition is likely to be developing?
    (A) acute pulmonary oxygenation failure
    (B) acute pulmonary oxygenation and ventilation failure
    (C) acute and chronic ventilation failure
    (D) chronic ventilation failure

35. Treatment of this condition would center on which of the following areas?
    (A) intubation and mechanical ventilation
    (B) PEEP (positive end expiratory pressure) or CPAP (continuous positive airway pressure) therapy
    (C) antibiotic and oxygen therapy
    (D) bronchodilator and IPPB (intermittent positive pressure, breathing) treatment

36. A sudden increase in pain in a patient admitted with duodenal ulcers may indicate that which condition is developing?
    (A) increase in bleeding
    (B) spreading of the ulcer to the pain-sensitive gastrum
    (C) perforation of the ulcer
    (D) pancreatic ulcer formation

Questions 37 and 38 refer to the following scenario.

A 73-year-old female in previously good health is admitted to your unit with complaints of intermittent chest pain for the past 6 hr. The chest pain is unrelated to activity, although it worsens if she "moves around during a spell." She has no shortness of breath but does complain of "swelling" of her feet during the day. A 12-lead ECG demonstrates ST-segment depression in I, aVL, V_5, and V_6. No Q waves exist in the ECG. Her finger oximeter reveals an SaO_2 value of 0.96 on room air.

37. Based on the preceding information, which condition is likely to be developing?
    (A) pulmonary emboli
    (B) angina
    (C) anterior MI (myocardial infarction)
    (D) left ventricular failure

38. Which treatment should be initially started for this condition?
    (A) furosemide (Lasix)
    (B) dobutamine
    (C) nitroglycerin
    (D) nifedipine

Questions 39 and 40 refer to the following scenario.

A 56-year-old, slightly overweight male is admitted to your unit with exacerbation of COPD (chronic obstructive pulmonary disease). A physical examination reveals that he is short of breath, is alert and oriented, and demonstrates inspiratory crackles and expiratory wheezes. He has circumoral cyanosis and pedal edema. Analysis of his blood gases reveals the following:

pH	7.34
PaO_2	52
$PaCO_2$	73
HCO_3^-	40
FIO_2	room air

39. Based on this information, what factor is altered which will change this patient's ability to breathe normally?
(A) PaO_2
(B) $PaCO_2$
(C) pH
(D) HCO_3^-

40. Which initial form of treatment is indicated in this patient?
(A) judicious oxygen therapy
(B) intubation and mechanical ventilation
(C) PEEP (positive end expiratory pressure) or CPAP (continuous positive airway pressure)
(D) diuretic therapy

41. Clinical symptoms of sepsis may vary, depending on the stage. Which of the following are not considered common septic symptoms?
(A) hypothermia
(B) hyperthermia
(C) bradycardia
(D) tachypnea

Questions 42 and 43 refer to the following scenario.

A 68-year-old male is admitted to your unit with severe abdominal pain radiating to the back. The pain does not subside with rest or position change. Oxygen therapy and sublingual nitroglycerin do not relieve the pain. He is diaphoretic with cool skin, but has no difficulty breathing. Breath sounds are clear. S_1 and S_2 are heard clearly and are the only heart sounds. His blood pressure is 172/100, pulse 114. His ECG shows a 1-mm ST-segment depression in V_1.

42. Based on the preceding information, which condition is likely to be developing?
(A) anterior MI (myocardial infarction)
(B) recalcitrant angina
(C) pulmonary emboli
(D) abdominal aortic aneurysm

43. Which treatment would most likely be employed in this patient?
(A) abdominal aortic aneurysm repair
(B) thrombolytic therapy
(C) intravenous nitroglycerin
(D) sedation

44. The "high airway pressure" alarm on the ventilator is activated, indicating a worsening of the patient's pulmonary dynamic compliance. Which of the following are not potential reasons for the pulmonary dynamic compliance (lung stiffness) to worsen?
(A) airway secretions
(B) mucous plugging
(C) accidental disconnection from the ventilation
(D) coughing

45. Initial symptoms of colon cancer typically include which of the following?
(A) epigastric cramping
(B) anorexia
(C) rectal bleeding
(D) ascites

46. A 20-year-old male is in your unit with a severe head injury following a motor vehicle accident. He has been in the unit for 24 hr. On your shift, his ICP (intracranial pressure) changes from 14 to 31. The physician states that the volume–pressure relationship in the brain may have reached a critical point. Which of the following statements best describes the volume–pressure relationship within the skull when brain compliance is decreased?
(A) Large increases in volume will cause small pressure increases.
(B) Large increases in pressure will cause small volume increases.
(C) Small increases in volume will cause small pressure increases.
(D) Small increases in volume will cause large pressure increases.

47. Maintaining the $PaCO_2$ at 25–30 mm Hg can be helpful in managing ICP (intracranial pressure) because of its effect on which of the mechanisms listed below?
(A) cerebral blood flow
(B) cerebral tissue edema
(C) production of CSF (cerebrospinal fluid)
(D) systemic blood pressure

48. A 50-year-old female returns from cardiac catheterization with a report of a complete obstruction of the left anterior descending artery. Which condition may result from this situation?
(A) superior vena caval syndrome
(B) anterior MI (myocardial infarction)
(C) inferior MI
(D) posterior MI

49. A patient admitted with the diagnosis of cardiogenic shock requires mechanical ventilation. Which form of ventilation would be most appropriate to reduce his work of breathing?
    (A) IMV (intermittent mandatory ventilation)
    (B) pressure support ventilation
    (C) assist control ventilation
    (D) PEEP (positive end expiratory pressure)

Questions 50 and 51 refer to the following scenario.

A 62-year-old female is in the intensive care unit following a cardiac arrest 2 days ago. She is responsive only to painful stimuli. Vital signs include a blood pressure of 86/56 and a pulse of 110. She is receiving mechanical ventilation on assist control of 10 breaths/min (with no spontaneous breathing), tidal volume 750 ml, FIO_2 0.40. Her urine output has decreased over the past 24 hr to 150 ml. The latest hemodynamic data are as follows:

PA	23/8
PAOP	7
CVP	2
cardiac output	3.7
cardiac index	2.2

Laboratory data are listed below:

	Serum	Urine
Na^+	146	11
K^+	3.6	
osmolality	288	1090
Cl^-	96	
creatinine	3	
BUN	60	

50. Based on the preceding information, which condition is likely to be developing?
    (A) hypovolemic prerenal azotemia
    (B) acute tubular necrosis
    (C) postrenal failure secondary to ureteral obstruction
    (D) hypernatremia-induced renal failure

51. Which of the following treatments would be indicated at this point?
    (A) diuretics
    (B) fluid bolus
    (C) norepinephrine (Levophed)
    (D) dobutamine

52. A 78-year-old female is admitted from the emergency room after being found unresponsive at home. She is hypotensive and requires mechanical ventilation to support her breathing. A pulmonary artery catheter is inserted to assist in identifying her primary problem. The initial ECG is unremarkable. At 0500, the physician requests that dobutamine administration be started to improve her hemodynamics. In the readings to be obtained at 0600, which parameters would be expected if the dobutamine has been effective?

	0400	0500
blood pressure	106/66	104/62
pulse	111	105
cardiac index	2.4	2.5
PA	34/23	32/21
PAOP	21	17
CVP	12	11

    (A) decreased pulmonary capillary wedge pressure and increased stroke volume
    (B) increased stroke volume and increased CVP
    (C) increased pulmonary artery pressure
    (D) decreased ejection fraction

53. A 59-year-old male is in your unit with pulmonary edema from an MI (myocardial infarction). He currently is on assist/control ventilation and is triggering the ventilator for a total rate of 32. In order to read his PAOP (pulmonary artery opening pressure) tracing accurately and avoid respiratory artifact, where is the best location on the waveform?
    (A) end inspiration
    (B) end expiration
    (C) initial expiration
    (D) initial inspiration

Questions 54 and 55 refer to the following scenario.

A 32-year-old female is admitted to your unit following a house fire in which she was rescued after losing consciousness. She has a 30% burn, with most of the burns on her back and legs.

54. Upon admission to the unit, which therapies are most likely to be initiated?
    (A) conservative fluid resuscitation
    (B) topical antimicrobial agents (e.g., silver sulfadiazine, Silvadene)
    (C) occlusive dry dressings
    (D) sedation and paralysis

55. Which test would be performed to assess the extent of her smoke inhalation?
    (A) chest roentgenography
    (B) measurement of carboxyhemoglobin level

(C) arterial blood gas analysis
(D) ventilation/perfusion lung scan

56. Which findings, due to increased dead space, are almost always present in a patient with a pulmonary embolism?
(A) tachypnea and tachycardia
(B) hyperventilation and hypercarbia
(C) decreased pH and hypoxemia
(D) increased respiratory rate and decreased tidal volume

Questions 57 and 58 refer to the following scenario.

A 61-year-old female is admitted to your unit from her physician's office for possible dehydration. The dehydration is the result of anorexia and low fluid intake during the last several days because of a "cold." The family states that she has shown behavioral changes and has been extremely lethargic during the last 2 days. She has lost 10 lb in the last week, probably because of an increased urine output, based on family history. Laboratory results reveal the following information:

Na^+	153
K^+	3.5
Cl^-	114
HCO_3^-	20
osmolality	367
glucose	503

57. Based on the preceding information, which condition is present?
(A) insulin reaction
(B) DKA (diabetic ketoacidosis)
(C) thyroid storm
(D) HHNK (hyperosmolar, hyperglycemic, nonketotic) coma

58. Treatment for this condition would center on which therapy?
(A) glucose bolus (50 ml of $D_{50}W$)
(B) insulin bolus and normal saline
(C) insulin drip without bolus
(D) thyroxine and glucocorticoids

59. A 62-year-old male is admitted to your unit with possible pericarditis. If pericarditis is present, which of the following symptoms would be present?
(A) S_3 or gallop rhythm
(B) split S_2
(C) pleural friction rub worsening on inspiration
(D) ST-segment elevation in most leads of the 12-lead ECG

60. Given the following blood gas values, identify which condition is present.

pH	7.23
Pao_2	85
$Paco_2$	26
HCO_3^-	16

(A) respiratory alkalosis alone
(B) metabolic acidosis alone
(C) combined respiratory and metabolic acidosis
(D) respiratory alkalosis and metabolic acidosis

61. A 59-year-old female with a history of alcoholism is admitted to your unit after being found unresponsive. During the next 24 hr, she develops decreased blood flow to her distal extremities, manifested by discoloration of her hands and feet. The physician believes that DIC (disseminated intravascular clotting) may be taking place. Which of the following tests may help confirm that DIC is present?
(A) measurement of platelet levels
(B) determination of bleeding time
(C) measurement of fibrinogen degradation product levels
(D) determination of plasminogen to plasmin converting time

62. Immunoglobulins are derived from which component of the white blood cell differential?
(A) B-cell lymphocytes
(B) T-cell lymphocytes
(C) segmented neutrophils
(D) monocytes

63. Hyperglycemia frequently presents with all of the following physical symptoms but one. Which of the following symptoms does NOT characterize hyperglycemic reactions?
(A) cool skin
(B) increased respirations
(C) increased urine output
(D) tachycardia

64. The PAOP (pulmonary artery opening pressure) estimates which of the following hemodynamic parameters?
(A) left ventricular end diastolic pressure
(B) mean pulmonary artery pressure
(C) cardiac output
(D) left ventricular end systolic pressure

65. Which of the following is the most accurate estimate of intrapulmonary shunting?

(Answers on pg. 616.)

(A) A-a (alveolar-arterial) gradient
(B) $PaCO_2$–$PERCO_2$ gradient
(C) respiratory index
(D) PaO_2/FIO_2 ratio

66. Major complications of pancreatic surgery include which of the following?
(A) overproduction of insulin
(B) stimulation of glucagon production
(C) inhibition of trypsin production
(D) leakage of digestive enzymes into the pancreas

67. A 73-year-old male with a history of CHF (congestive heart failure) is placed on an afterload-reducing drug. Which of the following measures would be used to assess the effectiveness of afterload reduction?
(A) PAOP (pulmonary artery opening pressure)
(B) CVP (central venous pressure)
(C) SVR (systemic vascular resistance)
(D) MAP (mean arterial pressure)

68. A 33-year-old female is admitted with the diagnosis of possible adrenal cortical tumor. Levels of which of the following hormones would NOT likely be altered in this situation?

(A) cortisol
(B) epinephrine
(C) aldosterone
(D) androgens

69. While interpreting a pulmonary capillary wedge pressure, you note the presence of giant V waves. Which of the following conditions can produce giant V waves on a hemodynamic waveform?
(A) mitral regurgitation
(B) left bundle branch block
(C) atrial septal defects
(D) hypovolemia

70. A 71-year-old male with the diagnosis of chronic lung disease has cyanosis of the nailbeds. How can a patient have cyanosis and still have adequate oxygen transport?
(A) He can if the oxyhemoglobin curve is shifted to the left.
(B) He can if the hemoglobin and cardiac output are adequate.
(C) He can if the FIO_2 is high enough to raise CaO_2 values.
(D) Oxygen transport cannot be adequate with the presence of cyanosis.

71. A 54-year-old female is in your unit with acute tubular necrosis. As a result of the acute renal failure, she has developed hyperkalemia. She does not yet have vascular access for dialysis to be initiated. Which of the following therapies could be used to treat the hyperkalemia prior to the use of dialysis?
(A) ammonium chloride resin
(B) Kayexalate
(C) calcium chloride—500 mg
(D) sodium chloride—500-ml fluid bolus

Questions 72 and 73 refer to the following scenario.

A 23-year-old male is in the intensive care unit following a closed head injury from a fight. During the second day of hospitalization, he develops a severe thirst and is consuming 1000 ml of water per shift. Urine output is 2000 ml per shift. An electrolyte analysis is obtained and reveals the following data:

Na^+	150
K^+	3.6
Cl^-	118
HCO_3^-	23
osmolality	324
glucose	178
urinary osmolality	304
urinary Na^+	61

72. Based on the preceding information, which condition is developing?
(A) hyperosmolar, nonketotic acidosis
(B) diabetes insipidus
(C) diabetic ketoacidosis
(D) thyroid storm

73. Which treatment would be indicated for this condition?
(A) insulin-glucose infusion
(B) DDAVP (desmopressin acetate)
(C) Hageman factor in intravenous form
(D) diuretics

Questions 74 and 75 refer to the following scenario.

A 49-year-old female is admitted to your unit with a history of primary pulmonary hypertension. Her pulmonary artery blood pressure is 70/46. She complains of a marked decrease in exercise capability and persistent shortness of breath. Her 12-lead ECG shows the following: 5-mm R wave in V_1 and V_2, 4-mm S wave in V_1. She has small Q waves in leads II, III, and aVF. Her underlying rhythm is sinus tachycardia.

74. Based on the preceding information, which condition is likely to be present?

(A) pulmonary edema

(B) non-Q-wave anterior–inferior MI (myocardial infarction)

(C) left ventricular hypertrophy

(D) right ventricular hypertrophy

75. Treatment for this condition would most likely include which of the following?
    (A) Mannitol and fluid restriction
    (B) oxygen therapy and dobutamine
    (C) vasodilators, e.g., protacyclin and calcium channel blockers
    (D) dopamine at 6 mcg/kg/min

76. The chest film with ARDS (adult respiratory distress syndrome) is typically described by which of the following terms?
    (A) hilar infiltrates
    (B) air bronchioles
    (C) white-out
    (D) bibasilar infiltrates

Questions 77 and 78 refer to the following scenario.

Two days after a lung resection in a 61-year-old, 78-kg male, the physician requests your advice on nutritional replenishment for the patient. He states that, before surgery, he lost "11 pounds." He is currently receiving 1000 ml of D_5W and 500 ml of NaCl per day. Bowel sounds are present and the patient states that he is hungry. He has the following vital signs:

blood pressure	118/70
pulse	88
respiratory rate	22
temperature	37.8°C

77. Based on the preceding information, how many calories is the patient receiving at the present time?
    (A) 170 kcal
    (B) 250 kcal
    (C) 500 kcal
    (D) 1000 kcal

78. Based on the preceding information, which action should be taken?
    (A) Start the patient on 1800 ml of a full-strength enteral preparation, e.g., Osmolite or Ensure.
    (B) Start the patient on hyperalimentation with 1500 ml of $D_{50}W$ with 10% amino acids.
    (C) No action is necessary; the current regimen is adequate in meeting nutritional needs.
    (D) No enteral feeding should be started, keep the patient on an NPO regimen for the first week and increase the D_5W volume to 2000 ml per day.

Questions 79 and 80 refer to the following scenario.

A 56-year-old male is admitted to your unit from the cardiac catheterization laboratory, where an angioplasty of the right coronary artery was performed. He currently has a balloon pump in place, set at an inflation ratio of 1:2. His cardiac output is 5.1, with a blood pressure of 142/82. After admission, he complains of a headache unrelieved by acetaminophen. During the next 24 hr, he is weaned off the balloon pump and it is removed. The headache, however, remains and is unrelieved by acetaminophen plus 30 mg of codeine.

79. Which of the following conditions is possibly developing?
    (A) ventricular aneurysm
    (B) pericardial tamponade
    (C) distal migration of a coronary thrombus into the head
    (D) intracerebral bleeding

80. Which of the following actions should be taken?
    (A) repeat of the cardiac catheterization
    (B) cessation of heparin
    (C) administration of thrombolytics
    (D) administration of a fentanyl drip for pain relief

81. Which component of the immune system has reduced effectiveness in AIDS (acquired immune deficiency syndrome) and/or when the drug cyclosporine is used?
    (A) B lymphocytes
    (B) T4 lymphocytes
    (C) T8 lymphocytes
    (D) neutrophils

82. Pulsus paradoxus is manifested by which of the following symptoms?
    (A) decrease in blood pressure on inspiration
    (B) increase in heart rate on inspiration
    (C) decrease in central venous pressure with the addition of PEEP (positive end expiratory pressure)
    (D) increase in blood pressure on inspiration

Questions 83 and 84 refer to the following scenario.

A 59-year-old female was admitted yesterday to your unit with the diagnosis of sepsis, accompanied by a fever (temperature 39°C). Over the past few hours, she has developed severe shortness of breath and anxiety. Her respiratory rate is 40 breaths/min and her breathing is labored. Lung sounds are present bilaterally with widespread crackles and scattered wheezes. A chest film indicates generalized opacity. Analysis of her blood gases indicates the following:

pH	7.46
$Paco_2$	30
Pao_2	49
Fio_2	0.60 via face mask

83. Based on the preceding information, which condition is likely to be developing?
    (A) severe pneumonia
    (B) ARDS (adult respiratory distress syndrome)
    (C) generalized atelectasis
    (D) cardiogenic pulmonary edema

84. Which of the following treatments would be most appropriate to treat the pulmonary disturbance?
    (A) increased oxygen therapy
    (B) sedation and diuretics
    (C) PEEP (positive end expiratory pressure) or CPAP (continuous positive airway pressure)
    (D) bronchodilators

85. Which of the following is responsible for fibrinolytic activity?
    (A) plasmin
    (B) thrombin
    (C) factor I
    (D) factor X

86. Which type of treatment would be preferred in reducing excessive bleeding in a patient with hemophilia A?
    (A) whole blood
    (B) platelets
    (C) factor IX
    (D) cryoprecipitate

87. A drug that acts to alter depolarization of cardiac muscle cells will act in which phase of the action potential?
    (A) phase 1
    (B) phase 2
    (C) phase 3
    (D) phase 0

88. A 67-year-old male is admitted to your unit following coronary artery bypass grafting. He is in the unit for 6 hr and is nearly rewarmed to normal body temperature. However, you note that his Svo_2 has fallen from 0.65 to 0.56 during your shift. Which of the following is LEAST likely to be responsible for the fall in the Svo_2 level?
    (A) decreased hemoglobin
    (B) decreased cardiac output

    (C) increased oxygen consumption
    (D) decreased Pao_2

89. Treating pancreatic cancer can be surgically attempted by means of which procedure?
    (A) pancreaticoantrectomy
    (B) islet cell transplant
    (C) pancreaticohepatic resection (Lewis procedure)
    (D) pancreatoduodenectomy (Whipple procedure)

Questions 90 and 91 refer to the following scenario.

A 38-year-old female is in the intensive care unit for treatment of hypotension related to sepsis. Her primary diagnosis is metastatic breast cancer. Her current vital signs are listed below:

blood pressure	88/58
pulse	118
respiratory rate	36
temperature	39°C

Earlier in the shift, you noted she had begun spontaneous bleeding from a central intravenous line. The physician ordered coagulation studies, which revealed the following:

platelets	60,000
prothrombin time	30
activated partial thromboplastin time	80
fibrin degradation products	70

90. Based on the preceding information, which condition is likely to be developing?
    (A) von Willebrand's syndrome
    (B) disseminated intravascular clotting
    (C) vitamin K deficiency
    (D) primary platelet dysfunction

91. Which treatment would most likely to be given for this condition?
    (A) fresh frozen plasma
    (B) cyroprecipitate
    (C) factor IX
    (D) intravenous vitamin K

92. Mitral valve papillary muscle rupture would initially present with which of the following signs or symptoms?
    (A) distended neck veins
    (B) systolic murmur
    (C) low PAOP (pulmonary arterial opening pressure)
    (D) pulsus paradoxus

93. In a patient with thick airway secretions, which of the following would best aid secretion removal?
    (A) stimulating the cough reflex
    (B) postural drainage
    (C) instillation of saline into the airway
    (D) increasing suction pressure to 300 mm Hg during endotracheal suctioning

94. A patient admitted to your unit after ingestion of a caustic acid solution could be expected to receive which treatment?
    (A) ipecac to induce vomiting
    (B) administration of ammonium chloride
    (C) gastric irrigation with large volumes of water
    (D) immediate exploratory laparotomy

95. Which of the following is/are consistent with symptoms of spinal shock?
    (A) loss of autonomic nervous control
    (B) loss of cranial nerve function
    (C) decreased level of consciousness
    (D) reflex paralysis below level of injury

96. Left ventricular failure alone presents with all of the symptoms listed below but one. Select the symptom that does NOT accompany simple left ventricular failure.
    (A) tachycardia
    (B) increased PAOP (pulmonary artery opening pressure)
    (C) increased CVP (central venous pressure)
    (D) shortness of breath

97. Which of the following sets of blood gases values is illustrative of pure respiratory acidosis?
    (A) pH 7.28, $PaCO_2$ 22, HCO_3^- 16
    (B) pH 7.38, $PaCO_2$ 62, HCO_3^- 36
    (C) pH 7.48, $PaCO_2$ 31, HCO_3^- 24
    (D) pH 7.22, $PaCO_2$ 62, HCO_3^- 25

98. You are caring for a 37-year-old female admitted with an intracerebral bleed. The nurse on the preceding shift tells you that a neurological examination was performed on your patient and that she had an abnormal "doll's eyes" test. Which of the following descriptions best describes an abnormal oculocephalic response to the "doll's eyes" test?
    (A) Bright light in one eye causes a constriction of the opposite pupil.
    (B) The eyes follow the direction of a quick turn of the head.
    (C) The eyes tend to remain opposite to the direction of the head turn.
    (D) The eyes develop nystagmus following instillation of cold water into the ear.

Questions 99 and 100 refer to the following scenario.

A 25-year-old female is admitted to your unit following a motor vehicle accident. She complains of abdominal pain although no external evidence of trauma exists. Her neurological examination is normal, although she appears anxious. Vital signs are blood pressure 86/54, pulse 118, respiratory rate 32. She has no specific abdominal pain although left upper quadrant pain is slightly more evident. Bowel sounds are distant but present. Her skin is cool and clammy. As you examine her, you note that her blood pressure falls to 72/48.

99. Based on the preceding information, which condition is likely to be developing?
    (A) vasovagal reaction to the accident situation
    (B) liver laceration
    (C) pancreatic hemorrhage
    (D) splenic rupture

100. Which treatment would be avoided in this situation?
    (A) fluid expansion with lactated Ringer's and monitoring of the blood pressure
    (B) placing a nasogastric tube and performing gastric lavage
    (C) preparing for an exploratory laparotomy
    (D) placement in Trendelenburg position

101. Interpret the following ECG rhythm strip.
    (A) ventricular tachycardia
    (B) ventricular fibrillation
    (C) atrial tachycardia
    (D) atrial flutter (figure on page 620)

Questions 102 and 103 refer to the following scenario.

A 55-year-old male is in your unit with the diagnosis of cardiomyopathy. His ejection fraction as measured during a cardiac catheterization is 19%. He is in the unit now with increasing shortness of breath, decreased urine output, and episodes of confusion. His admission ECG indicates ST-segment depression in leads V_1–V_4. He currently has a pulmonary artery catheter in place to help in the assessment of his hemodynamics. The following information is available from the catheter:

blood pressure	114/62
pulse	102
cardiac index	2.3
arterial pressure	42/26
PAOP	24
CVP	14

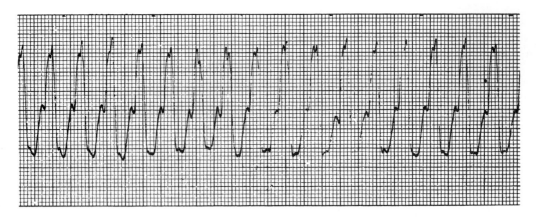

Figure for Question 101.

102. Based on the preceding information, which situation exists?
    (A) left ventricular failure
    (B) right ventricular failure
    (C) biventricular failure
    (D) anterior wall MI (myocardial infarction)

103. Which therapy is most likely to be effective in improving the ejection fraction in this patient?
    (A) dobutamine
    (B) oxygen therapy
    (C) dopamine
    (D) nitroglycerin

104. Nursing care for the immunosuppressed patient includes all of the following EXCEPT:
    (A) assessment of the mouth and throat
    (B) taking only rectal temperatures
    (C) avoiding live flowers and plants in the room
    (D) enteral as opposed to parenteral nutrition

105. Which of the following statements best describe the high mortality associated with the person who progresses from sepsis to septic shock?
    (A) Respiratory failure occurs too rapidly for antibiotics to work.
    (B) Cardiac failure occurs too rapidly for antibiotics to work.
    (C) Sepsis organisms are immune to antibiotics.
    (D) No treatments exist that address the primary problem in sepsis.

106. An inferior MI (myocardial infarction) is manifested on the 12-lead ECG in which of the following leads?
    (A) V_1 to V_4
    (B) I, aVL, V_5, V_6
    (C) V_{3R} to V_{6R}
    (D) II, III, and aVF

107. Which of the following is NOT an appropriate parameter to measure to determine adequacy for weaning from mechanical ventilation?
    (A) minute ventilation
    (B) tidal volume
    (C) peak inspiratory pressure
    (D) forced expiratory volume in 1 sec (FEV_1)

Questions 108 and 109 refer to the following scenario.

A 65-year-old male is admitted to your unit following a coronary artery bypass graft and valve replacement. During your shift, he complains of left-side chest pain. His lung sounds are clear, he does not complain of shortness of breath, and he has an SpO_2 value of 0.92 on 40% oxygen. His mediastinal chest tube has drained 10 ml on your shift. His hemodynamics are listed below.

blood pressure	112/70
pulse	112
cardiac index	2.0
arterial pressure	32/20
PAOP	19
CVP	19

108. Based on the preceding information, which condition is likely to be developing?
    (A) left ventricular failure
    (B) right ventricular failure
    (C) pericardial tamponade
    (D) pulmonary emboli

109. What would be the most appropriate therapy to treat this situation?
    (A) dobutamine
    (B) stripping of the mediastinal tube
    (C) thrombolytics
    (D) pericardiocentesis

Questions 110 and 111 refer to the following scenario.

A 31-year-old male is admitted to your unit with ARD (acute respiratory distress). He has lost weight over the past few weeks, has a generalized lymphadenopathy, and is febrile (39.5°C). He has been told in the past his blood tested positive for HIV (human immunodeficiency virus).

110. Based on the preceding information, what is the most likely cause of the ARD?
    (A) *Pneumocystis carinii* pneumonia
    (B) *Haemophilus influenzae* pneumonia
    (C) ARDS (adult respiratory distress syndrome)
    (D) Kaposi's sarcoma

111. Aside from oxygenation and ventilation support, treatment for this condition would most likely include which therapy?
    (A) aminoglycosides
    (B) ticarcillin
    (C) pentamidine
    (D) amphotericin

112. Right ventricular infarctions are best seen in which of the following leads?
    (A) V_1 to V_4
    (B) I, aVL, V_5, V_6
    (C) V_{3R} to V_{6R}
    (D) II, III, and aVF

113. A 31-year-old female is admitted to your unit following a motor vehicle accident in which she received crush injuries to the chest. She is currently intubated and on AMV (assist/control mechanical ventilation). Her PaO_2 is not responding to oxygen therapy so the physician decides to add PEEP (positive end expiratory pressure) to her therapy. In monitoring the effectiveness of the PEEP, which parameters should be present to indicate an appropriate response to the therapy?
    (A) drop in $PaCO_2$ levels
    (B) increase in PaO_2 and SaO_2
    (C) increase in pH
    (D) increase in MAP (mean airway pressure)

Questions 114 and 115 refer to the following scenario.

A 24-year-old female is admitted in an unresponsive condition to your unit. No overt signs of trauma are present. Vital signs include blood pressure 110/80, pulse 96, respiratory rate 21, and temperature 37.5°C. Shortly after admission to the unit, she has a generalized seizure. A subsequent head CT (computed tomography) scan is negative and a neurolog-

ical examination reveals no abnormalities. Laboratory serum data indicate the following:

Na^+	111
K^+	3.3
Cl^-	74
HCO_3^-	25
PaO_2	61
$PaCO_2$	34
pH	7.43

114. Based on the preceding information, which condition is likely to be the cause of the neurological symptoms?
    (A) hypoxemia
    (B) pontomedullary hemorrhage
    (C) hypokalemia
    (D) hyponatremia

115. Correction of the abnormal sodium level should be done slowly in order to avoid which of the following?
    (A) dehydration
    (B) cerebral injury
    (C) exacerbation of hypoxemia
    (D) spinal shock

116. Which of the following is an indication of an aberrantly conducted APC (atrial premature contraction) versus a PVC (premature ventricular contraction)?
    (A) rsR' in V_1
    (B) precordial concordancy
    (C) Rr' in V_1
    (D) extreme right axis deviation

117. Which of the following is the best indicator of alveolar ventilation?
    (A) PaO_2 levels
    (B) minute ventilation
    (C) $PaCO_2$ values
    (D) respiratory rate

Questions 118 and 119 refer to the following scenario.

A 71-year-old female returns to your unit from the cardiac catheterization laboratory. While in the cath lab, she was noted to have 70% obstruction of her left anterior descending artery, 95% obstruction of her circumflex artery, and 60% obstruction of her right coronary artery. An angioplasty was performed on her circumflex artery, which reduced the degree of obstruction to 30%.

118. If she were to develop a reocclusion of the circumflex artery, which type of MI (myocardial infarction) could occur?

(Answers on pg. 622.)

(A) anterior
(B) inferior
(C) lateral
(D) posterior

119. Which type of ECG changes are likely to occur in the first 24 hr postangioplasty?
(A) posterior hemiblocks
(B) left axis deviations
(C) bradycardias
(D) bundle branch blocks

Questions 120 and 121 refer to the following scenario.

Following a subtotal thyroidectomy, your patient develops an increased heart rate (120) and temperature (39.7°C). She becomes confused, disoriented, and agitated. Her blood pressure changes from 130/78 to 170/100. Breath sounds are equal, and a neurological examination is normal except for the presence of agitation and confusion. Analysis of her blood gases reveals the following:

pH	7.47
$PaCO_2$	32
PaO_2	90
FIO_2	room air

120. Based on the preceding information, which condition would you suspect is most likely to be developing?
(A) parathyroid storm
(B) cerebral hemorrhage
(C) pulmonary emboli
(D) thyroid storm

121. Which initial treatment would most likely be administered?
(A) calcium gluconate
(B) heparin
(C) Inderal (propranolol)
(D) thyroxine

122. A 22-year-old female is admitted to your unit for treatment of a supraventricular tachycardia. Which of the following medications may be employed to try to terminate this dysrhythmia?
(A) lidocaine
(B) bretylium
(C) epinephrine
(D) adenosine

123. PSV (pressure support ventilation) differs from IMV (intermittent mandatory ventilation) and AMV (assist/control mechanical ventilation) in which of the following ways?

(A) Volumes are delivered within pressure limits.
(B) Volumes are delivered within time limits.
(C) PSV is useful when the pulmonary compliance is at least 15 cm H_2O, whereas IMV and AMV can only be used at 10 cm H_2O.
(D) PSV requires a preset tidal volume.

124. A 39-year-old male is in your unit after being found in an unresponsive state in the city park. He currently responds to deep, painful stimuli. He has no identification and no past medical history, although his clothes have the odor of alcohol. His vital signs and laboratory data are as follows:

blood pressure	116/68
pulse	96
respiratory rate	29
temperature	36.6°C
Na^+	135
K^+	3.9
Cl^-	100
HCO_3^-	22
BUN	92
glucose	196
SGOT	652
alkaline phosphatase	155
lactate	14

Based on the preceding information, which condition is likely to be present?

(A) hepatic encephalopathy
(B) diabetic coma
(C) hepatorenal syndrome
(D) portacaval syndrome

125. A 43-year-old male is admitted to your unit following a motorcycle accident. He was thrown from the cycle and skidded 150 feet in gravel along the side of the road. He now has multiple contusions and abrasions, although his neurological examination is unremarkable. He does, however, develop a rhabdomyolysis with a resultant lactic acidosis. His current laboratory data are as follows:

pH	7.28
PaO_2	81
$PaCO_2$	33
HCO_3^-	19
lactate	4
Na^+	138
K^+	5.4
Cl^-	104

In this situation, the house officer wants to treat the potassium level of 5.4. What is the relationship between potassium and the lactic acidosis seen in this situation?

(A) K^+ decreases with large muscle injury
(B) K^+ increases with large muscle injury
(C) as pH decreases, K^+ decreases
(D) as pH increases, K^+ increases

126. Unstable angina is differentiated from stable angina by which of the following?
(A) chest pain at rest
(B) Q-wave development on the ECG
(C) ST-segment depression in affected leads
(D) chest pain relieved by nitroglycerin

Questions 127 and 128 refer to the following scenario.

A 52-year-old male with the diagnosis of lymphocytic leukemia is admitted to your unit with mild hypotension, hypoxemia, and shortness of breath. He is placed on AMV (assist/control mechanical ventilation), tidal volume (V_T) 750 ml, respiratory rate 12, total rate 33, FIO_2 0.70. He is very anxious and requires sedation to alleviate the anxiety. A pulmonary artery catheter is inserted and blood gases drawn. The following information is obtained:

blood pressure	108/66
pulse	116
cardiac output	4
cardiac index	2.3
PA	46/30
PAOP	10
CVP	10
PaO_2	56
$PaCO_2$	32
pH	7.36
HCO_3^-	23

127. Based on the preceding information, which condition is developing?
(A) noncardiogenic pulmonary edema
(B) cardiogenic pulmonary edema
(C) right ventricular failure causing pulmonary edema
(D) hypovolemia

128. Which strategy would be followed in the treatment of this patient?
(A) Administer fluids to increase the PAOP (pulmonary artery opening pressure).
(B) Give diuretics to keep the PAOP as low as possible.
(C) Give bicarbonate to treat the metabolic acidosis.
(D) Administer dopamine to support the failing left ventricle.

129. What is the cerebral perfusion pressure in a patient with the following information?

blood pressure	100/70
ICP	15
CVP	10
PAOP	8

(A) 40
(B) 55
(C) 60
(D) 65

130. A 46-year-old male is admitted to your unit with the diagnosis of an epidural hematoma following a motor vehicle accident. Which artery is usually involved when a head injury produces an epidural bleed?
(A) internal carotid
(B) middle meningeal
(C) anterior communicating
(D) parietal

131. For what does the first letter in DVI [pacemaker] stand?
(A) digital signal processing
(B) dual-chamber sensing mechanisms
(C) dual-chamber pacing
(D) diverse programmability features

132. A 30-year-old female is admitted to your unit with the diagnosis of possible pulmonary emboli. The following information is available to aid in the diagnosis:

pH	7.36
$PaCO_2$	32
PaO_2	77
HCO_3^-	23
dead space (V_T)	45%
End tidal CO_2 ($PETCO_2$)	20

Based on the preceding information, are enough data present to establish the diagnosis of pulmonary embolism?
(A) Yes, dead space measurements are definitive for pulmonary embolism.
(B) Yes, the $PaCO_2$–$PETCO_2$ gradient confirms a pulmonary embolism.
(C) No, a ventilation perfusion scan is needed.
(D) No, pulmonary angiography is the optimal method to confirm a pulmonary embolism.

133. Aldosterone production is stimulated by which event?
(A) renin-angiotensin release
(B) systemic hypertension
(C) hypernatremia
(D) parathyroid release

Questions 134 and 135 refer to the following scenario.

A 27-year-old female presents to the intensive care unit with hypotension and respiratory distress following initial chemotherapy for acute myelogenous leukemia. A pulmonary artery catheter is placed to help manage the hemodynamics. Vital signs and laboratory data are as follows:

blood pressure	94/62
pulse	113
respiratory rate	32
temperature	40°C
cardiac index	6.2
arterial pressure	27/11
PAOP	9
CVP	3
PaO_2	68
$PaCO_2$	34
pH	7.36
FIO_2	0.80
platelets	21,000
white blood cells	900
segmented neutrophils	30%
banded neutrophils	20%
lymphocytes	35%

134. Based on the preceding information, which condition is likely to be developing?
(A) ARDS (adult respiratory distress syndrome)
(B) CHF (congestive heart failure)
(C) graft-versus-host reaction
(D) systemic inflammatory response syndrome

135. Which nursing or medical intervention would NOT be necessary based on the preceding information?
(A) reverse isolation
(B) bleeding precautions
(C) administration of triple antibiotic coverage
(D) intubation

136. During your shift, a 79-year-old male who has been admitted for CHF (congestive heart failure) develops a bradycardia (ventricular escape rhythm). He becomes hypotensive and his level of consciousness decreases. Which of the following is a reason why a transcutaneous pace-

maker would be preferable to a transvenous pacemaker under this circumstance?
(A) better capture ability
(B) less painful
(C) easier to apply
(D) smaller-sized equipment

137. Cardiac contusion is best identified by which of the following techniques?
(A) creatine phosphokinase (CPK) MB isoenzyme analysis
(B) ECG
(C) chest roentgenography
(D) echocardiography

138. Physical assessment of the abdomen should take place in which sequence?
(A) inspection, deep palpation, light palpation, percussion
(B) deep palpation, light palpation, percussion, inspection
(C) light palpation, inspection, deep palpation, percussion
(D) inspection, light palpation, percussion, deep palpation

139. Which test is performed when giving platelets?
(A) human leukocyte matching
(B) indirect Coombs' test
(C) complement fixation studies
(D) histamine fixation

140. A patient with a C-6 fracture would most likely be able to perform which of the following movements?
(A) no movements of any kind
(B) movement from the waist up
(C) movement of only the shoulders and fingers
(D) some crude walking movements

141. A 62-year-old male is admitted to your unit with a diagnosis of non-Q-wave MI (myocardial infarction). He was transferred from another hospital, where he was admitted initially 2 days ago. In order to confirm the diagnosis of MI, which test would most likely be performed?
(A) creatine phosphokinase (CPK) MB isoenzyme analysis
(B) ECG
(C) echocardiogram
(D) troponin I analysis

142. A 27-year-old female is in your unit following a single right lung transplant. On your shift, she

complains of shortness of breath. Upon auscultation, you hear diminished breath sounds on the right. You are able to palpate crepitations (subcutaneous emphysema) in her neck and upper chest. Her pulse oximeter is reading 0.93, down from 0.99. Based on this information, which condition is likely to be developing?
(A) pulmonary emboli
(B) pleural rupture and hemothorax
(C) bronchial tear
(D) pneumopericardium

143. AQS wave in V_1 and a normal axis are associated with which conduction defect?
(A) left bundle branch block
(B) anterior hemiblock
(C) right bundle branch block
(D) posterior hemiblock

144. An upper motor neuron lesion presents with which of the following symptoms?
(A) hypertension and bradycardia
(B) muscle flaccidity
(C) muscle spasticity
(D) cognitive defects

145. Which antibody mediates hypersensitivity (allergic) reactions?
(A) IgG
(B) IgM
(C) IgA
(D) IgE

Questions 146 and 147 refer to the following scenario.

A 65-year-old female is admitted to your unit in an unresponsive state, with blood pressure 80/48, pulse 122, and skin that is cool and clammy to the touch. Her family states that she was healthy until after supper that evening, when she suddenly slumped over in her chair. A central line is inserted along with a pulmonary artery catheter. The catheter reveals the following information:

arterial pressure	42/25
PAOP	24
CVP	16
cardiac output	3.4
cardiac index	1.6

146. Based on the preceding information, which condition is likely to be developing?
(A) hypovolemic shock
(B) pericardial tamponade
(C) sepsis
(D) cardiogenic shock

147. Which medication would most effectively raise her blood pressure at this time?
(A) dopamine
(B) dobutamine
(C) nitroprusside
(D) furosemide (Lasix)

148. Following a code for a cardiopulmonary arrest on an 83-year-old male, the physician suspects that a flail chest injury may be present secondary to aggressive CPR (cardiopulmonary resuscitation). If flail chest is present, which of the following would be seen?
(A) paradoxical movement of portions of the chest with inspiration
(B) expansion of both the chest and the abdomen on inspiration
(C) outward expansion of at least two locations of the chest wall during expiration
(D) a cracking sound in the chest during breathing

149. An ICP (intracranial pressure) tracing with the presence of C waves at a pressure of 10 mm Hg indicates which of the following?
(A) cerebral hypoxia
(B) increasing ICP
(C) impending seizures
(D) normal ICP

150. A 61-year-old female is in your unit with the diagnosis of CHF (congestive heart failure). She develops a series of dysrhythmias, which include aberrantly conducted APCs (atrial premature contractions) with both left and right bundle branch block characteristics. Which lead is most likely to detect the left and right bundle branch block characteristics?
(A) lead avL
(B) lead II
(C) MCL_1 lead
(D) MCL_3 lead

151. Which category of drugs is most helpful in relieving unstable angina?
(A) preload reducers
(B) beta blockers
(C) parasympathetic inhibitors
(D) contractility agents

Questions 152 and 153 refer to the following scenario.

A 71-year-old female is in her fourth day in the intensive care unit with left lower lobe pneumonia. Her present antibiotic regimen includes gentamicin and imipenem. She is currently intubated and receiving mechanical ventilation with the following settings:

mode	IMV
V_T	750 ml
respiratory rate	12
total rate	27
FIO_2	0.60

Her blood pressure is stable at 128/84, and her urine output has been 750 ml over the past 24 hr. Her current laboratory data reveal the following information:

PaO_2	71
$PaCO_2$	44
pH	7.35
creatinine	2.4
BUN	40

152. Based on the preceding information, which type of organisms is the antibiotic therapy attempting to affect?
    (A) pulmonary gram-positive bacteria
    (B) pulmonary gram-negative bacteria
    (C) systemic fungi
    (D) systemic viruses

153. Which treatment is most likely to improve the intrapulmonary shunt in this situation?
    (A) addition of PEEP (positive end expiratory pressure)
    (B) normal saline bolus
    (C) changing antibiotics
    (D) diuretics

154. A 36-year-old male is in your unit with a diagnosis of cardiomyopathy. He is currently unresponsive to dobutamine therapy. Which other inotrope might be employed to improve his hemodynamics?
    (A) epinephrine
    (B) phenylephrine
    (C) digoxin
    (D) amrinone

155. Which of the following medications would be most likely to stimulate gastrointestinal motility?
    (A) lasix
    (B) epinephrine
    (C) atropine
    (D) dopamine

156. Which of the following interventions is most appropriate for pain relief due to unstable angina?

(A) home dobutamine
(B) IABP (intra-aortic balloon pump) use
(C) CABG (coronary artery bypass grafting)
(D) cardiac transplantation

Questions 157 and 158 refer to the following scenario.

A 65-year-old female is in your unit following surgery to repair a ruptured small intestine. She has been in the unit for 5 days and has developed respiratory distress requiring mechanical ventilation. She is currently arousable upon stimulation and is confused, but has no complaints other than incisional discomfort. She has the following vital signs and laboratory information:

blood pressure	94/58
pulse	114
respiratory rate	28
temperature	38.9°C
pH	7.33
PaO_2	77
$PaCO_2$	36
HCO_3^-	20
FIO_2	0.60
LDH	496
SGOT	517
white blood cells	23,000

157. Based on the preceding information, which condition is likely to be developing?
    (A) multisystem organ failure
    (B) renal failure
    (C) hepatic failure
    (D) meningeal irritation

158. Which of the following therapies is considered curative for this situation?
    (A) antibiotic therapy
    (B) mechanical ventilation and oxygenation support
    (C) administration of osmotic diuretics
    (D) No therapies are curative for this situation.

159. Hepatic encephalopathy is frequently preceded by which physical symptom?
    (A) Trousseau's sign
    (B) asterixis
    (C) positive Babinski (extensor plantar) reflex
    (D) Warner's sign

160. A 51-year-old male is admitted to your unit with shortness of breath, crackles scattered throughout both lung fields, 3+ pitting edema of the lower extremities, and an SpO_2 (pulse oximeter) value of 0.88. The following hemodynamic information is available:

cardiac index	2.6
PA	51/34
PAOP	13
CVP	19

Based on the preceding information, which condition is likely to be developing?
(A) left ventricular failure
(B) biventricular failure
(C) right ventricular failure
(D) ARDS (adult respiratory distress syndrome)

161. Thrombolytic therapy for MI (myocardial infarction) should be undertaken when which of the following criteria has been met?
(A) Q-wave formation to document presence of MI
(B) ST-segment depression in consecutive leads
(C) pain should be relieved by nitroglycerin
(D) pain should be less than 4 hr

162. A 32-year-old male is in your unit after sustaining a blunt trauma to the head. His pupillary response changes from one in which the pupils are bilaterally equal and responsive to one in which the left pupil is responsive but the right pupil is unresponsive to light and dilated. What does this pattern of responses indicate?
(A) central herniation
(B) uncal herniation
(C) anterior cord compression
(D) optic nerve compression

Questions 163 and 164 refer to the following scenario.

A 27-year-old female is admitted to your unit with the diagnosis of acute exacerbation of asthma. Wheezing is prominent thoughout both lungs. Breath sounds are equal and easily heard. Blood gas analysis and vital signs indicate the following:

PaO_2	76
$PaCO_2$	32
pH	7.44
blood pressure	134/76
pulse	110
respiratory rate	30

Shortly after admission, she complains of increasing shortness of breath. Listening to her lungs, you note that the wheezing and breath sounds have decreased. Blood gas values and vital signs are now as follows:

PaO_2	70
$PaCO_2$	43
pH	7.35
blood pressure	150/88
pulse	120
respiratory rate	38

163. Based on the preceding information, which condition is likely to be developing?
(A) pneumothorax secondary to increased mean airway pressures with auto-PEEP (positive end expiratory pressure) from the asthma
(B) pulmonary emboli
(C) worsening alveolar airflow
(D) right heart failure complicating the asthma situation

164. Which treatment would be least effective at this time?
(A) subcutaneous epinephrine
(B) postural
(C) intravenous theophylline
(D) intravenous atropine

165. A 34-year-old fireman is admitted to your unit following smoke inhalation injury. He states he was entering a room when a "ball of fire" exploded in front of him. During which time period would he be at greatest risk for developing pulmonary edema from the inhalation injury?
(A) during the first 2 hr
(B) 4 to 12 hr
(C) 12 to 36 hr
(D) >24 hr

166. IABP (intra-aortic balloon pump) therapy produces two direct physiological benefits. Identify these two benefits from the choices below.
(A) decreases preload and afterload
(B) increases coronary perfusion and decreases afterload
(C) increases coronary perfusion and decreases preload
(D) increases contractility and preload

167. Following abdominal aurtic arterial resection, which activity is most important for the nurse to perform in the first 12 hours?
(A) measuring O_S/O_T
(B) helping short-distance ambulation
(C) placing pt in prone position
(D) ST segment analysis

168. Based on the hypoxemic drive to breath concept, which of the following patients would be most at risk for developing respiratory depression with the administration of excessive oxygen therapy?
(A) chronic bronchitic patient with pH 7.34, PaO_2 56, $PaCO_2$ 68
(B) emphysematous patient with pH 7.37, PaO_2 56, $PaCO_2$ 35

(Answers cont'd.)

(C) asthmatic patient with pH 7.24, PaO_2 79, $PaCO_2$ 58

(D) COPD (chronic obstructive pulmonary disease) patient with pH 7.44, PaO_2 64, $PaCO_2$ 39

Questions 169 and 170 refer to the following scenario.

A 57-year-old male is admitted to your unit for investigation of the cause of an acute onset of abdominal pain. He has a history of alcohol abuse. He states that he has had abdominal pain for several days but that the pain became acutely worse today. Currently he states that he is in severe epigastric pain with radiation to the back. The abdomen is tender but no guarding is exhibited. Chvostek's and Trousseau's signs are present. Serum amylase is elevated.

169. Based on the preceding information, which condition is likely to be developing?
(A) acute pancreatitis
(B) bowel obstruction
(C) superior mesenteric artery occlusion
(D) abdominal aortic aneurysm

170. Which treatment would most likely be avoided in this condition?
(A) placing the patient on an NPO (nil per os; nothing by mouth) regimen
(B) starting nasogastric suction
(C) pain relief with meperidine (Demerol)
(D) surgery to remove the causative pancreatic area

171. The simultaneous use of nitroprusside and dobutamine is intended to work through which of the following actions?
(A) decrease preload and increase afterload
(B) increase contractility through reducing preload
(C) decrease SVR (systemic vascular resistance) and improve contractility
(D) increase cerebral perfusion pressure and baroreceptor stimulation

172. A 57-year-old female has been in your unit for two weeks and is diagnosed as having Multi-organ Dysfunctional Syndrome (MODS). On the 15th day she develops a fever that reaches 41°C. Which condition is likely to be developing?
(A) inflammatory response to multisystem organ failure
(B) continuation of MODS
(C) probable viral infection and infectious response
(D) bacterial inflammatory response

173. Which of the following is NOT a strong after-load-reducing agent?
(A) nicardipine
(B) labetalol
(C) nitroprusside
(D) dobutamine

Questions 174 and 175 refer to the following scenario.

Following head trauma from a hammer blow, a 45-year-old male is admitted to your unit after evacuation of a subdural hematoma. Initial postoperative neurologic checks reveal equally responsive pupils and appropriate limb movement. During your shift he begins to complain of headache and nausea. He is confused as to time and place. His respiratory rate increases to 24 from 18.

174. Which of the preceding signs is not an indication of increasing ICP (intracranial pressure)?
(A) nausea
(B) headache
(C) increased respiratory rate
(D) development of confusion

175. Which of the following nursing measures would help reduce the ICP (intracranial pressure)?
(A) keeping head elevated 15–30°
(B) turning the head to the right to aid choroid plexus absorption of CSF (cerebrospinal fluid)
(C) increasing the frequency of suctioning while administering 100% oxygen
(D) adding PEEP (positive end expiratory pressure) to reduce inflow of blood to the brain

Questions 176 and 177 refer to the following scenario.

A 71-year-old male is admitted to your unit with increasing shortness of breath. He has a history of COPD (chronic obstructive pulmonary disease). His current medications are Lasix (furosemide) (40 mg daily), potassium (40 mEq daily), and Theo-Dur (theophylline) (300 mg daily). He has dependent edema and distended neck veins. Crackles are heard throughout both lung fields. Analysis of his blood gases on admission reveals the following:

PaO_2	59
$PaCO_2$	54
pH	7.33
FIO_2	0.30

During your shift, he becomes hypotensive and a pulmonary artery catheter is placed. The catheter reveals the following:

cardiac index	2.2
PA	66/38
PAOP	13
CVP	20

176. Based on the preceding information, which condition is present?
    (A) cardiac tamponade
    (B) pulmonary hypertension
    (C) ARDS (adult respiratory distress syndrome)
    (D) biventricular failure

177. Which treatment would be most effective in reducing the pulmonary arterial occlusive pressure (PAOP)?
    (A) helium therapy
    (B) aminophylline
    (C) furosemide (Lasix)
    (D) vasodilators

178. When listening to a patient's lungs, you note that crackles are present throughout both lungs. The patient is not orthopneic and the lung sounds do not change with position. He has "swelling of the feet and hands." Distended jugular veins are present. Which of the following conditions could be present based on this information?
    (A) pulmonary disease (right ventricular failure)
    (B) cardiac disease (left ventricular failure)
    (C) aortic stenosis
    (D) arterial vascular disease

179. A patient admitted with hyperparathyroidism would most likely benefit from which of the following treatments?
    (A) thyroxine
    (B) vitamin K
    (C) fluid bolus with normal saline
    (D) calcium gluconate

180. You are caring for a 78-year-old female with exacerbation of CHF (congestive heart failure). The following data are available for assessment:

blood pressure	124/74
cardiac output	3.6
cardiac index	1.8
PAOP	16
CVP	12
stroke volume	33
stroke index	16
ejection fraction	31%

Give an example of a therapy that would be most effective in treating these hemodynamics.
    (A) dobutamine
    (B) dopamine

    (C) digitalis
    (D) 500 mg calcium chloride

181. A 61-year-old female develops ventricular fibrillation while you are watching the monitor. What is the first action you should take to re-establish stable hemodynamics in this situation? (Assume you have established pulselessness and called for help.)
    (A) defibrillate initially at 200 joules
    (B) start cardiopulmonary resuscitation
    (C) start a dopamine drip to increase blood pressure
    (D) give 10 mg epinephrine

182. In the same patient, you note the following electrolyte values on the first postoperative day:

serum Na^+	111
serum osmolality	272
urine Na^+	32
urine osmolality	322

Based on these values, which treatment would most likely be instituted?
    (A) normal saline bolus
    (B) fluid restriction or diuretics
    (C) increase free water intravenous rate (D_5W)
    (D) hyperventilation

Questions 183 and 184 refer to the following scenario.

A 48-year-old male is admitted to your unit following a cardiopulmonary arrest. He was admitted 2 days ago for investigation of a cerebral mass. He is currently being ventilated at an AMV (assist/control mechanical ventilation) rate of 12, with 10 spontaneous breaths in addition to the ventilator rate. Vital signs include blood pressure 142/86, pulse 104, temperature 37.1°C. Laboratory data reveal the following:

PaO_2	91
$PaCO_2$	32
pH	7.26
Na^+	141
K^+	4.9
Cl^-	101
HCO_3^-	17
glucose	38 mg/dl
oxygen transport	465 cc
creatinine	5
BUN	60

183. Based on the preceding information, which condition is present?
    (A) non-anion-gap acidosis
    (B) hyperkalemia-induced metabolic alkalosis

(Answers cont'd.)

(C) compensated metabolic alkalosis

(D) anion gap acidosis

184. Which therapy would be employed to help improve the level of consciousness in this patient?

(A) increase the F_{IO_2}

(B) give a glucose bolus

(C) increase HCO_3^-

(D) give 20 µg KCl

185. A 73-year-old male is transferred to your unit following a hypotensive episode on the floor. His original diagnosis is sepsis secondary to an above-the-knee amputation. The following laboratory data are available:

Na^+	142
K^+	4.1
Cl^-	103
HCO_3^-	17
glucose	123
BUN	38
lactate	15
pH	7.29
PaO_2	66
$PaCO_2$	29
F_{IO_2}	0.50

Based on the preceding information, the physician believes this patient to have cellular hypoxia. Which of the conditions listed are consistent with this diagnosis?

(A) increased intrapulmonary shunt (a/A ratio is 0.21)

(B) PaO_2 of 66

(C) $PaCO_2$ of 29

(D) lactate of 15

186. A 51-year-old male with chronic atrial fibrillation is admitted to your unit. Which of the following therapies may be employed to treat this condition?

(A) cardioversion at 200 joules

(B) adenosine

(C) digoxin

(D) radioablation

Questions 187 and 188 refer to the following scenario.

Following blunt trauma to the head, a 17-year-old male is admitted to your unit for observation. He is alert and oriented although anxious to leave. Over the next hour, you notice that he has ecchymotic development around both eyes. His level of consciousness is unchanged.

187. What is a common name for the above clinical picture?

(A) Battle's sign

(B) Homan's sign

(C) raccoon eyes

(D) mask eyes

188. Based on the preceding information, which condition may be developing?

(A) temporal skull fracture involving falx cerebri

(B) uncal herniation

(C) fracture of both eye orbits

(D) basilar skull fracture in the anterior fossa

189. A 54-year-old, obese male is admitted to your unit 2 days after right femoral–popliteal bypass surgery with a complaint of shortness of breath. Upon examination, you note that he is very anxious and appears dyspneic, although the difficulty in breathing is unaffected by position changes. Pulses in the legs are good, although the right leg is more edematous than the left. The right leg feels warmer to the touch than the left. His body temperature is 38.5°C. Analysis of his blood gases reveals the following:

PaO_2	63
$PaCO_2$	34
pH	7.46

Based on the preceding data, which condition is likely to be causing the shortness of breath?

(A) pulmonary emboli

(B) CHF (congestive heart failure)

(C) pneumonia

(D) initial stages of ARDS (adult respiratory distress syndrome)

190. Which measure would most likely improve his shortness of breath?

(A) place him in an upright position

(B) increase the frequency of deep breathing and coughing

(C) sedate him with morphine

(D) give a thrombolytic agent

191. Which of the following are therapies in the treatment of sepsis?

(A) fluids (not likely to be used)

(B) antibiotics

(C) monoclonal antibodies

(D) dopamine

192. A 69-year-old male is in your unit with a diagnosis of CHF (congestive heart failure). Dobutamine is started at 0800 in an attempt to improve his hemodynamics. From the following information, was the addition of dobutamine helpful?

	0400	0800	1200
blood pressure	108/72	90/62	94/66
pulse	112	92	102
cardiac index	2.1	2.1	2.2
PAOP	18	24	19
CVP	11	13	10
stroke volume	36	39	38

   (A) yes, based on the increased cardiac index
   (B) yes, based on the decreased PAOP
   (C) no, based on increased heart rate
   (D) no, based on the absence of improvement in stroke volume

193. A 21-year-old male is admitted following a motor vehicle accident in which he was thrown from the car. At the scene, he had a Glasgow Coma Scale score of 7. Currently he opens his eyes to painful stimuli, manifests unintelligible verbal responses, and has decorticate posturing (abnormal flexion). Based on his current responses, what is the present Glasgow Coma Scale score?
   (A) 3
   (B) 7
   (C) 10
   (D) 15

194. Beta cells in the pancreas are responsible for producing which of the following substances?
   (A) insulin
   (B) glucagon
   (C) trypsin
   (D) plasminogen

195. A 44-year-old male is in your unit following surgery for hepatic resection. During the fourth postoperative day, he develops a temperature of 39°C. His vital signs are as follows:

blood pressure	100/64
pulse	120
respiratory rate	32

Which of the following would be considered accurate statements regarding the elevation in the temperature?
   (A) Immediate reduction in the temperature is necessary.
   (B) The temperature elevation is dangerous.
   (C) The temperature elevation is predicting respiratory failure.
   (D) The temperature accounts for the heart rate change.

Questions 196 and 197 refer to the following scenario.

A 43-year-old secretary is directly admitted to your unit from her physician's office for evaluation of a recent onset of extremity paralysis. Her husband brought her to the physician when she could not move this morning. She had been feeling better after an episode of measles over a week ago but started feeling weak yesterday and today could not move. Examination reveals sensation and tingling in the legs and arms but no movement. She noticed that the symptoms started in her hands and feet and moved up her arms and legs.

196. Based on the preceding information, which condition is likely to be developing?
   (A) Guillain–Barré syndrome
   (B) myasthenia gravis
   (C) amyotrophic lateral sclerosis
   (D) multiple sclerosis

197. Which nursing measure should be taken at least daily to assess the adequacy of her ability to take a deep breath and maintain spontaneous breathing?
   (A) FEV_1 (forced expiratory volume in 1 sec)
   (B) vital capacity
   (C) dynamic compliance
   (D) oxygen gas diffusion testing

198. Intubation of the trachea has several potential complications. Which of the following is NOT a likely complication of attempting tracheal intubation?
   (A) vocal cord injury
   (B) right mainstem intubation
   (C) left mainstem intubation
   (D) esophageal intubation

199. Which of the following parameters is NOT effectively treated by continuous arteriovenous hemofiltration?
   (A) creatinine
   (B) serum volume
   (C) potassium
   (D) albumin

200. A cardiologist requests that you maintain the PAOP (pulmonary artery opening pressure) at 20 mm Hg, based on the patient's history of CHF (congestive heart failure). From the data given below, is this request valid?

	1600	1800	2000	2200
blood pressure	102/70	92/64	98/68	104/70
pulse	104	90	102	92
cardiac index	1.9	2.1	2.1	2.4
PA	44/25	32/18	39/24	49/26
PAOP	24	16	22	25
CVP	13	8	11	14
stroke index	18	23	21	24

(A) yes, based on the increased stroke index over time

(B) yes, based on the increased blood pressure over time

(C) no, since the PA have not stabilized

(D) no, since the PAOP near 20 does not have optimal stroke index

CONGRATULATIONS!

You have finished the exam. Review it to cover any problematic questions. Do not change any answers unless you are sure the change is necessary. Compare your results with the answers beginning on p. 635. Do not immediately grade your test. After reviewing the exam, take some time to relax before returning to grade your test and study any areas you missed. Note the areas in which you need improvement. This test is an approximation of the actual CCRN exam and should give you a rough idea of how you will do on the exam. Reread in the text any areas in which your success rate was less than 70%. We wish you luck in the actual exam. You are to be congratulated for taking the time and effort to prepare for it.

Comprehensive Practice Exam—1

1. _____   28. _____   55. _____   82. _____
2. _____   29. _____   56. _____   83. _____
3. _____   30. _____   57. _____   84. _____
4. _____   31. _____   58. _____   85. _____
5. _____   32. _____   59. _____   86. _____
6. _____   33. _____   60. _____   87. _____
7. _____   34. _____   61. _____   88. _____
8. _____   35. _____   62. _____   89. _____
9. _____   36. _____   63. _____   90. _____
10. _____ 37. _____   64. _____   91. _____
11. _____ 38. _____   65. _____   92. _____
12. _____ 39. _____   66. _____   93. _____
13. _____ 40. _____   67. _____   94. _____
14. _____ 41. _____   68. _____   95. _____
15. _____ 42. _____   69. _____   96. _____
16. _____ 43. _____   70. _____   97. _____
17. _____ 44. _____   71. _____   98. _____
18. _____ 45. _____   72. _____   99. _____
19. _____ 46. _____   73. _____   100. _____
20. _____ 47. _____   74. _____   101. _____
21. _____ 48. _____   75. _____   102. _____
22. _____ 49. _____   76. _____   103. _____
23. _____ 50. _____   77. _____   104. _____
24. _____ 51. _____   78. _____   105. _____
25. _____ 52. _____   79. _____   106. _____
26. _____ 53. _____   80. _____   107. _____
27. _____ 54. _____   81. _____   108. _____

109. _____
110. _____
111. _____
112. _____
113. _____
114. _____
115. _____
116. _____
117. _____
118. _____
119. _____
120. _____
121. _____
122. _____
123. _____
124. _____
125. _____
126. _____
127. _____
128. _____
129. _____
130. _____
131. _____

132. _____
133. _____
134. _____
135. _____
136. _____
137. _____
138. _____
139. _____
140. _____
141. _____
142. _____
143. _____
144. _____
145. _____
146. _____
147. _____
148. _____
149. _____
150. _____
151. _____
152. _____
153. _____
154. _____

155. _____
156. _____
157. _____
158. _____
159. _____
160. _____
161. _____
162. _____
163. _____
164. _____
165. _____
166. _____
167. _____
168. _____
169. _____
170. _____
171. _____
172. _____
173. _____
174. _____
175. _____
176. _____
177. _____

178. _____
179. _____
180. _____
181. _____
182. _____
183. _____
184. _____
185. _____
186. _____
187. _____
188. _____
189. _____
190. _____
191. _____
192. _____
193. _____
194. _____
195. _____
196. _____
197. _____
198. _____
199. _____
200. _____

Answers

1.	B	p23	28.	C	p23	55.	B	p591
2.	B	p93	29.	D	p567	56.	A	p207–208
3.	C	p33–34, 36	30.	C	p569	57.	B	p267
4.	A	p68	31.	D	p569–70	58.	B	p267
5.	C	p51–52	32.	D	p33, 34, 66	59.	D	p112
6.	A	p83	33.	A	p68	60.	D	p184
7.	A	p161	34.	A	p177	61.	C	p333–334
8.	B	p535	35.	C	p178	62.	A	p297
9.	C	p535	36.	C	p484	63.	A	p268
10.	B	p370	37.	B	p65	64.	A	p51
11.	D	p101–102	38.	C	p65	65.	D	p175
12.	D	p217	39.	B	p169	66.	D	p487
13.	B	p218	40.	A	p169	67.	C	p52–53
14.	D	p324	41.	C	p569	68.	B	p271
15.	D	p525	42.	D	p119–120	69.	A	p54
16.	B	p525	43.	A	p120	70.	B	p172
17.	D	p51–52	44.	C	p169–170	71.	B	p526
18.	C	p217	45.	C	p486	72.	B	p252
19.	B	p218	46.	D	p371	73.	B	p252
20.	C	p293	47.	A	p375	74.	D	p44–45
21.	B	p106	48.	B	p13	75.	C	p70, 83
22.	C	p106	49.	C	p193	76.	C	p199
23.	A	p49	50.	A	p534–535	77.	A	p463, 465
24.	D	p177	51.	B	p524	78.	A	p492
25.	B	p494	52.	A	p19	79.	D	p382
26.	C	p42	53.	B	p55	80.	B	p385, 388
27.	B	p51–52	54.	B	p587	81.	B	p326

82.	A	p12
83.	B	p199
84.	C	p201
85.	A	p305
86.	D	p310
87.	D	p8
88.	D	p172
89.	D	p487
90.	B	p333
91.	A	p335–336
92.	B	p11
93.	A	p191
94.	C	p576–577
95.	A	p398
96.	C	p50–51
97.	D	p184
98.	B	p406
99.	D	p488
100.	B	p489
101.	A	p108
102.	C	p51–52
103.	A	p19
104.	B	p324
105.	C	p569–570
106.	D	p34, 66
107.	D	p195
108.	C	p123

109. ___D___ p123
110. ___A___ p326
111. ___C___ p326
112. ___C___ p33, 66
113. ___B___ p190
114. ___D___ p525
115. ___B___ p525
116. ___A___ p108
117. ___C___ p177
118. ___C___ p13
119. ___C___ p69
120. ___D___ p261
121. ___C___ p261
122. ___D___ p99
123. ___A___ p194
124. ___A___ p478
125. ___B___ p526
126. ___A___ p65
127. ___A___ p199
128. ___B___ p201
129. ___D___ p370
130. ___B___ p381
131. ___C___ p78

132. ___D___ p208
133. ___A___ p273
134. ___D___ p566
135. ___D___ p178, 571
136. ___C___ p77
137. ___A___ p122
138. ___D___ p494
139. ___A___ p318
140. ___C___ p399
141. ___D___ p18
142. ___C___ p214
143. ___A___ p41–42
144. ___C___ p396
145. ___D___ p298
146. ___D___ p88
147. ___A___ p88
148. ___A___ p214
149. ___D___ p374
150. ___C___ p41–42
151. ___B___ p65
152. ___B___ p313, 570
153. ___A___ p190
154. ___D___ p19

155. ___C___ p449
156. ___C___ p65
157. ___A___ p572
158. ___D___ p572
159. ___B___ p476
160. ___C___ p82–83
161. ___D___ p68–69
162. ___B___ p405
163. ___C___ p178
164. ___B___ p186
165. ___C___ p591
166. ___B___ p88
167. ___D___ p120
168. ___A___ p168–169
169. ___A___ p479
170. ___D___ p480
171. ___C___ p83
172. ___B___ p570
173. ___D___ p22
174. ___C___ p375
175. ___A___ p383–384
176. ___B___ p20
177. ___C___ p83

178. ___A___ p83
179. ___C___ p257
180. ___A___ p19
181. ___A___ p109
182. ___B___ p525
183. ___D___ p531–532
184. ___B___ p269
185. ___D___ p53
186. ___C___ p102
187. ___C___ p380
188. ___D___ p380
189. ___A___ p208
190. ___A___ p209
191. ___C___ p570–571
192. ___D___ p48
193. ___B___ p378
194. ___A___ p265
195. ___D___ p294
196. ___A___ p413–414
197. ___B___ p171
198. ___C___ p192
199. ___D___ p542–543
200. ___D___ p48–49

Comprehensive Practice Exam—2

Questions 1 and 2 are based on the following scenario.

A 59-year-old female is in your unit with the diagnosis of CHF (congestive heart failure). She has a history of adult-onset diabetes that has been well controlled. Upon examination, you note she has crackles in her dependent lung areas. She has a II/VI systolic murmur. Her 12–lead ECG shows a left-axis deviation with an anterior hemiblock. A pulmonary artery catheter was placed yesterday following an unexplained episode of hypotension. The following hemodynamic and laboratory data are available:

blood pressure	92/64	pH	7.35
pulse	104	$Paco_2$	39
cardiac index	2.3	Pao_2	76
cardiac output	3.9	HCO_3^-	22
PA	32/20	Spo_2	0.95
PAOP	17	Fio_2	0.28 (2 L/min cannula)
CVP	9	Svo_2	0.58

1. Based on this information, what is likely happening?
   (A) exacerbation of the COPD (chronic obstructive pulmonary disease)
   (B) development of cor pulmonale
   (C) congestive heart failure
   (D) subendocardial MI (myocardial infarction)

2. Based on the above information, what would the best treatment be to improve the symptoms?
   (A) sedation and oxygen therapy
   (B) dobutamine
   (C) furosemide (Lasix) and nitroprusside
   (D) dopamine

Questions 3 and 4 refer to the following scenario.

A 42-year-old female is in the unit following a motor vehicle accident. She had a fractured left femur, lacerated liver, and pulmonary contusion. She is currently awake and oriented. She is receiving assisted ventilation in the assist/control (AMV) mode. Her chest film reveals a large left posterior lobe contusion. On postop day 2, her urine output decreases to 10 ml/h. She has the following urine and blood electrolyte information available:

Na^+	136	creatinine	3.0
K^+	4.4	BUN	67
Cl^-	101	Urinary Na^+	18
HCO_3^-	21	Urine osmolality	878

3. Based on the above information, what is the likely cause of the decreased urine output?
   (A) prerenal failure (azotemia)
   (B) ATN (acute tubular necrosis)
   (C) acute renal failure
   (D) postrenal obstruction due to rhabdomyolysis

4. Based on above information, what is the most likely treatment to improve the urine output?
   (A) renal dose domapine
   (B) a loop diuretic like furosemide (Lasix)
   (C) a proximal tubular diuretic like mannitol
   (D) fluid bolus of normal saline

5. A 33-year-old male is in the unit following a fall from a second-floor balcony. He has a fractured skull and right pneumothorax. He has developed acute respiratory failure, possibly secondary to ARDS (adult respiratory distress syndrome). He has an ICP intracranial pressure fiberoptic catheter in place to monitor his ICP. Because of refractory hypoxemia, the physician requests the PEEP be increased to 10 cm H_2O from 5. He has the following changes in vital signs after the addition of the PEEP:

	Before PEEP	After PEEP
blood pressure	116/70	100/62
pulse	92	88
ICP	10	19
PaO_2	54	76
$PaCO_2$	27	29

Based on the above information, what was the effect of the PEEP addition on cerebral oxygenation?

(A) oxygenation is improved based on the increased PaO_2

(B) no change since the $PaCO_2$ did not fall

(C) oxygenation is unchanged based on the similar blood pressures

(D) oxygenation is worsened due to drop in cerebral perfusion pressure (MAP—ICP).

6. Which therapy is most likely to reduce the ICP for a short-term benefit?

(A) a reduction in the $PaCO_2$

(B) increasing the PaO_2

(C) increasing the MAP (mean arterial pressure)

(D) adding desmopressin (DDAVP)

7. In the following ECG, what is the most significant abnormality?

(A) left bundle branch block

(B) anterior MI (myocardial infarction)

(C) posterior hemiblock

(D) inferior wall ischemia

8. Which of the following tests is helpful in distinguishing acute renal failure from prerenal problems, e.g., hypovolemia?

(A) fractional excretion of sodium (FeNa)

(B) BUN (blood urea nitrogen) levels

(C) creatinine levels

(D) serum potassium values

9. Which of the following blood gas levels reflects respiratory acidosis with compensating metabolic alkalosis?

	(A)	(B)	(C)	(D)
pH	7.25	7.34	7.54	7.35
$PaCO_2$	59	25	26	87
PaO_2	72	88	75	70
HCO_3^-	23	18	30	43

Questions 10 and 11 refer to the following scenario.

A 61-kg, 32-year-old female is admitted into the following an acute episode of unresponsive asthma. Upon physical exam, she is found to have generalized wheezing throughout both lung fields. She is short of breath and appears very anxious. In the emergency room, she has received 0.9 mg of subcutaneous epinephrine and a loading dose of 300 mg of aminophylline. Her first set of blood gas levels in the unit reveals the following:

pH	7.44
$PaCO_2$	32
PaO_2	91

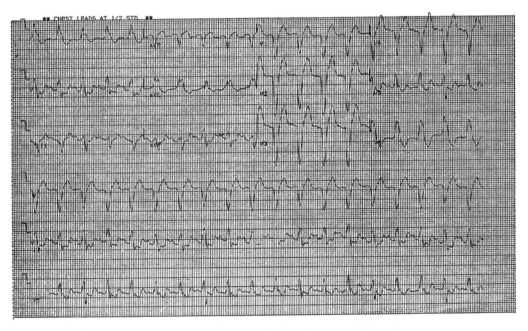

Figure for Question 7

HCO_3^-	25
FIO_2	0.40

10. Based on the above information, which of the following treatments might be helpful in improving her clinical symptoms?
(A) mast cell stablizers (e.g. cromolyn sodium)
(B) beta stimulants (e.g. albuterol)
(C) incentive spirometry
(D) racemic epinephrine

11. After 6 hours in the intensive care unit, she appears less anxious and is now somewhat drowsy. Her wheezing is still generalized, although it is now less intense. Her repeat blood gas levels indicate the following:

pH	7.32
$PaCO_2$	49
PaO_2	77
HCO_3^-	25
FIO_2	0.30

Based on the above information, what is likely happening?
(A) she is improving based on the reduction in wheezing
(B) she is improving based on the increased $PaCO_2$
(C) she is worsening based on the developing respiratory acidosis
(D) there is a slight worsening due to the reduction in the PaO_2

Questions 12 and 13 are based on the following scenario.

A 23-year-old male is in the ICU following a gunshot wound to the right chest. Postoperatively, left posterior and anterior chest tubes are inserted. He has a three-chamber closed chest drainage system (i.e., Pleuravac) for both air and fluid drainage. The physician requests 20 cm H_2O suction be applied. He presently has bubbling in the suction control chamber although the water seal chamber does not bubble.

12. Based on the above information, does he have a current pleural air leak?
(A) yes
(B) no
(C) as long as bubbling exists in the suction control chamber, a pleural leak is likely
(D) One cannot identify a pleural leak in a three chamber closed chest drainage system.

13. A radiology technician calls you into the room. It seems while maneuvering the chest x-ray machine near the bed, he knocked the chest unit down and ran over it, causing the water seal chamber to leak. When you come into the room, you can see no fluid remains in the water seal chamber. At this point what should you do?
(A) immediately clamp the chest tube and notify the physician
(B) leave the tube open to air and call the physician
(C) call the radiology department to report the technician
(D) place the end of the chest tube in a sterile water container and replace the chest unit

14. Following an angioplasty, a 55-year-old male returns to the critical care unit. Which of the following measures would be expected to be performed in the next 8 hr?
(A) sitting him up in the chair after 4 hr
(B) intermittent pressure over the insertion site
(C) monitoring for reperfusion dysrhythmias
(D) protomine sulfate infusions

15. Which of the following are common reperfusion changes on the 12-lead ECG?
(A) ST-segment prolongation
(B) delta-wave formation due to accessory path activation
(C) atrial fibrillation/flutter
(D) bradycardias

Questions 16 and 17 refer to the following scenario.

A 75-year-old female has been in the intensive care unit for 15 days following surgery for a fractured pelvis suffered in a motor vehicle accident. Her postoperative course has been complicated by acute respiratory failure. She currently is off mechanical ventilation but has been spiking intermittent fevers. She is receiving intravenous fluids (D_5W) at a rate of 75 ml/h. Her enteral feeding has been stopped for the past 48 hr because of a potential ileus. She has lost 5 lbs in the past 2 days. The following laboratory information is available:

Na^+	132	WBC	5100
K^+	3.6	segmented neutrophils	75%
Cl^-	102	banded neutrophils	10%
HCO_3^-	23	monocytes	10%
albumin	2.8	lymphocytes	5%

16. Normally, when should nutritional support be started?

(Answers cont'd.)

(A) as soon as possible

(B) no more than 3 days

(C) about 1 week without food does not harm patients

(D) no feeding until all infections are cleared

17. Based on the above laboratory data, which of the data is reflecting nutritional insufficiency?

(A) Na⁺ of 132

(B) albumin of 2.8

(C) weight change of 5 lbs

(D) Cl⁻ of 102

Questions 18 and 19 refer to the following scenario.

A 56-year-old male is in the unit following a motor vehicle accident. He had a fractured right humerus and ruptured spleen. He is extubated, alert, oriented, and in mild pain (18 hr postsurgery). He currently has the following vital signs:

| blood pressure | 96/56 | respiratory rate | 22 |
| pulse | 125 | temperature | 38.7 |

He has normal saline running at 100 ml/h. His urine output is 60 ml over the past 2 hr. The physician believes the patient may be developing hypovolemia secondary to the increased heart rate and reduced blood pressure.

18. Based on the information above, what condition is likely developing?

(A) hypovolemia as suggested by the physician

(B) tachycardia secondary to inflammation and surgery

(C) early stages of congestive heart failure

(D) sepsis

19. Given the above temperature, what therapy is necessary?

(A) observation and pain relief

(B) administration of platelets

(C) cooling blanket

(D) ice packets to axillae

Questions 20 and 21 refer to the following scenario.

A 73-year-old male is admitted to the unit from an oncology division. He has an admitting diagnosis of possible sepsis secondary to an unknown infectious source. His vital signs and laboratory data are listed below:

blood pressure	102/70
pulse	126
temperature	38.7
respiratory rate	30
WBC	2200
segmented neutrophils	55

banded neutrophils	10
lymphocytes	25
monocytes	7
eosinophils	1

20. Based on the above information, is the total granulocyte abnormal?

(A) yes, based on the total of segmented neutrophils

(B) no, based on the low total WBC count

(C) yes, based on the abnormal number of lymphocytes

(D) no, based on the segs/band ratio remaining in normal proportion

21. Which of the following aspects of the differential is abnormal?

(A) segmented neutrophils

(B) lymphocytes

(C) monocytes

(D) all are abnormal

22. A lateral wall MI (myocardial infarction) is most likely to involve which coronary artery?

(A) right coronary

(B) left main coronary

(C) left anterior descending

(D) circumflex

23. A 76-year-old female is in the unit with the diagnosis of CHF (congestive heart failure). The physician inserts a pulmonary artery catheter to aid in assessment of therapeutic treatments. One of the therapies she selects is dobutamine. With the addition of dobutamine to the treatment regimen, what change would you expect to see if the therapy were successful?

(A) increase in pulmonary artery pressure

(B) increase in systemic vascular resistance

(C) increase in stroke volume

(D) decrease in ventricular ejection fraction

24. A patient with the diagnosis of COPD (chronic obstructive pulmonary disease) is admitted to the unit with acute shortness of breath. Upon auscultation, you note he has generalized crackles. Based on the presence of crackles and shortness of breath, the physician orders 20 mg of furosemide (Lasix). Is this request appropriate?

(A) yes, the presence of crackles suggests fluid overload

(B) yes, because of the combined diuretic and bronchodilator effect of furosemide

(C) no, since furosemide is a beta antagonist which may promote bronchoconstriction in addition to its diuretic effect

(D) not enough information is available to justify furosemide since crackles may be due to airway disease, not fluid overload

25. A 61-year-old male is in the unit postoperatively for a small bowel resection secondary to cancer. During his fifth postoperative day, he develops a small amount of hematemesis. The physician diagnoses the bleeding as from a potential stress ulcer. Which of the following might would NOT be effective in controlling gastrointestinal bleeding?
(A) ranitidine
(B) cimetidine
(C) antibiotics
(D) aluminum gels

26. A clinical specialist in your unit tells you a new admission has a potential anterior septal myocardial infarction. Which leads would you examine to assess this type of injury pattern?
(A) I, avL
(B) II, III, avF
(C) V_1 to V_4
(D) V_5, V_6

27. Which ECG monitoring lead is most likely to detect a right bundle branch block?
(A) II
(B) avL
(C) MCL1
(D) MCLr3

Questions 28 and 29 are based on the following scenario.

A 45-year-old male is admitted to the unit following an emergent repair of a perforated gastric ulcer. On his third postoperative day, he develops shortness of breath and a temperature elevation to 38.9°C. He is started on broad-spectrum, triple antibiotic coverage and antipyretics as indicated. His condition does not improve over the next 24 hr and he develops hypotension (blood pressure 88/58) and tachycardia (pulse 122). The physician believes he is entering into septic shock.

28. Based on the above information, which therapy would be useful in supporting the hypotension due to septic shock?
(A) nicardipine
(B) dopamine at <5 μg/kg/min

(C) blood transfusion
(D) fluid bolus with normal saline

29. Which of the following has been proposed as a potential mediator in controlling the clinical effects of sepsis and may be effective in improving the above clinical status?
(A) steroids, such as methylprednisolone
(B) phenylephrine (Neo-Synephrine)
(C) broad-spectrum antibiotics
(D) monoclonal antibodies to tumor necrosis factor

Questions 30 and 31 refer to the following scenario.

A 71-year-old male is admitted to the unit with shortness of breath, orthopnea, and progressive reduction in exercise tolerance. He states he has "not ever been to a doctor." His lung sounds demonstrate crackles in most of his posterior lobes. A pulse oximeter indicates a value of 0.89. A pulmonary artery catheter is placed to help identify the origin of the shortness of breath. The following data are available:

blood pressure	118/70
pulse	110
respiratory rate	28
temperature	37.1
cardiac index	2.2
stroke index	20
PA	36/22
PAOP	20
CVP	6

30. Based on the above information, what condition is likely developing?
(A) left ventricular failure
(B) primary pulmonary hypertension
(C) sepsis
(D) noncardiogenic pulmonary edema

31. What therapy would most likely improve his symptoms?
(A) oxygen therapy
(B) furosemide (Lasix)
(C) dopamine
(D) gentamicin

Questions 32 and 33 are based on the following scenario.

A 32-year-old male construction worker is admitted to the unit following a fall from a scaffold. He suffered an epidural hematoma, which was surgically evacuated. He has a fiberoptic ICP (intracranial pressure) monitor in place. Currently, he is responsive to pain and has a Glasgow Coma Scale score of 10. His vital signs and laboratory data are as follows:

blood pressure	122/82
pulse	66
respiratory rate	17
ICP	11
SMA6	
Na^+	135
K^+	3.9
Cl^-	101
HCO_3^-	24
Glucose	110
Creatinine	1.1
ABGs	
pH	7.41
PaO_2	89
$PaCO_2$	38
FIO_2	0.40

During your shift, he becomes less responsive, with his Glasgow Coma Scale score changing to 6. His current vital signs are:

blood pressure	98/56
pulse	84
respiratory rate	25
ICP	14
SMA6	
Na^+	137
K^+	3.8
Cl^-	100
HCO_3^-	24
Glucose	99
Creatinine	1.1
ABGs	
pH	7.39
PaO_2	76
$PaCO_2$	35
FIO_2	0.40

32. Based on the above information, what is the most likely reason for the change in level of consciousness?
    (A) change in blood glucose
    (B) increase in ICP
    (C) reduction in cerebral perfusion pressure
    (D) reduction in the PaO_2

33. What would be the most effective therapy for improving the level of consciousness?
    (A) administration of 50 ml of $D_{50}W$
    (B) administration of an osmotic diuretic (e.g., mannitol)
    (C) increase mean arterial pressure (e.g., dopamine)
    (D) increase the $FIO2$ to 0.50

Questions 34 and 35 refer to the following scenario.

A 78-year-old female is in the unit following a change in level of consciousness. Her head CT (computed tomography) scan demonstrates a large subdural bleed. This is her third day in the unit. Presently, she is responsive only to painful stimuli. Her current vital signs and laboratory data are as follows:

blood pressure	144/84
pulse	85
respiratory rate	21
temperature	37.4
intake	3100
output	6340
urinary osmolality	288
serum osmolality	324
Na^+	152

34. Based on the above information, what condition is likely developing?
    (A) SIADH (syndrome of inappropriate secretion of the antidiuretic hormone)
    (B) myxedema coma
    (C) hyperthyroidism
    (D) diabetes insipidus

35. Which of the following is the most likely effective treatment for the above condition?
    (A) DDAVP (desmopressin acetate)
    (B) thyroxine
    (C) 500 ml of D_5W
    (D) propylthiouracil

36. A 42-year-old male is in the unit following a farm accident in which his chest was crushed by a tractor. He currently is intubated and is on mechanical ventilation. He has been unresponsive to oxygen therapy and PEEP. His peak airway pressures are elevated (60 cm H_2O). The physician decides to add PCIRV (pressure control inverse ratio ventilation). He states this will reduce his peak airway pressure and also allow for the reduction in PEEP. How can PCIRV raise the PaO_2 and SaO_2 if peak airway pressures and PEEP are reduced?
    (A) by increasing pleural pressures
    (B) through increasing alveolar gas exchange
    (C) by augmenting pulmonary blood flow
    (D) through a reduction in the ventilation/perfusion ratio

Questions 37 and 38 refer to the following scenario.

A 32-year-old male with a history of bisexual social behavior is admitted to the unit from the emergency room with the diagnosis shortness of breath of unknown origin. The emergency room physician has indicated that *Pneumocystis* pneumonia as one of the diagnoses which must be ruled out. The patient currently is short of breath and requires a F_{IO_2} of 50% via face mask. On 50% oxygen, his SpO_2 level is 0.90. He informs you this is his first hospitalization involving difficulty breathing.

37. Based on this information, what body fluid is considered potentially dangerous?
    (A) blood
    (B) sputum
    (C) tears
    (D) perspiration (sweat)

38. Which of the following therapies may help treat this condition?
    (A) penicillin derivatives
    (B) trimetaphan (Septra)
    (C) Imipenem
    (D) amikacin

39. Which of the following therapies has been shown to be of no benefit in improving the clinical course of patients with sepsis?
    (A) fluid bolus
    (B) vasopressors
    (C) inotropes
    (D) steroids

40. A 56-year-old female is in the unit with the diagnosis of sepsis secondary to a urinary tract infection. She presently has the following vital signs and hemodynamic data:

blood pressure	94/58
pulse	118
respiratory rate	34
temperature	39
cardiac output	8.8
PA	43/15
PAOP	12
CVP	3
SvO_2	0.78
cardiac index	5.1

    Based on this information, describe the adequacy of her oxygenation.
    (A) adequate, based on her cardiac output
    (B) adequate, based on her high SvO_2
    (C) inadequate, based on her high SvO_2
    (D) inadequate, based on her high cardiac index

41. If the cardiac output falls secondary to hypovolemia, what is the compensatory mechanism which serves to maintain the blood pressure?

    (A) increase in preload
    (B) increase in systemic vascular resistance
    (C) decrease in afterload
    (D) increase in blood viscosity

42. With the addition of PEEP and other forms of positive pressure ventilatory assistance, the potential exists to reduce the cardiac output. What is the mechanism for the reduction in cardiac output with these therapies?
    (A) increased mean airway pressure decreases thoracic blood flow
    (B) through stimulation of the atrial naturietic effect
    (C) through resisting the exit of air flow at the bronchial level, thereby causing a worsening of the intrapulmonary shunt
    (D) positive pressure ventilation blocks the natural passive return of blood to the heart

43. A 57-year-old is admitted to the unit with an acute exacerbation of congestive heart failure. In order to reduce the symptoms of CHF (congestive heart failure), the physician elects to administer preload reducing agents. Which of the following would be considered a preload reducing therapy?
    (A) nitroglycerin
    (B) tissue plasminogen activator (tPa)
    (C) norepinephrine (Levophed)
    (D) dopamine

44. A 31-year-old female is admitted to the unit with the diagnosis of acute gastrointestinal bleeding. She has a history of esophageal varices secondary to alcohol abuse. Which of the following may be used to treat this condition?
    (A) ranitidine
    (B) antibiotics
    (C) endoscopy with cauterization
    (D) transjugular intrahepatic portal shunt

45. Hepatitis B is transmitted through which of the following vectors?
    (A) blood
    (B) saliva
    (C) bile
    (D) sweat

46. Which of the following are NOT considered to improve long-term survival following myocardial infarction?
    (A) aspirin
    (B) beta blockers

(Answers cont'd.)

(C) prophylactic antidysrhythmia (antiarrhythmia) agents

(D) ACE (angiotensin converting enzyme) inhibitors

Questions 47 and 48 refer to the following scenario.

A 67-year-old female is admitted to the unit with the diagnosis of hypotension of unknown origin. She presently is unresponsive but is breathing spontaneously and is not intubated. Breath sounds are clear, urine output is 15 ml in 8 hr and her skin is cool. A pulmonary artery (Swan–Ganz) catheter is inserted to aid the interpretation of the situation. The following data are available:

blood pressure	86/54
pulse	118
respiratory rate	30
temperature	37.3
cardiac index	1.9
stroke index	16
PA	24/10
PAOP	6
CVP	3

47. Based on this information, what condition is likely developing?
(A) left ventricular failure
(B) biventricular failure (CHF)
(C) sepsis
(D) hypovolemia

48. What would the most likely therapy for this condition include?
(A) fluid bolus
(B) dobutamine
(C) dopamine
(D) furosemide (Lasix)

49. Which of the following is the most common cause for a reduction in the arterial P_{O_2}?
(A) reduced barometric pressure
(B) increased Pa_{CO_2} levels
(C) anatomic shunt
(D) intrapulmonary shunt

50. Multiorgan dysfunction syndrome (MODS) can affect any organ. Which of the following is the most commonly affected organ in MODS?
(A) liver
(B) kidney
(C) lungs
(D) brain

Questions 51 and 52 refer to the following scenario.

A 43-year-old male is admitted to the unit with chest pain following an episode of playing racketball. The chest pain has been present for about 90 min and has not been relieved by rest or position changes. His ECG demonstrates ST elevation in leads II, III, and avF. No Q waves are present.

51. Based on this information, what condition is likely developing?
(A) subendocardial myocardial infarction
(B) epicardial ischemia
(C) inferior wall myocardial infarction
(D) Prinzmetal's angina

52. Which therapy is most important to initiate at this time?
(A) oxygen therapy
(B) thrombolytic treatment
(C) inotropic therapy (dobutamine)
(D) afterload reduction

53. Prinzmetal's angina differs from most forms of angina through which characteristic?
(A) ST-segment elevation
(B) chest pain developing during exercise
(C) elevation of cardiac isoenzymes
(D) formation of Q waves on the 12-lead ECG

54. In conditions such as left ventricular failure and adult respiratory distress syndrome, an increase in extravascular lung water occurs. What is the primary clinical sign from any condition which causes an increase in extravascular lung water?
(A) increase in pulmonary interstitial osmotic pressure
(B) thickening of the alveolar membrane
(C) increase in mean alveolar pressure
(D) worsening Q_S/Q_T

55. A pH-tipped nasogastric tube is thought to aid in identification of passage of the tube through the gastrointestinal tract. What factor makes this concept possible?
(A) the pH of the stomach is not measurable
(B) the pH of the duodenum is alkaline
(C) the pH of the esophagus is alkaline initially, then acidic
(D) the colon pH is acidic

56. Which of the following substrates serve as the primary energy source for cerebral metabolism?
(A) proteins
(B) fats

(C) carbohydrates
(D) ketones

57. A 63-year-old male is in the unit after being transferred from the emergency room. He was found lying unresponsive in his apartment by his neighbor. His admitting diagnosis is reduced LOC (level of consciousness) of unknown origin. Based on this diagnosis, which of the following would be considered a potential cause of the decreased LOC?
(A) blood glucose level of less than 60
(B) cerebral perfusion pressure between 60 and 90 mm Hg
(C) urinary sodium of less than 20 mEq
(D) serum potassium of less than 3.5 mEq

58. Clinical estimation of left ventricular preload is assumed possible by utilizing which parameter?
(A) central venous pressure
(B) pulmonary artery occlusive pressure
(C) left ventricular stroke work index
(D) coronary sinus pressure

59. Cyanosis can be an unreliable sign of oxygenation. What is the mechanism that explains why cyanosis can be misleading?
(A) cyanosis is only present in patients with a reduced cardiac output
(B) cyanosis reflects capillary and arterial oxyhemoglobin levels, not tissue oxygenation
(C) bluish discoloration is not the only sign of cyanosis
(D) not everyone has blue hemoglobin components

Questions 60–61 refer to the following scenario

A 65-year-old male is in the unit after developing hypotension on the floor. He had a femoral-popliteal bypass surgery four days earlier and was doing well unitil yesterday. He began to complain of generalized malaise and has the following vital signs:

blood pressure	122/78
pulse	110
respiratory rate	27
temperature	38.1

His wound site is reddened but has no drainage. This morning, he was less oriented and hypotensive (blood pressure 88/54, pulse 114), prompting a transfer to the unit. He does not complain of any discomfort or shortness of breath. His lung sounds are clear and he has a pulse oximeter value of 99%.

A flow-directed pulmonary artery catheter is inserted to assist in the assessment of the cause of hypotension. The following data are available from the pulmonary artery catheter:

cardiac output	10.5
cardiac index	6.0
PA	22/11
PAOP	8
CVP	2

60. Based on the above information, what condition is likely developing?
(A) bleeding into the postoperative wound site
(B) left ventricular failure
(C) hypovolemia
(D) sepsis

61. Which treatment is likely to be instituted in the above scenario?
(A) exploratory opening and draining of the surgical wound
(B) broad-spectrum antibiotics
(C) dobutamine at 5 µg/kg/min
(D) fluid bolus with D_5W at 100 ml/h

62. Which of the following helps the diagnosis of adult respiratory distress syndrome?
(A) high temperatures
(B) tachycardia
(C) high Pa_{CO_2} levels
(D) resistive hypoxemia

63. A 76-year-old male is admitted with congestive heart failure secondary to systemic hypertension. The physician states she wants to initially attempt afterload manipulation to aid the congestive heart failure. Which of the following is NOT an afterload reducer which might help improve the CHF condition?
(A) nicardipine
(B) labetalol
(C) enalapril
(D) norepinephrine

64. In the patient with a cardiomyopathy, which of the following treatment options is likely to improve his cardiac output?
(A) dobutamine
(B) fluid bolus with hetastarch
(C) phenylephrine
(D) ranitidine

65. What is the likely reason for an increased cardiac output in a septic patient?
(A) decreased venous return
(B) decreased systemic vascular resistance

(Answers cont'd.)

(C) increased sympathetic catecholamine stimulation

(D) decreased parasympathetic stimulation

66. Which of the following therapies might help reduce the pulmonary hypertension associated with ARDS (adult respiratory distress syndrome)?
    (A) gentamicin (gram-negative antibiotic)
    (B) fluid challenge
    (C) ampicillin (gram-positive antibiotic)
    (D) nitric oxide

67. At what level of oxygen is oxygen toxicity thought to develop?
    (A) 30% for 4 hr
    (B) 40% for 12 hr
    (C) 50% for 24 hr
    (D) any FIO_2 greater than room air (21%) if exposed for more than 2 consecutive hours

68. Which of the following is the most important contributor to cardiac output?
    (A) systemic vascular resistance
    (B) stroke volume
    (C) ejection fraction
    (D) ventricular end diastolic volume

69. A 55-year-old male is admitted to the unit with the diagnosis of congestive heart failure. In order to increase his cardiac output without increasing his myocardial oxygen demand, which of the following therapies might be utilized?
    (A) nitroprusside
    (B) dobutamine
    (C) dopamine
    (D) amrinone

Questions 70 and 71 refer to the following scenario.

A 66-year-old male is admitted to the unit with the diagnosis of upper gastrointestinal bleeding. He presently is jaundiced, has a distended abdomen and appears cachectic. He has had a prior endoscopy for an earlier episode of gastrointestinal bleeding. He is confused as to time and place.

70. Based on the above information, which therapy is the most important to initiate to control the bleeding?
    (A) repeat endoscopy
    (B) intravenous H_2 blockers
    (C) surgical creation of a portocaval shunt
    (D) esophageal balloon (Sengstaken-Blakemore) tube

71. Which of the following symptoms would indicate a large bleed occurring from the gastric region, besides hematemesis?
    (A) epigastric pain
    (B) hypotension and tachycardia
    (C) right lower quadrant pain
    (D) sudden increase in liver enzymes

72. A 45-year-old male is in the unit with the diagnosis of acute respiratory failure secondary to refractory pneumonia. He is intubated and presently receiving 70% FIO_2 and +5 cm H_2O PEEP. He is on AMV (assisted mechanical ventilation) at a rate of 12 breaths/min and VT of 800 mL. He has the following blood gas levels on these settings:

pH	7.37
$PaCO_2$	40
PaO_2	51
HCO_3^-	23

    Vital signs at this time are blood pressure 122/78, pulse 88. Based on the above blood gas levels, the PEEP setting is increased to 10 cm H_2O. A repeat blood gas analysis reveals the following:

pH	7.35
$PaCO_2$	38
PaO_2	67
HCO_3^-	26

    Vital signs show blood pressure 104/62, pulse 109. Based on the information provided, has the change in PEEP been effective in improving oxygen delivery?
    (A) no, based on the change in blood pressure and heart rate
    (B) yes, based on the change in PaO_2
    (C) unable to tell without a pulse oximeter reading
    (D) unable to tell without a hemoglobin level

73. If a pulse oximeter reading (SpO_2) is 0.96, what is the likely value for the actual oxyhemoglobin (SaO_2) value, assuming no unusual conditions exist which might interfere with light absorption?
    (A) 0.90
    (B) 0.93
    (C) 0.96
    (D) 0.99

74. The most common cause for a myocardial infarction is:

(A) thrombosis around an atherosclerotic plaque
(B) excessive myocardial oxygen consumption
(C) obstruction of coronary artery from lipid accumulation
(D) decreased diastolic filling pressures

75. Which of the following is considered the most accurate measure for identifying if a myocardial infarction has occurred?
(A) 12-lead ECG
(B) cardiac isoenzymes
(C) two-dimensional echocardiography
(D) coronary angiography

Questions 76 and 77 refer to the following scenario.

A 71-year-old male is admitted to your unit with hypotension of unknown origin. He presently has a fiberoptic pulmonary artery catheter in place to determine the origin of the hypotension. At 1800, he is unresponsive with a Glasgow Coma Scale score of 4. His vital signs and pulmonary artery catheter information are as follows:

blood pressure	102/68
pulse	101
cardiac output	3.9
cardiac index	2.4
PA	42/22
PAOP	14
CVP	12
SvO_2	0.56

The physician requests that dobutamine be added to his treatment. One hour after the dobutamine, a repeat set of hemodynamics reveals the following:

blood pressure	104/66
pulse	106
cardiac output	4.4
cardiac index	2.6
PA	40/23
PAOP	14
CVP	13
SvO_2	0.56

76. Based on this information, why did the increase in cardiac output not produce an improvement in the SvO_2?
(A) SvO_2 reflects oxygenation, not the adequacy of hemodynamics.
(B) The increase in cardiac output was not adequate to meet cellular demands for oxygen.
(C) because the oxygen consumption decreased

(D) mainly because the SvO_2 reflects venous oxygen, not arterial flow, which is what is measured by cardiac output values

77. Based on the above information, what therapy would most likely be effective in improving cellular oxygenation?
(A) oxygen therapy
(B) increasing dobutamine
(C) adding norepinephrine (Levophed)
(D) adding bronchodilators

78. A 44-year-old male is admitted to the unit with the diagnosis of hypotension of unknown origin, although sepsis from possible pneumonia is a potential cause. He has no complaints of discomfort other than a persistent cough and low-grade fever (37.6°C). His lung sounds are clear except for a slight increase in sound in the left lingular area. His urine output is low and appears concentrated. Urinary electrolytes are not available yet. A pulmonary artery (Swan–Ganz) catheter is inserted to aid in assessment. The following data are available from the catheter:

cardiac output	9.2
cardiac input	5.3
PA	19/10
PAOP	7
CVP	1

While discussing these data with a new orientee, she states that these data indicate that the patient is hypovolemic, not septic. What information would help differentiate sepsis from hypovolemia and thereby help you explain to the new nurse how to interpret these data?
(A) whether urine is concentrated
(B) clear lung sounds
(C) high cardiac output with low PAOP
(D) low stroke volumes with high PAOP

Questions 79 and 80 refer to the following scenario.

A 78-year-old male is in the unit with potential MODS (multiorgan dysfunction syndrome). He currently is on mechanical ventilation with an FIO_2 of 0.70, PEEP of +8. The nurse on the previous shift cautioned that this patient rapidly desaturates with any movement. You note that when you suction his airway, his pulse oximetry reading drops from 92 to 81.

79. What is the likely cause of this reduction in saturation?
(A) drop in cardiac output

(Answers cont'd.)

(B) reduction in alveolar PO_2
(C) phrenic nerve stimulation
(D) vagal nerve stimulation

80. What treatment would most likely prevent the decrease in saturations?
(A) increase the expiratory time during the ventilator cycle
(B) hyperventilation
(C) use of lower suction pressures and open suction systems
(D) use of closed suction systems and 100% oxygen

Questions 81 and 82 refer to the following scenario.

A 76-year-old female is admitted to the unit from the emergency room with unexplained unresponsiveness. Her husband states that she had not been "feeling well" for the past few days and that this morning she became short of breath and confused. He called the emergency medical service, who brought her to the emergency room. Upon admission to your unit, she was unresponsive and intubated, with blood pressure of 76/44 and heart rate of 117. Her blood gas analysis reveals the following:

pH	7.30
$PaCO_2$	21
PaO_2	63
HCO_3^-	16
FIO_2	0.70

A pulmonary artery catheter was inserted to help assess her condition. The catheter revealed the following data:

cardiac index	1.5
PA	42/27
PAOP	25
CVP	15
SvO_2	0.45

81. Based on the above information, what condition is likely present?
(A) hypovolemic shock
(B) noncardiogenic shock
(C) cardiogenic shock
(D) neurogenic shock

82. What therapy is most likely to help improve her tissue oxygenation?
(A) dopamine
(B) dobutamine
(C) furosemide (Lasix)
(D) nitroprusside

83. An 85-year-old female in the unit with possible pulmonary embolism develops shortness of breath and hypotension (blood pressure 82/52) during your shift. Based on these symptoms, the physician is concerned with tissue oxygenation. Which of the following tests would be a good indicator of cellular hypoxia?
(A) arterial blood gas analysis, specifically PaO_2 levels
(B) pulse oximetry
(C) capnography
(D) SvO_2 levels

84. Systemic hypertension, which causes left ventricular weakness or dysfunction, produces which type of cardiac problem?
(A) high cardiac output failure
(B) systolic dysfunction
(C) diastolic dysfunction
(D) cardiac tamponade

Questions 85 and 86 refer to the following scenario.

A 23-year-old female is admitted to the unit with unknown origin of unresponsiveness. Her roommate states that while she was away for the weekend, her friend had stayed home. When she returned, she found her friend unresponsive. Currently, she has the following laboratory data and is scheduled for a head CT (computed tomography) scan. Her skin is warm to touch and she responds only to painful stimuli. Her urine output is about 17 ml for the past hour.

Na^+	148
K^+	4.9
Cl^-	111
HCO_3^-	14
glucose	655
serum posmolality	344
pH	7.19
$PaCO_2$	28
PaO_2	88

85. Based on the above information, what condition is likely developing?
(A) diabetes insipidus
(B) diabetic hyperosmolar coma
(C) diabetic ketoacidosis
(D) exacerbation of acute renal failure

86. Which of the following therapies would most likely be effective in treating the above condition?
(A) normal saline fluid bolus
(B) initiation of an insulin drip

(C) sodium bicarbonate drip
(D) fluid bolus of D_5W

87. Which of the following is a potential cause for the development of giant A waves in a CVP or PAOP waveform?
(A) ventricular septal defect
(B) aortic stenosis
(C) cardiac tamponade
(D) third degree heart block

88. An 81-year-old male is admitted with the diagnosis of right ventricular myocardial infarction. In an attempt to monitor therapy, right ventricular preload will need to be monitored. Which of the following parameters will therefore need to be monitored?
(A) pulmonary vascular resistance
(B) right ventricular stroke work index
(C) central venous pressure
(D) pulmonary capillary wedge pressure

89. Which of the following statements best describes the difference between assisted mandatory ventilation (AMV or assist/control) and pressure support ventilation (PSV)?
(A) AMV is able to deliver larger tidal volumes than PSV
(B) AMV gives more consistent tidal volumes than PSV
(C) AMV tidal volumes are based on inspiratory:expiratory ratios, unlike PSV
(D) PSV is more useful than AMV during weaning

90. Which of the following has the strongest effect on controlling the blood pressure?
(A) cardiac output
(B) systemic vascular resistance
(C) ventricular wall tension
(D) ejection fraction

91. Reverse isolation frequently is ineffective in preventing infections for which reason?
(A) autoinfection from resident pathogens on the skin and mucous membranes
(B) failure of the staff to wear masks
(C) presence of untrained personnel in intensive care units
(D) the overuse of antibiotic therapy

92. In the septic cascade, a variety of agents are released which alter vascular reactivity. All but one of the following cause vasoconstriction and reduce capillary blood flow. Which of the following is a vasodilator and may improve capillary blood flow in sepsis?

(A) tumor necrosis factor
(B) interleukin 1
(C) thromboxane A_2
(D) prostaglandin (PGE_1)

93. A 51-year-old female is admitted to the unit with the diagnosis of acute inferior wall myocardial infarction. Which type of dysrhythmia is she potentially likely to develop?
(A) second degree type 1 heart block
(B) second degree type 2 heart block
(C) third degree heart block
(D) idioventricular escape rhythm

94. A 67-year-old female is admitted to the unit following a cardiopulmonary arrest on a step-down unit. When she is admitted to the unit, she is unresponsive to verbal stimuli, but has dilation of her right pupil. Based on this response, what type of neurological condition is present?
(A) ureal herniation
(B) lower motor neuron impairment
(C) left cerebral infarct
(D) cerebellar infarct

95. When reading a pulmonary artery pressure waveform, the best location to avoid respiratory artifact is at which point?
(A) end inspiration
(B) end QRS complex
(C) during the trough (lowest point) of a spontaneous breath
(D) end expiration

96. Which of the physical signs are consistent with right ventricular failure, not left ventricular failure?
(A) dependent edema in the legs
(B) dependent crackles in the lungs
(C) systemic hypotension
(D) shortness of breath

Questions 97 and 98 refer to the following scenario.

A 81-year-old male admitted to the unit with the diagnosis of CVA (cerebrovascular accident). He has been unresponsive since admission and the family has requested no aggressive measures be performed regarding resuscitation. On your shift, you note his left pupil dilates and is unresponsive to light.

97. Based on this information, what condition is likely developing?

(Answers on pg. 654.)

(A) uncal herniation
(B) ventricular bleeding
(C) brain stem edema
(D) medullary compression

98. What nerve is likely involved in this situation?
(A) optic (cranial nerve II)
(B) oculomotor (cranial nerve III)
(C) vagal nerve (cranial nerve X)
(D) trigeminal nerve (cranial nerve VI)

99. A 71-year-old female is in the unit following a small bowel resection. On her second postoperative day, the physician requests weaning parameters to determine if she is ready to be removed from mechanical ventilation. Which of the following values would be indicators of likely successful spontaneous breathing and therefore successful weaning?
(A) respiratory rate of less than 30 with a tidal volume less than 2 ml/kg
(B) vital capacity less than 5 ml/kg
(C) PaO_2 of 60 with an FIO_2 of 0.50
(D) minute ventilation between 5 and 10 L/min

100. While starting an IV in a newly admitted 33-year-old male with the diagnosis of hepatitis, you accidently stick yourself with the needle. Which type of hepatitis would you be most at risk for developing?
(A) hepatitis A
(B) hepatitis B
(C) non-A, non-B hepatitis
(D) hepatitis D

101. A 55-year-old male is in the unit following an episode of hypotension during surgery for a ruptured bowel. His hypotension has resolved but he remains with an acidotic pH of a metabolic origin. Which of the following would be suggestive of a reason for the acidosis?
(A) anion gap of greater than 15
(B) low $PaCO_2$ level
(C) BUN: creatinine ratio of less than 15:1
(D) BUN level of 35

Questions 102 and 103 refer to the following scenario.

A 66-year-old male post MI (myocardial infarction) develops second-degree heart block with a rate of 44 and a blood pressure of 86/52. Along with this rhythm, he has occasional PVCs.

102. Which of the following would be considered an effective therapy for this situation?

(A) lidocaine
(B) flecainide
(C) atropine
(D) dopamine

103. Assume the initial therapies have failed and the physician elects to place an external pacemaker. What nursing consideration will be required with the use of the external pacemaker?
(A) warning the patient about the extreme pain he might experience
(B) disconnecting all IVs during the procedure
(C) resetting all IV infusion pumps after the pacemaker is activated
(D) potential need for sedation of the patient

Questions 104 and 105 refer to the following scenario.

A 77-year-old female is in the unit following a fall down a flight of stairs. She suffered a fracture of her right femur and left humerus along with a ruptured spleen. Postoperatively, she is in the unit for hemodynamic stabilization before being discharged to the floor. During the first 2 postoperative days, her vital signs are stable, and she is alert and oriented; besides requiring medication for pain, she is in no overt distress. During the third postoperative day, she begins to complain of shortness of breath and pain in her left chest. The pain does not change with respiration. Oxygen therapy is initiated (face mask at 30%) and sublingual nitroglycerin is given. No improvement in symptoms is noted. A stat ECG shows no ischemic changes. A blood gas analysis reveals the following:

pH	7.45
$PaCO_2$	31
PaO_2	76
HCO_3^-	24
FIO_2	.30

Auscultation of her lungs reveals they are clear except for a few crackles in the right posterior area.

104. Based on this information, what condition is likely developing?
(A) left ventricular failure
(B) right ventricular failure
(C) pulmonary emboli
(D) ARDS (adult respiratory distress syndrome)

105. Based on the information above, which therapy is most likely to help improve her symptoms?
(A) increase the FIO_2 to 50%
(B) use of thrombolytic therapy (e.g., tPA or streptokinase)

(C) addition of heparin

(D) intravenous nitroglycerin

106. In a hypotensive patient who is normovolemic, which of the following agents would NOT be used to raise the blood pressure?
(A) dopamine
(B) norepinephrine
(C) phenylephrine
(D) amiodarone

Questions 107 and 108 refer to the following scenario.

During your shift, you notice the urine output decreases to 75 ml on a 58-year-old COPD (chronic obstructive pulmonary disease) patient. He has a history of pulmonary hypertension and 45 pack-year history of smoking. The following information available to you:

Na^+	121
K^+	3.6
Cl^-	88
HCO_3^-	22
creatinine	2.0
BUN	27
osmolality	267
urinary osmolality	319
urinary Na^+	32

107. Based on this information, what condition is likely developing?
(A) prerenal failure (azotemia)
(B) acute renal failure
(C) diabetes insipidus
(D) inappropriate secretion of the antidiuretic hormone

108. What treatment plan would you consider?
(A) vasopressin
(B) fluid bolus
(C) diuretics
(D) DDAVP (desmopressin acetate)

109. A 54-year-old male is admitted to the unit with the diagnosis of hepatic failure. Which of the following disturbances could you expect to see in a patient with this diagnosis?
(A) increase in glucose levels
(B) excessive bleeding tendencies
(C) increase in serum proteins
(D) decrease in erythropoietin levels

110. Following an automobile accident, a 20-year-old female is admitted to the unit for observation. She has possible blunt chest trauma although no overt injuries are present. In attempting to establish whether myocardial injury has occurred, which of the following tests would be most useful?
(A) CPK isoenzymes
(B) 12-lead ECG
(C) chest roentgenography
(D) transesophageal echocardiography

111. Therapies designed to improve the cardiac performance in a patient with cardiomyopathy can be monitored by several measures. Which of the measures below would indicate a positive response to treatment in a patient with a cardiomyopathy?
(A) increased PAOP
(B) increased ejection fraction
(C) increased left ventricular end diastolic volume
(D) decreased stroke volume

112. Which of the following tests is most diagnostic for a pulmonary embolism?
(A) arterial blood gas analysis
(B) pulmonary angiography
(C) chest roentgenography
(D) ventilation/perfusion scans

113. Which of the clinical symptoms are INCONSISTENT with the diagnosis of sepsis?
(A) hypo- or hyperthermia
(B) tachycardia
(C) warm extremities
(D) development of skin rashes

114. A 48-year-old male is admitted to the unit with the diagnosis of anterior wall myocardial infarction. During your shift, he develops ventricular fibrillation and requires resuscitation. Which of the following medications would be administered first during the ventricular fibrillation situation?
(A) dopamine
(B) lidocaine
(C) epinephrine
(D) sodium bicarbonate

Questions 115 and 116 are based on the following scenario.

A 20-year-old female is in the unit following chemotherapy and radiation treatments for lymphoma treatment. She presently is markedly short of breath, with the following information available:

blood pressure	98/64
pulse	133
respiratory rate	41

temperature	39
PaO$_2$	66
FIO$_2$	0.80 (face mask)
pH	7.33
PaCO$_2$	30
HCO$_3^-$	20
WBC	1800

She has crackles throughout both lung fields, a strong pulse, and warm, moist skin.

115. Based on the above information, what condition is likely developing?
    (A) systemic response to immunosuppression
    (B) pulmonary capillary leak syndrome (ARDS)
    (C) myocardial infarction
    (D) pneumonia

116. Which therapy is most likely to immediately improve her symptoms and reduce her distress?
    (A) antibiotic therapy
    (B) diuretic, like furosemide (Lasix)
    (C) intubation and sedation
    (D) increasing the oxygen to 100%

Questions 117 and 118 refer to the following scenario.

A 47-year-old female is admitted to the unit following an attempted suicide through an overdose of acetaminophen and aspirin. During the initial 24 h, she requires intubation for decreased level of consciousness. Her ventilator settings are placed in a AMV (assisted mechanical ventilation) mode with a tidal volume of 750 ml and rate of 12. She has markedly elevated liver enzymes and develops compartment syndrome bilaterally in her lower legs. The compartment syndrome requires fasciotomy to relieve the pressure. On the second day after admission, she is alert and appears oriented. During your shift, she begins to indicate that she is having difficulty breathing. Her pulse oximetry reading changes from 0.98 to 0.86 on a FIO$_2$ of 0.30. The physician requests the FIO$_2$ be increased to 0.50 and orders a stat chest film. The SpO$_2$ changes from 0.86 to 0.89 and the chest film shows diffuse infiltrates throughout her lungs. The physician requests the FIO$_2$ be increased to 0.70, which results in the SpO$_2$ changing from 0.89 to 0.90.

117. Based on the above information, what condition is likely developing?
    (A) pulmonary hemorrhage
    (B) ARDS (adult respiratory distress syndrome)
    (C) pulmonary emboli
    (D) unilateral pulmonary edema

118. Which therapy is most likely to improve the arterial hypoxemia produced by the above situation?
    (A) increasing the FIO$_2$ to 100%
    (B) changing from AMV to PSV (pressure support ventilation)
    (C) performing a therapeutic bronchoscopy
    (D) adding PEEP (positive end expiratory pressure)

119. Tissue plasminogen activator (tPA) works by which mechanism?
    (A) blocking the production of thromboxane A$_2$
    (B) stimulating the process of fibrin degradation
    (C) stimulating endothelial ion activation
    (D) accelerating the release of arachidonic acid

120. Interpret the following dysrhythmia:
    (A) atrial fibrillation
    (B) sinus tachycardia with block
    (C) atrial tachycardia with block
    (D) atrial flutter with block

121. A 38-year-old male is admitted to the unit with change in behavior. Upon admission, he is confused as to date and place but knows his name and family members. He has no known medical history, smokes one pack of cigarettes per day and drinks six cans of beer per day, more on weekends. He has the following laboratory data:

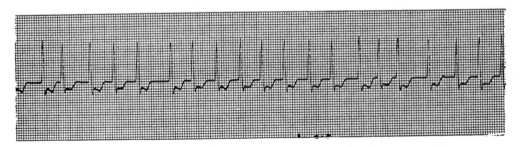

Figure for Question 120

Na⁺	134
K⁺	5.8
Cl⁻	99
HCO₃⁻	14
SGPT	2914
ammonia	86
SGOT	458
alkaline phosphate	352
bilirubin	35

Based on the above information, what condition is likely developing?
(A) cholecystitis
(B) hyperkalemic alkalosis
(C) acute renal failure
(D) hepatic encephalopathy

Questions 122 and 123 refer to the following scenario.

A 33-year-old male is admitted to the unit with complaints of progressive muscular weakness. He states he noticed the symptoms started in his arms and legs and have "worked upward from his toes and hands to now involve (his) arms and legs." He has noted a persistent shortness of breath over the past 24 h.

122. Based on this information, what clinical condition is likely developing?
(A) muscular dystrophy
(B) multiple sclerosis
(C) generalized myositis
(D) Guillain-Barré

123. Which of the following is most likely to improve the clinical symptoms exhibited by this patient?
(A) plasmapheresis
(B) steroids
(C) Dilantin
(D) electrotherapy

Questions 124 and 125 refer to the following scenario:

A 77-year-old female is in the unit with the diagnosis of congestive heart failure. She presently is not short of breath but complains of orthopnea. She is on a 40% high-humidity face mask with a pulse oximetry (SpO₂) value of 0.95. Inspiratory crackles are present along her posterior lobe. In the hemodynamic parameters listed below, you note a change in some parameters between 0400 and 0500.

	0400	0500
blood pressure	100/60	102/56
pulse	110	108
respiratory rate	25	27
cardiac index	2.4	2.3
stroke index	22	21
PA	39/19	43/24
PAOP	16	22
CVP	10	13

124. Based on the above information, has any clinically significant change in hemodynamics occurred?
(A) yes, the PAOP has risen
(B) yes, the stroke index has fallen
(C) no, the changes are generally within the range seen with normal measurement error
(D) no, the decrease in stroke index has been matched by an increase in blood pressure

125. Based on the change in hemodynamics, what treatment would be indicated?
(A) no treatment would be indicated
(B) dobutamine
(C) furosemide (Lasix)
(D) dopamine

126. Which of the following components of the immune system provide the initial response to an infection?
(A) neutrophils
(B) lymphocytes
(C) monocytes
(D) eosinophils

127. During the initial response to an antigen, one component of the immune system is responsible for stimulating the immune system to start producing antibodies. Which of the following components of the immune system is considered to stimulate antibody production?
(A) segmented neutrophils
(B) T4 lymphocytes
(C) T8 lymphocytes
(D) immunoglobulin G (IgG)

128. The combination therapy of dobutamine and nitroprusside is designed to improve hemodynamics by which action?
(A) increasing contractility and preload
(B) increasing afterload and contractility
(C) reducing afterload and increasing cardiac/stroke index
(D) reducing preload and increasing cardiac/stroke index

Questions 129 and 130 refer to the following scenario:

129. While helping a new orientee pull a patient up in bed, you notice after she lowers the side rail that the low pressure alarm on the ventilator is activated. When the low pressure alarm is activated, what is likely occurring?

(Answers on pg. 654.)

(A) the patient has secretions in the endotracheal tube

(B) the ventilator is not meeting the expected resistance to give a breath

(C) the endotracheal tube is out of place

(D) the inspiratory time has decreased to a point where the programmed inspiratory pressure is not being met

130. After this event, the orientee is concerned that she would not have known what to do if you had not been in the room. What would be the best course of action to treat low pressure if the cause were not immediately evident?

(A) suction the endotracheal tube

(B) increase the F_{IO_2} from the ventilator

(C) increase the V_T from the ventilator and call respiratory therapy for assistance

(D) remove the ventilator and use a manual resuscitator (e.g., Ambu bag) until assistance arrived

131. What is the maximal time post-MI (myocardial infarction) that thrombolytics are considered to be effective?

(A) 1–2 hr

(B) 3–4 hr

(C) less than 6 hr

(D) any time within the first 24 hr

132. A 61-year-old male has a 2-day history of abdominal pain with nausea and vomiting. He has intermittent chest pain which is unrelieved by nitrates, changing position, or rest. He has a history of congestive heart failure and underwent a CABG (coronary artery bypass graft) 2 years ago. Currently he has a urine output of 15 ml/h. He has had a urine output of 200 ml over the past 24 hr. Presently, he has the following vital signs, laboratory data, and hemodynamic information:

blood pressure	88/56
pulse	114
respiratory rate	32
cardiac output	3.7
cardiac index	2.4
PA	20/8
PAOP	6
CVP	2
Na^+	153
K^+	3.6
Cl^-	120
HCO_3^-	19
creatinine	2.2

glucose	154
BUN	35
serum osmolality	320
urinary osmolality	845
urinary Na^+	34
urinary creatinine	48

Based on the above information, what is the condition likely developing?

(A) prerenal hypoperfusion (azotemia) due to hypovolemia

(B) prerenal azotemia from left ventricular failure

(C) acute renal failure

(D) post renal obstruction

Questions 133 and 134 refer to the following scenario.

A 41-year-old female is admitted to the unit with abdominal pain and hypotension. She states the pain is severe and unremitting, is primarily epigastric and "goes into her back." She has the following laboratory data:

Na^+	140
K^+	4.3
Cl^-	104
HCO_3^-	21
glucose	531
WBC	13,300
BUN	48
amylase	464
calcium	6.6 mg/dl

133. Based on the above information, what condition is likely developing?

(A) hyperglycemic reaction

(B) perforation of gastric ulcer

(C) pancreatitis

(D) hepatic inflammation

134. Which of the following treatments would most likely be effective in helping improve her comfort level?

(A) initiation of NPO (*nil per os*) status

(B) surgical intervention

(C) administration of meperidine (Demerol) for pain relief

(D) intubation and sedation

Questions 135 and 136 refer to the following scenario.

A 34-year-old male is admitted to the unit following surgical repair of a lacerated liver from a motor vehicle accident. During your shift and during postoperative day 1, his blood pressure falls from 134/84 to 88/56 and his heart rate increases from 78 to 122. His skin is cool and clammy, and he denies shortness of breath although he is slightly confused. Heart sounds are normal and lungs are clear.

135. Based on these changes, what condition is likely developing?
     (A) left ventricular failure
     (B) hypovolemia secondary to bleeding
     (C) parasympathetic response due to vagal stimulation
     (D) hypotension secondary to lack of protein production due to hepatic failure

136. Which of the following would be most effective in rapidly increasing the blood pressure in this situation?
     (A) dobutamine
     (B) dopamine
     (C) 500 ml of 6% hetastarch
     (D) 500 ml of normal saline

137. During monitoring of a 63-year-old male with acute respiratory failure, you note his $Petco_2$ (end tidal Pco_2) value to be 33. Assuming a normal correlation between the end tidal and arterial CO_2 exists, what would the approximate $Paco_2$ value be if the $Petco_2$ is 33 mm Hg?
     (A) 29
     (B) 33
     (C) 37
     (D) 41

Questions 138 and 139 refer to the following scenario.

Following a code on a 56-year-old male, you notice his breath sounds are decreased on the left. His pulse oximeter is reading 0.98 on an Fio_2 of 0.50. The right lung has good breath sounds with a few coarse crackles. His blood pressure is 142/84 and his pulse is 94. He is presently unresponsive to verbal stimuli.

138. Based on the above information, what condition is likely present?
     (A) right bronchial intubation
     (B) mucus plug of the left mainstem bronchus
     (C) left pneumothorax
     (D) ventilator malfunction

139. Which test is most likely to detect the cause of the difference in breath sounds?
     (A) arterial blood gases
     (B) ventilator perfusion scan
     (C) chest roentgenography
     (D) capnography and end tidal CO_2 analysis

140. A patient is admitted to the unit with the diagnosis of low cardiac output secondary to myocardial injury. The physician elects to insert a intra-aortic balloon pump (IABP) in order to improve his clinical situation. Which of the following is considered a major advantage of IABP?
     (A) reduction in afterload
     (B) reduction in pulmonary artery pressures
     (C) increased perfusion to the lower extremities
     (D) reduction in cardiac injury patterns

141. The AIDS virus and the antirejection drug cyclosporine both act to inhibit one aspect of the immune system. Which part of the immune system is blocked by both the AIDS virus and cyclosporine?
     (A) plasma cells
     (B) killer T cells
     (C) T4 lymphocytes
     (D) B cell lymphocytes

142. Which of the following are considered major risk factors for the development of sepsis?
     (A) sex (males develop sepsis more than females)
     (B) age (above 65 years)
     (C) prior use of steroids
     (D) presence of coagulopathies

Questions 143 and 144 refer to the following scenario.

A 49-year-old male is in the unit following a CABG (coronary artery bypass graft). He has failed conventional methods of weaning from mechanical ventilation and has been in the unit for 2 weeks. During report, the nurse on the shift prior to you states she is concerned over the lack of activity and the potential for development of deep venous thrombosis (DVT).

143. Which of the following would be a sign of the presence of emboli due to DVT?
     (A) cerebral bleeding
     (B) loss of pedal pulses
     (C) decreased temperature of affected leg
     (D) pulmonary emboli

144. Which of the following would be considered an effective therapy to treat an arterial obstruction?
     (A) elevated leg position
     (B) surgury
     (C) increased fluid intake
     (D) avoiding the left side-lying position

145. Inflation of the IABP (intra-aortic balloon pump) should coincide with which of the following hemodynamic events?
(A) end ventricular diastole
(B) peak V-wave point
(C) dicrotic notch
(D) anacrotic notch

146. Which of the following is unlikely to help alter the course of a patient with ARDS (adult respiratory distress syndrome) and sepsis?
(A) antibiotics
(B) positive end expiratory pressure
(C) steroids
(D) maintaining low airway pressure

147. A 77-year-old female is in the unit following an episode of angina which precipitated an episode of CHF (congestive heart failure). She has a pulmonary artery catheter in place which reveals her initial set of information. A second set of hemodynamics indicates her status following the initiation of nitroglycerin. Based on the data, was the nitroglycerin effective in improving her hemodynamics?

	Initial Values	Postnitroglycerin Values
blood pressure	114/76	112/72
pulse	106	92
cardiac index	2.4	2.4
PA	40/23	35/20
PAOP	22	17
CVP	12	9

(A) yes, based on the reduced PAOP and increased stroke index
(B) no, since the cardiac index did not improve
(C) no, based on the decrease in blood pressure
(D) yes, based on the stable cardiac index

Questions 148 and 149 refer to the following scenario.

A 45-year-old male is admitted to the unit with the diagnosis of status asthmaticus. He requires intubation and is placed on mechanical ventilation in the AMV (assisted mechanical ventilation) mode with a V_T of 850 and respiratory rate of 10. He is, however, very anxious and is triggering the ventilator at a rate of 40 breaths/min. His FIO_2 is 0.40 and no PEEP is present. He has the following set of blood gas values at this time:

pH	7.34
$PaCO_2$	30
PaO_2	54
HCO_3^-	18

He is attempting to pull the endotracheal tube out because he is anxious and confused. The physician requests the administration of 10 mg of Versed (midazolam). After receiving this, the patient's respiratory rate changes from 40 to 10. His pulse oximeter now reads 0.95.

148. At this point, what should be done to monitor his status?
(A) arterial blood gas analysis
(B) continued monitoring of his SpO_2 values
(C) electrolyte analysis to search for the cause of the metabolic acidosis
(D) No further assessment is necessary at this point since the respiratory rate has fallen to desirable levels.

149. With the administration of Versed, the respiratory rate decreased from 40 to 10. What is the possible effect of this change in respiratory rate?
(A) development of a metabolic acidosis
(B) development of a respiratory acidosis
(C) No major effect will occur as long as the SpO_2 is normal.
(D) No major effect will occur as long as the ventilator rate is maintained at least at 10.

150. Treatment of CHF (congestive heart failure) consists of unloading the heart with preload-reducing drugs. Which of the following would be a type of preload-reducing agent?
(A) furosemide (Lasix)
(B) epinephrine
(C) dopamine
(D) trimethaphan

151. A 34-year-old female is in the unit for 2 days for coma of unknown origin. She was admitted from her home with her family stating she has been "sick for a few days." Upon admission, she was unresponsive and required intubation in the emergency room. She presently has a Glasgow Coma Scale score (GCS) of 3. Her pupils are fixed and unresponsive. Her body temperature is 38. She currently is on a ventilator in the assist/control mode, with a ventilator rate of 12 and total rate of 15. The physician wants to obtain an EEG (electroencephalogram) to help establish brain death. Given the above information, does the EEG provide new information regarding outcome?
(A) yes, it will provide definitive evidence of brain death
(B) yes, while it will not alone support brain death it will confirm brain death in the presence of a GCS of 3.

(C) no, clear evidence is already present

(D) no, since not enough time has passed for brain death criteria to be initiated

152. Assume you have a patient with the following hemodynamic values. Give an example of a medication combination which would be most effective in treating these hemodynamics.

blood pressure	124/74
pulse	109
cardiac index	1.8
PA	33/20
PAOP	17
CVP	12

(A) dobutamine and furosemide (Lasix)

(B) captopril and dopamine

(C) Lasix and norepinephrine

(D) digitalis and nitroprusside

Questions 153 and 154 refer to the following scenario.

A 71-year-old male is admitted to the unit following an exacerbation of COPD. He currently is short of breath but is not orthopneic. He has generalized expiratory wheezing and diffuse crackles. He appears to be slightly malnourished and underweight. He is on oxygen at 40 via a Venturi face mask. His admission blood gas analysis reveals the following information:

pH	7.34
$PaCO_2$	42
PaO_2	87
HCO_3^-	26

153. The physician states that he has a large intrapulmonary shunt. If you wanted to estimate this patient's intrapulmonary shunt, which test would allow this estimate?

(A) V_D/V_T (dead space/tidal volume ratio)

(B) EVLW (extravascular lung water)

(C) $PaCO_2/PetCO_2$ gradient

(D) PaO_2/FIO_2 ratio

154. Status asthmaticus is not likely to respond to which therapy?

(A) aminophylline

(B) sympathetic stimulants

(C) steroids

(D) sedation

155. Following an abdominal aortic aneurysm repair, a 55-year-old male is admitted to the unit for postoperative management. Which of the following would be factors to consider for potential complications following this type of surgery?

(A) decreased urine output

(B) cerebral hemorrhage

(C) cyanosis of the feet

(D) pulmonary emboli

156. A 55-year-old male in the unit has been diagnosed as septic secondary to a hepatic abscess. The physician has requested a fluid bolus of normal saline to be given to support his hemodynamics. What is the rationale for this therapy?

(A) to offset the loss of preload secondary to vasodilation

(B) to increase afterload secondary to vasodilation

(C) to raise the capillary osmotic pressure

(D) to compensate for the reduction in hemoglobin carrying capacity

157. In sepsis, one substrate which is normally not used for energy becomes preferentially catabolized. From the choices below, select this substrate.

(A) fats

(B) carbohydrates

(C) phospholipids

(D) proteins

158. A 31-year-old female with a history of mental retardation is admitted to the unit following respiratory arrest. She has a disorder which causes excessive parasympathetic tone. What will be the primary pulmonary effect of the increased parasympathetic tone?

(A) decreased level of consciousness

(B) bradycardia

(C) excessive airway reactivity

(D) increased coughing

159. Increased secretions and mucous plugging will potentially result in which clinical condition?

(A) congestive heart failure

(B) atelectasis

(C) increased physiologic dead space

(D) chronic lung disease

Questions 160 and 161 refer to the following scenario.

A 56-year-old male is in the unit following an episode of shortness of breath. Upon physical examination, he is found to be short of breath, has 3+ pitting edema of both lower legs, and has generalized crackles throughout both lung fields. His vital signs are as follows:

blood pressure	136/82
pulse	113
respiratory rate	36
temperature	37.7

A pulmonary artery catheter reveals the following information:

cardiac index	2.7
PA	56/38
PAOP	14
CVP	18

160. Based on these symptoms, what condition is likely present?
(A) right ventricular failure
(B) left ventricular failure
(C) biventricular failure
(D) sepsis induced respiratory failure

161. Which therapy would most likely help improve these symptoms?
(A) helium therapy
(B) furosemide (Lasix)
(C) prostaglandin (PGE_1)
(D) aminophylline

Questions 162 and 163 refer to the following scenario.

A 64-year-old male is admitted to the unit with shortness of breath. He has not ever been to a physician since he states "I've never been sick." He states he has smoked about one pack of unfiltered cigarettes since he was a teenager. He has marked inspiratory wheezing with scattered coarse crackles. He is coughing large amounts of yellowish-green sputum and states he normally coughs mostly in the morning. The change in color of the sputum from white to the present discoloration occurred within the past 2 days. His blood gas analysis reveals the following information:

pH	7.35
$PaCO_2$	48
PaO_2	57
HCO_3^-	25

162. Based on the above information, what condition is likely present?
(A) reactive airway disease
(B) small (oat) cell cancer
(C) pneumonia
(D) ARDS (adult respiratory distress syndrome)

163. Which therapy is most likely to immediately help improve his symptoms?
(A) antibiotics
(B) theophylline

(C) beta stimulants
(D) steroids

164. When the pH falls with a metabolic acidosis, what is the response of other electrolytes?
(A) potassium increases
(B) sodium falls
(C) bicarbonate increases
(D) chloride decreases

Questions 165 and 166 refer to the following scenario.

Following a code, a 77-year-old female is admitted to the unit for management. She is awake and alert but states her chest is "sore." During your shift, you note her blood pressure decreases from 118/78 to 98/66 during spontaneous breathing. Upon auscultation, her heart sounds are muffled and distant, although S_1 and S_2 are audible. She does not indicate any discomfort exits. A 12-lead ECG is free of any injury pattern although the voltage (ECG height) is diminished.

165. Based on the above information, what condition is likely developing?
(A) pericardial tamponade
(B) congestive heart failure
(C) pericarditis
(D) Prinzmetal's angina

166. The most effective treatment for this condition is:
(A) pericardiocentesis
(B) aspirin
(C) beta blockade
(D) nitroglycerin

167. A 44-year-old female is in the unit following a pulmonary resection of her left lower lobe from primary large-cell cancer. She is recovering uneventfully although on the postoperative day 3 she is still intubated. Following a series of coughs, she indicates she feels short of breath and is becoming anxious. When you listen to her you notice a sound like air rushing out the back of her throat. The low pressure and low volume alarms on the ventilator now go off. Based on this information, what is likely occuring?
(A) pneumothorax
(B) tracheal tear
(C) malpositioning of the endotracheal tube
(D) tearing of the balloon on the endotracheal tube

168. Which of the following are considered most helpful in determining the presence or absence of status epilepticus?

(A) electroencephalogram (EEG)
(B) magnetic resonance imaging
(C) skull roentgenography
(D) cerebral angiography

169. A 49-year-old male is in the unit following a two-story fall from an apartment window. He has a fractured skull, is unresponsive, and has equal but dilated, unresponsive pupils. The physician wants to reduce the ICP (intracranial pressure) rapidly, based on the potential for elevation of the ICP. Which of the following therapies would be effective in reducing the ICP rapidly?
(A) hyperoxygenation
(B) hyperventilation
(C) use of an osmotic diuretic (mannitol)
(D) use of a loop diuretic (furosemide; Lasix)

Questions 170 and 171 refer to the following scenario.

A 49-year-old male is admitted to the unit with persistent chest pain. He complains of chest pain which is unrelieved by rest and worsens upon inspiration. He states the pain has been present for about 24 hr. His ECG demonstrates ST elevation in leads I, II, III, avL, avF, and V_1–V_5. Auscultation of the heart and lungs reveals no overt abnormalities.

170. Based on this information, what condition is likely developing?
(A) anterior/lateral MI
(B) inferior/anterior MI

(C) pericardial tamponade
(D) pericarditis

171. What would be the most effective treatment in this situation?
(A) thrombolytics
(B) afterload reduction
(C) steroids
(D) analgesics

172. Interpret the following 12-lead ECG.
(A) inferior MI (myocardial infarction)
(B) anterior MI
(C) lateral ischemia
(D) subendocardial MI

173. A 49-year-old male in the unit with cirrhosis is sightly hypotensive (blood pressure 96/58) and tachycardiac (pulse 113 beats/min). He has marked ascites which results in his feeling "sort of having a hard time breathing." Based on this information, what would most likely be done to improve his comfort level?
(A) paracentesis
(B) use of semi-Fowler's position
(C) administration of 25 g intravenous albumin
(D) peritoneal dialysis

174. A 28-year-old female is admitted to the unit with the diagnosis paroxysmal of supraventricular tachycardia. Physical measures to slow the heart rate have failed. The physician elects to try a rapid-acting pharmacologic therapy in an

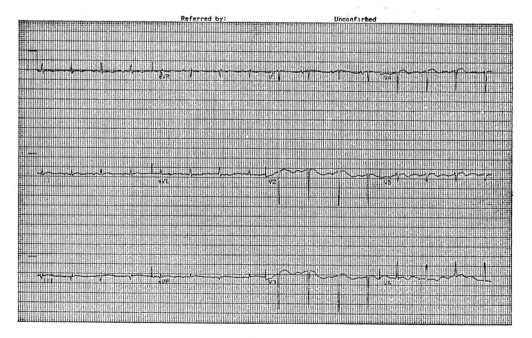

Figure for Question 172

attempt to break the tachycardia. Which of the following could be utilized for this therapy?
(A) esmolol
(B) lidocaine
(C) isoproterenol
(D) encainide

175. A 51-year-old male is admitted to the unit following a pancreatectomy. Which of the following therapies will need to be administered to replace the loss of pancreatic function?
(A) insulin
(B) alpha-1 antitrypsin
(C) exogenous bilirubin
(D) bicarbonate

176. A 76-year-old female is admitted to the unit with the chief complaint of nausea, vomiting, and cramping pain in the epigastric region. Her abdomen is distended and is hyperresonant upon percussion. Bowel sounds are distant. Based on this information, what condition is likely developing?
(A) perforation of the small intestine
(B) obstruction of the small intestine
(C) pancreatitis
(D) obstruction of the large intestine

177. Which of the following are characteristic of left bundle branch block?
(A) Q waves in V_1
(B) R waves in leads II, III, avF
(C) narrow, notched QRS in V_5, V_6
(D) rsR', complex in V_1

178. A 66-year-old male is in the unit following a CABG (coronary artery bypass grafting). Postoperatively his recovery has been complicated by a low urine output and fluid retention. He is to be started on CRRT. Which of the following will be effectively treated by this therapy?
(A) fluid removal
(B) addition of potassium
(C) elimination of creatinine
(D) elimination of excessive protein

179. Large R-wave progression V_1 and V_2 leads might indicate which of the following?
(A) left ventricular hypertrophy
(B) right ventricular hypertrophy
(C) pericardial tamponade and pericarditis
(D) loss of ventricular muscle mass

180. During the measurement of cardiac output, you note the cardiac output values fluctuate as follows:

1st measurement	5.1
2nd measurement	3.3
3rd measurement	3.7
4th measurement	4.8

The average cardiac output based upon these readings is 3.93 L/min. A new nurse asks if the variation seen in the above reasons are normal. When explaining the variations, which of the following would be considered accurate statements regarding the thermodilution cardiac output technique.
(A) All values should be within 1% of each other.
(B) The first reading is the most accurate.
(C) Dysrhythmias do not affect the cardiac output readings.
(D) The Fick equation is used to check the accuracy of the thermodilution cardiac output.

181. Right ventricular hypertrophy is characterized by which of the following?
(A) large Q waves in I and avL
(B) larger R wave than S wave in V_1
(C) larger R wave than S wave in V_6
(D) Q wave in V_3R

182. A 79-year-old female is admitted from a nursing home with the diagnosis of hypotension. She has the following clinical and laboratory data available:

blood pressure	88/50
pulse	116
respiratory rate	30
temperature	38
SpO_2	.94
Na^+	156
K^+	4.7
Cl^-	120
HCO_3^-	21
albumin	3.6
urinary Na^+	33
urinary osmolality	643

Her lung sounds are clear, her heart sounds fast but normal, and she has dark, concentrated urine. Based on this information, what condition is likely developing?
(A) acute renal failure
(B) dehydration
(C) left ventricular failure
(D) acute nutritional failure

183. Which therapy would most likely help this condition?

(A) fluid bolus of 500 ml D_5W
(B) Na^+ restriction
(C) dobutamine
(D) hyperalimentation

Questions 184 and 185 refer to the following scenario.

A 76-year-old male is admitted from the emergency room complaining of persistent, although intermittent, chest pain. His pain started on Friday (3 days ago) and has been intermittent since that time. The pain is severe at times and is unrelieved by rest or position. He did not want to come to the hospital since he did not want to bother his physician over the weekend. His admission ECG shows a large R wave in V_1 and V_2 with 2-mm ST depression in II, III, and avF.

184. Based on this information, what condition is likely present?
(A) anterior MI (myocardial infarction)
(B) posterior MI
(C) inferior ischemia
(D) pericarditis

185. Which cardiac isoenzymes might be useful in identifying whether a myocardial infarction has occurred?
(A) CPK-MB of 12
(B) CPK-MM greater than CPK-MB
(C) troponin I of .3
(D) CPK total of 80

186. Which of the following would be indications for initiating ICP (intracranial pressure) monitoring?
(A) closed head injury
(B) cerebellar infarction
(C) preoperative management of brain tumors
(D) brain stem ischemia monitoring

187. Which statement regarding thrombolytic therapy is true?
(A) Tissue plasminogen activators (tPA) are the most reliable thrombolytic in lysing coronary thrombi.
(B) Streptokinase is the most reliable thrombolytic in lysing coronary thrombi.
(C) Aspirin and heparin can effectively lyse most coronary thrombi.
(D) All thrombolytics act with the same effectiveness.

Questions 188 and 189 refer to the following scenario.

A 47-year-old male is admitted to the unit following a house fire. He made repeated efforts to enter his house to evacuate his three children who were trapped in the house. He was rescued by fire department personnel after he had collapsed in the house.

He presently is admitted with second-degree burns over 30% of his body, primarily involving his arms, face, and back. He is awake but in considerable pain. He does not complain of any shortness of breath and his pulse oximeter registers a value of 100%.

188. Based on this information, what laboratory test would be useful?
(A) coagulation profile
(B) urine electrolytes to rule out rhabdomyolysis
(C) serum albumin levels
(D) carboxyhemoglobin levels

189. Which of the following therapies will most likely be employed to help treat the above burn wounds?
(A) magnesium maleate ointment
(B) nitroglycerin ointment
(C) silver sulfadiazine ointment
(D) silver/iodine patches

190. A 67-year-old female is admitted to the unit with atrial fibrillation. On her echocardiogram, she is noted to have a large mural thrombus. Of the conditions listed below, which of the following would not be a potential complication of this atrial thrombus?
(A) pulmonary emboli
(B) CVA (cerebrovascular accident)
(C) loss of pulse in either hand
(D) loss of pulse in lower legs

191. Interpret the following dysrhythmia:
(A) atrial flutter
(B) atrial tachycarda
(C) atrial fibrillation
(D) second-degree type 2 heart block (figure on page 662)

Questions 192 and 193 refer to the following scenario.

A 71-year-old male is in the unit following (CABG) coronary bypass graft surgery. His initial postoperative recovery is uneventful and he is extubated 8 hr after returning to the unit. At 0400, you note his mediastinal chest tube has drained 200 ml in the past hour. He has the following hemodynamics at 0400:

blood pressure	102/70
pulse	88
ICP	2.5
PA	26/12
PAOP	11
CVP	5
SpO_2	0.99
FIO_2	0.30

His lung sounds are clear and he does not complain of any change in his discomfort level.

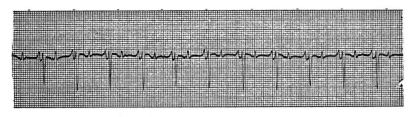

Figure for Question 191.

192. Based on this situation, what condition is likely to be present?
    (A) normal postoperative mediastinal drainage
    (B) mediastinal bleeding indicating major postoperative bleeding is occurring
    (C) developing hemothorax
    (D) cardiac tamponade

193. If the condition above were clinically significant, what clinical indicator would be present?
    (A) orthopnea
    (B) decreased stroke volume/index
    (C) increased ejection fraction
    (D) decreased SpO_2

Questions 194 and 195 are based on the following scenario.

A 34-year-old female is admitted to the unit with the diagnosis of possible pulmonary embolism. She tells you she had a "slight" pneumonia about 1 month ago. Currently, she complains of shortness of breath and inspiratory right-sided chest pain. Her respiratory rate is 34 and minute ventilation is 14 L/min. Blood gas analysis reveals the following:

pH	7.52
$PaCO_2$	25
PaO_2	88
HCO_3^-	24
FIO_2	0.28

194. Based on the above information, which of the above is consistent with the diagnosis of pulmonary emboli?
    (A) history of pneumonia
    (B) PaO_2 of 88 on 28% oxygen
    (C) HCO_3^- of 24
    (D) minute ventilation of 14 L/min

195. If a pulmonary embolism is present, what happens to the physiologic dead space of the lung?
    (A) remains normal
    (B) increases
    (C) decreases
    (D) initially elevates, then falls

196. In cardiac tamponade, which of the following clinical indicators may be present?
    (A) severe, unrelenting left-sided chest pain
    (B) CVP is greater than the PAOP
    (C) increased stroke volume/index
    (D) pulsus paradoxus

197. A 54-year-old male is to be transferred from the unit pending his morning blood gas analysis. He was initially admitted to the unit with the diagnosis of COPD (chronic obstructive pulmonary disease) with an acute exacerbation. He presently is alert and oriented, although he has mild shortness of breath and has peripheral cyanosis and "clubbing" of his fingernails. His blood gas values are as follows:

pH	7.35
$PaCO_2$	89
PaO_2	62
HCO_3^-	41

Based on the above information, what should be done?
    (A) consider intubation and mechanical ventilation
    (B) high-flow oxygen therapy and discharge from the unit
    (C) keep in the unit and start nasal CPAP (continuous positive airway pressure)
    (D) proceed with discharge from the unit

198. When administering an ACE (angiotensin converting enzyme) inhibitor (such as captopril or enalapril), which of the following would be montored to assess the effectiveness of the therapy?
    (A) PAOP (pulmonary artery opening pressure)
    (B) CVP (central venous pressure)
    (C) heart rate
    (D) SVR (systemic vascular resistance)

Questions 199 and 200 refer to the following scenario.

A 66-year-old male is admitted to the unit with the diagnosis of an acute anginal episode. He currently has the following vital signs:

blood pressure	168/104
pulse	82
respiratory rate	28
temperature	37.3

His skin is cool and he is diaphoretic. He currently denies having any chest pain.

199. In order to effectively reduce his chest pain, which of the following therapies would be most effective in relieving the chest pain?

(A) nitroglycerin
(B) lasix
(C) dobutamine
(D) dopamine

200. What is the likely precipitating mechanism of the anginal episode?
(A) increased myocardial oxygen consumption
(B) reduced left ventricular stroke work index
(C) increased end diastolic and opening pressures
(D) increased systemic oxygen consumption

Comprehensive Practice Exam—2

1. _____   28. _____   55. _____   82. _____
2. _____   29. _____   56. _____   83. _____
3. _____   30. _____   57. _____   84. _____
4. _____   31. _____   58. _____   85. _____
5. _____   32. _____   59. _____   86. _____
6. _____   33. _____   60. _____   87. _____
7. _____   34. _____   61. _____   88. _____
8. _____   35. _____   62. _____   89. _____
9. _____   36. _____   63. _____   90. _____
10. _____   37. _____   64. _____   91. _____
11. _____   38. _____   65. _____   92. _____
12. _____   39. _____   66. _____   93. _____
13. _____   40. _____   67. _____   94. _____
14. _____   41. _____   68. _____   95. _____
15. _____   42. _____   69. _____   96. _____
16. _____   43. _____   70. _____   97. _____
17. _____   44. _____   71. _____   98. _____
18. _____   45. _____   72. _____   99. _____
19. _____   46. _____   73. _____   100. _____
20. _____   47. _____   74. _____   101. _____
21. _____   48. _____   75. _____   102. _____
22. _____   49. _____   76. _____   103. _____
23. _____   50. _____   77. _____   104. _____
24. _____   51. _____   78. _____   105. _____
25. _____   52. _____   79. _____   106. _____
26. _____   53. _____   80. _____   107. _____
27. _____   54. _____   81. _____   108. _____

109. _____	132. _____	155. _____	178. _____
110. _____	133. _____	156. _____	179. _____
111. _____	134. _____	157. _____	180. _____
112. _____	135. _____	158. _____	181. _____
113. _____	136. _____	159. _____	182. _____
114. _____	137. _____	160. _____	183. _____
115. _____	138. _____	161. _____	184. _____
116. _____	139. _____	162. _____	185. _____
117. _____	140. _____	163. _____	186. _____
118. _____	141. _____	164. _____	187. _____
119. _____	142. _____	165. _____	188. _____
120. _____	143. _____	166. _____	189. _____
121. _____	144. _____	167. _____	190. _____
122. _____	145. _____	168. _____	191. _____
123. _____	146. _____	169. _____	192. _____
124. _____	147. _____	170. _____	193. _____
125. _____	148. _____	171. _____	194. _____
126. _____	149. _____	172. _____	195. _____
127. _____	150. _____	173. _____	196. _____
128. _____	151. _____	174. _____	197. _____
129. _____	152. _____	175. _____	198. _____
130. _____	153. _____	176. _____	199. _____
131. _____	154. _____	177. _____	200. _____

Answers—2

1.	C	p52	28.	D	p570	55.	B	p450	82.	A	p53
2.	B	p19	29.	C	p570	56.	C	p369	83.	D	p53
3.	A	p535	30.	A	p52	57.	A	p369	84.	B	p82
4.	D	p549	31.	B	p20–21	58.	B	p51–52	85.	C	p267
5.	D	p370	32.	C	p372	59.	B	p181	86.	B	p267
6.	A	p375	33.	C	p372	60.	D	p49	87.	D	p54
7.	A	p41–42	34.	D	p252	61.	B	p570	88.	C	p51
8.	A	p535–536	35.	A	p252	62.	D	p199	89.	B	p193–194
9.	D	p178	36.	B	p195	63.	D	p22	90.	B	p49
10.	B	p186	37.	A	p325	64.	A	p111–112	91.	A	p322
11.	C	p178	38.	B	p326	65.	B	p49	92.	D	p567
12.	B	p219	39.	D	p571	66.	D	p201	93.	A	p68
13.	D	p639	40.	C	p54	67.	C	p189	94.	A	p404
14.	C	p69	41.	B	p91	68.	B	p48	95.	D	p55
15.	D	p69	42.	A	p190	69.	A	p83	96.	A	p83
16.	A	p465	43.	A	p21	70.	D	p470	97.	A	p404
17.	B	p492	44.	D	p470	71.	B	p468	98.	B	p364
18.	B	p49	45.	A	p474	72.	A	p190	99.	D	p195
19.	A	p49	46.	C	p70	73.	B	p187	100.	B	p474
20.	A	p324	47.	D	p93	74.	A	p66	101.	A	p531
21.	D	p292	48.	A	p93	75.	B	p66	102.	C	p73
22.	D	p13	49.	D	p174	76.	B	p53	103.	D	p77
23.	C	p197	50.	C	p174–175	77.	B	p53	104.	C	p208
24.	D	p197	51.	C	p34, 66	78.	C	p569	105.	B	p209
25.	C	p467–468	52.	B	p68	79.	B	p191	106.	D	p23
26.	C	p34, 66	53.	A	p65	80.	D	p191	107.	B	p535
27.	C	p42	54.	D	p569	81.	C	p87–88	108.	C	p525

109. ___B___ p478
110. ___D___ p122
111. ___B___ p19
112. ___B___ p208
113. ___D___ p566
114. ___C___ p109
115. ___B___ p199
116. ___C___ p201
117. ___B___ p199
118. ___D___ p201
119. ___B___ p 305
120. ___A___ p102
121. ___D___ p428
122. ___D___ p413
123. ___A___ p415
124. ___C___ p48–49
125. ___A___ p48–49
126. ___A___ p292
127. ___B___ p297
128. ___C___ p19, 21
129. ___B___ p192
130. ___D___ p198
131. ___B___ p68

132. ___A___ p535
133. ___C___ p478–480
134. ___C___ p480
135. ___B___ p93
136. ___C___ p93–94
137. ___C___ p188
138. ___A___ p191
139. ___C___ p191
140. ___A___ p88
141. ___C___ p326, 332
142. ___B___ p569
143. ___D___ p121
144. ___B___ p121
145. ___C___ p89
146. ___C___ p201, 571
147. ___A___ p21
148. ___A___ p178
149. ___B___ p178
150. ___A___ p20–21
151. ___C___ p388
152. ___A___ p19–21
153. ___D___ p174–175
154. ___D___ p205

155. ___A___ p120
156. ___A___ p520
157. ___D___ p571
158. ___B___ p361
159. ___B___ p174
160. ___A___ p82–83
161. ___B___ p83–84
162. ___C___ p202
163. ___C___ p203
164. ___A___ p526
165. ___A___ p123
166. ___A___ p123
167. ___C___ p192
168. ___A___ p423
169. ___C___ p375
170. ___D___ p112
171. ___D___ p112
172. ___A___ p34
173. ___B___ p477
174. ___A___ p99
175. ___A___ p457
176. ___B___ p483
177. ___A___ p41–42

178. ___A___ p543
179. ___B___ p45
180. ___D___ p60–61
181. ___B___ p42–45
182. ___B___ p93
183. ___A___ p93
184. ___B___ p35
185. ___A___ p66, 68
186. ___A___ p372
187. ___D___ p68
188. ___D___ p591
189. ___C___ p590
190. ___A___ p208
191. ___B___ p100
192. ___A___ p117
193. ___B___ p48
194. ___D___ p208
195. ___B___ p208
196. ___D___ p123
197. ___D___ p178
198. ___D___ p21
199. ___A___ p68
200. ___A___ p65

Index

Note: Italicized letters following page numbers indicate figures (f) and tables (t).